MODELL'S
DRUGS IN CURRENT USE
AND NEW DRUGS
2004

ABOUT THE EDITORS

Milagros Fernandez, PharmD, received her bachelor of science in pharmacy from Arnold and Marie Schwartz College of Pharmacy and Health Sciences of Long Island University and her doctor of pharmacy from St. John's University College of Pharmacy and Health Professions. Dr. Fernandez is currently the lead pharmacist for general medicine at New York–Presbyterian Hospital. Prior to her current position, Dr. Fernandez worked as a target drug monitoring/staff pharmacist specializing in renal dosing of antibiotics and histamine$_2$ receptor antagonists for 5 years. She is a member of the Education Committee and Quality Improvement Committee at New York–Presbyterian Hospital. Her professional affiliations include the American Society of Health-System Pharmacists and the New York State Council of Health-System Pharmacists. Her primary areas of interest are infectious diseases, oncology, and ambulatory care.

Lydia Calix, BS Pharm, RPh, received her bachelor of science in pharmacy from Arnold and Marie Schwartz College of Pharmacy and Health Sciences of Long Island University. Ms. Calix is currently a staff pharmacist for the Division of IV/TPN/Oncology at New York–Presbyterian Hospital. Her professional affiliations include the American Society of Health-System Pharmacists.

FIFTIETH EDITION

MODELL'S DRUGS IN CURRENT USE AND NEW DRUGS 2004

Milagros Fernandez, PharmD
Lydia Calix, BS Pharm, RPh,
Editors

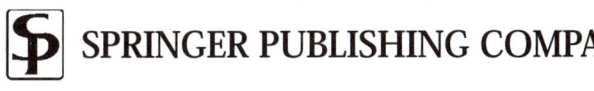 SPRINGER PUBLISHING COMPANY

No part of this publication may be reproduced, stored in a retrieval system, or transmitted in any form or by any means, electronic, mechanical, photocopying, recording, or otherwise, without the prior permission of Springer Publishing Company, Inc.

Copyright © 2004
SPRINGER PUBLISHING COMPANY, INC.
536 Broadway   New York, New York 10012
ALL RIGHTS RESERVED.

Library of Congress Catalog Card Number: 72-622-911

International Standard Book Number: 0-8261-7094-3

International Standard Serial Number: 1044-0704

Printed in the United States by Maple-Vail Book Manufacturing Group.

Acquisitions Editor: Shoshana Bauminger
Production Editor: Sara Yoo
Cover design by Joanne Honigman

We try to keep the information on the drugs in Part II as current as possible, but there is an inevitable lag between our publisher's deadline for copy and publication of the book. In addition, new drugs are often approved near the end of the calendar year, so it is not always possible to include drugs that were introduced toward the end of the preceding year.

The Editor and Publisher have made every attempt to check dosages and nursing content for accuracy. Because the science of pharmacology is continually advancing, our knowledge base continues to expand. Therefore we recommend that the reader always check product information for changes in dosage or administration before administering any medication. This is particularly important with new or rarely used drugs.

The Publisher shall not be liable for any special, consequential, or exemplary damages resulting, in whole or in part, from the readers' use of, or reliance on, the information contained in this book.

CONTENTS

Preface		vii
PART I	Drugs in Current Use (an alphabetical listing)	1
PART II	New Drugs	347
	Alinia™	374
	Avandamet™	385
	Benicar®	377
	Duac™	359
	Elitek™	383
	Eloxatin™	378
	Faslodex®	368
	Forteo™	392
	Hepsera™	351
	Humira™	349
	Inspra™	362
	Lexapro™	364
	Metaglip™	371
	Orfadin®	375
	Pegasys®	380
	Relpax®	360
	Reminyl®	369
	Remodulin™	394
	Strattera™	353
	Subutex®	355
	Suboxone®	357
	VFend®	396
	Xyrem®	389
	Zelnorm™	391
	Zetia™	366
PART III	Glossary of Side Effects	401
PART IV	References	409

PREFACE

The publication of the fiftieth edition continues a longstanding commitment to provide timely, concise information about the newest therapeutic agents with a new drugs section. To facilitate understanding the side effects of drugs, a dictionary of the most common side effects is also available. The format in this edition is expanded to three sections, with Part I consisting of an alphabetical listing of the drugs currently in use, Part II giving special attention to the drugs that have been recently introduced (most within the past year) in the United States, and Part III defining side effects. The new drugs are described in greater detail to provide readers with more information about the most current medications.

The purpose of Part I is to provide useful and concise information concerning drugs in current use. The primary trade names, uses, and preparations are provided for each of the medications included in this section. More detailed information, including precautionary statements regarding adverse reactions, is included for those agents that are most frequently used in current therapy, as well as for the relatively new drugs that have been introduced over the last several years, but prior to the introduction of the agents included in Part II.

The drugs included in Part I and Part II are listed alphabetically by their generic names. Common trade names and synonyms are included, but the listing of the trade names of many of the medications available from multiple companies is not complete. Trade names are followed by the symbol®.

Although the emphasis of *Drugs in Current Use* continues to be on the properties and uses of individual therapeutic agents, a number of combination products are also listed. The combination products selected for inclusion are the most frequently used and those about which questions are most frequently asked of health professionals.

PREFACE

Dosage information is provided for the new drugs listed in Part II. However, in view of the many factors that will influence dosage determinations for a particular patient, this information is not provided for the agents listed in Part I, and the product labeling or other more comprehensive references should be consulted.

The focus of *Drugs in Current Use* is on those agents used for therapeutic purposes. Thus, most agents used for diagnostic purposes, biological products such as vaccines, and ingredients in pharmaceutical formulations that are not pharmacologically active have not been included.

This reference is designed to provide rapid access to what is considered to be the most pertinent information regarding the drugs used in current therapy. However, such a publication cannot be all-inclusive, and the product literature and/or more comprehensive references should be consulted for prescribing purposes or when additional information is needed.

MILAGROS FERNANDEZ, **PharmD**
LYDIA CALIX, **RPh**

PART I

Drugs in Current Use

A

A-200 PYRINATE®, see Pyrethrins

ABACAVIR—Ziagen®

Description/Actions: Indicated in the treatment of HIV-1 infection, in combination with other antiretroviral agents.

Precautions/Adverse Reactions: Abacavir is contraindicated in patients with a known sensitivity to the drug. Hypersensitivity reactions have been seen in about 5% of the adult and pediatric patients taking abacavir. Because these reactions are potentially fatal, patients developing symptoms of hypersensitivity (which may include fever, rash, fatigue, nausea, vomiting, diarrhea, or abdominal pain) should immediately discontinue the drug and seek medical attention. Abacavir should never be restarted after a hypersensitivity reaction because more severe symptoms will recur within hours and may include life threatening hypotension and death. Hypersensitivity reactions may occur at any time during treatment, but usually appear in the first 6 weeks of use.

Discontinue if clinical or lab findings of lactic acidosis or hepatotoxicity occur (risk is higher in women, in the obese, or with prolonged exposure to nucleosides). Use cautiously in liver disease and the elderly. Do not add as a single agent to a failing regimen. Not recommended in pregnancy (Category C) or for nursing mothers.

Adverse reactions may include nausea, vomiting, diarrhea, anorexia, insomnia, headache, fever, rash, hypersensitivity reactions including anaphylaxis (may be fatal), lactic acidosis, severe hepatomegaly with steatosis, mild hyperglycemia, and elevated triglycerides. Changes in body fat have been seen in some patients taking antiretroviral therapy. These changes may include increased amounts of fat in the upper back and neck, breast, and around the trunk. Loss of fat from legs, arms, and face may also occur.

Administration: Oral.

Patient Care Implications: Inform patients about the signs and symptoms of hypersensitivity reactions and the actions to take if it occurs. Provide the patient with a Medication Guide and a Warning Card and instruct the patient to carry the card with him/her.

Preparations: Tablets, 300 mg. Oral solution, 20 mg/ml in strawberry-banana flavor.

ABACAVIR, LAMIVUDINE, AND ZIDOVUDINE—Trizivir™

Description/Actions: Trizivir™ is indicated for the treatment of HIV infection (either alone or in combination with other antiretroviral agents). This combination of antiretroviral is believed to act synergistically to inhibit reverse transcriptase through the incorporation of the nucleoside analogue and DNA chain termination.

Precautions/Adverse Reactions: Usage is contraindicated in patients with a hypersensitivity to abacavir, lamivudine, or any other formulation components. Do not restart patients who have had a hypersensitivity reaction to abacavir, a component of Trizivir™; life-threatening and fatal reactions have been reported. Patients must be monitored for possible fatal hypersensitivity reactions with abacavir. Patients exhibiting symptoms of fever, skin rash, fatigue, respiratory symptoms and/or gastrointestinal symptoms should discontinue therapy immediately and call for medical attention. Trizivir™ should be permanently stopped if hypersensitivity cannot be ruled out, even when other diagnoses are possible. Do not restart following a hypersensitivity reaction to abacavir because more severe symptoms will recur within hours and may include life-threatening hypotension and death. Fatal hypersensitivity reactions have occurred following the reintroduction of abacavir in patients whose therapy was interrupted, serious reactions have occurred within hours. If Trizivir™ is to be restarted following an interruption in therapy, first evaluate the patient for previously unsuspected symptoms of hypersensitivity; therapy should not be reinstated if hypersensitivity is suspected or if hypersensitivity cannot be ruled out. Lactic acidosis and severe hepatomegaly with steatosis have been reported. Use caution in patients at risk for hepatomegaly and steatosis, such as patients with hepatic dysfunction, prior liver diseases, prolonged use with a nucleoside, and obesity. Use with caution in patients with bone marrow compromise, myopathy, and myositis; bone marrow suppression and myopathy have been associated with prolonged use of zidovudine. Pregnancy Category C. No well-controlled studies in pregnant women. Trizivir™ should be used during pregnancy only if the potential benefits outweigh the risks. Some components are excreted in breast milk and with the concomitant risk for postnatal HIV transmission, breast-feeding is not recommended. Not recommended for pediatric patients, in patients < 40 kg, those requiring dosage adjustments or creatinine clearance ≤ 50 ml/minute. Should not be administered concomitantly with abacavir, lamivudine, or zidovudine.

Some adverse effects are increased triglycerides, nausea, vomiting, diarrhea, loss of appetite/anorexia, insomnia, hypersensitivity, pancreatitis, and increased GGT. Changes in body fat have been seen in some patients taking antiretroviral therapy. These changes may include increased amounts of fat in the upper back and neck, breast, and around the trunk. Loss of fat from legs, arms, and face may also occur. *Drug Interactions:* Probenecid increases the effect of zidovudine. Ribavirin decreases the effect of zidovudine.

Ganciclovir, interferon-alpha, and other bone marrow suppressive or cytotoxic agents may increase the hematologic toxicity of zidovudine.

Administration: Oral.

Patient Care Implications: Inform patient to take exactly as prescribed and educate patient of the potential hypersensitivity reactions associated with Trizivir™. Patient should carry the warning card which comes with this medicine.

Preparations: Tablet: Abacavir 300 mg, lamivudine 150 mg, and zidovudine 300 mg.

ABBOKINASE®, see Urokinase

ABCIXIMAB—ReoPro®

Platelet aggregation inhibitor.

Description/Actions: Inhibits platelet aggregation by preventing binding of fibrinogen and other adhesive molecules to receptor sites on activated platelets. Indicated as an adjunct to percutaneous transluminal coronary angioplasty (PTCA) or arthrectomy for the prevention of acute cardiac ischemic complications in patients at high risk for abrupt closure of the treated coronary vessel. Is used in conjunction with heparin and aspirin.

Warnings: Contraindicated in situations in which a significant risk of bleeding complications exists, when intravenous dextran is used before or during PTCA and in individuals with known hypersensitivity to any component of the product or to murine proteins.

Administration: Intravenous.

Preparations: Vials (5 ml) 2 mg/ml. Vials should be stored in refrigerator; but not frozen. Do not shake vials.

ABELCET®—Amphotericin B lipid complex

ABREVA®, see Docosanol 10% Cream

ACARBOSE—Precose®

Oral antidiabetic agent (alpha-glucosidase inhibitor).

Description/Actions: Reduces blood sugar by inhibiting alpha glucosidase enzymes in the GI tract resulting in delayed glucose absorption. Indicated as an adjunct to diet in non-insulin-dependent diabetes mellitus (NIDDM). Administered alone or with sulfonylurea oral hypoglycemic agents, insulin or metformin.

Warnings: Risk of hypogycemia is increased when used with oral hypoglycemic agents. Treat mild-to-moderate hypoglycemia with oral glucose (e.g., glucose tablets). Adverse reactions include flatulence, diarrhea, and abdominal pain. Contraindicated in ketoacidosis, cirrhosis, inflammatory bowel disease, chronic ulceration, partial or predisposition to intestinal obstruction, chronic intestinal disease with marked disorders of digestion or absorbency, and in conditions that may deteriorate from increased intestinal gas formation.

Administration: Oral. Take with first bite of each main meal.

Preparations: Scored tablets, 25, 50, and 100 mg.

ACCOLATE®, see Zafirlukast

ACCURETIC®, see Quinapril/ Hydrochlorothiazide

ACCUPRIL®, see Quinapril

ACCUTANE®, see Isotretinoin

ACEBUTOLOL HYDROCHLORIDE—Sectral®

Antihypertensive and antiarrhythmic agent.

Description/Actions: A cardioselective beta-adrenergic blocking agent possessing mild intrinsic sympathomimetic activity. Indicated for the treatment of hypertension, and may be used alone or in combination with other agents, usually a thiazide diuretic. Is also indicated in the management of ventricular premature beats.

Warnings: Contraindicated in patients with persistently severe bradycardia, second- and third-degree heart block in the absence of a functioning artificial pacemaker, overt cardiac failure, and cardiogenic shock. Adverse reactions include fatigue, dizziness, headache, nausea, dyspepsia, arthralgias, and myalgias. Use is best avoided in patients with bronchospastic diseases and therapy in diabetic patients must be closely monitored.

Administration: Oral. Patients should be cautioned about the interruption or discontinuation of therapy.

Preparations: Capsules, 200 and 400 mg.

ACETAMINOPHEN—Panadol®, Tempra®, Tylenol®

Analgesic/antipyretic.

Description/Actions: Used in the treatment of mild to moderate pain, and fever.

Warnings: Overdosage may result in hepatotoxicity; acetylcysteine is used as the antidote.

Administration: Oral and rectal.

Preparations: Tablets/capsules/caplets, 80, 160, 325, 500, and 650 mg. Controlled-release caplets, 650 mg. Chewable tablets, 80 mg. Granules, 80 mg. Liquid, 160 mg/5 ml, 500 mg/15 ml, and 100 mg/ml. Drops, 100 mg/ml. Suppositories, 120, 325, and 650 mg.

ACETAZOLAMIDE—Diamox®

Description/Actions: Carbonic anhydrase inhibitor indicated in the treatment of glaucoma, edema, certain convulsive disorders, and for the prevention or relief of symptoms associated with acute mountain sickness.

Preparations: Tablets, 125 and 250 mg. Controlled release capsules, 500 mg. Vials (sodium salt), 500 mg.

ACETIC ACID—VoSol®

Description/Actions: Anti-infective agent used as a bladder irrigant, for otic infections, and certain dermatologic conditions.

Preparations: Solution (bladder irrigation), 0.25%. Otic solution (VoSol®), 2%.

ACETOHEXAMIDE—Dymelor®

Description/Actions: First-generation sulfonylurea hypoglycemic agent indicated in the treatment of non-insulin-dependent diabetes mellitus.

Preparations: Tablets, 250 and 500 mg.

ACETOHYDROXAMIC ACID—Lithostat®

Description/Actions: Adjunctive therapy in certain urinary tract infections. Inhibits the bacterial enzyme urease, thereby inhibiting the hydrolysis of urea and production of ammonia in urine infected with urea-splitting organisms.

Preparations: Tablets, 250 mg.

ACETOPHENAZINE MALEATE—Tindal®

Description/Actions: Phenothiazine antipsychotic agent indicated for psychotic disorders.

Preparations: Tablets, 20 mg.

ACETYLCARBROMAL—Paxarel®

Description/Actions: Central nervous system depressant used as a sedative and hypnotic.

Preparations: Tablets, 250 mg.

ACETYLCYSTEINE—Mucomyst®

Description/Actions: Mucolytic agent indicated as adjunctive therapy in patients with abnormal or viscid mucous secretions in various pulmonary disorders. Also indicated in the management of acetaminophen overdosage.

Preparations: Vials (solution of sodium salt), 10% and 20%. Administered by nebulization or direct instillation, or enterally. Usually administered via nasogastric tube as noxious taste causes regurgitation.

ACETYLSALICYLIC ACID, see Aspirin

ACHROMYCIN V®, see Tetracycline

ACIPHEX®, see Rabeprazole

ACLOVATE®, see Alclometasone

ACRIVASTINE/PSEUDOEPHEDRINE HYDROCHLORIDE—Semprex-D®

Antihistamine/decongestant combination.

Description/Actions: Indicated for the relief of symptoms associated with seasonal allergic rhinitis.

Warnings: Contraindicated in patients with severe hypertension, severe coronary artery disease, and in patients taking a monoamine oxidase inhibitor. Adverse reactions preclude driving and operating machinery until response is ascertained. Avoid CNS-acting drugs including alcohol. Patients should be advised against the concurrent use with nonprescription antihistamines and/or decongestants.

Administration: Oral.

Preparations: Capsules, 8 mg of acrivastine and 60 mg of pseudophedrine hydrochloride.

ACTH, see Corticotropin

ACTHAR®, see Corticotropin

ACTIG®, see Fentanyl

ACTIGALL®, see Ursodiol

ACTIMMUNE®, see Interferon gamma-1b

ACTINEX®, see Masoprocol

ACTISITE®, see Tetracycline hydrochloride

ACTIVASE®, see Alteplase, recombinant

ACTIVELLA™, combination of norethindrone acetate and estradiol

ACTONEL®, see Risedronate

ACTOS®, see Pioglitazone

ACTRON®, see Ketoprofen

ACULAR®, see Ketorolac

ACYCLOVIR—Zovirax®

Description/Actions: Antiviral agent indicated in the treatment of genital herpes infections, varicella (chickenpox) infections, varicella zoster (shingles) infections, herpes simplex encephalitis, and mucosal and cutaneous herpes simplex (HSV-1 and HSV-2) infections in immunocompromised patients.

Preparations: Capsules, 200 mg. tablets, 800 mg. Suspension, 200 mg/5 ml. Ointment, 5%. Vials (sodium salt), 500 and 1000 mg (administered by IV infusion).

ADAGEN®, see Pegademase bovine

ADALAT®, see Nifedipine

ADALAT CC®, see Nifedipine

ADALIMUNAB—Humira™

ADAPALENE—Differin®

Description/Actions: A synthetic analogue, alcohol-free topical gel indicated in the treatment of acne vulgaris.

Warning: Do not use on cuts, abrasions, or broken eczematous or sunburned skin. Avoid contact with eyes, lips, angles of the nose, and mucous membranes. Minimize exposure to sun and UV light. Increased irritation may occur in extreme weather (e.g., wind, cold). Reduce frequency or discontinue if prolonged or severe irritation occurs. Do not use concomitantly with other topical irritants. Adverse reactions include erythema, scaling, dryness, pruritis, burning, and acne flares.

Administration: Apply a thin film to affected areas once daily at bedtime after washing.

Preparations: 0.1% gel, topical (alcohol free), 15, 45 g. 0.1% topical solution, 30 ml.

ADEFOVIR DIPIVOXIL—Hepsera™

ADENOCARD®, see Adenosine

ADENOSINE—Adenocard®

Antiarrhythmic agent.

Description/Actions: Slows conduction through the AV node of the heart and reestablishes normal heart rhythm. Has a rapid onset of action and a very short duration of action. Indicated for the conversion to sinus rhythm of paroxysmal supraventricular tachycardia (PSVT), including those associated with accessory bypass tracts (Wolff-Parkinson-White syndrome).

Warnings: Contraindicated in second- or third-degree AV block (except in patients with a functioning artificial pacemaker), sick sinus syndrome (except in patients with a functioning artificial pacemaker), atrial flutter, atrial fibrillation, and ventricular tachycardia. Adverse reactions include myocardial conduction abnormalities, facial flushing, headache, shortness of breath/dyspnea, chest pressure, lightheadedness, and nausea. Action may be potentiated by dipyridamole. Caution must be exercised in patients receiving carbamazepine concurrently because a higher degree of heart block may be produced. Actions of adenosine may be competitively antagonized by methylxanthines such as theophylline and caffeine.

Administration: Administered as a rapid bolus IV injection over a 1- to 2-second period. To be certain the solution reaches the systemic circulation, it should be administered either directly into a vein or, if given into an IV line, it should be given as proximal as possible and followed by a rapid saline flush.

Preparations: Vials, 6 mg/2 ml. The product should not be refrigerated as crystallization may occur.

ADIPEX®, see Phentermine

ADRENALIN®, see Epinephrine

ADRIAMYCIN PFS®, see Doxorubicin

ADRIAMYCIN RDF®, see Doxorubicin

ADRUCIL®, see Fluorouracil

ADVAIR™ DISKUS®, combination of Fluticasone and Salmeterol

ADVICOR™, see Niacin and Lovastatin

ADVIL®, see Ibuprofen

AEROBID®, see Flunisolide

AEROSPORIN®, see Polymyxin B

AFRIN®, see Oxymetazoline

AFRINOL®, see Pseudoephedrine

AGGRASTAT®, see Tirofiban

AGRYLIN®, see Anagrelide

AKINETON®, see Biperiden

AKNE-MYCIN®, see Erythromycin base (topical)

ALAMAST®, see Pemirolast

ALBAMYCIN®, see Novobiocin

ALBENZA®, see Albendazole

ALBENDAZOLE—Albenza®

Description/Actions: Anthelmintic indicated for treatment of cystic hydatid disease of the liver, lung, and peritoneum caused by the larval form of the dog tapeworm (*Echonococcus granulosus*) and for parenchymal neurocysticercosis from active lesions caused by larval forms of the pork tapeworm (*Taenia solium*). Also indicated in the treatment of ascariasis, hookworm, strongyloidiasis, giardiasis, and microsporidiosis in patients with HIV.

Warnings: In treating neurocysticercosis during the 1st week of therapy administer steroid and anticonvulsant therapy concurrently to prevent cerebral hypertension. The most common adverse drug reactions are alterations in LFTs, abdominal pain, and nausea and vomiting. Monitor LFTs prior and during therapy. If enzymes significantly increase, discontinue the albendazole. Therapy can be reinstituted when enzymes have returned to pretreatment levels. Monitor white blood cells (WBC) as reversible reductions in total WBCs have been noted.

Administration: Oral.

Preparations: Tablets, 200 mg.

ALBUMIN (HUMAN)—Albuminar®, Buminate®, Plasbumin®

Description/Actions: Plasma protein fraction indicated as supportive treatment in patients in shock, or patients with burns, hepatic cirrhosis, nephrosis, and certain other conditions.

Preparations: Vials, 5% and 25%, administered by IV infusion.

ALBUMINAR®, see Albumin

ALBUTEROL—Proventil®, Proventil HFA Inhaler®, Ventolin®, Ventolin®, HFA, Volmax®

Bronchodilator.

Description/Actions: Stimulates beta 2-adrenergic receptors. Indicated for the relief of bronchospasm in patients with reversible obstructive airway disease and for the prevention of exercise-induced bronchospasm.

Warnings: Adverse reactions include nervousness, tremor, headache, tachycardia, and palpitations. Should be used cautiously in patients with cardiovascular disorders. Concurrent use with other adrenergic (sympathomimetic) agents will have additive adrenergic effects. Must be used with caution in patients being treated with a tricyclic antidepressant or monoamine oxidase inhibitor because the action of albuterol may be increased. Beta-adrenergic blocking agents and albuterol may inhibit the effect of each other.

Administration: Oral and oral inhalation.

Preparations: Tablets, 2 and 4 mg. Controlled-release tablets, 4 and 8 mg. Capsules for inhalation, 200 ug. Syrup, 2 mg/5 ml. Metered-dose inhaler. (HFA inhaler is chloroflurocarbon free). Solution for inhalation.

ALCLOMETASONE DIPROPIONATE—Aclovate®

Topical corticosteroid.

Description/Actions: Indicated for relief of the inflammatory and pruritic manifestations of corticosteroid-responsive dermatoses.

Warnings: Adverse reactions include itching, burning, erythema, dryness, irritation, and papular rashes. Children may absorb proportionally larger amounts of the drug and thus be more susceptible to the development of systemic effects.

Administration: Topical.

Preparations: Cream and ointment, 0.05%.

ALCOHOL—Ethyl alcohol

Description/Actions: Antiseptic, astringent, and solvent when applied topically. Also used intravenously as a source of calories.

Preparations: Solution (topical), 70%. Bottles (intravenous), 5% and 10% with 5% dextrose in water.

ALDACTONE®, see Spironolactone

ALDARA®, see Imiquimod

ALDESLEUKIN—Proleukin®

Antineoplastic agent.

Description/Actions: A human recombinant interleukin-2 product (rIL-2) produced by recombinant DNA technology using a genetically engineered *E. coli* strain containing an analogue of the human interleukin-2 gene. Indicated for the treatment of adults (18 years of age and older) with metastatic renal cell carcinoma.

Warnings: Contraindicated in patients with organ allografts and in patients who do not have normal cardiac and pulmonary functions as defined by thallium stress testing and formal pulmonary function testing. Many adverse reactions are associated with capillary leak syndrome which results in hypotension and reduced organ perfusion. Pressor agents may be necessary to sustain blood pressure and the use of dopamine to help maintain organ perfusion. Other adverse reactions include renal dysfunction with oliguria/anuria, pulmonary congestion, dyspnea, respiratory failure, mental status changes, seizure, myocardial ischemia, myocarditis, gastrointestinal bleeding, intestinal perforation/ileus, sinus tachycardia, nausea, vomiting, diarrhea, anemia, thrombocytopenia, pruritus, erythema, fever and/or chills, pain, fatigue, and edema. It should be monitored closely. Hematologic tests (including CBC, differential and platelet counts), blood chemistries (including electrolytes, renal and hepatic function tests), and chest X-rays should be conducted prior to beginning treatment and then daily during drug administration. Use is associated with an increased risk of disseminated infection, including sepsis and bacterial endocarditis; therefore, preexisting infections should be adequately treated prior to starting therapy. Patients with indwelling central lines should be evaluated for antibiotic prophylaxis against *Staphylococcus aureus*.

Administration: Intravenous.

Preparations: Vials, 22 million units (1.3 mg).

ALDOMET®, see Methyldopa

ALDORIL® Combination of methyldopa and hydrochlorothiazide

ALENDRONATE SODIUM— Fosamax®

Bone resorption inhibitor.

Description/Actions: Inhibits resorption of bone by inhibiting osteoclast activity. Indicated in the prevention and treatment of osteoporosis in postmenopausal women and treatment of Paget's disease of the bone.

Warnings: Should not be used in patients whose creatinine clearance is less than 35 ml/minute, or during pregnancy and lactation. Adverse reactions include headache, GI symptoms, rash, and musculoskeletal pain.

Administration: Oral. Administer first thing in the morning with 6–8 oz of plain water 30 minutes prior to other medication, beverages, or food. (Must also avoid lying down for at least 30 minutes after the dose is administered.)

Preparations: Tablets, 5, 10, 35, and 70 mg.

ALESSE®—Levonorgestrel

10 mg ethinyl estradiol, 20 μg low dose combination oral contraceptive.

ALEVE®, see Naproxen sodium

ALFENTA®, see Alfentanil

ALFENTANIL HYDROCHLORIDE—Alfenta®

Opioid analgesic/anesthetic.

Description/Actions: Indicated (1) as an analgesic adjunct given in incremental doses in the maintenance of anesthesia with barbiturate/nitrous oxide/ oxygen, (2) as an analgesic administered by continuous infusion with nitrous oxide/ oxygen in the maintenance of general anesthesia, and (3) as a primary anesthetic agent for the induction of anesthesia in patients undergoing general surgery in which endotracheal intubation and mechanical ventilation are required. Has an almost immediate onset of action and a short duration of action.

Warnings: Skeletal muscle rigidity of the chest wall, trunk, and extremities is one of the most common adverse reactions; the incidence may be reduced by the appropriate use of a neuromuscular blocking agent. Respiratory depression including delayed respiratory depression and respiratory arrest have been reported, and the monitoring of the patient must be continued well after surgery; caution must be exercised in patients with pulmonary disease or those with potentially compromised respiration. Other adverse reactions include cardiovascular effects (e.g., bradycardia, hypotension, arrhythmias), nausea, vomiting, and dizziness. When administered with other central nervous system depressants the dose of one or both agents should be reduced. It can produce dependence and has the potential for being abused; is included in Schedule II under the provisions of the Controlled Substances Act.

Administration: Intravenous.

Preparations: Ampules (2, 5, 10, and 20 ml) containing the equivalent of 500 ug. of alfentanil base in each ml.

ALFERON N®, see Interferon alfa-n3

ALGLUCERASE—Ceredase®

Agent for Gaucher disease.

Description/Actions: Is a modified form of the enzyme glucocerebrosidase. Indicated for use as long-term enzyme replacement therapy for patients with a confirmed diagnosis of Type 1 Gaucher's disease who exhibit signs and symptoms that are severe enough to result in one or more of the following conditions: moderate to severe anemia; thrombocytopenia with bleeding tendency; bone disease; significant hepatomegaly or splenomegaly.

Warnings: Adverse reactions include fever, chills, abdominal discomfort, nausea, vomiting, and discomfort, burning, and swelling at the site of venipuncture.

Administration: Intravenous. Is administered by IV infusion over 1–2 hours. Dosage should be individualized for each patient.

Preparations: Vials, 10 units/ml and 80 units/ml.

ALITRETINOIN—Panretin®

Description/Actions: Alitretinoin is a retinoid indicated in the treatment of cutaneous AIDS related Kaposi's sarcoma (KS) lesions.

While response may be seen in as little as 2 weeks, the average response time is 4–8 weeks and some patients may need as many as 14 weeks before a response is seen.

Precautions/Adverse Reactions: Not indicated for use when systemic anti-KS therapy is needed. Do not place occlusive dressings over the lesions after applications of the medication. Use cautiously in the elderly and on T-cell lymphoma, as there is an increased risk of dermal toxicity. Minimize exposure to sun and UV light. Pregnancy Category D. Instruct patients to use adequate contraception. Avoid concomitant use of DEET. May cause fetal harm if absorbed by a pregnant woman.

Adverse reactions include rash (e.g., erythema, scaling), pain, pruritis, exfoliative dermatitis, skin disorders (e.g., excoriation, scab, eschar), paresthesia, edema, inflammation.

Administration: Topical.

Patient Care Implications: Instruct patients that a light dressing may be applied over the gel but not to place an occlusive dressing over it. Minimize sun and UV light exposure and do not use bug repellants that contain DEET. Let patients know that local reactions are common and may improve with use as a tolerance develops.

Preparations: Gel, 0.1%.

ALKERAN®, see Melphalan

ALLEGRA®, see Fexofenadine Hydrochloride

ALLEGRA-D®—Combination agent hydrochloride and fexofenadine hydrochloride and pseudoephredrine (Antihistamine and sympathomimetic)

ALLOPURINOL—Lopurin®, Zyloprim®

Agent for gout.

Description/Actions: A xanthine oxidase inhibitor indicated in the management of (1) gout; (2) patients with leukemia, lymphoma, and malignancies who are receiving cancer therapy that causes elevations of serum and urinary uric acid levels; and (3) patients with recurrent calcium oxalate calculi.

Warnings: Adverse reactions include hypersensitivity reactions, and therapy should be discontinued at the first appearance of rash or other signs of an allergic response. Will increase the action of azathioprine and mercaptopurine, and the dosage of these agents should be reduced to one-third to one-quarter the usual dose when allopurinol is administered concomitantly.

Administration: Oral.

Preparations: Tablets, 100 and 300 mg.

ALMOTRIPTAN MALEATE—AXERT™

Description/Actions: Almotriptan is indicated for the acute treatment of migraine with or without aura in adults.

Precautions/Adverse Reactions: Almotriptan should not be given to patients with risk factors for coronary artery disease until a thorough cardiovascular evaluation is performed. Significant elevations in blood pressure, including hypertensive crisis, have been reported on rare occasions in patients with and without a history of hypertension. Sensations of tightness, pain, pressure and heaviness in the precordium, throat, neck, and jaw have been reported after treatment with Axert. If a patient does not respond to the first dose of almotriptan, the diagnosis of migraine headache should be reconsidered. Pregnancy Category C. No adequate or well-controlled studies in pregnant women. Almotriptan should be used during pregnancy only if the potential benefit justifies the potential risk to the fetus. Excretion in human breast milk is unknown. Safety and efficacy in pediatrics have not been established. The most common adverse effects observed during treatment with almotriptan include nausea, somnolence, headache, paresthesia, and dry mouth. Serious and fatal cardiac events including coronary artery vasospasm, transient myocardial ischemia, myocardial infarction, ventricular tachycardia, and ventricular fibrillation have occurred. These events are extremely rare, and most have occurred in patients with risk factors predictive of coronary artery disease.

Administration: Oral.

Patient Care Implications: Patients should be instructed to report any sensations of tightness, pain, pressure, or heaviness in the chest, throat, neck, or jaw.

If patient does not respond to the first dose of almotriptan, the diagnosis of migraine should be reconsidered.

Preparations: Tablets, 6.25 and 12.5 mg.

ALOCRIL®, see Nedocromil Sodium

ALOMIDE®, see Lodoxamide tromethamine

ALORA®, see Estradio

ALOSESTRON HYDROCHLORIDE—Lotronex®

Description/Actions: A potent and selective antagonist of the serotonin 5-HT3 receptor type indicated for the treatment of irritable bowel syndrome in women whose predominant bowel symptom is diarrhea.

Administration: Oral.

Preparations: Tablets. 1 mg.

ALPHAGAN®, see Brimonidine Tartrate

ALPHA1-ANTITRYPSIN, see Alpha$_1$-Proteinase Inhibitor

ALPHA1-PROTEINASE INHIBITOR (HUMAN)— Prolastin®

Agent for alpha1-proteinase inhibitor deficiency.

Description/Actions: Also known as alpha$_1$-antitrypsin, it is indicated for chronic replacement therapy in individuals having congenital deficiency of alpha$_1$-proteinase inhibitor with clinically demonstrable panacinar emphysema.

Warnings: Preparation is purified from large pools of fresh human plasma obtained from many donors, and the presence of hepatitis viruses in such pools must be assumed. It is, therefore recommended that patients be immunized against hepatitis B.

Administration: Intravenous.

Preparations: Vials, with the activity, in milligrams, stated on the label of each vial.

ALPRAZOLAM—Xanax®

Benzodiazepine antianxiety agent.

Description/Actions: A CNS depressant indicated for the management of anxiety disorders or the short-term relief of the symptoms of anxiety. Anxiety associated with depression is also responsive. Also indicated in the treatment of panic disorder.

Warnings: Contraindicated in patients with acute narrow-angle glaucoma. Adverse reactions include drowsiness and other CNS effects; patients should be cautioned regarding activities such as driving and operating machinery, as well as interactions with other CNS-acting drugs including alcohol. Can cause dependence and is included in Schedule IV.

Administration: Oral.

Preparations: tablets, 0.25, 0.5, 1, and 2 mg.

ALPROSTADIL—Caverject®, Edex®, Prostin VR Pediatric®, Prostaglandin E$_1$, PGE$_1$

Description/Actions: Prostaglandin indicated (Prostin VR Pediatric®) for palliative therapy to temporarily maintain the patency of the ductus arteriosus until corrective or palliative surgery can be performed in neonates who have congenital heart defects and who depend upon the patent ductus for survival. Also indicated (Caverject®) for the diagnosis and treatment of male erectile dysfunction due to neurologic, vascular, psychological, or mixed causes.

Administration: Intravenous infusion (Prostin VR Pediatric®) and into an area along the shaft of the penis known as the corpus cavernosum (Caverject®).

Preparations: Ampules, 500 µg (Prostin VR Pediatric®). Vials, 5, 10, 20, and 40 µg (Caverject®). 2 injection starter pack (1 inj. device and supplies edex.)

ALREX®, see Loteprednol Etabonate

ALTACE®, see Ramipril

ALTEPLASE, RECOMBINANT—
Activase®

Fibrinolytic agent.

Description/Actions: Is a form of the body's natural tissue plasminogen activator (TPA) that promotes the conversion of plasminogen to plasmin, which is fibrinolytic. Indicated for the management of acute myocardial infarction in adults for the lysis of thrombi obstructing coronary arteries, the improvement of ventricular function, and reduction of the incidence of congestive heart failure. Also indicated for the management of acute massive pulmonary embolism and acute ischemic stroke. Alteplase is also indicated to restore patency of occluded catheters.

Warnings: Contraindicated in patients with active bleeding, history of cerebrovascular accident, recent (within 2 months) intracranial or intraspinal surgery or trauma, intracranial neoplasm, arteriovenous malformation or aneurysm, known bleeding diathesis, or severe uncontrolled hypertension. Serious bleeding reactions (i.e., internal and/or surface bleeding) may occur and appropriate precautions must be taken. Intramuscular injections should be avoided. Intracranial bleeding has occurred in some patients. The coronary thrombolysis produced by the drug may result in arrhythmias associated with reperfusion.

Administration: Intravenous infusion.

Preparations: Vials, 20 mg (11.6 million IU) and 50 mg (29 million IU). Powder for injection, 2 mg.

ALternaGEL®, see Aluminum hydroxide gel

ALTRETAMINE—Hexalen®

Antineoplastic agent.

Description/Actions: A synthetic cytotoxic agent that must be metabolized for its cytotoxic effect to develop. Indicated for use as a single agent in the palliative treatment of patients with persistent or recurrent ovarian cancer following first-line therapy with a cisplatin and/or alkylating agent-based combination.

Warnings: Should not be used in patients with preexisting severe bone marrow depression or severe neurologic toxicity. Adverse reactions include nausea, vomiting, peripheral neuropathy, and CNS symptoms (e.g., mood disorders, ataxia, dizziness, vertigo). Neurologic examinations should be performed regularly. May cause myelosuppression (e.g., leukopenia, thrombocytopenia) and peripheral blood counts should be monitored at least monthly, prior to the initiation of each course of the drug. May cause fetal damage if administered during pregnancy. If a nursing mother is to be treated with the drug it is recommended that breast-feeding be discontinued. Concurrent use with a monoamine oxidase inhibitor may cause severe orthostatic hypotension. Activity may be increased by the concurrent use of cimetidine.

Administration: Oral. The total daily dose should be given as 4 divided doses after meals and at bedtime.

Preparations: Capsules, 50 mg.

ALUDROX®, see Aluminum and magnesium hydroxides

ALUMINUM ACETATE

Description/Actions: Astringent used as a wet dressing (e.g., Burow's solution) for relief of inflammatory conditions of the skin.

Preparations: Solution.

ALUMINUM AND MAGNESIUM HYDROXIDES—Aludrox®, Maalox®

Description/Actions: Antacid indicated for hyperacidity associated with ulcers and other GI conditions.

Preparations: Liquid and tablets.

ALUMINUM CARBONATE GEL, BASIC—Basaljel®

Description/Actions: Antacid indicated for hyperacidity associated with ulcers and other GI conditions. Also indicated for the management of hyperphosphatemia or for use with a low phosphate diet to prevent formation of phosphate urinary stones.

Preparations: Capsules, tablets, and suspension.

ALUMINUM HYDROXIDE GEL— Amphojel®, ALternaGEL®

Description/Actions: Antacid indicated for hyperacidity associated with ulcers and other GI conditions.

Preparations: Capsules, tablets, suspension.

ALUMINUM PHOSPHATE GEL— Phosphaljel®

Description/Actions: Indicated to reduce fecal excretion of phosphates.

Preparations: Suspension.

ALUPENT®, see Metaproterenol

ALURATE®, see Aprobarbital

AMANTADINE HYDROCHLORIDE— Symmetrel®

Antiviral agent and antiparkinson agent.

Description/Actions: Indicated in the prevention and treatment of respiratory tract illness caused by influenza A virus strains. Also indicated for parkinsonism and drug-induced extrapyramidal reactions.

Warnings: Adverse reactions include orthostatic hypotensive episodes, urinary retention, depression, psychosis, and congestive heart failure.

Administration: Oral.

Preparations: Capsules, 100 mg. Syrup, 50 mg/5 ml.

AMARYL, see Glimepiride

AMBENONIUM CHLORIDE— Mytelase®

Description/Actions: Anticholinesterase indicated for the treatment of myasthenia gravis.

Preparations: Tablets, 10 mg.

AMBIEN®, see Zolpidem tartrate

AMCINONIDE—Cyclocort®

Description/Actions: Corticosteroid indicated in the topical treatment of corticosteroid-responsive dermatoses.

Preparations: Cream, ointment, and lotion, 0.1%.

AMERGE®, see Naratriptan

AMICAR®, see Aminocaproic acid

AMIDATE®, see Etomidate

AMIFOSTINE—Ethyol

Cytoprotective agent (for cisplatin).

Description/Actions: Reduces renal toxicity due to cumulative effects of cisplatin in patients being treated for ovarian cancer or non-small-cell lung cancer.

Warnings: Should not be used in patients with hypotension or dehydration. Adverse effects most commonly seen are hypotension, nausea, and vomiting.

Administration: Intravenous.

Preparations: Powder for injection, 500 mg/vial (with 500 mg mannitol).

AMIKACIN SULFATE—Amikin®

Aminoglycoside antibiotic.

Description/Actions: Indicated in the treatment of serious infections caused by gram-negative bacteria including *Pseudomonas aeruginosa.* Is also effective in the treatment of staphylococcal infections.

Warnings: May cause nephrotoxicity, ototoxicity, and neurotoxicity, and the concurrent or serial use of other nephrotoxic or ototoxic agents should be avoided.

Administration: Intravenous and intramuscular. Clinical response and dosage should be closely monitored.

Preparations: Vials, 100 and 500 mg, and 1 g. Syringes, 500 mg.

AMIKIN®, see Amikacin

AMILORIDE HYDROCHLORIDE—Midamor®

Description/Actions: Diuretic (potassium-sparing) indicated as adjunctive treatment with thiazide or other potassium-depleting diuretics in patients with congestive heart failure or hypertension. Should be administered with food.

Preparations: Tablets, 5 mg.

AMINOACETIC ACID—Glycine

Description/Actions: Anti-infective for urological irrigation. Has also been used in conjunction with antacids.

Preparations: Solutions (for irrigation), 1.5%.

AMINOCAPROIC ACID—Amicar®

Description/Actions: Coagulant that inhibits fibrinolysis. Useful in enhancing hemostasis when fibrinolysis contributes to bleeding.

Preparations: Tablets, 500 mg. Syrup, 250 mg/ml. Vials (for IV use) 250 mg/ml.

AMINOLEVULINIC ACID HYDROCHLORIDE—Levulan Kerastick® for Topical Solution

Description/Actions: Used with BLU-U Blue Light Photodynamic Therapy Illuminator for treatment of non-hyperkeratotic actinic keratoses of the face or scalp.

Precautions/Adverse Reactions: Levulan Kerastick for Topical Solution plus blue light illumination is contraindicated in patients with cutaneous photosensitivity at wavelengths of 400–450 nm, porphyria or known allergies to porphyrins, and in patients with known sensitivity to any of the components of the Levulan Kerastick for Topical Solution. Transient local symptoms following photodynamic therapy include stinging and/or burning, itching, erythema, and edema. After application, patients should avoid exposure of the photosensitive treatment sites to sunlight or bright indoor light during the period prior to blue light treatment. Sunscreens will not protect the patient against photosensitivity reactions. Care should be taken not to apply Levulan Kerastick to perilesional skin.

Administration: The recommended treatment frequency is one application of Levulan Topical Solution and one dose of illumination per treatment site per 8-week treatment session. Application of the product to target lesions with Levulan Kerastick is followed 14–18 hours later by illumination with blue light using the BLU-U Blue Light Photodynamic Therapy Illuminator.

Patient Care Implications: This product is not intended for application by patients or unqualified medical personnel.

Preparations: Levulan Kerasticks for Topical Solution, 20%.

AMINOPHYLLINE—Theophylline ethylenediamine, Phyllocontin®

Description/Actions: Bronchodilator indicated for the management of bronchial asthma, chronic bronchitis, and emphysema. Has been used as a diuretic and in certain cardiovascular disorders.

Preparations: Tablets, 100 and 200 mg. Controlled-release tablets, 225 mg. Liquid, 105 mg/5 ml. Suppositories, 250 and 500 mg. Ampules and vials, 250 mg.

AMINOSALICYLATE SODIUM—
Para-aminosalicylate sodium, PAS sodium

Description/Actions: Antitubercular agent indicated for tuberculosis in combination with other antitubercular agents.

Preparations: Tablets, 500 mg. Powder.

AMINOSALICYLIC ACID, see Aminosalicylate sodium

AMIODARONE HYDROCHLORIDE—
Cordarone®

Antiarrhythmic agent.

Description/Actions: A class III antiarrhythmic agent indicated for documented life-threatening, recurrent ventricular fibrillation and for recurrent, hemodynamically unstable ventricular tachycardia. Use when those conditions have not responded to treatment with other antiarrhythmic agents or when alternative drugs were not tolerated. Is often effective in patients with serious ventricular arrhythmias that are refractory to other agents.

Warnings: Contraindicated in patients with severe sinus-node dysfunction, causing marked sinus bradycardia; second- and third-degree AV block, and when episodes of bradycardia have caused syncope (except when used in conjunction with a pacemaker). Adverse reactions include pulmonary toxicity that may be fatal, proarrhythmic events, GI effects, neurologic effects (e.g., fatigue, tremor), ocular effects (e.g., visual halos, blurred vision), hepatic dysfunction, hepatitis, cholestatic hepatitis, cirrhosis, epididymitis, vasculitis, pseudotumor cerebri, thrombocytopenia, angioedema, bronchiolitis obliterans organizing pneumonia (possibly fatal), pleuritis, pancreatitis, toxic epidermal necrolysis, myopathy, hemolytic anemia, aplastic anemia, pancytopenia, neutropenia, and dermatologic effects (e.g., photosensitivity reactions).

May interact with and increase the activity of digoxin, warfarin, diltiazem, and other antiarrhythmic agents. Orally has variable absorption. Slow onset of action and long duration of action make dosing and monitoring of therapy difficult. IV administration results in complete bioavailability. Contains the preservative benzyl alcohol, which has been associated with a fatal "gasping syndrome" in neonates. Oral use during pregnancy has been associated with neonatal congenital goiter/hypothyroidism and hyperthyroidism.

Administration: Oral/IV.

Preparations: Tablets, 200 mg. Injection, 50 mg/ml in 3 ml ampules.

AMITRIPTYLINE HYDROCHLORIDE—Elavil®, Endep®

Tricyclic antidepressant.

Description/Actions: Indicated for the relief of symptoms of depression.

Warnings: Should not be given concomitantly with a monoamine oxidase inhibitor. Is not recommended for use during the acute recovery phase following myocardial infarction. Use cautiously in patients with history of seizure, urinary retention, glaucoma, cardiovascular disease, suicidal tendencies, surgery, ECT, psychosis, hyperthyroidism, diabetes and liver dysfunction. Adverse reactions include CNS effects, and patients should be cautioned regarding activities such as driving and operating machinery, as well as interactions with other CNS-acting drugs including alcohol. Other adverse reactions include anticholinergic effects (e.g., dry mouth, blurred vision), GI effects (e.g., nausea, vomiting), and cardiovascular effects (e.g., orthostatic hypotension). Caution should be exercised in patients with cardiovascular disorders. May reduce the action of guanethidine and guanadrel.

Administration: Oral and intramuscular.

Preparations: Tablets, 10, 25, 50, 75, 100, and 150 mg. Vials, 10 mg/ml.

AMLEXANOX 5%—Aphthasol®

Antiinflammatory

Description/Actions: Oral adhesive paste indicated in the treatment of canker sores.

Warnings: Not for use in immunocompromised patients. Discontinue if rash or contact mucositis occurs. Pregnancy Category B. Use cautiously in nursing mothers. Adverse reactions include transient local pain, burning and/or stinging. Instruct patients to consult health care provider if ulcer does not heal after 10 days.

Administration: Topical.

Preparations: 5 g tubes of 5% adhesive oral paste.

AMLODIPINE BESYLATE— Norvasc®

Antihypertensive and antianginal agent.

Description/Actions: Is a calcium channel blocking agent that causes a reduction in peripheral vascular resistance and a lowering in blood pressure. Indicated for the treatment of hypertension. Also indicated for the treatment of chronic stable angina and vasospastic angina (Prinzmetal's or variant angina).

Warnings: Adverse reactions include edema, flushing, palpitation, dizziness, fatigue, somnolence, nausea, and abdominal pain.

Administration: Oral.

Preparations: Tablets, 2.5, 5, and 10 mg.

AMMONIA, AROMATIC SPIRIT— Aromatic ammonia spirit

Description/Actions: Respiratory stimulant used by inhalation to treat or prevent fainting.

Preparations: Inhalant and solution.

AMMONIATED MERCURY

Description/Actions: Anti-infective agent used for the topical treatment of certain skin infections and conditions such as psoriasis.

Preparations: Ointment, 5% and 10%.

AMMONIUM CARBONATE

Description/Actions: Respiratory stimulant used in the preparation of aromatic ammonia spirit and as a source of ammonia in smelling salts.

AMMONIUM CHLORIDE

Description/Actions: Expectorant, diuretic, and acidifying agent. Used orally as an expectorant, diuretic, and to acidify the urine, and intravenously in the treatment of certain hypochloremic states and metabolic alkalosis.

Preparations: Tablets, 500 mg and 1 g. Vials and bottles, 0.4 mEq/ml and 5 mEq/ml.

AMMONIUM LACTATE—Lac-Hydrin®

Description/Actions: Emollient indicated in treatment of dry skin and ichthyosis vulgaris. Transient stinging or burning, erythema, peeling, eczema, petechiae, dryness, and hyperpigmentation may occur.

Administration: Apply and rub into affected areas twice daily.

Preparations: Lotion and cream, 12%.

AMOBARBITAL SODIUM—Amytal sodium®

Description/Actions: Barbiturate sedative-hypnotic indicated for the treatment of anxiety and convulsive disorders, for preanesthetic sedation, and in narcoanalysis and narcotherapy.

Preparations: Vials, 250 and 500 mg.

AMOXAPINE—Asendin®

Description/Actions: Antidepressant (dibenzoxazepine) indicated for the relief of symptoms of depression, and for depression accompanied by anxiety or agitation.

Preparations: Tablets, 25, 50, 100, and 150 mg.

AMOXICILLIN—Amoxil®, Polymox®, Trimox®

Penicillin antibiotic.

Description/Actions: Is bactericidal and exhibits activity that is most similar to that of ampicillin. Indicated for the treatment of infections caused by susceptible strains of *Escherichia coli, Haemophilus influenzae, Proteus mirabilis, Neisseria gonorrhoeae,* streptococci, and non-penicillinase-producing staphylococci. Is commonly used in the treatment of respiratory tract infections, otitis media, urinary tract infections, and uncomplicated gonorrhea.

Warnings: Contraindicated in patients with a history of allergic reaction to any of the penicillins. Adverse reactions include hypersensitivity reactions, rash, urticaria, nausea, vomiting, and diarrhea.

Administration: Oral. May be administered without regard to meals.

Preparations: Capsules, 250 and 500 mg. Chewable tablets, 125, 250, and 875 mg.

AMOXICILLIN/CLAVULANATE POTASSIUM—Augmentin®, Augmentin® XR

Penicillin antibiotic with beta-lactamase inhibitor.

Description/Actions: Clavulanic acid inhibits beta-lactamase enzymes and protects amoxicillin from degradation by these enzymes; the spectrum of action of amoxicillin is extended to include many gram-positive and gram-negative bacteria, including *Moraxella catarrhalis.* Indicated for the treatment of lower respiratory infections, otitis media, sinusitis, skin and skin-structure infections, and urinary tract infections.

Warnings: Contraindicated in patients with a history of allergic reaction to any of the penicillins. Adverse reactions include hypersensitivity reactions, rash, urticaria, nausea, vomiting, and diarrhea. Incidence of GI effects is higher than when amoxicillin is administered alone. Due to clavulanic acid component, 2 Augmentin 250 mg are not equivalent to 1 Augmentin 500 mg.

Administration: Oral. May be administered without regard to meals.

Preparations: Tablets, 250, 500, and 875 mg with 125 mg potassium clavulanate, and 1g with 62.5 mg potassium clavulanate. Chewable tablets, 125 mg amoxicillin with 31.25 mg of clavulanic acid, 200 mg amoxicillin, with 28.5 mg clavulanic acid, 250 mg amoxicillin with 62.5 mg of clavulanic acid, and 400 mg amoxicillin with 57 mg of clavulonic acid. Powder for oral suspension, 125 mg amoxicillin with 31.25 mg clavulonic acid/5 ml; 200 mg amoxicillin with 28.5 mg clavulanic acid/5ml; and 400 amoxicillin with 57 mg clavulanic acid/5 ml; and 600 mg amoxicillin with 42.9 mg clavulonic acid/5 ml.

AMPHETAMINE SULFATE

Description/Actions: Central nervous system stimulant indicated in the treatment of narcolepsy, attention deficit disorder in children, and exogenous obesity.

Preparations: Tablets, 5 and 10 mg.

AMPHOJEL®, see Aluminum hydroxide gel

AMPHOTEC®—Amphotericin B cholesteryl sulfate, also, AMBISOME®—Amphotericin B liposome for injection

Antifungal.

Description/Actions: Indicated in patients with aspergillosis who are intolerant or refractory to conventional dosage form of Amphotericin B. Empiric treatment of presumed fungal infections in febrile neutropenic patients.

Administration: Intravenous infusion after dilution. An intravenous bolus of 0.25 mg/kg is administered 10–60 minutes.

Preparations: Vials, 100 mg with single-use filter needle.

AMPHOTERICIN B—Fungizone®

Description/Actions: Antifungal agent indicated for the intravenous treatment of systemic fungal infections, topical treatment of cutaneous candidal infections and oral suspension for oral candidiasis.

Warnings: Be fully familiar with the use of this product. Administer under close supervision; cardiopulmonary resuscitation facilities should be available. Monitor serum creatinine, liver function, serum electrolytes (esp. magnesium and potassium), and CBC.

Preparations: Vials, 50 mg. Oral suspension, 100 mg/ml. Cream, ointment, and lotion, 3%.

AMPICILLIN—Omnipen®, Polycillin®, Principen®, Totacillin®

AMPICILLIN SODIUM

Penicillin antibiotic.

Description/Actions: Is bactericidal. Indicated for the treatment of infections caused by susceptible strains of *Escherichia coli, Haemophilus influenzae, Neisseria gonorrhoeae, Neisseria meningitidis, Proteus mirabilis, Salmonella* species, *Shigella*, streptococci, and nonpenicillinase-producing staphylococci. Is used in the treatment of urinary tract infections, respiratory tract infections, and uncomplicated gonorrhea. Used intravenously in the treatment of meningitis and septicemia caused by susceptible organisms.

Warnings: Contraindicated in patients with a history of allergic reaction to any of the penicillins. Adverse reactions include hypersensitivity reactions, rash, urticaria, nausea, vomiting, and diarrhea.

Administration: Oral, intravenous, and intramuscular. When administered orally, it is best administered apart from meals.

Preparations: Capsules, 250 and 500 mg. Powder for oral suspension, 125, 250, and 500 mg/5 ml (when reconstituted). Vials, ampicillin sodium equivalent to 125, 500 mg, 1, 2, and 10 g of ampicillin per vial.

AMPICILLIN SODIUM/ SULBACTAM SODIUM— Unasyn®

Penicillin antibiotic with beta-lactamase inhibitor.

Description/Actions: A combination of ampicillin and a beta-lactamase inhibitor, sulbactam. By irreversibly binding to beta-lactamase enzymes that are produced by certain bacteria, sulbactam protects ampicillin against inactivation by these enzymes, thereby extending the spectrum of ampicillin to include many bacteria that are resistant to it when it is given alone. Indicated for intraabdominal, gynecological, and skin structure infections caused by susceptible bacteria. Among the bacteria that are susceptible are beta-lactamase producing strains of *Acinetobacter calcoaceticus, Bacteroides* species (including *B. fragilis*), *Enterobacter* species, *Escherichia coli, Klebsiella* species (including *K. pneumoniae*), *Proteus mirabilis,* and *Staphylococcus aureus.*

Warnings: Contraindicated in patients with a known hypersensitivity to any of the penicillins. Adverse reactions include diarrhea, rash, pain at the intramuscular and intravenous injection sites, and thrombophlebitis. Should not be used in patients with mononucleosis because of the likelihood of a nonallergic skin rash developing.

Administration: Intravenous and intramuscular. The coadministration of lidocaine significantly decreases the incidence of local pain following intramuscular injection.

Preparations: Vials and piggyback bottles containing 1.5 g (1 g ampicillin sodium plus 0.5 g sulbactam sodium) and 3 g (2 g ampicillin sodium plus 1 g sulbactam sodium).

AMPRENAVIR—Agenerase®

Description/Actions: Amprenavir is an HIV protease inhibitor indicated as a combination agent with other antiretroviral agents in the treatment of HIV infection.

Precautions/Adverse Reactions: Amprenavir is contraindicated in concomitant use with several other drugs. Prescribers need to verify the patient's drug profile and consult product literature before prescribing. The capsules and solution are not interchangeable on a mg to mg basis. Use cautiously in patients with sulfa allergy and the elderly. Reduce the dose in patients with hepatic dysfunction. Monitor diabetics for hyperglycemia and fat redistribution and hemophiliacs for spontaneous bleeding. Pregnancy Category C. Use in nursing mothers not recommended.

Adverse reactions include GI upset, rash (e.g., Stevens-Johnson), paresthesia, and depression.

Administration: Oral.

Patient Care Implications: Instruct patients to continue to use appropriate barrier precautions when engaging in sexual activity to prevent spread of the disease. Patients taking amprenavir should be instructed not to use hormonal contraceptives because some birth control pills have been found to decrease the concentration of amprenavir therefore, patients receiving hormonal contraceptives should be instructed to use alternative contraceptive measures during therapy with amprenavir. Let the patient know this drug is not a cure, but can keep the infection under control.

Tell the patient to avoid taking the drug with a high fat meal. Do not take additional vitamin E supplements, as this drug supplies enough. Do not switch between capsules and oral solution without consulting the physician.

Preparations: Capsules, 50 and 150 mg (contain Vitamin E). Oral solution, 15 mg/ml grape-bubblegum-peppermint flavor (contains vitamin E).

AMYL NITRITE

Description/Actions: Antianginal agent administered by inhalation for the relief of acute angina pectoris.

Preparations: Inhalant, 0.18 and 0.3 ml.

AMYTAL®, see Amobarbital

ANADROL-50®, see Oxymetholone

ANAFRANIL®, see Clomipramine hydrochloride

ANAGRELIDE—Agrylin®

Description/Actions: Indicated in the treatment of essential thrombocythemia. Reduces platelet counts at therapeutic doses and at higher doses inhibits platelet aggregation as well. Does not affect WBC counts or coagulation parameters at therapeutic doses although it may have clinically insignificant effect on RBC parameters.

Warnings: Use cautiously in cardiovascular disease, hepatic or renal dysfunction. Adverse reactions include headache, palpitations, tachycardia, anorexia, edema, pain, dizziness, dyspnea, rash, paresthesia, tachycardia, anorexia, CHF, MI, malaise, cardiomyopathy, cardiomegaly, complete heart block, atrial fibrillation, CVA, pericarditis, pulmonary infiltrates/ fibrosis, hypertension, pancreatitis, ulcer, and seizures. Instruct patients to report signs/symptoms of hepatic, renal, or cardiac dysfunction.

Administration: 0.5 mg 4 times daily or 1 mg twice daily for at least 1 week. Then adjust to the lowest effective dosage required to reduce and maintain platelet count < 600,000/mcl.

Preparations: Capsules, 0.5 and 1 mg.

ANAKINRA—KINERET™

Description/Actions: Anakinra is indicated for the reduction in signs and symptoms of moderately to severely active rheumatoid arthritis in patients 18 years of age and older who have failed one or more disease-modifying antirheumatic drugs (DMARDs).

Precautions/Adverse Reactions: Anakinra is contraindicated in patients with a known sensitivity to *E. coli* derived proteins, to anakinra, or to any components of the drug. It has been associated with an increased incidence of serious infections; administration should be discontinued if the patient develops a serious infection. Treatment should not be started in patients with active infections. Safety and efficacy in patients with chronic infections or immunosuppressed patients have not been evaluated. When used with tumor necrosis factor (TNF)–blocking agents, preliminary data suggested a higher rate of serious infections. When given with etanercept, neutropenia was observed.

Anakinra interferes with normal immune response mechanisms to new antigens such as vaccines; therefore, vaccination may not be effective. Live vaccines should not be given concurrently with anakinra. Pregnancy Category B. No controlled trials in pregnant women. Use only if clearly needed. It is not known whether anakinra is secreted in breast milk; use caution in nursing women. Safety and efficacy in juvenile rheumatoid arthritis have not been established. The most common adverse reactions were injection site reactions (typically lasts 14–28 days), serious infection (stop drug), neutropenia, headache, nausea, diarrhea, sinusitis, and influenza-like symptoms.

Administration: Geriatrics and adults: 100 mg once a day by subcutaneous injection. Administer at same time each day.

Patient Care Implications: Rotate injection sites; injection should be given at least 1 inch away from previous site. Discard any unused portion; anakinra contains no preservative. Do not shake. Neutrophil counts should be obtained prior to treatment and repeated monthly for 3 months, and thereafter quarterly for a period up to 1 year. Instruct patient in the importance of proper disposal of syringe, and caution against reuse of needles, syringes, and drug. Should be stored in rerigerator. Do not freeze. Protect from light.

Preparations: Injection, prefilled 1 ml glass syringe with 27 gauge needle: 100 mg/0.67 ml.

ANAPROX®, see Naproxen sodium

ANAPROX DS®, see Naproxen sodium

ANASPAZ, see Hyoscyamine

ANASTROZOLE—Arimidex®

Antiestrogen.

Description/Actions: Exerts antineoplastic effect and is indicated for the treatment of advanced breast cancer in postmenopausal women with disease progression after tamoxifen therapy and for the adjuvant treatment of postmenopausal women with hormone receptor positive early breast cancer.

Warnings: Contraindicated in pregnancy. Asthenia, GI disturbances, headache, hot flashes, pain, dyspnea, rash, dry mouth, peripheral edema, depression, parenthesia, and vaginal bleeding may occur. Anastrozole may be associated with rash, including very rare cases of mucocutaneous disorders such as erythema multiforme and Stevens-Johnson Syndrome.

Administration: Oral, 1 mg once daily.
Preparations: Tablets, 1 mg.

ANCEF®, see Cefazolin

ANCOBON®, see Flucytosine

ANDRODERM®, see Testosterone

ANDROGEL®, see Testosterone Gel

ANECTINE®, see Succinylcholine

ANGIOMAX™, see Bivalirudin

ANISINDIONE—Miradon®

Description/Actions: Anticoagulant (indandione) indicated for the prophylaxis and treatment of conditions such as venous thrombosis and pulmonary embolism.

Preparations: Tablets, 50 mg.

ANISOTROPINE METHYLBROMIDE

Description/Actions: Anticholinergic agent indicated as adjunctive therapy in the management of peptic ulcer.

Preparations: Tablets, 50 mg.

ANISTREPLASE—Eminase®

Thrombolytic agent.

Description/Actions: Also known as anisoylated plasminogen streptokinase activator complex (APSAC). Promotes the conversion of plasminogen to plasmin, which is fibrinolytic. Indicated for acute management of coronary thrombosis (myocardial infarction). Treatment should be initiated as soon as possible after the onset of AMI symptoms.

Warnings: Contraindicated in patients who are hypersensitive to the drug or to streptokinase. Is also contraindicated in patients with active internal bleeding, history of cerebrovascular accident, recent intracranial or intraspinal surgery or trauma, intracranial neoplasm, arteriovenous malformation, or aneurysm, known bleeding diathesis, or severe, uncontrolled hypertension. Serious bleeding reactions (e.g., internal bleeding and/or superficial or surface bleeding) may occur and appropriate precautions must be taken. Concurrent use of heparin anticoagulation may contribute to the bleeding. Warfarin, aspirin, and dipyridamole may increase the risk of bleeding if administered prior to anistreplase therapy. Intramuscular injections should be avoided during treatment with anistreplase. Other adverse reactions include hypotension and allergic-type reactions.

Administration: Intravenous.

Preparations: Vials, 30 units.

ANSAID®, see Flurbiprofen

ANSPOR®, see Cephradine

ANTABUSE®, see Disulfiram

ANTAGON®, see Ganirelix

ANTEPAR®, see Piperazine citrate

ANTHRA-DERM®, see Anthralin

ANTHRALIN—Anthra-Derm®, Dithranol

Description/Actions: Used in the topical management of psoriasis and certain other dermatologic disorders.

Preparations: Cream and ointment, 0.1%, 0.2%, 0.25%, 0.4%, 0.5%, and 1%.

ANTILIRIUM®, see Physostigmine

ANTIMINTH®, see Pyrantel pamoate

ANTISPAS®, see Dicyclomine

ANTITHROMBIN III (HUMAN)—ATnativ®

Coagulation inhibitor.

Description/Actions: Is identical with heparin cofactor I, a factor that is necessary for heparin to exert its anticoagulant effect. Inactivates thrombin and the activated forms of Factors IX, X, XI, and XII. Indicated for the treatment of patients with hereditary antithrombin III deficiency in connection with surgical or obstetrical procedures or when they suffer from thromboembolism.

Warnings: The anticoagulant effect of heparin is increased by concurrent treatment with antithrombin III and the dosage of heparin should be reduced.

Administration. Intravenous. Plasma antithrombin III levels should be measured preceding and 30 minutes after the dose until the patient is stabilized, and thereafter measured once a day immediately before the next infusion.

Preparations: Infusion bottles, 500 international units.

ANTIVERT®, see Meclizine

ANTURANE®, see Sulfinpyrazone

ANZEMET®, see Dolasetron Mesylate

APHTHASOL®, see Amlexanox 5%

A.P.L.®, see Chorionic gonadotropin

APRACLONIDINE HYDROCHLORIDE—Iopidine®

Ocular laser surgical agent.

Description/Actions: An alpha adrenergic agonist which, when instilled into the eye, reduces intraocular pressure. Indicated (1% solution) to control or prevent postsurgical elevations in intraocular pressure that occur in patients after argon laser trabeculoplasty or argon laser iridotomy. Also indicated (0.5% solution) for short-term adjunctive therapy in patients on maximally tolerated medical therapy who require additional intraocular pressure reduction.

Warnings: Adverse reactions include upper lid elevation, conjunctival blanching, and mydriasis.

Administration: Ophthalmic.

Preparations: Ophthalmic solution, containing the equivalent of 0.5% and 1% apraclonidine base.

APRESOLINE®, see Hydralazine

APROBARBITAL—Alurate®

Description/Actions: Barbiturate sedative-hypnotic indicated for the treatment of anxiety and insomnia.

Preparations: Elixir, 40 mg/5 ml.

APROTININ—Trasylol®

Antifibrinolytic agent.

Description/Actions: Is a natural protease inhibitor that inhibits fibrinolysis and decreases bleeding, and reduces the need for donor blood or blood products. Indicated for prophylactic use to reduce perioperative blood loss and the need for blood transfusion in patients undergoing cardiopulmonary bypass in the course of repeat coronary artery bypass graft (CABG) surgery. Is also indicated in selected cases of primary CABG surgery where the risk of bleeding is especially high or where transfusion is unavailable or unacceptable.

Warnings: Adverse reactions include anaphylactic reactions, renal dysfunction, and abnormal liver function tests. All patients should first receive a test dose to assess the potential for allergic reactions. Patients who experience any allergic reaction to the test dose should not receive further administration of the drug. Particular caution is necessary when administering aprotinin (even test doses) to patients who have received the drug in the past. In reexposure cases, an antihistamine should be administered intravenously shortly before the loading dose. May inhibit the effects of fibrinolytic agents. May be administered concurrently with heparin; however, aprotinin prolongs the activated clotting time (ACT) and some patients may require additional heparin, even in the presence of ACT levels that appear to represent adequate anticoagulation.

Administration: Intravenous. Is administered through a central line and other drugs should not be administered using the same line. A 1 ml (10,000 Kallikrein Inhibitor Units [KIU]) test dose should be administered at least 10 minutes before the loading dose. The loading dose is given slowly over 20–30 minutes after induction of anesthesia but prior to sternotomy. When the loading dose is complete, it is followed by the constant infusion dose, which is continued until surgery is complete and the patient leaves the operating room. A "pump prime" dose is added to the priming fluid of the cardiopulmonary bypass circuit, by replacement of an aliquot of the priming fluid, prior to the institution of the cardiopulmonary bypass.

Preparations: Vials 1,000,000 and 2,000,000 Kallikrein Inhibitor Units (KIU). One million units represents 140 mg of the drug.

AQUA MEPHYTON®, see Phytonadione

AQUACARE®, see Urea

AQUASOL A®, see Vitamin A

AQUASOL E®, see Vitamin E

ARA-C, see Cytarabine

ARALEN®, see Chloroquine

ARAMINE®, see Metaraminol

ARANESP™, see Darbepoetin Alfa

ARDEPARIN—Normiflo®

Antithrombolic

Description/Actions: Antithrombolic indicated in the prevention of postop deep vein thrombosis in patients undergoing elective knee replacement.

Warnings: Contraindicated in severe hemorrhagic diathesis, active major bleeding; Type II thrombocytopenia associated with a positive in vitro test for antiplatelet antibody associated with ardeparin sodium, heparin, or pork allergy.

Use cautiously in neuraxial anesthesia and postop indwelling epidural catheter or spinal puncture (risk of epidural or spinal hematoma), asthma, heparin-induced thrombocytopenia, bleeding disorders, severe renal dysfunction (monitor carefully if serum Cr≥2 mg/dl), severe uncontrolled hypertension, acute bacterial endocarditis, acute ulceration and angiodysplastic GI disease, bleeding diathesis, non-hemorrhagic stroke, invasive procedures, recent brain, spinal, or eye surgery.

Adverse reactions include hemorrhage, hematoma, thrombocytopenia, local reactions (e.g., hematoma, pain), fever, allergic reaction, GI upset, constipation, rash, pruritus, edema, dizziness, insomnia, and anemia.

Administration: SQ injection.

Preparations: 5,000 anti-Xa units in 0.5 ml.

10,000 anti-Xa units in 0.5 ml.

ARDUAN®, see Pipecuronium bromide

AREDIA®, see Pamidronate disodium

ARGATROBAN

Description/Actions: Argatroban is an anticoagulant used in the prophylaxis or the treatment of thrombosis in adults with heparin-induced thrombocytopenia (HIT). Argatroban is also indicated for use during percutaneous coronary intervention (PTCI) in patients who have HIT or those who are at risk for HIT.

Precautions/Adverse Reactions: Argatroban is contraindicated in patients with active major bleeding, or in patients hypersensitive to this product or any of its product formulations. Since hemorrhage can occur with Argatroban, it should be used with extreme caution in patients with disease states or circumstances associated with increased risk of bleeding. Use caution in patients with hepatic impairment, initiate with a lower dose and titrate to desired effect. Concurrent use with warfarin will cause increased prolongation of the PT and INR greater than that of warfarin alone. Safety and efficacy for use with other thrombolytic agents have not been established. All parental anticoagulants should be discontinued before administration of Argatroban. Pregnancy Category B. No adequate and well-controlled studies have been done in pregnant women. Argatroban should be used in pregnant women only if clearly needed. It is not known if this drug is excreted in human milk; not recommended for nursing women. Safety and efficacy have not been established in children < 18 years of age.

Some adverse effects are gastrointestinal bleed, genitourinary bleed and hematuria, hypotension, decrease in hemoglobin and hematocrit, fever, pain, diarrhea, nausea, and vomiting.

Administration: Intravenous.

Conversion to oral anticoagulant: Because there may be a combined effect on the INR when Argatroban is combined with warfarin, loading doses of warfarin should not be used. Warfarin therapy should be started at the expected daily dose.

Patient Care Implications: This medication can only be administered by intravenous infusion; vials must be diluted to 1 mg/ml prior to infusion and must not be mixed with other medications. Monitor aPTT, hemoglobin, and hematocrit. Inform patients to report any unusual bleeding or bruising while receiving Argatroban.

Preparations: Solution for injection: 100 mg/ml (2.5 ml) vials. Each vial contains 250 mg Argatroban.

ARGININE HYDROCHLORIDE— R-Gene®

Description/Actions: Diagnostic agent administered intravenously in the evaluation of pituitary function.

Preparations: Solution, 10%.

ARICEPT®, see Donepezil Hydrochloride

ARISTOCORT®, see Triamcinolone

ARIMIDEX, see Anastrozole

ARISTOSPAN®, see Triamcinolone hexacetonide

ARIXTRA®, see Fondaparinux

AROMASIN®, see Exemestane

AROMATIC SPIRIT OF AMMONIA, see Ammonia, aromatic spirit

ARSENIC TRIOXIDE—Trisenox®

Description/Actions: Indicated for induction of remission and consolidation in patients with acute promyelocytic leukemia who are refractory to, or have relapsed from retinoid and anthracycline chemotherapy and whose acute promyelocytic leukemia is characterized by the presence of the t(15;17) translocation or PML-RAR-alpha gene expression.

Precautions/Adverse Reactions: Arsenic trioxide is contraindicated in anyone with a known hypersensitivity to arsenic or to any component of the product. Arsenic trioxide should be administered only under the supervision of a physician who is experienced in the management of acute leukemia. May cause a syndrome known as retinoic acid acute promyelocytic leukemia (RA-APL) or APL differentiation syndrome. This syndrome can be fatal and requires prompt therapy with high dose dexamethasone. Arsenic trioxide may cause prolongation of the QT interval and complete atrioventricular block. It may lead to torsade de pointes which can be fatal. The extent of the QT interval prolongation, coadministration of drugs known to prolong the QT interval, a history of torsade de pointes, preexisting QT interval prolongation, congestive heart failure, administration of potassium wasting diuretics or other conditions that result in hypokalemia or hypomagnesemia are risk factors for the development of torsade de pointes. Baseline EKG (12 lead), serum potassium, magnesium, calcium, and creatinine values should be obtained prior to the initiation of therapy with arsenic trioxide. Electrolyte abnormalities should be corrected prior to the start of therapy. Potassium and magnesium levels should be kept at 4 mEq/dL and 1.8 mEq/dL respectively during treatment with arsenic trioxide. A QT_c interval > 500 msec should be corrected prior to the start of therapy with arsenic. If during therapy, the QT_c interval exceeds 500 msec, the patient should be reassessed and corrective action taken. If at any point, syncope or rapid or irregular heartbeat develops, the patient should be hospitalized for monitoring. Hyperleukocytosis is possible during therapy with arsenic. Use cautiously in patients with renal insufficiency. Use caution when coadministering with other drugs known to prolong the QT interval or to cause electrolyte disturbances. Pregnancy Category D. No adequate or well-controlled studies in pregnant women. May cause fetal harm. Excreted in human breast milk; not recommended in nursing women. Limited data in 5–16 year olds. No efficacy or safety data in children < 5 years of age.

Most serious adverse effects seen in patients treated with arsenic trioxide include: APL differentiation syndrome (22.5%), QT_c interval prolongation (38%), hyperleukocytosis (50%), and EKG abnormalities. Adverse reactions occurring in ≥ 10% of patients include fatigue, fever, edema, rigors, chest pain, injection site, weakness, weight gain, nausea, anorexia, diarrhea, vomiting, abdominal pain, sore throat, constipation, loose stools, dyspepsia, hypokalemia, hypomagnesemia, headache, insomnia, paresthesia, dizziness, tremors, cough, dyspnea, epistaxis, hypoxia, pleural effusion, postnasal drip, wheezing, decreased breath sounds, crepitations, rales, dermatitis, pruritis, ecchymosis, dry skin, erythema, increased sweating, tachycardia, palpitations, sinusitis, herpes simplex, upper respiratory tract infections, arthralgias, myalgias, pain, anemia, thrombocytopenia, neutropenia, hypotension, hypertension, flushing, pallor, anxiety, depression, eye irritation, blurred vision, and vaginal hemorrhage.

Administration: Intravenous.

Patient Care Implications: Chemotherapeutic agent—handle and dispose of properly.

Baseline, then twice weekly serum electrolytes, coagulation, and hematologic parameters. Baseline and weekly EKG (12 lead).

Preparations: Solution for injection: 10 mg/10 ml, 10 ml glass single-use ampules.

ARTANE®, see Trihexyphenidyl

ARTHROPAN®, see Choline salicylate

ARTHROTEC®—Combination agent diclotenac sodium and misoprostol

ARTICAINE HYDROCHLORIDE AND EPINEPHRINE—
Septocaine™

Description/Actions: Used as an anesthesia agent for infiltration and nerve block anesthesia in clinical dentistry. The onset of anesthesia occurs within 1 to 6 minutes after injection and the duration of complete anesthesia is approximately 1 to 2.5 hours.

Precautions/Adverse Reactions: This medication is contraindicated in patients with a hypersensitivity to Septocaine™/local anesthetics of the amide type or to sodium metabisulfite. Intravascular injections should be avoided; accidental intravascular injection may be associated with convulsions, followed by CNS or cardiorespiratory depression and respiratory arrest. Product contains epinephrine, which may cause local tissue necrosis or systemic toxicities. To avoid serious adverse effects and high plasma levels, use the lowest effective dose. Pregnancy Category C. Articaine should only be used during pregnancy if the potential benefit justifies a potential risk to the fetus.

Some adverse effects are headache, dizziness, anxiety, agitations, paresthesia, pain (body as a whole), and hypersensitivity reactions.

Administration: Injection.

Patient Care Implications: Dental practitioners and/or clinicians using local anesthetics should be trained in diagnosis and management of emergencies that may arise from the utilization of these agents. Systemic absorption of local anesthetics may produce CNS and cardiovascular effects; careful monitoring of cardiovascular and respiratory status of the patient should be performed.

Preparations: Injection: Articaine hydrochloride 4% with epinephrine (as bitartrate), 1: 100,000 (1.7 ml cartridges).

ASA, see Aspirin

ASACOL®, see Mesalamine

ASCORBIC ACID, see Vitamin C

ASENDIN®, see Amoxapine

A-SPAS®, see Dicyclomine

ASPARAGINASE—Elspar®

Description/Actions: Antineoplastic agent indicated in the treatment of acute lymphocytic leukemia.

Preparations: Vials, 10,000 IU.

ASPERCREME®, see Trolamine salicylate

ASPIRIN—Acetylsalicylic acid, ASA, Bayer aspirin®, Easprin®, Ecotrin®, Empirin®, ZORprin®

Analgesic/antipyretic and anti-inflammatory agent.

Description/Actions: A salicylate used in the treatment of mild to moderate pain, fever, and arthritic and other disorders associated with inflammation. Also indicated for reducing the risk of stroke in male patients with recurrent ischemic attacks, and to reduce the risk of death and/or nonfatal myocardial infarction in patients with a previous infarction or unstable angina pectoris.

Warnings: Contraindicated in patients known to be hypersensitive to salicylates or in individuals with the syndrome of nasal polyps, angioedema, and bronchospastic reactivity to aspirin. May cause GI effects, and use should be avoided in patients with active GI tract disease and closely supervised in patients with a previous history of such disorders. Other adverse reactions include rash, tinnitus, interference with hemostasis, aspirin intolerance, and salicylism. May interact with and increase the effect of anticoagulants, hypoglycemic agents, and methotrexate. May reduce the effect of probenecid and sulfinpyrazone.

Discontinue the drug 7–10 days before elective surgical procedures. Use in children or teenagers with influenza or chicken pox may be associated with the development of Reye's syndrome. Use during pregnancy is best avoided, especially in the third trimester.

Administration: Oral and rectal. Enteric-coated and controlled-release formulations should be swallowed intact.

Preparations: Tablets, 81, 325, and 500 mg. Enteric-coated tablets/capsules, 325, 500, 650, and 975 mg. Controlled-release tablets, 650, and 800 mg. Suppositories, 60, 130, 200, 325, and 650 mg.

ASTELIN®, see Azelastine Hydrochloride

ASTRAMORPH PF®, see Morphine.

ATACAND HCT™, Combination of Candesartan and hydrochlorothiazide

ATARAX®, see Hydroxyzine

ATENOLOL—Tenormin®

Antihypertensive and antianginal agent.

Actions and Uses: A cardioselective beta-adrenergic blocking agent indicated in the management of hypertension, angina pectoris, and myocardial infarction.

Warnings: Contraindicated in patients with sinus bradycardia, heart block greater than first degree, cardiogenic shock, and overt cardiac failure. Adverse reactions include dizziness, fatigue, bradycardia, postural hypotension, and nausea. Use is best avoided in patients with bronchospastic diseases, and therapy in diabetic patients must be closely monitored.

Administration: Oral and intravenous. Patients should be cautioned about the interruption or discontinuation of therapy; exacerbation of angina pectoris has occurred following the abrupt cessation of therapy and, when therapy is to be discontinued, the dosage should be gradually reduced over a period of 1 to 2 weeks.

Preparations: Tablets, 25, 50, and 100 mg. Ampules, 5 mg/10 ml.

ATIVAN®, see Lorazepam

ATnativ®, see Antithrombin III (Human)

ATOVAQUONE—Mepron®

Antiprotozoal agent.

Description/Actions: Indicated for the treatment of mild to moderate *Pneumocystis carinii* pneumonia (PCP) and prevention of PCP in patients who are intolerant to trimethoprim-sulfamethoxazole.

Warnings: Adverse reactions include rash, nausea, vomiting, diarrhea, headache, fever, insomnia, and elevation of liver enzymes.

Administration: Oral. Should be taken with meals. Patients should be advised of the importance of administering the drug with meals.

Preparations: Suspension, 750 mg/5 ml.

ATOVAQUONE AND PROGUANIL HYDROCHLORIDE— Malarone™

Description/Actions: Fixed combination antimalarial agent, indicated for the prevention or treatment of acute, uncomplicated *P. falciparum* malaria, including in areas where chloroquine resistance has been reported.

Precautions/Adverse Reactions: Usage is contraindicated in patients with hypersensitivity to atovaquone, proguanil, or any formulation components and for the prophylaxis of *P. falciparum* malaria in patients with severe renal impairment (creatinine clearance < 30 ml/min). Malarone™ is not indicated for severe or complicated manifestations of malaria. Absorption of atovaquone may be diminished in patients who have diarrhea or vomiting, parasitemia should be closely monitored in these patients and treatment with an antiemetic should be considered. Recrudescent infections or infections following chemoprophylaxis with this medication should be treated with an alternative agent(s). Not for use in patients < 11 kg. Delayed cases of *P. falciparum* may occur after stopping prophylaxis with Malarone™, therefore travelers returning from endemic areas who experience febrile illnesses should be investigated for malaria. Do not administer with other proguanil-containing products; concomitant treatment with tetracycline, metoclopramide, rifampin, or rifabutin with atovaquone has been associated with decreased bioavailability or plasma levels of atovaquone. Pregnancy Category C. Use in pregnant women only if the potential benefit outweighs the possible risk to the fetus. Excretion of atovaquone in breast milk is unknown; proguanil is excreted in small quantities; exercise caution when administering to nursing women.

Some adverse effects are abdominal pain, nausea, vomiting, diarrhea, headache, dizziness, and myalgia.

Administration: Oral.

Patient Care Implications: The daily dose should be given at the same time each day with food or a milky drink. If vomiting occurs within 1 hour of administration, repeat the dose.

Preparations: Tablet: atovaquone 250 mg and proguanil hydrochloride 100 mg. Tablet pediatric: atovaquone 62.5 mg and proguanil hydrochloride 25 mg.

ATRACURIUM BESYLATE—
Tracrium®

Description/Actions: Nondepolarizing skeletal muscle relaxant administered intravenously as an adjunct to general anesthesia, to facilitate endotracheal intubation, and to provide skeletal muscle relaxation during surgery or mechanical ventilation.

Preparations: Ampules and vials, 10 mg/ml.

ATROMID-S®, see Clofibrate

ATROPINE SULFATE

Description/Actions: Anticholinergic, mydriatic, and cycloplegic agent used parenterally in a number of conditions including peptic ulcer, biliary and ureteral colic, bronchial spasm, and parkinsonism, to lessen the degree of AV heart block, to restore cardiac rate and arterial pressure during anesthesia in certain situations, and as preanesthetic medication. Used via ophthalmic administration for cycloplegic refraction, or for pupil dilation in certain acute ocular inflammatory conditions.

Preparations: Ampules, vials, and syringes, 0.05, 0.1, 0.3, 0.4, 0.5, 0.8, 1, and 1.2 mg/ml. Tablets, 0.4 mg. Hypodermic tablets, 0.3, 0.4, and 0.6 mg. Ophthalmic solution, 0.5%, 1%, 2%, and 3%. Ophthalmic ointment, 0.5%, and 1%.

ATORVASTATIN—Lipitor®

Description/Actions: An HMG-CoA reductase inhibitor indicated as an adjunct to diet for the reduction of elevated total and LDL-cholesterol levels in patients with primary hypercholesterolemia and mixed dyslipidemia. Atorvastatin is also indicated for the treatment of heterozygous familial hypercholesterolemia in adolescent boys and post-menarchal girls aged 10–17 and as an adjunct to diet to reduce total cholesterol, low density lipoprotein cholesterol and apolipoprotein B levels if after an adequate trial of diet, LDL-C levels are ≥ 190 mg/dL or LDL-C levels are ≥ 160 mg/dL and there is a positive family history of premature cardiovascular disease or two or more other cardiovascular risk factors are present in the patient.

Warnings: Contraindicated in active liver disease, unexplained peristent elevated serum transaminases, and pregnancy. Monitor liver function before and during therapy. Reduce or discontinue dose if serum transaminase levels > 3 times the upper limit of normal persist. Use cautiously in patients with chronic alcohol ingestion. Discontinue if myopathy or elevated CPK levels occur. Suspend therapy if predisposition to development of renal failure secondary to rhabdomyolysis develops. Adverse reactions include constipation, flatulence, dyspepsia, abdominal pain, headache, myalgia, arthralgia, rash, asthenia, and elevated serum transaminases.

Administration: Initially 10 mg once daily. Range 10–80 mg once daily.

Preparations: Tablets, 10, 20, and 40 mg.

ATROVENT®, see Ipratropium

AUGMENTIN®, see Amoxicillin/ clavulanate potassium

AURANOFIN—Ridaura®

Antiarthritic Agent.

Description/Actions: An orally administered gold-containing formulation indicated in the management of rheumatoid arthritis in adult patients who have had an insufficient therapeutic response to one or more nonsteroidal anti-inflammatory drugs or who are intolerant of such drugs.

Warnings: Adverse reactions include loose stools or diarrhea, abdominal pain, nausea, vomiting, rash, pruritus, stomatitis, proteinuria. A complete blood count (CBC) with differential and platelet count, urinalysis, and physical examination of the mouth and skin should be done at least monthly during therapy.

Administration: Oral.

Preparations: Capsules, 3 mg.

AUREOMYCIN®, see Chlortetracycline

AUROTHIOGLUCOSE—Solganal®

Description/Actions: Gold formulation administered intramuscularly in the treatment of rheumatoid arthritis.

Preparations: Vials, 50 mg/ml.

AVAPRO®, see Irbesartan

AVC®, see Sulfanilamide

AVELOX®, see Moxifloxacin Hydrochloride

AVENTYL®, see Nortriptyline

AVITA®, see Tretinoin

AVLOSULFON®, see Dapsone

AVODART™, see Dutasteride

AVONEX®, see Interferon beta-1A

AXERT™, see Almotriptan Maleate

AXID®, see Nizatidine

AZACTAM®, see Aztreonam

AZATADINE MALEATE— Optimine®

Description/Actions: Antihistamine indicated for the treatment of perennial and seasonal allergic rhinitis and chronic urticaria.

Preparations: Tablets, 1 mg.

AZATHIOPRINE—Imuran®

Description/Actions: Immunosuppressant indicated as an adjunct for the prevention of rejection in renal homotransplantation, and in the management of severe rheumatoid arthritis that has not responded satisfactorily to other agents.

Preparations: Tablets, 50 mg. Vials (sodium salt), 100 mg.

AZELAIC ACID—Azelex®
Topical antibacterial.

Description/Actions: Exerts antibacterial and keratolytic activity when applied topically. Indicated for treatment of mild to moderate inflammatory acne vulgaris.

Warnings: Not recommended for use in children. Monitor patients with dark complexion for hypopigmentation. Discontinue if sensitivity or severe irritation develops. Pruritis, burning, stinging, tingling, exacerbation of acne, hypopigmentation, contact dermatitis, vitiligo, depigmentation, and hypertrichosis may occur.

Administration: Massage thin film on clean, dry affected areas twice daily. Wash hands after application. If persistent irritation occurs, may decrease to once daily.

Preparations: 20% topical cream.

AZELASTINE HYDROCHLORIDE—Astelin®, Optivar™

Description/Actions: Antihistamine indicated in the treatment of seasonal allergic rhinitis symptoms including rhinorrhea. A nasal spray formulation of an H_1 antagonist.

Ophthalmic preparation used for the treatment of itching of the eye associated with seasonal allergic conjunctivities in children ≥ 3 years of age and adults.

Warnings: May potentiate CNS depression of other drugs or alcohol. Adverse reactions include bitter taste, somnolence, headache, weight increase, myalgia, nasal burning, sneezing, and nausea.

Administration: Two sprays in each nostril twice daily. Opthalmic: Instill 1 drop into affected eye(s) twice daily.

Preparations: Aqueous nasal spray 137 mg/actuation, ophthalmic solution, 0.05%.

AZELEX®, see Azelaic Acid

AZITHROMYCIN—Zithromax®, Z-Pak®, Zitromax® Tri-Pak
Azalide antibiotic.

Description/Actions: Inhibits protein synthesis and usually exhibits a bacteriostatic action against gram-positive and gram-negative bacteria. Indicated for upper respiratory tract infections, lower respiratory tract infections, and uncomplicated skin and skin structure infections caused by susceptible organisms. Also indicated for nongonococcal urethritis and cervicitis caused by *Chlamydia trachomatis*. Used to treat acute otitis media.

Warnings: Contraindicated in patients with a known hypersensitivity to any of the macrolide antibiotics. Adverse reactions include diarrhea/loose stools, nausea, vomiting, abdominal pain, and vaginitis. Aluminum- and magnesium-containing antacids may reduce the rate of absorption, and the two agents should not be administered at the same time.

Administration: Oral (should be administered at least one hour before or 2 hours after a meal) and intravenous.

Preparations: Tablets 250 (scored), 500, and 600 mg. Oral suspension 100 mg/5 ml, and 200 mg/5 ml. Single-dose packets for oral suspension, 1 g. Vials for IV infusion after reconstitution, 500 mg/vial. Tablet (3x500mg).

AZMACORT®, see Triamcinolone acetonide

AZO-STANDARD®, see Phenazopyridine hydrochloride

AZT, see Zidovudine

AZTREONAM—Azactam®
Monobactam antibiotic.

Description/Actions: Indicated for urinary tract infections, lower respiratory tract infections, septicemia, skin and skin-structure infections, intraabdominal infections, and gynecologic infections caused by susceptible gram-negative bacteria. Among the organisms that are susceptible to the drug are *Pseudomonas aeruginosa, Haemophilus influenzae, Escherichia coli, Klebsiella pneumoniae, Proteus mirabilis, Serratia* species, *Enterobacter* species, and *Citrobacter* species. It is also indicated as adjunctive therapy to surgery in the management of infections caused by susceptible organisms.

Warnings: It has only a weak potential to cause hypersensitivity reactions or to demonstrate cross-reactivity with the penicillins and cephalosporins. Adverse reactions include diarrhea, nausea and/or vomiting, rash, phlebitis/thrombophlebitis following intravenous administration, discomfort at the injection site following intramuscular administration, and superinfection with gram-positive bacteria such as enterococci.

Administration: Intravenous and intramuscular.

Preparations: Vials, 500 mg, 1 and 2 g. Intravenous infusion bottles, 500 mg, 1 and 2 g.

B

BACAMPICILLIN HYDROCHLORIDE—Spectrobid®

Description/Actions: Penicillin antibiotic. Is a prodrug that is hydrolyzed to ampicillin following administration. Indicated in the treatment of respiratory tract, urinary tract, and dermatologic infections caused by susceptible bacteria, and also in the management of gonorrhea. Tablets may be given without regard to meals, but the suspension should be administered apart from meals.

Preparations: Tablets, 400 mg. Powder for oral suspension, 125 mg/5 ml when reconstituted.

BACITRACIN

Anti-infective agent that is primarily active against gram-positive bacteria such as staphylococci. Most often used topically.

Preparations: Ointment and ophthalmic ointment, 500 units/g. Vials (for parenteral administration), 10,000 and 50,000 units.

BACLOFEN—Lioresal®

Description/Actions: Muscle relaxant and antispastic agent indicated for the alleviation of signs and symptoms of spasticity resulting from multiple sclerosis, and also in the management of certain spinal cord injuries and diseases. Intrathecal baclofen is indicated for use in the management of severe spasticity of cerebral and spinal origin.

Precautions/Adverse Reactions: Abrupt discontinuation of intrathecal baclofen, regardless of the cause, has resulted in sequelae that include high fever, altered mental status, exaggerated rebound spasticity, and muscle rigidity, which in rare cases has advanced to rhabdomyolysis, multiple organ-system failure, and death.

Preparations: Tablets, 10 and 20 mg.

Ampules (for intrathecal use), 10 mg/5 ml and 10 mg/20 ml.

BACTRIM®, see Trimethoprim-sulfamethoxazole

BACTROBAN®, see Mupirocin

BAKING SODA, see Sodium bicarbonate

BAL, see Dimercaprol

BALSALAZIDE—Colazal™

Description/Actions: Balsalazide is an anti-inflammatory agent used in the treatment of mild to moderate active ulcerative colitis.

Precautions/Adverse Reactions: Balsalazide is contraindicated in patients with hypersensitivity to salicylates or to any of the components of balsalazide or its metabolites. Patients with pyloric stenosis may have prolonged gastric rentention of balsalazide capsules. Reports during clinical trials indicate that balsalazide may exacerbate symptoms of colitis. Because other mesalamine products have shown renal toxicity, balsalazide should be used with caution, and with careful monitoring, by persons with a history of or with current renal disease. The safety and efficacy has not been established beyond 12 weeks of therapy and in children. Pregnancy Category B. No adequate and well-controlled studies have been done in pregnant women. Balsalazide should be used in pregnant women only if clearly needed. It is not known whether balsalazide is excreted in breast milk. Caution should be used in administering to nursing women. Some adverse effects are headache, abdominal pain, nausea, diarrhea, vomiting, arthralgia, respiratory infections, and hepatotoxicity.

Administration: Oral.

Patient Care Implications: Do not chew or open capsules. Report abdominal pain, unresolved diarrhea, or severe headache to prescriber.

Preparations: Capsule: 750 mg.

BARIUM SULFATE

Description/Actions: Diagnostic agent used in the X-ray examination of the gastrointestinal tract.

BASALJEL®, see Aluminum carbonate gel, basic

BASILIXIMAB—Simulect®

Description/Actions: Basiliximab is an immunosuppressive agent. It is indicated for the prophylaxis of acute organ rejection in patients receiving renal transplantation when used as part of an immunosuppressive regimen that includes cyclopsporine and corticosteroids.

Precautions/Adverse Reactions: It is not known whether basiliximab will have a long-term effect on the ability of the immune system to respond to antigens first encountered during basiliximab-induced immunosuppression. Readministration after an initial course of therapy has not been studied in humans.

Adverse effects include GI symptoms such as diarrhea, constipation, vomiting, abdominal pain, and dyspepsia.

Administration: Intravenous.

Patient Care Implications: Immunosuppressive therapy places patients at greater risk of developing an infection. Instruct patients in the measures to reduce the risk of infection as well as signs and symptoms that should be reported promptly to the prescriber. Basiliximab is used as a part of an immunosuppressive regimen of corticosteroids and cyclopsorine.

Preparations: Single-use vial containing 20 mg.

BAYER ASPIRIN®, see Aspirin

BECAPLERMIN—Regranex®

Description/Actions: Indicated as an adjunct to good ulcer care in the treatment of lower extremity diabetic neuropathic ulcers that extend into the subcutaneous tissue or beyond and have an adequate blood supply.

Warnings: Contraindicated in neoplasia at the application site. Not for use in wounds that close by primary intention, in pregnancy (category C), and in nursing mothers.

Adverse reactions include erythematous rash.

Administration: Topical.

Preparations: 0.01% gel in 15 g tubes.

BECLOMETHASONE DIPROPIONATE—Beclovent®, Vanceril®, Beconase®, Beconase AQ®, Qvar™, Vancenase®, Vancenase AQ®, Double Strength®, Vanceril®, Double strength

Description/Actions: Corticosteroid administered by oral inhalation (Beclovent®, Vanceril®) or nasal spray in patients who require chronic treatment with corticosteroids to control the symptoms of bronchial asthma. Also administered by nasal inhalation for the relief of symptoms of seasonal or perennial rhinitis.

Preparations: Aerosol, 42 and 84 μg per actuation. Nasal spray (Beconase AQ®, Vancenase AQ®), 84 μg/spray. Oral inhaler (Qvar™), 40 mcg and 80 mcg/inhalation.

BECLOVENT®, see
  Beclomethasone dipropionate

BECONASE®, see
  Beclomethasone dipropionate

BECONASE AQ®, see
  Beclomethasone dipropionate

BEEPEN VK®, see Penicillin V potassium

BELLADONNA

Description/Actions: Anticholinergic. Contains atropine, hyoscyamine and scopolamine alkaloids and has been used in the treatment of gastrointestinal disorders and parkinsonism.

Preparations: Tincture of belladonna.

BENADRYL®, see
  Diphenhydramine

**BENAZEPRIL
  HYDROCHLORIDE**—Lotensin®

Antihypertensive agent.

Description/Actions: An angiotensin-converting enzyme (ACE) inhibitor that is a prodrug. Following oral administration, is converted to its active metabolite, benazeprilat. Indicated for the treatment of hypertension and may be used alone or in combination with a thiazide diuretic.

Warnings: Adverse reactions include headache, dizziness, fatigue, cough, and nausea. May cause an elevation in serum potassium levels; the risk of hyperkalemia is increased in patients also taking a potassium-sparing diuretic, a potassium supplement, and/or a potassium-containing salt substitute. May cause symptomatic postural hypotension. There have been infrequent reports of angioedema of the face, extremities, lips, tongue, glottis, and larynx, especially following the first dose. Patients should be told to report immediately any symptoms suggesting angioedema and to stop taking the drug. When used during the second and third trimesters of pregnancy, ACE inhibitors have been reported to be associated with the development of neonatal hypertension, renal failure, and skull hypoplasia; use during pregnancy should be avoided. May increase serum lithium levels and concurrent therapy should be closely monitored. Monitor renal function especially in the elderly.

Administration: Oral.

Preparations: Tablets, 5, 10, 20, and 40 mg.

BENDROFLUMETHIAZIDE—
  Naturetin®

Description/Actions: Thiazide diuretic indicated as adjunctive therapy in the treatment of edema and in the management of hypertension.

Preparations: Tablets, 2.5, 5, and 10 mg.

BENEMID®, see Probenecid

BENOQUIN®, see Monobenzone

BENOXINATE HYDROCHLORIDE

Description/Actions: Local anesthetic sometimes employed to provide anesthesia in certain ophthalmic procedures.

BENTYL®, see Dicyclomine

BENYLIN COUGH®, see
  Diphenhydramine hydrochloride

BENYLIN DM®, see Dextromethorphan

BENZALKONIUM CHLORIDE—Zephiran®

Description/Actions: Anti-infective agent used topically as an antiseptic, in the irrigation of certain tissues, and in the preoperative preparation of the skin. Also used as a preservative (e.g., in ophthalmic solutions) and in the sterile storage of instruments.

Preparations: Solution and tincture, 1:750. Concentrate (to be diluted), 17%.

BENZATHINE PENICILLIN G—Bicillin®, Permapen®

Description/Actions: Penicillin antibiotic that has a long duration of action following intramuscular administration. Indicated in infections caused by highly susceptible organisms such as streptococci. Also used in the prevention of recurrent rheumatic fever and in the treatment of syphilis.

Preparations: Vials, 300,000 units/ml. Syringes, 600,000, 1,200,000, and 2,400,000 units.

BENZEDREX®, see Propylhexedrine

BENZOCAINE—Ethyl aminobenzoate, Zilabrace®, Ziladent®

Description/Actions: Local anesthetic administered topically in dermatologic disorders, locally to provide oral and mucosal anesthesia, and orally as an adjunct in a weight reduction regimen.

Preparations: Cream, ointment, solution, and lotion, 0.5% to 20%. Gel, 6% and 10%. Candy and gum (in weight-reduction regimen), 6 mg.

BENZOIC ACID

Description/Actions: Anti-infective agent used topically in the treatment of fungal infections, usually in combination with salicylic acid in an ointment formulation known as Whitfield's ointment (6% benzoic acid and 3% salicylic acid).

BENZOIN

Description/Actions: Protectant used topically to protect the skin against irritants and to coat sores. Tincture and compound benzoin tincture have sometimes been placed in boiling water as steam inhalants to provide an expectorant and soothing action in certain respiratory conditions.

Preparations: Tincture.

BENZONATATE—Tessalon®

Description/Actions: Antitussive indicated for the symptomatic relief of cough.

Preparations: Capsules, 100 mg.

BENZPHETAMINE HYDROCHLORIDE—Didrex®

Description/Actions: Anorexiant indicated in the management of exogenous obesity as a short-term adjunct in a regimen of weight reduction based on caloric restriction.

Preparations: Tablets, 25 and 50 mg.

BENZTHIAZIDE—Exna®

Description/Actions: Thiazide diuretic indicated in the treatment of edema in the management of hypertension.

Preparations: Tablets, 50 mg.

BENZTROPINE MESYLATE—Cogentin®

Antiparkinson agent.

Description/Actions: Exhibits anticholinergic activity, and is indicated for the treatment of parkinsonism and the control of drug-induced extrapyramidal reactions.

Warnings: Adverse reactions include dry mouth, nausea, vomiting, blurred vision, tachycardia, confusion, nervousness, and urinary retention.

Administration: Oral, intravenous, and intramuscular.

Preparations: Tablets, 0.5, 1, and 2 mg. Ampules, 1 mg/ml.

BEPRIDIL HYDROCHLORIDE— Vascor®

Antianginal agent.

Description/Actions: A calcium channel-blocking agent that is indicated for the treatment of chronic stable angina (classic effort-associated angina) in patients who have failed to respond optimally to, or are intolerant of, other antianginal medications. May be used alone or in combination with beta-blockers and/or nitrates.

Warnings: Contraindicated in patients with a history of serious ventricular arrhythmias, sick sinus syndrome or second- or third-degree AV block except in the presence of a functioning ventricular pacemaker, hypotension, uncompensated cardiac insufficiency, congenital QT interval prolongation, and in patients taking other drugs that prolong QT interval. May cause proarrhythmic effects including serious ventricular arrhythmias. May prolong the QT interval and the QTc interval which has been associated with the development of torsadesdepointes–type ventricular tachycardia. The risk of this reaction is increased by the presence of antecedent bradycardia, hypokalemia, and the use of potassium-depleting diuretics. If the concurrent use of a diuretic is needed, a potassium-sparing diuretic should be used if possible. Any potassium deficiency should be corrected before bepridil therapy is initiated and serum potassium levels should be monitored periodically. Other adverse reactions include nausea, diarrhea, dyspepsia, GI distress, dizziness, asthenia, and nervousness. Agranulocytosis has been reported rarely. Other agents that may prolong the QT interval (e.g., quinidine, procainamide, tricyclic antidepressants) should not be used concurrently because of a greater potential for ventricular arrhythmias. Concurrent use with digoxin may result in an increase in serum digoxin levels and therapy should be closely monitored.

Administration. Oral.

Preparations: Tablets, 200, 300, and 400 mg.

BERACTANT—Survanta®

Agent for respiratory distress syndrome.

Description/Actions: A pulmonary surfactant of bovine origin that contains phospholipids, neutral lipids, fatty acids, and surfactant-associated proteins, to which colfosceril palmitate, palmitic acid, and tripalmitin are added to standardize the composition and to mimic the surface tension lowering properties of natural lung surfactant. Replenishes surfactant and restores surface activity to the lungs. Indicated for the prevention and treatment of respiratory distress syndrome in premature infants.

Warnings: Adverse reactions include bradycardia and oxygen desaturation. May rapidly affect oxygenation and lung compliance.

Administration: Intratracheal. If settling has occurred during storage, swirl the vial gently (do not shake) to redisperse. Is stored refrigerated and, before administration, should be warmed by standing at room temperature for at least 20 minutes or warmed in the hand for at least 8 minutes. Is administered intratracheally by instillation through a 5 French end-hole catheter inserted into the infant's endotracheal tube. Each dose is divided into 4 quarter-doses, and each quarter-dose is administered with the infant in a different position.

Preparations: Vials, 200 mg phospholipids/8 ml.

BETADINE®, see Povidone-Iodine

38 • BETAGAN®

BETAGAN®, see Levobunolol

BETAMETHASONE, BETAMETHASONE SODIUM PHOSPHATE, BETAMETHASONE ACETATE—Celestone®

Corticosteroid.

Description/Actions: Indicated in a wide range of endocrine, rheumatic, allergic, dermatologic, respiratory, hematologic, neoplastic, and other disorders.

Preparations: Tablets, 0.6 mg. Syrup, 0.6 mg/5 ml. Vials (solution), 4 mg as the sodium phosphate per ml. Vials (suspension), 6 mg as the sodium phosphate and acetate per ml.

BETAMETHASONE BENZOATE—Uticort®

Topical corticosteroid.

Preparations: Cream, lotion, and gel, 0.025%.

BETAMETHASONE DIPROPIONATE—Diprosone®, Maxivate®

Topical corticosteroid.

Preparations: Cream, ointment, and lotion, 0.05%.

Topical aerosol, 0.1%.

BETAMETHASONE DIPROPIONATE AUGMENTED—Diprolene®, Diprolene AF®

Topical corticosteroid.

Description/Actions: Specially formulated vehicle increases penetration and potency. Indicated for the short-term treatment of the inflammatory and pruritic manifestations of moderate to severe corticosteroid-responsive dermatoses.

Warnings: Is highly potent and is more likely than less potent analogs to cause systemic effects including suppression of the hypothalamic-pituitary-adrenal (HPA) axis. Treatment period should be limited to 2 weeks and the total dosage should not exceed 45 g per week. Occlusive dressings should not be used.

Administration: Topical.

Preparations: Cream, ointment, and lotion, 0.05%.

BETAMETHASONE VALERATE—Luxig®, Valisone®

Topical corticosteroid.

Description/Actions: Indicated for relief of the inflammatory and pruritic manifestations of corticosteroid-responsive dermatoses.

Warnings: Adverse reactions include burning, itching, irritation, dryness, and a potential for systemic effect.

Administration: Topical.

Preparations: Cream, ointment, and lotion, 0.1%. Foam (Luxig®) 0.12%.

Reduced-strength cream 0.01%.

BETAPACE®, see Sotalol hydrochloride

BETAPACE AF™, see Sotalol hydrochloride

BETAPEN VK®, see Penicillin V potassium

BETASERON®, see Interferon beta-1b

BETAXOLOL HYDROCHLORIDE—Betoptic®, Betoptic S®, Kerlone®

Antihypertensive agent and agent for glaucoma.

Description/Actions: A cardioselective beta-adrenergic blocking agent indicated in the treatment of hypertension, and for ophthalmic administration in the treatment of chronic open-angle glaucoma and ocular hypertension.

Warnings: Contraindicated in patients with sinus bradycardia, second- and third-degree AV block in the absence of a functioning artificial pacemaker, overt cardiac failure, or cardiogenic shock. Adverse reactions include fatigue, dizziness, and bradycardia, and, when administered in the ophthalmic dosage forms, transient stinging during instillation. Use is best avoided in patients with bronchospastic diseases, and therapy in diabetic patients must be closely monitored.

Administration: Oral and ophthalmic. Patients should be cautioned about the interruption or discontinuation of oral therapy; exacerbation of angina pectoris has occurred following the abrupt cessation of therapy and when therapy is to be discontinued, the dosage should be gradually reduced over a period of 2 weeks.

Preparations: Tablets (Kerlone), 10 and 20 mg. Ophthalmic suspension (Betoptic S), 0.25%. Ophthalmic solution (Betoptic), 0.5%.

BETAXON®, See Levobetaxolol HCl ophthalmic suspension 0.5%

BETHANECHOL CHLORIDE— Urecholine®

Description/Actions: Cholinergic agent indicated for the treatment of acute postoperative and postpartum nonobstructive urinary retention, and for neurogenic atony of the urinary bladder with retention.

Preparations: Tablets, 5, 10, 25, and 50 mg. Vials, 5 mg/ml.

BETIMOL®, see Timolol

BETOPTIC®, see Betaxolol

BEXAROTENE—Targretin®

Descriptoin/Actions: Indicated for the treatment of cutaneous manifestations of cutaneous T-cell lymphoma in patients who are refractory to at least one prior systemic therapy.

Precautions/Adverse Reaction: Targretin capsules are contraindicated in patients with a known hypersensitivity to bexarotene or other components of the product. Targretin should not be given to a pregnant woman or a woman who intends to become pregnant. Targretin can induce major lipid abnormalities, biochemical evidence of or clinical hypothyroidism, and leukopenia so laboratory values should be followed and dosages adjusted as needed. Caution should be used in patients with a known hypersensitivity to retinoids, hepatic insufficiency, or diabetes mellitus. Retinoids have been associated with photosensitivity, and patients should be advised to minimize exposure to sunlight and artificial UV light while receiving Targretin capsules. Other adverse effects include headache, asthenia, infections, abdominal pain, rash, dry skin, nausea, diarrhea, vomiting, anorexia, peripheral edema, and insomnia.

Administration: Oral with meal.

Preparations: Capsules, 75 mg.

BEXTRA™, see Valdecoxib

BIAXIN®, see Clarithromycin

BIAXIN XL®, see Clarithromycin Extended-Release Tablets

BICALUTAMIDE—Casodex®

Antineoplastic, antiandrogen hormone.

Description/Actions: Antagonizes the effects of androgen (action is usually against a more potent androgen) at the cellular level. Indicated in the treatment of metastatic prostate carcinoma in conjunction with luteinizing hormone releasing hormone (LHRH) analogs (goserelin, leuprolide).

Warnings: May cause moderate to severe hepatic impairment. Monitor hepatic function and prostate specific antigen (PSA). Adverse reactions include weakness, constipation, nausea, diarrhea, back pain, pelvic pain, hot flashes, and generalized pain.

Administration: Oral, 50 mg once daily (must be given concurrently with LHRH analog).

Preparations: Tablets, 50 mg.

BICILLIN®, see Benzathine penicillin G

BICITRA®, see Sodium citrate and Citric Acid

BICNU®, see Carmustine

BILTRICIDE®, see Praziquantel

BIMATOPROST—LUMIGAN®

Description/Actions: Bimatoprost is indicated for the reduction of elevated intraocular pressure in patients with open-angle glaucoma or ocular hypertension who are intolerant of other intraocular pressure–lowering medications or failed treatment with another intraocular pressure–lowering drug.

Precautions/Adverse Reactions: Pregnancy Category C. No adequate and well-controlled studies in pregnant women. Excretion in human breast milk is unknown. Safety and efficacy in children have not been established. The most common side effects observed in patients treated with bimatoprost include conjunctival hyperemia, growth of eyelashes and ocular pruritis. Other side effects occurring less frequently include ocular dryness, visual disturbances, ocular burning, eye pain, eye discharge, tearing, photophobia, allergic conjunctivitis, and intraocular inflammation. Systemic side effects have been reported and include infections, headaches, abnormal liver function tests, asthenia and hirsutism.

Administration: Recommended adult dose: 1 drop in the affected eye(s) once daily in the evening.

Patient Care Implications: Remove contact lenses prior to using, and wait 15 minutes before reinserting. Contains benzalkonium chloride as a preservative. If more than one ophthalmic drug is being used, the drugs should be administered at least 5 minutes apart. Patients should be advised to avoid contamination of the solution. Patients should be informed that if only one eye is treated, cosmetic diferences between the eyes may occur.

Preparations: Ophthalmic solution, 0.03% in 2.5 ml, 5 ml, and 7.5 ml.

BIPERIDEN—Akineton®

Description/Actions: Antiparkinson agent indicated for the treatment of parkinsonism and the control of extrapyramidal disorders secondary to neuroleptic drug therapy.

Preparations: Tablets (as the hydrochloride), 2 mg. Ampules (as the lactate), 5 mg.

BISACODYL—Dulcolax®

Description/Actions: Laxative indicated for acute constipation, chronic constipation, preparation for x-rays, preoperative preparation, and other situations.

Preparations: Tablets, 5 mg. Suppositories, 5 and 10 mg.

BISMUTH SUBCARBONATE

Description/Actions: Antacid included in some combination formulations.

BISMUTH SUBSALICYLATE— PeptoBismol®

Description/Actions: Antidiarrheal/antacid and analgesic used in the management of nausea, gas pains, abdominal cramps, and diarrhea. Has been used in the prevention and treatment of traveler's diarrhea. Also indicated in regimens for the treatment of gastrointestinal disorders caused by *Helicobacter pylori*.

Preparations: Chewable tablets, 262 mg. Suspension, 262 mg/15 ml and 524 mg/15 ml.

BISOPROLOL FUMARATE— Zebeta®

Antihypertensive agent.

Description/Actions: Is a cardioselective beta-adrenergic blocking agent that is indicated for the treatment of hypertension.

Warnings: Contraindicated in patients in cardiogenic shock, or with overt cardiac failure, second- and third-degree heart block, or marked sinus bradycardia. Adverse reactions include headache, fatigue, dizziness, diarrhea, and cold extremities. Use is best avoided in patients with bronchospastic diseases and therapy in diabetic patients must be closely monitored.

Administration: Oral. When therapy is to be discontinued, the dosage should be gradually reduced over a period of one week.

Preparations: Tablets, 5 and 10 mg. Also available in combination formulations (Ziac) with hydrochlorothiazide that contain 2.5, 5, and 10 mg of bisoprolol fumarate with 6.25 mg of the diuretic.

BITOLTEROL MESYLATE— Tornalate®

Description/Actions: Bronchodilator used by oral inhalation for prophylactic and therapeutic use for bronchial asthma and for reversible bronchospasm.

Preparations: Metered dose inhaler, 0.37 mg per actuation. Inhalation solution, 0.2%

BIVALIRUDIN—Angiomax™

Description/Actions: Angiomax™ is used in conjunction with aspirin as an anticoagulant in patients with unstable angina undergoing percutaneous transluminal coronary angioplasty (PTCA).

Precautions/Adverse Reactions: Bivalirudin is contraindicated in patients with active major bleeding and hypersensitivity to bivalirudin or any of its formulation components. Safety and effectiveness have not been established when used in conjunction with platelet inhibitors other than aspirin (i.e., glycoprotein IIb/IIIa inhibitors) in patients with unstable angina who are not undergoing PTCA, in patients with other acute coronary syndromes, and in pediatrics. Since hemorrhage can occur with bivalirudin, exercise caution when utilizing in patients with disease states associated with increased risk of bleeding. Pregnancy Category B. Safety and efficacy for use in pregnant women have not been established. Use during pregnancy only if clearly needed. It is not known if bivalirudin is excreted in human milk; use with caution in nursing women.

Some adverse effects are bleeding, hypotension, back pain, headache, nausea, and vomiting.

Administration: Intravenous.

Patient Care Implications: For IV administration only. Do not mix with other medications. In patients with renal impairment monitor the ACT. Inform patient to report any unusual bleeding or bruising while on Angiomax™.

Preparations: Powder for injection. Each vial delivers 250 mg of Angiomax™.

BLENOXANE®, see Bleomycin

BLEOMYCIN SULFATE— Blenoxane®

Description/Actions: Antineoplastic agent indicated for parenteral use as a palliative treatment in the management of squamous cell carcinomas, lymphomas, and testicular carcinoma.

Preparations: Vials, 15 and 30 units.

BLOCADREN®, see Timolol

BONINE®, see Meclizine

BONTRIL®, see Phendimetrazine

BORIC ACID

Description/Actions: Antiseptic used topically for conditions associated with irritation of the skin, and for the treatment of irritated and inflamed eyelids.

Preparations: Ointment and ophthalmic ointment, 5% and 10%.

BOSENTAN—TRACLEER™

Description/Actions: Bosentan is indicated for the treatment of pulmonary artery hypertension in patients with WHO class III or IV symptoms to improve exercise ability and to decrease the rate of clinical worsening.

Precautions/Adverse Reactions: Because of a high potential for liver injury effects and the risk associated with use in pregnancy, bosentan is available only through a distribution program directly from the manufacturer (866-228-3546). It is not available through wholesalers or individual pharmacies. Bosentan is contraindicated in persons hypersensitive to bosentan or any component of the medication. It is associated with significant transaminase elevations, indicating a potential for serious hepatic injury. Avoid use in moderate to severe hepatic impairment; caution should be exercised in patients with mild liver function impairment. Pregnancy Category X. Based on animal studies, bosentan is likely to produce major birth defects. CYP3A3/4 inhibitors and cyclosporine may increase bosentan concentration. An increased risk of elevated liver aminotransferases were observed when given with glyburide. Most common adverse reactions include headache, flushing, increased serum transaminases (reversible), lower limb edema, nasopharyngitis, dyspepsia, hypotension, pruritus, and fatigue. Safety and efficacy in pediatric patients not established.

Administration: Oral.

Patient Care Implications: Pregnancy must be excluded before starting treatment and prevented thereafter by use of reliable contraception. Hormonal contraceptives (oral, injectable, and implanted) may not be reliable in the presence of bosentan and should not be used as the sole contraceptive method. Liver aminotransferase levels must be measured prior to initiation of treatment and then monthly. In patients developing elevated levels, dosage adjustment and monitoring of ALT/AST levels should be followed as per manufacturer's recommendations. If liver aminotransferase elevations are accompanied by clinical symptoms of iver injury (such as nausea, vomiting, fever, abdominal pain, jaundice, unusual lethargy, or fatigue) or increases in bilirubin ≥ 2 × ULN, treatment should be stopped. Hemoglobin levels should be monitored after 1 and 3 months of treatment, then every 3 months. Tablets should be administered morning and evening with or without food.

Preparations: Film-coated tablets: 62.5 and 125 mg.

BOTOX®, see Botulinum toxin type A

BOTULINUM TOXIN TYPE A— Botox®

Agent for muscle disorders.

Description/Actions: Is produced from a culture of *Clostridium botulinum* and, following injection into eye muscles, inhibits the release of acetylcholine resulting in a localized reversible muscle paralysis. Indicated for the treatment of strabismus and blepharospasm associated with dystonia, including benign essential blepharospasm or seventh cranial nerve disorders. Is also being evaluated in a number of other muscle disorders.

Warnings: Adverse reactions when used in the treatment of strabismus include spatial disorientation, double vision, ptosis, vertical deviation, and retrobulbar hemorrhages resulting from needle penetrations into the orbit. Adverse reactions when used in the treatment of blepharospasm include ptosis, irritation/tearing, ecchymosis, rash, and local swelling of the eyelid skin.

Administration: Ocular injection. In the treatment of strabismus the drug is injected using electromyographic guidance to facilitate placement within the target muscle. Paralysis of the injected muscles lasts for 2 to 6 weeks. In the treatment of blepharospasm the drug is injected into the orbicularis oculi without electromygraphic guidance. Each treatment lasts approximately 3 months.

Preparations: Vials, 100 units.

BRETHAIRE®, see Terbutaline

BRETHINE®, see Terbutaline

BRETYLIUM TOSYLATE—
Bretylol®

Description/Actions: Antiarrhythmic agent indicated for parenteral use in the prophylaxis and treatment of ventricular fibrillation and also in the treatment of life-threatening ventricular arrhythmias that have not responded to other agents.

Preparations: Ampules, vials, and syringes, 500 mg.

BRETYLOL®, see Bretylium

BREVIBLOC®, see Esmolol

BREVITAL®, see Methohexital

BRICANYL®, see Terbutaline

BRIMONIDINE TARTRATE—
Alphagan® Alphagan®P

Description/Actions: Antiglaucoma agent used to lower intraocular pressure in patients with open-angle glaucoma or ocular hypertension.

Warning: Use cautiously in severe cardiovascular diseases, hepatic or renal impairment, depression, cerebral disease, Raynaud's phenomenon, orthostatic hypertension, and thromboangiitis obliterans. Contraindicated with concomitant MAOI use. Adverse reactions include xerostomia, ocular hyperemia, burning/stinging, headache, blurred vision, foreign body sensation, fatigue/drowsiness, conjunctival follicles, ocular allergic reactions, ocular pruritus, corneal staining/erosion, photophobia, eyelid erythema, ocular ache/pain/dryness, tearing, upper respiratory symptoms, eyelid edema, conjunctival blanching, abnormal vision, and muscular pain.

Administration: One drop in affected eye(s) every 8 hours. Remove soft contact lenses before instillation and for 15 minutes after dose administration.

Preparations: 0.15% and 0.2% ophthalmic solution.

BRINZOLAMIDE—Azopt®

Description/Actions: Indicated for the treatment of elevated intraocular pressure in patients with ocular hypertension or open angle glaucoma.

Precautions/Adverse Reactions: Use not recommended in severe renal or hepatic impairment. Discontinue if serious systemic, ocular (e.g., conjunctivitis, lid edema) or hypersensitivity reactions occur.

Brinzolamide is a sulfonamide and while administered topically, it is absorbed systemically. Therefore, the same types of reactions attributable to sulfonamides may occur with topical application. Advise patients that if serious or unusual ocular or systemic reactions occur they should discontinue the use of the medication and call the prescriber. Pregnancy Category C.

Adverse reactions include blurred vision, bitter/sour taste, blepharitis, dermatitis, dry eye, foreign body sensation, headache, hyperemia, ocular discharge, pain, discomfort or itching, keratitis, rhinitis, and possible systemiclike sulfa reactions.

Administration: One drop of ophthalmic suspension in the affected eye 3 times daily

Patient Care Implications: Instruct patients to remove contact lenses prior to administration and to leave out for

15 minutes after application of the medication. Tell patients to shake the medication well prior to use. Separate use of this agent with other topical ocular medications by a minimum of 10 minutes.

Preparations: 1% ophthalmic suspension (contains benzalkonium chloride) in a dropper vial with a controlled dispensing tip. 5, 10, and 15 mL

BROMOCRIPTINE MESYLATE— Parlodel®

Description/Actions: Dopamine receptor agonist indicated for the treatment of dysfunctions associated with hyperprolactinemia (e.g., amenorrhea, infertility), acromegaly, and parkinsonism. Is an ergot derivative.

Preparations: Tablets, 2.5 mg. Capsules, 5 mg.

BROMODIPHENHYDRAMINE HYDROCHLORIDE

Description/Actions: Antihistamine included in some combination formulations.

BROMPHENIRAMINE MALEATE—Dimetane®

Description/Actions: Antihistamine indicated for the management of allergic disorders.

Preparations: Tablets, 4 mg. Controlled-release tablets, 8 and 12 mg. Elixir, 2 mg/5 ml. Vials, 10 mg/ml.

BRONKAID MIST, see Epinephrine

BRONKEPHRINE®, see Isoetharine

BRONKOMETER®, see Isoetharine

BRONKOSOL®, see Isoetharine

BUCLADIN-S®, see Buclizine

BUCLIZINE HYDROCHLORIDE— Bucladin-S®

Description/Actions: Antiemetic indicated in the management of nausea, vomiting, and dizziness associated with motion sickness.

Preparations: Tablets, 50 mg.

BUDESONIDE—Pulmicort Respules™, Pulmicort Turbuhaler®, Rhinocort®

Corticosteroid.

Description/Actions: Pulmicort is a potent adrenocortical steroid with locally acting anti-inflammatory and immune modifier properties. Use of aerosolized steroids may decrease the requirement for or avoid use of systemic glucocorticoids and delay pulmonary damage that occurs from chronic asthma. Pulmicort is indicated in the maintenance and prophylactic treatment of asthma including patients who require systemic corticosteroids and those who may benefit from systemic dose reduction/elimination.

Warnings: Contraindicated in acute asthma/status asthmaticus. Use cautiously in active untreated infections, patients with diabetes, glaucoma, underlying immunosuppression, systemic glucocorticoid therapy, pregnancy, nursing mothers, and children < 6.

Adverse reactions include headache, dysphonia, hoarseness, oropharyngeal fungal infections, bronchospasm, cough, wheezing, dry mouth, esophageal candidiasis, dyspepsia, gastroenteritis, back pain, and flulike symptoms.

Administration: Oral inhalation.

Preparations: 160 mcg/actuation powder in a 200 dose turbohaler, inhalation solution, 0.25 mg/2 ml and 0.5 mg/2 ml.

BUMETANIDE—Bumex®

Diuretic.

Description/Actions: Is a loop diuretic indicated for the treatment of edema associated with congestive heart failure, hepatic disease, and renal disease, including the nephrotic syndrome.

Warnings: Is contraindicated in anuria, and in patients in hepatic coma or in states of severe electrolyte depletion until the condition is improved or corrected. May cause volume and electrolyte depletion. Potential for hypokalemia warrants periodic measurement of serum potassium levels. Concurrent use with lithium is best avoided because of an increased risk of lithium toxicity. Parenteral administration is best avoided in patients receiving aminoglycoside antibiotics because of an increased risk of ototoxicity.

Administration: Oral, intravenous, and intramuscular.

Preparations: Tablets, 0.5, 1, and 2 mg. Ampules and vials, 0.25 mg/ml.

BUMEX®, see Bumetanide

BUMINATE®, see Albumin

BUPIVACAINE HYDROCHLORIDE—Marcaine®

Description/Actions: Local anesthetic administered by injection for the production of local or regional anesthesia or analgesia for surgery, dental and oral surgery procedures, diagnostic and therapeutic procedures, and for obstetrical procedures. A formulation is also available for the production of subarachnoid block (spinal anesthesia).

Preparations: Ampules and vials, 0.25%, 0.5%, and 0.75%, and in combination with epinephrine. Ampules for spinal anesthesia, 15 mg.

BUPRENEX®, see Buprenorphine

BUPRENORPHINE HYDROCHLORIDE—Buprenex®

Analgesic.

Description/Actions: Demonstrates both opiate agonist and antagonist actions, and is indicated for the relief of moderate to severe pain.

Warnings: Adverse reactions include sedation, dizziness, and vertigo; caution should be exercised in patients also receiving other CNS depressants. Is less likely than many other potent analgesics to cause dependence and is included in Schedule V. May precipitate withdrawal symptoms in patients who are physically dependent on other opiates. Respiratory depression produced by buprenorphine is only partially reversed by naloxone and doxapram may be used. Excreted in human breast milk. Nursing is not recommended.

Administration: Intravenous and intramuscular.

Preparations: Ampules, 0.3 mg.

BUPROPION HYDROCHLORIDE— Wellbutrin®, 2 g bar®, Wellbutrin® SR, Zyban™

Antidepressant.

Description/Actions: Indicated for the treatment of depression and as an aid to smoking cessation treatment.

Warnings: Contraindicated in patients undergoing abrupt discontinuation of alcohol or sedatives, including benzodiazepines. Contraindicated in patients with seizure disorders, and also in patients with a current or prior diagnosis of bulimia or anorexia nervosa because of a higher incidence of seizures noted in such patients when treated with bupropion. Concurrent use with a monoamine oxidase inhibitor is contraindicated and at least 14 days should elapse between discontinuation of an MAOI and initiation of treatment with bupropion. Adverse reactions most commonly encountered include nausea, vomiting, hallucinations, constipation, dry mouth, agitation, insomnia, headache, migraine, and tremor. Some patients experience weight loss. Patients should be cautioned regarding activities such as driving and operating machinery, as well as interactions with other CNS-acting drugs including alcohol. Extreme caution should be exercised in patients with a history of seizures or other predisposition toward seizure, and in patients treated with other medications (e.g., antipsychotics) that may lower seizure threshold. Is extensively metabolized and its activity may be changed by other medications known to affect hepatic enzyme systems (e.g., phenobarbital, cimetidine).

Administration: Oral. Because of a greater risk of seizures, no single dose should exceed 150 mg and the total daily dosage should not exceed 450 mg. Consecutive 150 mg doses should be separated by an interval of at least 6 hours, and consecutive 100 mg doses by an interval of at least 4 hours. For smoking cessation, treat for 7–12 week; avoid bedtime dosing. Patients should aim to stop smoking within 1–2 weeks after starting bupropion. May be used with transdermal nicotine (quit smoking when starting nicotine).

Preparations: Tablets, 75 and 100 mg. Sustained release tabs, 100, 150, and 200 mg.

BUROW'S SOLUTION, see
Aluminum acetate

BuSpar®, see Buspirone

BUSPIRONE HYDROCHLORIDE—BuSpar®

Antianxiety agent.

Description/Actions: Indicated for the management of anxiety disorders or the short-term relief of the symptoms of anxiety.

Warnings: Adverse reactions include dizziness, headache, nervousness, lightheadedness, excitement, and nausea. Buspirone is less likely than other antianxiety agents to cause effects such as sedation; however, because its CNS effects in any individual patient are usually not predictable, patients should be cautioned about engaging in activities such as operating an automobile or machinery. The concurrent use with other CNS-active drugs should be closely monitored, and the consumption of alcoholic beverages is best avoided. The drug should not be used concomitantly with a monoamine oxidase inhibitor because of the possibility of blood pressure elevations.

Administration: Oral.

Preparations: Tablets, 5, 10, and 15 mg.

BUSULFAN—Myleran®

Description/Actions: Antineoplastic agent indicated for the palliative treatment of chronic myelogenous leukemia.

Preparations: Tablets, 2 mg.

BUTABARBITAL SODIUM—Butisol sodium®

Description/Actions: Barbiturate sedative-hypnotic indicated for the treatment of anxiety and insomnia.

Preparations: Tablets, 15, 30, 50, and 100 mg. Elixir, 30 mg/5 ml.

BUTALBITAL

Description/Actions: Barbiturate sedative used in combination with analgesics in the management of muscle-contraction headaches.

BUTAMBEN PICRATE—Butesin picrate®

Description/Actions: Local anesthetic indicated for the temporary relief of pain due to minor burns.

Preparations: Ointment, 1%.

BUTENAFINE HYDROCHLORIDE—Mentax®

Description/Actions: Antifungal agent indicated in the treatment of tinea corporis, tinea cruris, interdigital tinea pedis, and tinea (pityriasis) versicolor due to *Malassezia furfur* (formerly *Pityrosporum orbiculare*).

Warnings: Avoid eyes, nose, mouth, and mucous membranes. Do not occlude area of application. Discontinue if irritation develops and confirm diagnosis. Use cautiously in patients with hypersensitivity to allylamines. Adverse reactions include burning/stinging, worsening of condition, and other local irritation.

Administration: Apply to affected area and immediately surrounding area according to the following guidelines:

Tinea pedis: once daily for 4 weeks.

Tinea corporis, cruris: once daily for 2 weeks.

If no improvement within 4 weeks, reconfirm diagnosis.

Preparations: 1% cream.

BUTESIN PICRATE®, see Butamben picrate

BUTISOL®, see Butabarbital

BUTOCONAZOLE NITRATE—
Femstat®

Imidazole antifungal agent.

Description/Actions: Indicated for the treatment of vulvovaginal mycotic infections caused by *Candida* species.

Warnings: Use during the first trimester of pregnancy should be avoided. Adverse reactions include vulvar/vaginal burning and/or vulvar itching.

Administration: Vaginal.

Preparations: Vaginal cream, 2%.

BUTORPHANOL TARTRATE—
Stadol®, Stadol NS®

Description/Actions: Analgesic also possessing narcotic antagonist activity. Indicated for parenteral use in the relief of moderate to severe pain, for preoperative or preanesthetic medication, as a supplement to balanced anesthesia, and for the relief of prepartum pain. Also indicated for nasal use in the management of pain (including postoperative analgesia).

Preparations: Vials and syringes, 1 mg/ml and 2 mg/ml. Nasal spray, 10 mg/ml.

BUTYL METHOXYDIBENZOYL-METHANE/PADIMATE O—
Photoplex®

Sunscreen.

Description/Actions: A combination of padimate O, which is highly protective against shortwave ultraviolet radiation [UVB (290-320 nm)], and butyl methoxydibenzoylmethane, which protects against long-wave ultraviolet radiation [UVA (320-400 nm)]. The combination of the two agents has been designated as a "broad" or "full" spectrum sunscreen. Indicated to provide protection against the acute (e.g., sunburn) and long-term (e.g., photoaging, skin cancer) risks associated with UVA and UVB light exposure.

Warnings: Contraindicated in patients with a history of allergy to para-aminobenzoic acid, sulfonamides, benzocaine, or aniline dyes. The formulation may stain some fabrics.

Administration: Topical.

Preparations: Lotion containing butyl methoxydibenzoylmethane in a 3% concentration and padimate O in a 7% concentration.

C

CABERGOLINE—Dostinex®

Description/Actions: Dopamine agonist indicated in treatment of hyperprolactinemic disorders, either idiopathic or due to pituitary tumors.

Warnings: Not for pregnancy-induced hypertension or postpartum lactation inhibition or suppression. Use cautiously in hepatic dysfunction. Contraindicated in uncontrolled hypertension and previous sensitivity to ergot alkaloids. Monitor prolactin levels monthly, until normalized.

Administration: Initially 0.25 mg twice weekly. Dose may be increased at 4-week intervals by 0.25 mg twice weekly. Maximum dose is 1 mg twice weekly.

Preparations: Scored tablets, 0.5 mg.

CAFERGOT®, Combination of ergotamine tartrate and caffeine

CAFFEINE—NoDoz®

Description/Actions: **Central nervous system stimulant** used as an aid in staying awake and as an adjunct to analgesics in the management of pain.

Preparations: Tablets, 100 and 200 mg. Controlled-release capsules, 200 and 250 mg.

CAFFEINE AND SODIUM BENZOATE

Description/Actions: **Central nervous system stimulant** that has been administered parenterally as a diuretic, as a stimulant in acute circulatory failure, in the treatment of poisoning, and to alleviate headaches following spinal puncture.

Preparations: Ampules, 250 mg/ml (equal parts caffeine and sodium benzoate).

CALAMINE

Description/Actions: **Protectant** applied topically in the treatment of dermatologic conditions associated with itching, pain, and irritation.

Preparations: Lotion, 8% with 8% zinc oxide.

CALAN®, see Verapamil

CALAN SR®, see Verapamil

CALCIFEDIOL—Calderol®

Description/Actions: **Vitamin D derivative** indicated in the management of metabolic bone disease or hypocalcemia associated with chronic renal failure in patients undergoing renal dialysis.

Preparations: Capsules, 20 and 50 μg.

CALCIBIND®, see Sodium cellulose phosphate

CALCIJEX®, see Calcitriol

CALCIMAR®, see Calcitonin—Salmon

CALCIPOTRIENE—Dovonex®

Agent for psoriasis.

Description/Actions: Is a synthetic analogue of vitamin D_3 that is indicated for the topical treatment of moderate plaque psoriasis.

Warnings: Contraindicated in patients with demonstrated hypercalcemia or evidence of vitamin D toxicity. Is also contraindicated for use on the face. Adverse reactions include burning, itching, skin irritation, and hypercalcemia. If an elevation in serum calcium outside the normal range should occur, treatment should be discontinued until normal calcium levels are restored.

Administration: Topical.

Preparations: Cream, ointment, scalp solution, 0.005%.

CALCITONIN—SALMON—Calcimar®, Miacalcin©

Description/Actions: **Hormone** indicated for the parenteral treatment of symptomatic Paget's disease of bone, hypercalcemia, and postmenopausal osteoporosis.

Preparations: Vials, 200 IU/ml. Nasal spray, 200 units/spray.

CALCITRIOL—Calcijex®, Rocaltrol®

Description/Actions: **Vitamin D derivative** indicated in the management of hypocalcemia and the resultant metabolic bone disease in patients undergoing chronic renal dialysis. Is also indicated in the management of hypocalcemia in patients with hypoparathyroidism.

Preparations: Capsules, 0.25 and 0.5 μg. Ampules, 1 μg/ml and 2 μg/ml.

CALCIUM ACETATE—PhosLo®

Description/Actions: **Phosphate binding agent** indicated for the control of hyperphosphatemia in end stage renal failure.

Preparations: Tablets, 667 mg.

CALCIUM CARBONATE—
Caltrate®, Os-Cal®, Tums®, Viactiv®

Description/Actions: Antacid and source of calcium used in the treatment of gastrointestinal conditions, and in the treatment of hypocalcemic disorders and in situations in which calcium intake is inadequate.

Preparations: Chewable tablets, 350, 500, 750, and 850 mg. Tablets, 1.25 and 1.5 g. Calcium carbonate 500 mg in combination with vitamin D 100 units, vitamin K 400 µg in soft chewable tablets (Viactiv®).

CALCIUM CHLORIDE

Description/Actions: Source of calcium and is administered intravenously in the treatment of hypocalcemic disorders. Also used IV in the treatment of magnesium intoxication, certain hyperkalemic conditions, and cardiac resuscitation.

Preparations: Ampules, vials, and syringes, 10%.

CALCIUM DISODIUM VERSENATE®, see Edetate calcium disodium

CALCIUM GLUCEPTATE

Description/Actions: Source of calcium and is administered parenterally in the treatment of hypocalcemic disorders and certain other conditions.

Preparations: Ampules and vials, 1.1 g/5 ml.

CALCIUM GLUCONATE

Description/Actions: Source of calcium and is administered orally and intravenously in the treatment of hypocalcemic disorders and in situations in which calcium intake is inadequate.

Preparations: Tablets, 500 and 650 mg, 1 g. Ampules and vials, 10%.

CALCIUM LACTATE

Description/Actions: Source of calcium used in the treatment of hypocalcemic disorders and in situations in which calcium intake is inadequate.

Preparations: Tablets, 325 and 650 mg.

CALCIUM PHOSPHATE, TRIBASIC—Tricalcium phosphate, Posture®

Description/Actions: Source of calcium used in the treatment of hypocalcemic disorders and in situations in which calcium intake is inadequate.

Preparations: Tablets, 300 and 600 mg.

CALCIUM UNDECYLENATE—
Caldesene®

Description/Actions: Antifungal agent applied topically in the management of dermatologic fungal infections.

Preparations: Powder, 10%.

CALDEROL®, see Calcifediol

CALDESENE®, see Calcium undecylenate

CALFACTANT—Infasurf®

Description/Actions: Indicated for the prevention of respiratory distress syndrome (RDS) in premature infants < 29 weeks of gestational age at high risk for RDS and for treatment ("rescue") of premature infants 72 hours of age who develop RDS and require endotracheal intubation. Calfactant prophylaxis should be administered as soon as possible, preferably 30 minutes after birth.

Precautions/Adverse Reactions: Calfactant is for intratracheal use only. Reflux of the calfactant into the endotracheal tube, cyanosis, bradycardia or airway obstruction have occurred during the dosing procedures. These events require stopping the calfactant administration and taking appropriate measures to relieve the condition. After the patient is stable, dosing can proceed with proper monitoring.

The administration of lung surfactants often rapidly improves oxygenation and lung compliance. Following administration of calfactant, monitor patients carefully so that oxygen therapy and ventilatory support can be modified in response to changes in respiratory status.

The most common adverse reactions associated with calfactant therapy are cyanosis, airway obstruction, bradycardia, reflux of surfactant into the endotracheal tube, requiring manual ventilation and reintubation. These events were generally transient and not associated with serious complication or death.

Administration: Administer through an endotracheal tube.

Preparations: Single-dose vials, 6 mL

CALTRATE®, see Calcium carbonate

CAMPHOR

Description/Actions: Analgesic and antipruritic. Is used in topically applied formulations used in the management of various dermatologic conditions.

CAMPHORATED OPIUM TINCTURE, see Paregoric

CANCIDAS®, see Caspofungin acetate

CANDESARTAN—Atacand®

Description/Actions: Candesartan is an angiotensin II antagonist that is selective for the AT1 receptor subtype. It is indicated in the treatment of hypertension as monotherapy or in combination with other antihypertensive agents.

Precautions/Adverse Reactions: Correct hypovolemia before starting therapy or monitor patients closely. Use cautiously in patients with renal impairment, severe CHF, renal artery stenosis, and the elderly. Pregnancy Category C in the first trimester, Category D in second and third trimesters. Use not recommended in nursing mothers.

Adverse reactions include back pain, dizziness, upper respiratory tract infection, pharyngitis, and rhinitis.

Administration: Oral.

Patient Care Implications: Instruct patients that following recommended measures for control of hypertension (e.g. exercise, smoking cessation, weight control, dietary measures) will facilitate the action of the medication and does not eliminate the need for these measures. Warn patients that dehydration may enhance the effects of the drugs and to avoid prolonged sun and heat exposure. Caution patient to make position changes slowly to decrease the risk of orthostatic hypotension. Remind patients to continue taking the medication even if feeling well as medication controls but does not cure hypertension.

This agent may not be as effective in Black patients and use of monotherapy in this population needs to be carefully assessed for effectiveness.

Preparations: Tablets, 4, 8, 16, and 32 mg.

CANTIL®, see Mepenzolate

CAPASTAT®, see Capreomycin

CAPECITABINE—Xeloda®

Description/Actions: Antineoplastic agent indicated in the treatment of patients with metastatic breast cancer resistant to both pacitaxel and an anthracycline—containing chemotherapy regimen or resistant to pacitaxel and for whom further anthracycline therapy is not indicated. Capecitabine is also indicated as first-line treatment for patients with metastatic colorectal carcinoma when treatment with fluoropyrimidine therapy alone is preferred.

Approved for use in combination with docetaxel for the treatment of metastatic breast cancer.

Warnings: Contraindicated in patients with hypersensitivity to 5-fluruoracil. Use cautiously in patients with renal or hepatic impairment and carefully monitor function during therapy. The concomitant administration of capecitabine and warfarin has resulted in altered coagulation parameters (INR or prothrombin time) and/or bleeding, including death. These events occurred in patients with and without liver metastasis. Patients receiving capecitabine and warfarin should have their anticoagulant response monitored closely and the anticoagulant dose adjusted accordingly.

Adverse effects include diarrhea which can be severe. Provide supportive treatment to minimize dehydration and electrolyte imbalance. Other adverse effects are hand and foot syndrome (plantar erythrodyesthesia or chemotherapy, induced acral erythema), cardiotoxicity (MI, angina, dysrhythmias, cardiogenic shock, sudden death, ECG changes), hyperbilirubinemia, anemia, neutropenia, thrombocytopenia, nausea, vomiting, stomatitis, and others.

Administration: 2500 mg/m^2/day orally in two divided doses (~12 hours apart) at the end of a meal for 2 weeks followed by a 1-week rest period given as 3-week cycles.

Preparations: Tablets, 150 and 500 mg.

CAPOTEN®, see Captopril

CAPOZIDE®, Combination of captopril and hydrochlorothiazide

CAPREOMYCIN SULFATE— Capastat®

Description/Actions: Antitubercular agent used for the intramuscular treatment of tuberculosis, in conjunction with other antitubercular agents.

Preparations: Vials, 1 g.

CAPSAICIN—Zostrix®, Zostrix-HP®

Description/Actions: Topical analgesic indicated for the relief of neuralgias that may accompany herpes zoster infections, diabetic neuropathy, or follow surgery.

Preparations: Cream, 0.025% and 0.075%.

CAPTOPRIL—Capoten®

Antihypertensive agent and agent for treatment of heart failure.

Description/Actions: Is an angiotensin-converting enzyme (ACE) inhibitor. Indicated for the treatment of hypertension, and in patients with congestive heart failure who have not responded adequately to treatment with diuretics and digitalis. Also indicated to improve survival following myocardial infarction in clinically stable patients with left ventricular dysfunction. Also indicated for the treatment of diabetic nephropathy.

Warnings: Adverse reactions include cough, rash, pruritus, dysgeusia, hypotension, hyperkalemia, proteinuria, and nephrotic syndrome. Neutropenia and agranulocytosis have occurred, and patients should be advised to report promptly any indication of infection (e.g., sore throat, fever) that may be a sign of neutropenia. Use during pregnancy should be avoided.

Administration: Oral. Food reduces absorption and the drug should be given one hour before meals.

Preparations: Tablets, 12.5, 25, 50, and 100 mg.

CARAC™, see Fluorouracil

CARAFATE®, see Sucralfate

CARBACHOL—Isopto Carbachol®, Miostat®

Description/Actions: Cholinergic and miotic agent indicated for ophthalmic administration (Isopto Carbachol®) to lower intraocular pressure in the treatment of glaucoma, and for intraocular administration (Miostat®) to provide miosis during surgery.

Preparations: Ophthalmic solution (Isopto-Carbachol®, 0.75%, 1.5%, 2.25%, and 3%. Solution for intraocular administration (Miostat®), 0.01%.

CARBAMAZEPINE—Carbatrol®, Tegretol®

Anticonvulsant and agent for trigeminal neuralgia.

Description/Actions: Indicated in the following conditions in patients who have not responded satisfactorily to treatment with other agents such as phenytoin, phenobarbital, or primidone: (1) partial seizures with complex symptomatology, (2) generalized tonic-clonic seizures (grand mal), and (3) mixed seizure patterns that include the above, or other partial or generalized seizures. Also indicated in the treatment of pain associated with trigeminal neuralgia and glossopharyngeal neuralgia.

Warnings: Is structurally related to the tricyclic antidepressants and should not be used in patients with a history of hypersensitivity to any of these agents. May cause serious hematologic reactions and should not be used in patients with a history of serious bone marrow depression. Patients should be advised to report immediately signs and symptoms of a potential hematologic problem, such as sore throat, fever, ulcers in the mouth, and easy brusing. Other adverse reactions include: dizziness, drowsiness, nausea, vomiting, and dermatologic effects. Concurrent use with a monoamine oxidase inhibitor is not recommended.

Administration: Oral.

Preparations: Tablets, 200 mg. Extended release 100, 200, 300, and 400 mg. Chewable tablets, 100 mg. Suspension, 100 mg/5 ml.

CARBAMIDE PEROXIDE—Urea peroxide, Debrox®, Gly-Oxide®

Description/Actions: Antiseptic and cleansing agent administered in the mouth for the treatment and prevention of minor oral inflammation such as canker sores, and in the ear to soften and remove earwax.

Preparations: Solution, 6.5% (otic use) and 10% (oral use).

CARBATROL®, see Carbamazepine

CARBENICILLIN INDANYL SODIUM—Geocillin®

Description/Actions: Penicillin antibiotic indicated in the oral treatment of urinary tract and prostatic infections caused by susceptible bacteria.

Preparations: Tablets, equivalent to 382 mg of carbenicillin.

CARBIDOPA—Lodosyn®

Description/Actions: Inhibits the peripheral decarboxylation of levodopa and is used in combination with that agent in the treatment of parkinsonism.

Preparations: Tablets, 25 mg.

CARBINOXAMINE MALEATE

Description/Actions: Antihistamine used in combination with other medications.

CARBOCAINE®, see Mepivacaine

CARBOL-FUCHSIN SOLUTION— Castellani paint

Description/Actions: Antifungal formulation used topically in the management of dermatologic fungal infections. Fuchsin is a dye and causes staining.

Preparations: Solution containing phenol and resorcinol in addition to fuchsin.

CARBOLIC ACID, see Phenol

CARBON DIOXIDE

Description/Actions: Respiratory stimulant used by inhalation in conjunction with oxygen.

Preparations: Gas, available in mixtures with oxygen.

CARBOPLATIN—Paraplatin®

Antineoplastic agent.

Description/Actions: A platinum compound related to cisplatin. Indicated for the palliative treatment of patients with ovarian carcinoma recurrent after prior chemotherapy, including patients who have been previously treated with cisplatin. Also indicated for the initial treatment of advanced ovarian carcinoma.

Warnings: Should not be used in patients with severe bone marrow depression or significant bleeding. Thrombocytopenia, neutropenia, leukopenia, and anemia are often experienced and therapy must be closely monitored. Serious allergic reactions may occur. Other adverse reactions include nausea, vomiting, abdominal pain, diarrhea, constipation, peripheral neuropathies, abnormal hepatic and renal function tests, electrolyte changes, alopecia, and cardiovascular, respiratory, genitourinary, and mucosal effects. Concomitant treatment with aminoglycosides has resulted in increased renal and/or audiologic toxicity. The drug may cause fetal harm when administered during pregnancy.

Administration: Intravenous infusion (lasting 15 minutes or longer). Carboplatin reacts with aluminum, causing precipitate formation and loss of potency; therefore, needles or intravenous sets containing aluminum parts that may come in contact with the drug must not be used for the preparation or administration of carboplatin.

Preparations: Vials, 50, 150, and 450 mg.

CARBOPROST TROMETHAMINE—Hemabate®

Description/Actions: Abortifacient administered intramuscularly for the termination of pregnancy during the period from 13 to 20 gestational weeks. Also indicated for the treatment of postpartum hemorrhage due to uterine atony that has not responded to conventional management.

Preparations: Ampules, 250 µg carboprost and 83 µg tromethamine per ml.

CARBOWAX®, see Polyethylene glycol

CARDENE®, see Nicardipine

CARDENE IV®, see Nicardipine

CARDILATE®, see Erythrityl tetranitrate

CARDIOQUIN®, see Quinidine polygalacturonate

CARDIZEM®, see Diltiazem

CARDIZEM CD®, see Diltiazem

CARDIZEM SR®, see Diltiazem

CARDURA®, see Doxazosin mesylate

CARISOPRODOL—Rela®, Soma®

Description/Actions: Skeletal muscle relaxant indicated as an adjunct to rest, physical therapy, and other measures for the relief of discomfort associated with acute, painful musculoskeletal conditions.

Preparations: Tablets, 350 mg.

CARMUSTINE—BiCNU®

Description/Actions: Antineoplastic agent administered intravenously as palliative therapy for brain tumors, multiple myeloma, Hodgkin's disease, and non-Hodgkin's lymphomas.

Preparations: Vials, 100 mg.

L-CARNITINE—Carnitor®, Vitacarn®

Agent for carnitine deficiency.

Description/Actions: Indicated in the treatment of primary systemic carnitine deficiency.

Warnings: Adverse reactions include nausea, vomiting, abdominal cramps, diarrhea, and patient body odor. Reducing the dosage often decreases or eliminates the GI effects or drug-related odor.

Administration: Oral.

Preparations: Tablets, 330 mg. Enteral liquid, 100 mg/ml.

CARNITOR®, see L-Carnitine

CARTEOLOL HYDROCHLORIDE—Cartrol®, Ocupress®

Antihypertensive agent and agent for glaucoma.

Actions and Uses: A nonselective beta-adrenergic blocking agent with intrinsic sympathomimetic activity. Indicated in the treatment of hypertension, and for ophthalmic administration in the treatment of chronic open-angle glaucoma and intraocular hypertension.

Warnings: Contraindicated in patients with bronchial asthma, cardiogenic shock, severe bradycardia, and second and third degree atrioventricular conduction block in the absence of a functioning artificial pacemaker. Adverse reactions include weakness, tiredness, fatigue, and muscle cramps. Use is best avoided in patients with bronchospastic diseases and therapy in diabetic patients must be closely monitored.

Administration: Oral and ophthalmic. Patients should be cautioned about the interruption or discontinuation of therapy; exacerbation of angina pectoris has occurred following the abrupt cessation of therapy and, when therapy is to be discontinued, the dosage should be gradually reduced over a period of 1 to 2 weeks.

Preparations: Tablets (Cartrol), 2.5 and 5 mg. Ophthalmic solution (Ocupress), 1%.

CARTROL®, see Carteolol

CARVEDILOL—Coreg®

Description/Actions: A noncardioselective beta-blocker/alpha blocker indicated for the treatment of mild or moderate heart failure (NYHA class II or III) and hypertension.

Warnings: Contraindicated in patients with bronchial asthma or related bronchospastic conditions, second- or third-degree AV block, sick sinus syndrome, severe bradycardia (unless paced), cardiogenic shock, severe bradycardia, and a history of carvedilol associated hepatic injury.

Use cautiously in peripheral vascular disease, nonallergic bronchospasm, diabetes, hyperthyroidism, hepatic dysfunction, prinzemetal's angina, pheochromocytoma, and anesthesia . Monitor renal function in ischemic heart disease, diffuse vascular disease, underlying renal insufficiency and/or if systolic BP < 100 mmHg. Avoid abrupt cessation. Pregnancy Category C. Use not recommended in nursing mothers.

Adverse reactions include bradycardia, orthostatic hypotension, edema, AV block, GI upset, hyperglycemia, increased weight, dizziness, and others.

Administration: Oral.

Preparations: Tablets, 3.125, 6.25, 12.5, and 25 mg.

CASANTHRANOL

Description/Actions: Laxative included in combination formulations indicated for constipation.

CASCARA SAGRADA

Description/Actions: Laxative used in the treatment of constipation.

Preparations: Tablets, 325 mg. Aromatic fluid extract.

CASODEX®, see Bicalutamide

CASPOFUNGIN ACETATE—
Cancidas®

Description/Actions: Caspofungin acetate, an antifungal, is indicated for the treatment of invasive aspergillosis in patients who are refractory to or intolerant to amphotericin B, lipid formulations of amphotericin B, and, or itraconazole. Cancidas® has not been studied as initial therapy for invasive aspergillosis. Cancidas® is also indicated for the treatment of esophageal candidiasis.

Precautions/Adverse Reactions: Contraindicated in patients with hypersensitivity to caspofungin or to any component of the product. Concomitant use of caspofungin acetate with cyclosporine is not recommended. Concurrent use has resulted in elevations of hepatic transaminases. Use only if the potential benefit outweighs the potential risk to the patient. Safety on duration of therapy exceeding 2 weeks is limited; however, treatment appears to be well tolerated. Monitoring of tacrolimus blood concentrations is recommended when used concurrently with caspofungin acetate. Dosage adjustments may be necessary.

Dosage of caspofungin acetate may need to be increased when administered concurrently with the enzyme inducers/mixed inducer/inhibitors such as efavirenz, nelfinavir, nevirapine, phenytoin, rifampin, dexamethasone, or carbamazepine. The exact mechanism of the interaction is unknown. Pregnancy Category C. Caspofungin acetate has been shown to be embryotoxic in rats and rabbits. There are no adequate and well-controlled studies in pregnant women. Use in pregnancy only if the potential benefit justifies the potential risk to the fetus. Excretion in human breast milk is unknown. Safety and efficacy in pediatric patients has not been established. Adverse reactions noted in > 10% of patients treated include headache, fever, increased hepatic transaminases, increased alkaline phosphatase and phlebitis/thrombophlebitis. Less frequently observed adverse reactions include rash, pruritis, flushing, chills, edema, nausea, vomiting, diarrhea, pain, myalgias, decreased serum potassium, decreased total serum protein, decreased hemoglobin, hematocrit, platelets, white blood cell count and decreased serum albumin levels. Possible histamine mediated symptoms have been reported during clinical trials.

Administration: Intravenous.

Patient Care Implications: Infuse slowly over at least 1 hour. Monitor patient during infusion. Do not use diluents containing dextrose. Do not mix or co-infuse with other medications. Reconstituted vials may be stored at room temperature for up to 1 hour prior to the preparation of the patient infusion solution. Diluted product is stable for 24 hours at room temperature. Vials should be stored in the refrigerator.

Preparations: Powder for injection: 70 mg and 50 mg single-use vials.

CASTELLANI PAINT, see Carbolfuchsin solution.

CASTOR OIL

Description/Actions: Laxative indicated for the treatment of constipation and preparation of the colon for X-ray and endoscopic examination.

Preparations: Liquid. Emulsions, 36%, 60%, 67%, and 95%.

CATAPRES®, see Clonidine

CATAPRES-TTS®, see Clonidine

CATHFLO™ ACTIVASE®, see Alteplase recombinant

CAVERJECT®, see Alprostadil

CCNU®, see Lomustine

CECLOR®, see Cefaclor

CEDAX®, see Ceftibuten

CeeNU®, see Lomustine

CEFACLOR—Ceclor®

Second-generation cephalosporin antibiotic.

Description/Actions: Spectrum of action includes many gram-positive and gram-negative bacteria. Indicated in upper and lower respiratory infections, otitis media, urinary tract infections, and skin and skin-structure infections caused by susceptible organisms.

Warnings: Must be used cautiously in penicillin-sensitive patients and use should be avoided in patients with a history of immediate and/or severe reactions to penicillin.

Administration: Oral. May be administered without regard to meals.

Preparations: Capsules, 250 and 500 mg. Extended release tablets, 375 and 500 mg. Powder for oral suspension, 125, 187, 250, and 375 mg/5 ml when reconstituted.

CEFADROXIL—Duricef®, Ultracef®

First-generation cephalosporin antibiotic.

Description/Actions: Spectrum of action includes many gram-positive and gram-negative bacteria. Indicated in pharyngitis and tonsillitis, urinary tract infections, and skin and skin-structure infections caused by susceptible organisms.

Warnings: Must be used cautiously in penicillin-sensitive patients and use should be avoided in patients with a history of immediate and/or severe reactions to penicillin.

Administration: Oral. May be administered without regard to meals.

Preparations: Capsules, 500 mg. Tablets, 1 g. Powder for oral suspension, 125, 250, and 500 mg/5 ml when reconstituted.

CEFADYL®, see Cephapirin

CEFAMANDOLE NAFTATE—Mandol®

Second-generation cephalosporin antibiotic.

Description/Actions: Active against many gram-positive and gram-negative bacteria. Indicated for lower respiratory infections, urinary tract infections, peritonitis, septicemia, skin and skin-structure infections, and bone and joint infections caused by susceptible organisms. May also be used for surgical prophylaxis.

Warnings: Must be used cautiously, if at all, in penicillin-sensitive patients and use should be avoided in patients with a history of immediate and/or severe reactions to penicillin. Therapy in patients at risk of bleeding reactions must be closely monitored. Disulfiram-like reactions may occcur following the consumption of alcoholic beverages.

Administration: Intravenous and intramuscular.

Preparations: Vials, 500 mg, 1, 2, and 10 g of cefamandole activity.

CEFANEX®, see Cephalexin

CEFAZOLIN SODIUM—Ancef®, Kefzol®, Zolicef®

First-generation cephalosporin antibiotic.

Description/Actions: Active against many gram-positive and gram-negative bacteria. Indicated for respiratory tract infections, genitourinary tract infections, skin and skin-structure infections, biliary tract infections, bone and joint infections, septicemia, and endocarditis caused by susceptible organisms. Is often used for surgical prophylaxis.

Warnings: Must be used cautiously, if at all, in penicillin-sensitive patients and use should be avoided in patients with a history of immediate and/or severe reactions to penicillins.

Administration: Intravenous and intramuscular.

Preparations: Vials, 250 and 500 mg, 1, 5, and 10 g of cefazolin.

CEFDINIR—Omnicef®

Description/Actions: Third-generation cephalosporin indicated in the treatment of susceptible community acquired pneumonia, acute exacerbations of chronic bronchitis, acute maxillary sinusitis, pharyngitis, tonsillitis and uncomplicated infections of the skin and skin structures.

Warnings: Use cautiously in patients with compromised renal or hepatic function, poor nutritional state, elderly or debilitated, and history of GI disease (esp. colitis). Monitor prothrombin time. Contraindicated in patients with known allergy to cephalosporins. Adverse reactions include rash, pseudomenbranous colitis and superinfection.

Administration: Dosing is every 12 hours or once every 24 hours for a duration of 5–10 days depending on the infection

Preparations: Capsules, 300 mg; suspension, 125 mg/5 ml.

CEFDITOREN PIVOXIL— SPECTRACEF™

Description/Actions: Cefditoren pivoxil is indicated for the treatment of mild to moderate infections in adults and adolescents (12 years of age or older) that are caused by susceptible strains of the designated microorganisms in the following conditions: acute bacterial exacerbations of chronic bronchitis, pharyngitis/tonsillitis, and uncomplicated skin and skin-structure infections.

Precautions/Adverse Reactions: Cefditoren causes renal excretion of carnitine; therefore, it is contraindicated in patients with carnitine deficiency or inborn errors of metabolism that may result in clinically significant carnitine deficiency. Cefditoren tablets contain sodium caseinate, a milk protein, and should not be administered to patients with milk protein hypersensitivity. Use caution when using in patients with a history of hypersensitivity reactions to penicillins or to other beta-lactam antibiotics. Pseudomembranous colitis may occur and may range in severity from mild to life-threatening. Cefditoren is not recommended when prolonged antibiotic treatment is necessary. Cefditoren may be associated with a fall in prothrombin time. Coadministration with aluminum/magnesium-containing antacids is not recommended. Coadministraion of cefditoren and famotidine is not recommended. The coadministration of cefditoren and probenecid resulted in increased plasma concentrations of cefditoren. Pregnancy Category B. No adequate and well-controlled studies in pregnant women. Use during pregnancy only if the potential benefit justifies the potential risk to the fetus. Excretion in human breast milk is unknown. Safety and efficacy in pediatric patients < 12 years have not been established. Most common adverse effects noted in patients receiving cefditoren include diarrhea, nausea, headache, abdominal pain, vaginal moniliasis, dyspepsia, vomiting, decreased hematocrit, hematuria, increased urine white blood cells, and increased glucose. In addition, adverse reactions seen with cephalosporin antibiotics including allergic reactions, anaphylaxis, drug fever, Stevens-Johnson syndrome, serum sickness–like reactions, erythema multiforme, toxic epidermal necrolysis, colitis, renal dysfunction including cholestasis, aplastic anemia, hemolytic anemia, hemorrhage, superinfection, and seizures have been observed with cefditoren. Prolonged prothrombin time, positive direct Coombs' test, false-positive test for urinary glucose, elevated alkaline phosphatase, elevated bilirubin, elevated LDH, increased creatinine, pancytopenia, neutropenia, and agranulocytosis may also occur.

Administration: Oral.

58 • CEFEPIME

Patient Care Implications: Take with meals. Avoid concomitant use of antacids or histamine$_2$ receptor antagonists. Not recommended when prolonged antibiotic therapy is needed.

Preparations: Tablets, 200 mg.

CEFEPIME—Maxipime®

Description/Actions: Fourth-generation cephalosporin indicated in treatment of susceptible uncomplicated or complicated urinary tract infections including pyelonephritis, uncomplicated skin and skin structure infections, and moderate to severe pneumonia, complicated intraabdominal infection in adults (in conjunction with metronidazole) and empiric therapy in febrile neutropenia.

Warnings: Use cautiously in patients with compromised renal or hepatic function, poor nutritional state, elderly or debilitated, and history of GI disease (esp. colitis). Monitor prothrombin time. Contraindicated in patients allergic to cephalasporins. Adverse reactions include local reactions to IV infusion (e.g., pain, phlebitis, inflammation), rash, pseudomembranous colitis, and superinfection.

Administration: IV infusion over 30 minutes or IM every 12 hours for 7–10 days.

Preparations: Powder for reconstitution, 500 mg, 1 and 2 g.

CEFIXIME—Suprax®

Antibiotic.

Description/Actions: An orally-administered, third-generation cephalosporin antibiotic that is especially active against gram-negative bacteria. Indicated in the treatment of otitis media, pharyngitis and tonsillitis, acute bronchitis and acute exacerbations of chronic bronchitis, uncomplicated gonorrhea, and uncomplicated urinary tract infections caused by susceptible bacteria. Among the bacteria that are susceptible are *Branhamella (Moraxella) catarrhalis, Escherichia coli, Haemophilus influenzae, Neisseria gonorrhoeae, Proteus mirabilis, Streptococcus pneumoniae, and Streptococcus pyogenes.*

Warnings: Must be used cautiously in penicillin-sensitive patients and use should be avoided in patients with a history of immediate and/or severe reactions to penicillin. Adverse reactions include diarrhea, loose or frequent stools, abdominal pain, nausea, dyspepsia, flatulence, headache, dizziness, pruritus, and rash.

Administration: Oral. The suspension formulation should be used in the treatment of otitis media. Because the suspension formulation provides higher peak blood levels than the tablet when administered at the same dose, patients should not be switched from the suspension to the tablets. May be administered without regard to meals.

Preparations: Tablets, 200 and 400 mg. Powder for oral suspension, 100 mg/5 ml when reconstituted.

CEFIZOX®, see Ceftizoxime

CEFMETAZOLE SODIUM— Zefazone®

Second-generation cephalosoporin antibiotic.

Description/Actions: Active against many aerobic and anaerobic gram-positive and gram-negative bacteria; spectrum of action includes *Bacteroides fragilis.* Indicated in the treatment of urinary tract, lower respiratory tract, skin and skin structure, and intraabdominal infections caused by susceptible bacteria. Is also indicated for surgical prophylaxis.

Warnings: Must be used cautiously, if at all, in penicillin-sensitive patients and use should be avoided in patients with a history of immediate and/or severe reactions to penicillin. Adverse reactions include diarrhea, nausea, epigastric pain, bleeding, allergic reactions, rash, pruritus, superinfection, pain and/or swelling at the injection site, thrombophlebitis, and prolonged prothrombin time. Prothrombin time should be monitored for patients at risk. Disulfiram-like reactions may occur when alcohol is ingested within 24 hours of cefmetazole administration.

Administration: Intravenous.

Preparations: Vials, 1 and 2 g.

CEFOBID®, see Cefoperazone

CEFONICID SODIUM—Monocid®

Second-generation cephalosporin antibiotic.

Description/Actions: Active against many gram-positive and gram-negative bacteria. Indicated for lower respiratory tract infections, urinary tract infections, septicemia, and bone and joint infections caused by susceptible organisms. May also be used for surgical prophylaxis.

Warnings: Must be used cautiously, if at all, in penicillin-sensitive patients and use should be avoided in patients with a history of immediate and/or severe reactions to penicillin.

Administration: Intravenous and intramuscular. Long duration of action permits once-daily dosing in many infections.

Preparations: Vials, 500 mg, 1 and 10 g of cefonicid.

CEFOPERAZONE SODIUM—
   Cefobid®

Third-generation cephalosporin antibiotic.

Description/Actions: Highly active against many gram-negative bacteria and also effective against some gram-positive bacteria; spectrum of action includes *Pseudomonas aeruginosa.* Indicated for respiratory tract infections, peritonitis and other intraabdominal infections, septicemia, skin and skin-structure infections, urinary tract infections, and pelvic inflammatory disease and other female genital tract infections caused by susceptible organisms.

Warnings: Must be used cautiously, if at all, in penicillin-sensitive patients and use should be avoided in patients with a history of immediate and/or severe reactions to penicillin. Therapy in patients at risk of bleeding reactions must be closely monitored. Is excreted via biliary mechanisms to a greater extent than are other cephalosporins, and use is associated with a higher incidence of diarrhea. Disulfiram-like reactions may occur following the consumption of alcoholic beverages.

Administration: Intravenous and intramuscular.

Preparations: Vials, 1, 2, and 10 g of cefoperazone.

CEFOTAN®, see Cefotetan

CEFOTAXIME SODIUM—
   Claforan®

Third-generation cephalosporin antibiotic.

Description/Actions: Highly active against many gram-negative bacteria and also effective against some gram-positive bacteria. Indicated for lower respiratory tract infections, bacteremia/septicemia, skin and skin-structure infections, intraabdominal infections, bone and/or joint infections, and central nervous system infections caused by susceptible organisms. May also be used for surgical prophylaxis.

Warnings: Must be used cautiously, if at all, in penicillin-sensitive patients and use should be avoided in patients with a history of immediate and/or severe reactions to penicillins.

Administration: Intravenous and intramuscular.

Preparations: Vials, 1, 2, and 20 g of cefotaxime.

CEFOTETAN DISODIUM—
   Cefotan®

Second-generation cephalosporin antibiotic.

Description/Actions: Active against many gram-positive and gram-negative bacteria; spectrum of action includes *Bacteroides fragilis.* Indicated for urinary tract

60 • CEFOXITIN SODIUM

infections, lower respiratory tract infections, skin and skin-structure infections, gynecologic infections, intraabdominal infections, and bone and joint infections caused by susceptible organisms. May also be used for surgical prophylaxis.

Warnings: Must be used cautiously, if at all, in penicillin-sensitive patients and use should be avoided in patients with a history of immediate and/or severe reactions to penicillin. Disulfiram-like reactions may occur when alcohol is ingested within 72 hours of cefotetan administration. Prothrombin times should be monitored in patients at risk of bleeding reactions.

Administration: Intravenous and intramuscular.

Preparations: Vials, 1, 2, and 10 g of cefotetan activity.

CEFOXITIN SODIUM—Mefoxin®
Second-generation cephalosporin antibiotic.

Description/Actions: Active against many gram-positive and gram-negative bacteria; spectrum of action includes *Bacteroides fragilis*. Indicated for lower respiratory tract infections, genitourinary infections, intraabdominal infections, gynecological infections, septicemia, bone and joint infections, and skin and skin-structure infections caused by susceptible organisms. May also be used for surgical prophylaxis.

Warnings: Must be used cautiously, if at all, in penicillin-sensitive patients and use should be avoided in patients with a history of immediate and/or severe reactions to penicillins.

Administration: Intravenous and intramuscular.

Preparations: Vials, 1, 2, and 10 g of cefoxitin.

CEFPODOXIME PROXETIL—Vantin®
Third-generation cephalosporin antibiotic.

Description/Actions: Is a prodrug that is converted to its active metabolite, cefpodoxime. Inhibits bacterial cell wall synthesis and exhibits a bactericidal action against many gram-positive and gram-negative bacteria. Indicated for upper respiratory tract infections, lower respiratory tract infections, uncomplicated skin and skin structure infections, and uncomplicated urinary tract infections (cystitis) caused by susceptible organisms. Also indicated for acute, uncomplicated urethral and cervical gonorrhea, and acute, uncomplicated anorectal infections in women due to *Neisseria gonorrhoeae*.

Warnings: Must be used cautiously in penicillin-sensitive patients and use should be avoided in patients with a history of immediate and/or severe reactions to penicillins. Adverse reactions include diarrhea, nausea, abdominal pain, vomiting, vaginal fungal infections, rash, and headache. Absorption may be reduced by the concomitant administration of an antacid or histamine H_2-receptor antagonist.

Administration: Oral. Tablet formulation should be administered with food.

Preparations: Tablets, 100 and 200 mg. Powder for oral suspension, 50 mg/5 ml and 100 mg/5 ml.

CEFPROZIL—Cefzil®
Second-generation cephalosporin antibiotic.

Description/Actions: Inhibits bacterial cell wall synthesis and exhibits a bactericidal action against many gram-positive and gram-negative bacteria. Indicated for upper respiratory tract infections (including pharyngitis and tonsilitis), lower respiratory tract infections, and uncomplicated skin and skin structure infections caused by susceptible organisms.

Warnings: Must be used cautiously in penicillin-sensitive patients and use should be avoided in patients with a history of immediate and/or severe reactions to penicillins. Adverse reactions include diarrhea, nausea, vomiting, abdominal pain, rash, eosinophilia, vaginitis, and superinfection.

Administration: Oral.

Preparations: Tablets, 250 and 500 mg. Powder for oral suspension, 125 mg/5 ml and 250 mg/5 ml.

CEFTAZIDIME—Ceptaz®, Fortaz®, Tazicef®, Tazidime®

Third-generation cephalosporin antibiotic.

Description/Actions: Highly active against many gram-negative bacteria and also effective against some gram-positive bacteria; spectrum of action includes *Pseudomonas aeruginosa.* Indicated for lower respiratory tract infections, skin and skin-structure infections, urinary tract infections, bacterial septicemia, bone and joint infections, gynecological infections, intraabdominal infections, and central nervous system infections caused by susceptible organisms.

Warnings: Must be used cautiously, if at all, in penicillin-sensitive patients and use should be avoided in patients with a history of immediate and/or severe reactions to penicillin. Adverse reactions include hyperbilirubinemia, jaundice, renal impairment, urticaria, pain at injection site, anaphylaxis, and rare severe allergic reactions such as cardiopulmonary arrest. Myoclonia and coma have been reported in patients with renal insufficiency.

Administration: Intravenous and intramuscular.

Preparations: Vials, 500 mg, 1, 2, and 6 g. Ceptaz formulation contains L-arginine instead of sodium carbonate, and does not release carbon dioxide following reconstitution as the other formulations do.

CEFTIBUTEN—Cedax®

Third-generation cephalosporin.

Description/Actions: Indicated in susceptible mild to moderate acute bacterial exacerbations of chronic bronchitis, acute bacterial otitis media, and pharyngitis/tonsillitis.

Warnings: May cause GI upset, headache, dizziness. Adjust dosing in renal impairment. Must be used cautiously in penicillin sensitive patients and use should be avoided in patients with a history of immediate and/or severe reactions to penicillin.

Administration: Oral. Suspension should be taken on an empty stomach. Capsules may be taken regardless of food intake.

Preparations: Capsules, 400 mg. Suspension, 90 mg/5 ml.

CEFTIN®, see Cefuroxime axetil

CEFTIZOXIME SODIUM—Cefizox®

Third-generation cephalosporin antibiotic.

Description/Actions: Highly active against many gram-negative bacteria and also effective against some gram-positive bacteria. Indicated for lower respiratory tract infections, urinary tract infections, gonorrhea, pelvic inflammatory disease, intraabdominal infections, septicemia, skin and skin-structure infections, bone and joint infections, and meningitis caused by susceptible organisms.

Warnings: Must be used cautiously, if at all, in penicillin-sensitive patients and use should be avoided in patients with a history of immediate and/or severe reactions to penicillins.

Administration: Intravenous and intramuscular.

Preparations: Vials, 1, 2, and 10 g of ceftizoxime.

CEFTRIAXONE SODIUM—Rocephin®

Third-generation cephalosporin antibiotic.

Description/Actions: Highly active against many gram-negative bacteria and also effective against some gram-positive bacteria. Indicated for lower respiratory tract infections, skin and skin-structure infections, urinary tract infections, gonorrhea, including pharyngeal gonorrhea, pelvic inflammatory disease, septicemia, bone and joint infections, intraabdominal infections, and meningitis caused by susceptible organisms. May also be used for surgical prophylaxis.

Warnings: Must be used cautiously, if at all, in penicillin-sensitive patients and use should be avoided in patients with a history of immediate and/or severe reactions to penicillins.

Administration: Intravenous and intramuscular. Long duration of action permits once-daily dosing in most infections.

Preparations: Vials, 250 and 500 mg, 1, 2, and 10 g of ceftriaxone.

CEFUROXIME AXETIL—Ceftin®

Second-generation cephalosporin antibiotic.

Description/Actions: Spectrum of action includes many gram-positive and gram-negative bacteria. Indicated in pharyngitis and tonsillitis, otitis media, lower respiratory tract infections, urinary tract infections, gonorrhea, and skin and skin-structure infections caused by susceptible organisms.

Warnings: Must be used cautiously in penicillin-sensitive patients and use should be avoided in patients with a history of immediate and/or severe reactions to penicillin.

Administration: Oral. Tablets may be administered without regard to meals but the suspension should be administered with food.

Preparations: Tablets, 125, 250, and 500 mg. Powder for oral suspension, 125 mg/5ml and 250 mg/5 ml.

CEFUROXIME SODIUM—
Kefurox®, Zinacef®

Second-generation cephalosporin antibiotic.

Description/Actions: Active against many gram-positive and gram-negative bacteria. Indicated for lower respiratory tract infections, urinary tract infections, skin and skin-structure infections, septicemia, bone and joint infections, meningitis, and gonorrhea caused by susceptible organisms. May also be used for surgical prophylaxis.

Warnings: Must be used cautiously, if at all, in penicillin-sensitive patients and use should be avoided in patients with a history of immediate and/or severe reactions to penicillins.

Administration: Intravenous and intramuscular.

Preparations: Vials, 750 mg, 1.5 and 7.5 g of cefuroxime.

CEFZIL®, see Cefprozil

CELECOXIB—Celebrex®

Description/Actions: An NSAID Cox-2 inhibitor indicated in the treatment of rheumatoid arthritis, osteoarthritis, management of acute pain and treatment of primary dysmenorrhea.

Precautions/Adverse Reactions: Celecoxib is contraindicated in aspirin or sulfa allergy and the third trimester of pregnancy.

Use is not recommended in severe renal or hepatic impairment. Discontinue if liver impairment develops after initiation. Use cautiously in fluid retention, heart failure, hypertension, asthma, dehydration, debilitated, and the elderly. Monitor for GI ulcer/bleed. The risk of ulcer is increased if patient is otherwise at high risk, with extended drug treatment, high doses, history of GI bleed, or ulcer.

Adverse reactions include GI upset, edema, pharyngitis, increase in liver tests (ALT/AST), and GI ulcer/bleed.

Administration: Oral.

Patient Care Implications: Instruct patients not to exceed dosing guidelines and not to independently increase the dose as this will increase the risk of serious adverse events. If pain relief is not achieved, call the doctor for other treatment options. If stomach discomfort is experienced, promptly call the doctor.

Preparations: Capsules, 100, 200, and 400 mg.

CELESTONE®, see Betamethasone

CELEXA®, see Citalopram Hydrobromide

CELLCEPT®, see Mycophenolate mofetil.

CELONTIN®, see Methsuximide

CENTRAX®, see Prazepam

CEPACOL®, see Cetylpyridinium

CEPHALEXIN—Cefanex®, Keflex®

CEPHALEXIN HYDROCHLORIDE—Keftab®

First-generation cephalosporin antibiotic.

Description/Actions: Spectrum of action includes many gram-positive and gram-negative bacteria. Indicated in respiratory tract infections, otitis media, skin and skin-structure infections, bone infections, and genitourinary tract infections caused by susceptible organisms.

Warnings: Must be used cautiously in penicillin-sensitive patients and use should be avoided in patients with a history of immediate and/or severe reactions to penicillin.

Administration: Oral. May be administered without regard to meals.

Preparations: Capsules and tablets, 250 and 500 mg, 1 g. Powder for oral suspension, 125 and 250 mg/5 ml when reconstituted, and formulation for pediatric use, 100 mg/ml when reconstituted.

CEPHALOTHIN SODIUM—Keflin®

Description/Actions: First-generation cephalosporin antibiotic indicated for the parenteral treatment of infections caused by susceptible organisms.

Preparations: Vials, 1, 2, 4, and 20 g.

CEPHAPIRIN SODIUM—Cefadyl®

First-generation cephalosporin antibiotic

Description/Actions: indicated for the parenteral treatment of infections caused by susceptible organisms.

Preparations: Vials, 500 mg, 1, 2, 4, and 20 g.

CEPHRADINE—Anspor®, Velosef®

First-generation cephalosporin antibiotic.

Description/Actions: Active against many gram-positive and gram-negative bacteria. Indicated for the oral treatment of respiratory tract infections, otitis media, skin and skin-structure infections, and urinary tract infections caused by susceptible organisms. May also be administered parenterally for these infections as well as for bone infections and septicemia caused by susceptible organisms. May be used parenterally for surgical prophylaxis.

Warnings: Must be used cautiously, if at all, in penicillin-sensitive patients and use should be avoided in patients with a history of immediate and/or severe reactions to penicillins.

Administration: Oral, intravenous, and intramuscular. May be administered orally without regard to meals.

Preparations: Capsules, 250 and 500 mg. Powder for oral suspension, 125 and 250 mg/5 ml when reconstituted. Vials, 250 and 500 mg, 1, 2, and 4 g.

CEPHULAC®, see Lactulose

CEPTAZ®, see Ceftazidime

CEREBYX®, see Fosphenytoin

CEREDASE®, see Alglucerase

CEREZYME®, see Imiglucerase

CERUBIDINE®, see Daunorubicin

CETIRIZINE AND PSEUDOEPHEDRINE— ZYRTEC-D 12 HOUR™

Description/Actions: Zyrtec-D 12 Hour™ is indicated for the relief of nasal and nonnasal symptoms associated with seasonal or perennial allergic rhinitis in adults and children 12 years of age and older.

Precautions/Adverse Effects: Zyrtec-D 12 Hour™ is contraindicated in patients with narrow-angle glaucoma or urinary retention, and in patients receiving monoamine oxidase inhibitor (MAOI) therapy or within 14 days of stopping therapy. Also contraindicated in patients with severe hypertension or severe coronary artery disease and in those who have shown hypersensitivity or idiosyncrasy to its components, to adrenergic agents, or to other drugs of similar chemical structure. Manifestations of patient idiosyncrasy to adrenergic agents include insomnia, dizziness, weakness, tremor and arrhythmias. Pseudoephedrine produces peripheral effects similar to those of ephedrine and central effects similar to, but less intense than, amphetamines. It has the potential for excitatory side effects. Sympathomimetic amines should be used judiciously and sparingly in patients with hypertension, diabetes mellitus, ischemic heart disease, increased intraocular pressure, hyperthyroidism, renal impairment, or prostatic hypertrophy. Use with caution in patients older than 60 years of age; there is a decrease in cetirizine clearance that may be related to decreased renal function. The elderly are more likely to experience side effects. In general, dosing in the elderly should be cautious, because of the greater frequency of decreased hepatic, renal, or cardiac function, and of concomitant disease or other drug therapy. Zyrtec-D 12 Hour™ is not recommended in patients < 12 years. Most common adverse reactions were somnolence, headache, fatigue, and dry mouth. Pregnancy Category C. No adequate, well-controlled studies in pregnant women. Use only if benefit justifies potential risk to fetus. Both cetirizine and pseudoephedrine are excreted in milk; use in nursing mothers is not recommended.

Administration: Oral.

Patient Care Implications: May be taken with or without food. Because of somnolence, caution should be exercised when driving a car or operating potentially dangerous machinery. Concurrent use with alcohol or other CNS depressants should be avoided because of additional decrease in alertness and additional impairment of CNS performance that may occur. Tablet should be swallowed whole; do not break, crush, or chew.

Preparations: Tablet, extended release: cetirizine hydrochloride, 5 mg, and pseudoephedrine hydrochloride, 120 mg.

CETIRIZINE HYDROCHLORIDE— Zyrtec®

Description/Actions: Antihistamine indicated for the treatment of seasonal rhinitis, for the relief of symptoms associated with perennial allergic rhinitis in adults and children 6 months of age and older and for the treatment of the uncomplicated skin manifestations of chronic idiopathic urticaria in adults and children 6 months of age or older.

Warnings: Contraindicated in hydroxyzine sensitivity. Use cautiously in hepatic or renal dysfunction. Use by nursing mothers is not recommended. Potentiates CNS depression with alcohol and other CNS depressants. Adverse reactions include somnolence, fatigue, dry mouth, and dizziness.

Administration: Oral. Adjust dose in hepatic or renal impairment.

Preparations: Tablets, 5 and 10 mg, syrup 1 mg/ml

CETRORELIX ACETATE— Cetrotide®

Description/Actions: Indicated for the inhibition of premature LH surges in women undergoing controlled ovarian stimulation. The extent and duration of LH inhibition is dose dependent. Effects are reversible upon discontinuation of cetrorelix.

Precautions/Adverse Reactions: Contraindicated in patients with a known hypersensitivity to cetrorelix acetate, extrinsic peptide hormone, or mannitol. Known hypersensitivity to Gn-RH or any other Gn-RH analogs. Contraindicated in pregnancy and lactation. Caution is advised when administered to patients with a hypersensitivity to Gn-RH. Carefully monitor patients after the first injection. A severe anaphylactic reaction was observed in one patient after 7 months of treatment with cetrorelix for an indication other than infertility. Should only be prescribed by fertility specialists. No formal drug interaction studies have been performed. Pregnancy Category X. Cetrorelix is contraindicated in pregnant women. Animal studies have shown fetal resorption and loss of implantation. These results would also be expected in pregnant women. Excretion in human breast milk is unknown; therefore, cetrorelix should not be used by nursing mothers. Adverse reactions occurring in ≥ 1% of patients include ovarian hyperstimulation syndrome (3.5%), nausea, headache, increased alkaline phosphatase and increased liver enzymes. Local site reactions such as redness, erythema, bruising, itching, swelling, and pruritis have been reported; however, they were usually mild and transient. Congenital anomalies and stillbirths have been reported.

Administration: SQ injection.

Patient Care Implications: Instruct patient and or caregiver on the proper administration of cetrorelix. Store drug in refrigerator.

Preparations: Injection: 0.25 mg vial and 3 mg vial each with one prefilled glass syringe, sterile water for injection, one 20 gauge needle, one 27 gauge needle, and two alcohol pads.

CETYLPYRIDINIUM CHLORIDE— Cepacol®

Description/Actions: Antiseptic included in formulations used in minor sore throat and in conditions in which there is minor irritation of the mouth or throat.

Preparations: Lozenges, 0.07%. Mouthwash, 0.05%.

CEVIMELINE HYDROCHLORIDE—Evoxac®

Description/Actions: Cholinergic agonist indicated in the treatment of symptoms of dry mouth in patients with Sjogren's syndrome.

Precautions/Adverse Reaction: Cevimeline is contraindicated in patients with uncontrolled asthma, known hypersensitivity to cevimeline, and when miosis is undesirable (e.g., in acute iritis and in narrow-angle glaucoma). Cevimeline should be used with caution in patients with cardiovascular disease, controlled asthma, chronic bronchitis, chronic obstructive pulmonary disease, or a history of nephrolithiasis or cholelithiasis. Caution should be advised while driving at night or performing hazardous activities in reduced lighting. Adverse effects include excessive sweating, nausea, rhinitis, diarrhea, excessive salivation, urinary tract infection, asthenia, flushing, and polyuria.

Administration: Oral.

Preparations: Capsules, 30 mg.

CHARCOAL, ACTIVATED

Description/Actions: Adsorbent used for relief of intestinal gas, diarrhea, and GI distress. Also used as an antidote in the treatment of poisoning by many drugs and chemicals.

Preparations: Capsules, 260 mg. Liquid. Powder.

CHEMET®, see Succimer

CHIBROXIN®, see Norfloxacin

CHILDREN'S ADVIL®—see Ibuprofen

CHILDREN'S MOTRIN®—see Ibuprofen

CHLORAL HYDRATE

Description/Actions: Sedative-hypnotic used in the treatment of insomnia and as an anesthetic adjunct for reduction of anxiety preoperatively.

Preparations: Capsules, 250 and 500 mg. Syrup, 500 mg/5 ml. Suppositories, 324, 500, and 648 mg.

CHLORAMBUCIL—Leukeran®

Description/Actions: Antineoplastic agent indicated in the treatment of chronic lymphocytic leukemia, malignant lymphomas including lymphosarcoma, giant follicular lymphoma, and Hodgkin's disease.

Preparations: Tablets, 2 mg.

CHLORAMPHENICOL— Chloromycetin®

Description/Actions: Antibiotic with a broad spectrum of activity that has been used in the treatment of systemic, dermatologic, ophthalmic, and otic infections. Is of greatest value in systemic infections caused by *Salmonella typhi, Haemophilus influenzae* (e.g., meningitis), and rickettsial organisms.

Preparations: Vials (as the sodium succinate), 1 g. Ophthalmic solution (0.5%) and ointment (1%). Otic solution, 0.5%.

CHLORDIAZEPOXIDE—Librium®, Libritabs®

Benzodiazepine antianxiety agent.

Description/Actions: A CNS depressant indicated for the management of anxiety disorders or for the short-term relief of symptoms of anxiety, withdrawal symptoms of acute alcoholism, and preoperative apprehension and anxiety.

Warnings: Adverse reactions include drowsiness and other CNS effects; patients should be cautioned regarding activities such as driving and operating machinery, as well as interactions with other CNS-acting drugs including alcohol. Can cause dependence and is included in Schedule IV.

Administration: Oral, intravenous, and intramuscular.

Preparations: Capsules (as the hydrochloride) and tablets, 5, 10, and 25 mg. Ampules (as the hydrochloride), 100 mg.

CHLORESIUM®, see Chlorophyll

CHLORHEXIDINE GLUCONATE—Hibiclens®, Hibistat®, Peridex®

Description/Actions: Antiseptic and cleanser indicated for topical use as a skin wound cleanser and general skin cleanser, as a surgical scrub, for patient preoperative showering and bathing, as a patient preoperative skin preparation, and as a health care personnel handwash or germicidal hand rinse. Also used as an oral rinse (Peridex®) for the treatment of gingivitis.

Preparations: Skin cleanser, 4%. Germicidal hand rinse, 0.5%. Oral rinse, 0.12%.

CHLORMEZANONE—Trancopal®

Description/Actions: Antianxiety agent indicated for the treatment of mild anxiety and tension states.

Preparations: Tablets, 100 and 200 mg.

CHLOROMYCETIN®, see Chloramphenicol

CHLOROPHYLL-Chloresium®, Derifil®

Description/Actions: Deodorizing agent used topically to reduce malodors in wounds, burns, and other dermatologic conditions, and orally for the control of fecal and urinary odor associated with incontinence and ostomy conditions, body odors, and odor of surface lesions.

Preparations: Solution, 0.2%. Ointment, 0.5%. Tablets, 100 mg.

CHLOROPROCAINE HYDROCHLORIDE—Nesacaine®, Nesacaine-CE®

Description/Actions: Local anesthetic indicated for the production of local anesthesia by infiltration and peripheral nerve block. Formulation without preservatives (Nesacaine-CE®) may also be used by central nerve block, including lumbar and caudal epidural blocks.

Preparations: Vials, 1% and 2%. Vials (Nesacaine-CE), 2% and 3%.

CHLOROQUINE—Aralen®

Description/Actions: Antimalarial agent and amebicide. Indicated for acute attacks of malaria and prophylaxis against malaria. Also indicated for the treatment of extraintestinal amebiasis.

Preparations: Tablets (as the phosphate), 500 mg. Vials (as the dihydrochloride), 50 mg/ml.

CHLOROTHIAZIDE—Diuril®

Description/Actions: Thiazide diuretic indicated as adjunctive therapy in edema and in the management of hypertension.

Preparations: Tablets, 250 and 500 mg. Suspension, 250 mg/5 ml.

CHLOROTRIANISENE—Tace®

Description/Actions: Estrogen indicated for the treatment of postpartum breast engorgement, moderate to severe vasomotor symptoms associated with the menopause, atrophic vaginitis, kraurosis vulvae, and female hypogonadism. Also used as palliative therapy of advanced prostatic carcinoma.

Preparations: Capsules, 12, 25, and 72 mg.

CHLORPHENESIN CARBAMATE—Maolate®

Description/Actions: Skeletal muscle relaxant indicated as an adjunct to rest, physical therapy, and other measures for relief of discomfort associated with acute, painful musculoskeletal conditions.

Preparations: Tablets, 400 mg.

CHLORPHENIRAMINE MALEATE—Chlor-Trimeton®, Teldrin®

Antihistamine.

Description/Actions: Indicated in the treatment of various allergic disorders.

Warnings: Adverse effects include drowsiness and other CNS effects; patients should be cautioned regarding activities such as driving and operating machinery, as well as interactions with other CNS-acting drugs including alcohol.

Administration: Oral, intravenous, intramuscular, and subcutaneous.

Preparations: Tablets, 2 and 4 mg. Controlled-release tablets and capsules, 8 and 12 mg. Syrup, 2 mg/5 ml. Vials, 10 mg/ml.

CHLORPROMAZINE—Thorazine®

Description/Actions: Phenothiazine antipsychotic and antiemetic agent. Indicated in the management of psychotic disorders, to control nausea and vomiting, as a preoperative medication, as an adjunct in the treatment of tetanus, for relief of intractable hiccups, to control the manifestations of the manic type of manic-depressive illness, and for acute intermittent porphyria. Also indicated for the treatment of certain severe behavioral problems in children, and in the short-term treatment of certain hyperactive children.

Preparations: Tablets, 10, 25, 50, 100, and 200 mg. Controlled-release capsules, 30, 75, 150, 200 and 300 mg. Syrup (as the hydrochloride), 10 mg/5 ml. Oral concentrate (as the hydrochloride), 30 and 100 mg/ml. Suppositories, 25 and 100 mg. Ampules and vials (as the hydrochloride), 25 mg/ml.

CHLORPROPAMIDE—Diabinese®

Sulfonylurea hypoglycemic agent.

Description/Actions: Indicated as an adjunct to diet to lower the blood glucose in patients with non-insulin-dependent diabetes mellitus whose hyperglycemia cannot be controlled by diet alone.

Warnings: May cause hypoglycemia and patients should be advised to contact their physician if symptoms of hypoglycemia develop. Adverse reactions include nausea, vomiting, diarrhea, pruritus, and rash. Oral hypoglycemic agents have been suggested to be associated with increased cardiovascular mortality as compared with treatment by diet alone or diet plus insulin. May cause disulfiram-like reactions following the consumption of alcoholic beverages. Therapy in patients also receiving a beta-adrenergic blocking agent should be monitored closely.

Administration: Oral.

Preparations: Tablets, 100 and 250 mg.

CHLORPROTHIXENE

Description/Actions: Antipsychotic agent indicated for the management of manifestations of psychotic disorders.

Preparations: Tablets, 10, 25, 50 and 100 mg. Oral concentrate (as the lactate and hydrochloride), 100 mg chlorprothixene/5 ml. Ampules (as the hydrochloride), 25 mg chlorprothixene/2 ml.

CHLORTETRACYCLINE— Aureomycin®

Description/Actions: Tetracycline antibiotic used in the treatment of dermatologic and ocular infections.

Preparations: Ointment, 3%.

CHLORTHALIDONE—Hygroton®

Diuretic and antihypertensive agent.

Description/Actions: Action is similar to that of the thiazide diuretics. Indicated in the management of hypertension, and as adjunctive therapy in edema associated with congestive heart failure, hepatic cirrhosis, and corticosteroid and estrogen therapy. Is also useful in edema due to various forms of renal dysfunction such as nephrotic syndrome.

Warnings: May cause hypokalemia and serum potassium levels should be determined periodically. Concurrent use with lithium is best avoided because of an increased risk of lithium toxicity. May cause hyperglycemia and hyperuricemia, and therapy in patients having diabetes or gout should be closely monitored.

Administration: Oral.

Preparations: Tablets, 25, 50, and 100 mg.

CHLOR-TRIMETON®, see Chlorpheniramine

CHLORZOXAZONE—Paraflex®, Parafon Forte DSC®

Description/Actions: Skeletal muscle relaxant indicated as an adjunct to rest, physical therapy, and other measures for the relief of discomfort associated with acute, painful skeletal muscle conditions.

Preparations: Tablets, 250 mg.

CHOLECALCIFEROL—Vitamin D_3

Description/Actions: A form of vitamin D used as a supplement to treat or prevent vitamin D deficiency.

Preparations: Tablets 400 and 1000 IU.

CHOLEDYL®, see Oxtriphylline

CHOLESTYRAMINE—Questran®, Questran Light®

Description/Actions: Antihyperlipidemic agent indicated as adjunctive therapy to diet for the reduction of elevated serum cholesterol in patients with primary hypercholesterolemia. Also indicated for the relief of pruritus associated with partial biliary obstruction.

Preparations: Powder and packets, 4 g/9 g of powder. (Questran). Powder and packets, 4 g/5 g of powder (Questran Light with aspartame). Chewable bar, 4 g.

CHOLINE MAGNESIUM TRISALICYLATE—Trilisate®

Description/Actions: Salicylate analgesic/anti-inflammatory agent indicated in the treatment of rheumatoid arthritis, osteoarthritis, and acute painful shoulder.

Preparations: Tablets, 500 and 750 mg., 1 g of salicylate. Liquid, 500 mg salicylate/5 ml.

CHOLINE SALICYLATE— Arthropan®

Description/Actions: Salicylate analgesic/anti-inflammatory agent used in the treatment of conditions associated with mild to moderate pain and/or inflammation.

Preparations: Liquid, 870 mg/5 ml.

CHOLINE THEOPHYLLINATE, see Oxtriphylline

CHOLOXIN®, see Dextrothyroxine

CHORIONIC GONADOTROPIN— A.P.L.®, Follutein®

Description/Actions: Hormone indicated for intramuscular use for cryptorchidism not due to anatomic obstruction, selected cases of male hypogonadism secondary to pituitary failure, and induction of ovulation and pregnancy in the anovulatory, infertile woman in selected situations.

Preparations: Vials, 5000, 10,000, and 20,000 units.

CHYMODIACTIN®, see Chymopapain

CHYMOPAPAIN—Chymodiactin®

Description/Actions: Proteolytic enzyme indicated for intradiscal injection for the treatment of documented herniated lumbar intervertebral discs in patients whose symptoms and signs have not responded to adequate periods of conservative therapy.

Preparations: Vials, 4000 units.

CICLOPROX—Penlac Nail Lacquer®

Description/Actions: Synthetic antifungal agent intended for topical use on fingernails, toenails, and immediately adjacent skin.

Precautions/Adverse Reactions: Penlac nail lacquer is contraindicated in individuals who have shown hypersensitivity to any of its components. Adverse reactions include periungual erythema of the proximal nail fold, nail shape change, nail irritation, ingrown toenail, and nail discoloration.

Administration: Apply one time each day, at bedtime or at least 8 hours before bathing or showering.

Patient Care Implications: If reactions suggesting sensitivity or chemical irritation should occur with the use of Penlac Nail Lacquer, treatment should be discontinued and appropriate therapy instituted.

Preparations: Topical solution, 8%, 6.6 ml.

CICLOPIROX OLAMINE—Loprox®

Description/Actions: Antifungal agent indicated for the topical treatment of

70 • CIDOFOVIR

tinea pedis, tinea cruris, tinea corporis, candidiasis, and tinea versicolor.

Preparations: Cream and lotion, 1%.

CIDOFOVIR—Vistide®

Description/Actions: Nucleoside analogue indicated in the treatment of cytomegalovirus (CMV) retinitis in patients with AIDS.

Warnings: Not recommended for use in patients with CrCl of < 55 ml/min. Contraindicated in severe sulfa or probenecid allergy and within 7 days of discontinuing other nephrotoxic agents (e.g., aminoglycosides, foscarnet, IV pentamidine, NSAIDs, vancomycin). Do not exceed recommended dose as this may increase the risk of nephrotoxicity. Women should use effective contraception during and 1 month after therapy. Men should use barrier contraception during and 3 months after therapy. Monitor serum creatinine, urine protein, WBC, with differential before each dose; monitor intraocular pressure, visual acuity, and ocular symptoms periodically. Use cautiously in the elderly. Adverse reactions include elevated serum creatinine, proteinuria, neutropenia, ocular hypotony, metabolic acidosis, GI disturbances, fever, asthenia, rash, headache, alopecia, infection, chills, and dyspnea. Contraindicated in severe probenecid or other sulfa allergy. Not for intraocular injection.

Administration: Give as an IV infusion over 1 hr. Pretreat with oral probenecid and hydrate with normal saline as per manufacturer's guidelines. Induction is 5 mg/kg once weekly for 2 consecutive weeks. Maintenance is 5 mg/kg once every 2 weeks. Adjust dosing for preexisting renal dysfunction or if function deteriorates during treatment as per manufacturer's recommendations.

Preparations: Solution for IV infusion after dilution, 75 mg/5 ml.

CILOSTAZOL—Pletal®

Description/Actions: Cilostazol is a quinolone derivative that is indicated in treatment of intermittent claudication. The medication preferentially enhances blood flow to the femoral arteries with a subsequent improvement in the patient's ability to walk distances.

Precautions/Adverse Reactions: In clinical trails other PDE III inhibitors have caused a decreased survival compared to placebo in patients with class III-IV heart failure, so this product is contraindicated in CHF of any severity. Use cautiously in patients with severe underlying heart disease and moderate to severe hepatic dysfunction. Pregnancy Category C. Use not recommended in nursing mothers.

Adverse reactions include headache, diarrhea, abnormal stools, palpitations, peripheral edema, dizziness, and tachycardia.

Administration: Oral. Take 1/2 hour before or 2 hours after breakfast and dinner.

Patient Care Implications: Instruct patients to avoid grapefruit juice. Take on an empty stomach. Instruct patients in the signs and symptoms of heart failure and to promptly report these symptoms to the prescriber. Patients should use this medication in combination with an exercise regimen of walking as prescribed by their health care provider.

Preparations: Tablets, 50 and 100 mg.

CILOXAN®, see Ciprofloxacin

CIMETIDINE—Tagamet®, Tagamet HB®

Antiulcer agent.

Description/Actions: A histamine H2 receptor antagonist that inhibits gastric acid secretion. Indicated in (1) short-term treatment of active duodenal ulcer, (2) maintenance therapy for duodenal ulcer patients at reduced dosage after healing of active ulcer, (3) short-term treatment of active benign gastric ulcer, (4) the treatment of erosive gastroesophageal reflux disease, (5) the treatment of pathological hypersecretory conditions (e.g., Zollinger-Ellison syndrome), and (6) the prevention of upper gastrointestiinal bleeding in critically ill patients. Available without a prescription (Tagamet HB®) to relieve heartburn and acid indigestion.

Warnings: Adverse reactions include diarrhea, rash, dizziness, somnolence, and confusional states. Has a weak antiandrogenic effect and has caused gynecomastia and impotence, particularly when used in high doses and/or for long periods.

Administration: Oral, intravenous, and intramuscular.

Preparations: Tablets, 100 (Tagamet HB®) 200, 300, 400, and 800 mg. Liquid (as the hydrochloride), 300 mg/5 ml. Vials and syringes (as the hydrochloride), 300 mg/2 ml. Plastic containers, 300 mg/50 ml.

CIPRO®, see Ciprofloxacin

CIPRO HC OTIC®—Combination agent ciprofloxacin and hydrocortisone (quinolone antibiotic and steroid)

CIPRO IV®, see Ciprofloxacin

CIPROFLOXACIN HYDROCHLORIDE—Ciloxan®, Cipro®, Cipro IV®

Anti-infective agent.

Description/Actions: A fluoroquinolone antibacterial agent with a broad spectrum of action. Indicated for lower respiratory tract, urinary tract, skin and skin structure, and bone and joint infections, urethral/cervical gonococcal infections, typhoid fever, infectious diarrhea, complicated intraabdominal infections (used with metranidazole), and ocular infections caused by susceptible bacteria. IV form is indicated in empicic therapy of febrile neutropenia and nosocomial pneumonia.

Warnings: Contraindicated in patients with a known hypersensitivity to the drug and is also best avoided in patients with a history of hypersensitivity to other fluoroquinolone/ quinolone derivatives. It should not be used in children or pregnant women because it and related drugs have been shown to cause arthropathy and damage to the weight-bearing joints in immature animals. Adverse reactions include nausea, vomiting, diarrhea, abdominal discomfort, headache, dizziness, restlessness, and rash. Because the drug may cause CNS effects, patients should be cautioned about engaging in activities that require mental alertness and coordination, and the drug should be used cautiously in patients with epilepsy or other CNS disorders. Concurrent use of ciprofloxacin and theophylline has resulted in elevated plasma concentrations of theophylline and a corresponding increase in the risk of adverse effects with this agent.

Administration: Oral, intravenous, and ophthalmic.

Preparations: Tablets, 250, 500, and 750 mg. Oral suspension, 5% (250 mg/5 ml) and 10% (500 mg/5 ml) microcapsules for suspension after reconsitution in strawberry flavor. Vials, 200 and 400 mg. Ophthalmic solution, 0.3% (Ciloxan).

CISPLATIN—Platinol®

Description/Actions: Antineoplastic agent indicated for intravenous use as palliative therapy for metastatic testicular tumors, metastatic ovarian tumors, and advanced bladder cancer.

Preparations: Vials, 10 and 50 mg.

CITALOPRAM HYDROBROMIDE—Celexa®

Description/Actions: An antidepressant in the SSRI category. Indicated in the treatment of depression, obsessive-compulsive disorder, panic disorder, chronic schizophrenia (adjuvant treatment) and dementia.

Precautions/Adverse Reactions: Use is

72 • CITANEST®

contraindicated within 14 days of use of MAOIs. Use cautiously in patients with a history of seizures or mania/hypomania, hepatic or severe renal impairment, recent MI, or unstable heart disease. Reevaluate use frequently for patients with suicidal tendencies or undergoing ECT. Category C pregnancy. Use in children and nursing mothers not recommended.

Adverse reactions include GI upset, dry mouth, somnolence, insomnia, increased sweating, anorexia, rhinitis, sexual dysfunction, agitation, fatigue, arthralgia, myalgia, hyponatremia, and SIADH.

Administration: Oral.

Patient Care Implications: Monitor mood changes and notify therapist if patient demonstrates signififcant increase in anxiety, nervousness, or insomnia. Assess for suicidal tendencies, especially during early therapy. Restrict the amount of drug available to patient.

Preparations: Scored tablets, 10, 20, and 40 mg. Oral solution, 10 mg/5 mL.

CITANEST®, see Prilocaine

CITRATE OF MAGNESIA, see Magnesium citrate

CITROVORUM FACTOR, see Leucovorin calcium.

CITRUCEL®, see Methylcellulose

CLADRIBINE—Leustatin®

Antineoplastic agent.

Description/Actions: Also known as 2-chlorodeoxyadenosine or 2-CdA, it crosses lymphocyte cell membranes and is metabolized to a triphosphate derivative that disrupts cell metabolism and is cytotoxic to both actively dividing and resting cells. Indicated for the treatment of active hairy cell leukemia.

Warnings: May cause myelosuppression (neutropenia, thrombocytopenia, anemia) and peripheral blood counts should be performed, particularly during the first 4 to 8 weeks following initiation of therapy. Caution should be exercised if cladribine is to be administered in conjunction with or following other drugs known to cause myelosuppression. Fever is often experienced (most often in neutropenic patients) and infection may develop; empiric antibiotic therapy should be initiated as necessary. Other adverse reactions include nausea, decreased appetite, vomiting, diarrhea, abnormal breath sounds, cough, fatigue, headache, injection site reactions, purpura, and rash. Women of childbearing age should be advised to avoid becoming pregnant.

Administration: Intravenous. Administered as a single course of treatment by continuous intravenous infusion for 7 consecutive days.

Preparations: Vials, 10 mg (1 mg/ml).

CLAFORAN®, see Cefotaxime sodium.

CLARITHROMYCIN—Biaxin®

Macrolide antibiotic.

Description/Actions: Is converted, in part, to an active metabolite, 14-hydroxyclarithromycin. Inhibits protein synthesis and its spectrum of action includes many gram-positive and gram-negative bacteria, as well as organisms such as *Mycoplasma pneumoniae*. Indicated for upper respiratory tract infections, lower respiratory tract infections, and uncomplicated skin and skin structure infections caused by susceptible organisms. Is also used in combination with other agents for the treatment of disseminated infection due to *Mycobacterium avium* complex and in treatment of active duodenal ulcer associated with *H. pylori* infection in combination with omeprazole.

Warnings: Contraindicated in patients with a known hypersensitivity to any of the macrolide antibiotics. Prescribers should review drugs profile to avoid interaction with contraindicated drugs. Adverse reactions include diarrhea, nausea, abnormal taste, dyspepsia, abdominal pain or discomfort, and headache. Should not be used in pregnant women unless no alternative therapy is appropriate. Concurrent use with terfenadine should be avoided. May increase serum concentrations of theophylline, carbamazepine, and other drugs that are metabolized via liver enzyme systems; concurrent therapy should be closely monitored.

Administration: Oral.

Preparations: Tablets, 250 and 500 mg. Granules for oral suspension, 125 mg/5 ml and 250 mg/5 ml when reconstituted.

CLARITHROMYCIN EXTENDED-RELEASE—Biaxin XL®

Description/Actions: A macrolide antibiotic in extended-release form.

Precautions/Adverse Reactions: Contraindicated in patients with a known hypersensitivity to any of the macrolide antibiotics. Adverse reactions include diarrhea, nausea, abnormal taste, dyspepsia, abdominal pain or discomfort, and headache. Should not be used in pregnant women unless no alternative therapy is appropriate. Concurrent use with terfenadine should be avoided. May increase serum concentrations of theophylline, carbamazepine, and other drugs that are metabolized via liver enzyme systems; concurrent therapy should be closely monitored. Concurrent use with terfenadine, pimozide, cisapride, and astemizole should be avoided.

Administration: Oral.

Preparations: Extended-release tablet, 500 mg.

CLARITIN®, see Loratadine

CLARITIN-D®, Combination of loratidine and pseudoephedrine

CLEMASTINE FUMARATE—Tavist®

Antihistamine.

Description/Actions: Indicated for the relief of symptoms associated with allergic rhinitis, and for the relief of mild, uncomplicated allergic skin manifestations of urticaria and angioedema.

Warnings: Contraindicated in nursing mothers and in patients being treated with a monoamine oxidase inhibitor. Should not be used to treat lower respiratory tract symptoms including asthma. Adverse reactions include drowsiness and other CNS effects; patients should be cautioned regarding activities such as driving and operating machinery, as well as interactions with other CNS-acting drugs including alcohol. Exhibits anticholinergic activity and must be used with caution in patients with conditions such as narrow-angle glaucoma.

Administration: Oral.

Preparations: Tablets, 1.34 and 2.68 mg. Syrup, 0.67 mg/5 ml.

CLEOCIN®, see Clindamycin

CLIDINIUM BROMIDE—Quarzan®

Description/Actions: Anticholinergic agent indicated as adjunctive therapy in peptic ulcer disease.

Preparations: Capsules, 2.5 and 5 mg.

CLIMARA®, see Estradiol

CLINDAMYCIN—Cleocin®, Cleocin T®

Description/Actions: Antibiotic indicated for the treatment of infections caused by susceptible anaerobic bacteria including *Bacteroides fragilis,* and for the treatment of infections caused by susceptible gram-positive cocci. Topical solution, gel, and lotion formulations are indicated in the treatment of acne. Vaginal cream is indicated in the treatment of bacterial vaginosis.

Preparations: Capsules (as the hydrochloride), 75, 150, and 300 mg. For oral solution (as the palmitate), 75 mg clindamycin/5 ml. Ampules and vials

CLINORIL®

(as the phosphate), 150 mg clindamycin/ml. Topical solution, gel, and lotion (as the phosphate), 1%. Vaginal cream, 2%.

CLINORIL®, see Sulindac

CLIOQUINOL—
Iodochlorhydroxyquin, Vioform®

Description/Actions: Anti-infective agent used in the topical management of inflamed conditions of the skin (e.g., eczema, athlete's foot).

Preparations: Cream and ointment, 3%.

CLOBETASOL PROPIONATE—
Olux™, Temovate®

Topical corticosteroid.

Description/Actions: Indicated for the short-term treatment of inflammatory and pruritic manifestations of moderate to severe corticosteroid-responsive dermatoses.

Warnings: Is highly potent and is more likely than are less potent analogs to cause systemic effects including suppression of the hypothalamic-pituitary-adrenal (HPA) axis. Treatment period should be limited to 2 weeks, and not more than 50 g of the cream or ointment should be used per week. Occlusive dressings should not be used.

Administration: Topical.

Preparations: Cream and ointment, 0.05% Topical (scalp) foam.

CLOFAZIMINE—Lamprene®

Antileprosy agent.

Description/Actions: Exerts a slow bactericidal effect on *Mycobacterium leprae.* Indicated in the treatment of lepromatous leprosy, including dapsone-resistant lepromatous leprosy and lepromatous leprosy complicated by erythema nodosum leprosum.

Warnings: The drug is a dye and will cause pink to brownish-black pigmentation of the skin within a few weeks of treatment. It will also cause discoloration of the cconjunctivae, lacrimal fluid, sweat, sputum, urine, and feces. Other dermatologic reactions include ichthyosis, dryness, rash, and pruritus; the application of oil to the skin may help alleviate some of these effects. Many patients experience adverse gastrointestinal effects, such as abdominal and epigastric pain, diarrhea, nausea, vomiting, and gastrointestinal intolerance; taking the medication with meals may reduce the occurrence of these effects. There have been rare reports of bowel obstruction, gastrointestinal bleeding, and splenic infarction.

Administration: Oral.

Preparations: Capsules, 50 and 100 mg.

CLOFIBRATE—Atromid-S®

Description/Actions: Antihyperlipidemic agent indicated for primary dysbetalipoproteinemia (Type III hyperlipidemia) that does not respond adequately to diet. May be considered for the treatment of selected patients with very high serum triglyceride levels (Types IV and V).

Preparations: Capsules, 500 mg.

CLOMID®, see Clomiphene

CLOMIPHENE CITRATE—
Clomid®, Milophene®, Serophene®

Description/Actions: Ovulation stimulant indicated for the treatment of ovulatory dysfunction in patients desiring pregnancy, and whose partners are fertile and potent. Unlabeled uses include male infertility, menstrual abnormalities, gynecomastia, fibrocystic breast disease, regulation of cycles in patients using rhythm methods of contraception, endometrial hyperplasia, and persistent lactation.

Preparations: Tablets, 50 mg.

CLOMIPRAMINE HYDROCHLORIDE—Anafranil®

Antiobsessional agent.

Description/Actions: A tricyclic antidepressant that acts primarily by inhibiting the reuptake of serotonin. Indicated for the treatment of obsessions and compulsions in patients with obsessive-compulsive disorder.

Warnings: Should not be given in combination, or within 14 days of treatment with a monoamine oxidase inhibitor. Is also contraindicated during the acute recovery period after a myocardial infarction. Adverse reactions include CNS effects and patients should be cautioned regarding activities such as driving and operating machinery, as well as interactions with other CNS-acting drugs including alcohol. Other adverse reactions include dry mouth, blurred vision, nausea, dyspepsia, increased appetite, weight gain, sweating, orthostatic hypotension, and sexual dysfunction.

Administration: Oral. During the initial titration, clomipramine should be given in divided doses with meals to reduce gastrointestinal side effects. After titration, the total daily dose may be given once daily at bedtime to minimize daytime sedation.

Preparations: Capsules, 25, 50, and 75 mg.

CLONAZEPAM—Klonopin®

Description/Actions: Benzodiazepine anticonvulsant indicated in the treatment of the Lennox-Gastaut syndrome (petit mal variant), akinetic and myoclonic seizures and panic disorder. May also be useful in absence seizures (petit mal).

Preparations: Tablets, 0.5, 1, and 2 mg.

CLONIDINE HYDROCHLORIDE— Catapres®, Catapres-TTS®

Antihypertensive agent.

Description/Actions: Is a centrally acting alpha-adrenergic receptor agonist indicated in the treatment of hypertension.

Warnings: Adverse reactions include drowsiness and other CNS effects; patients should be cautioned regarding activities such as driving and operating machinery, as well as interactions with other CNS-acting drugs including alcohol. Other adverse reactions include dry mouth, headache, dizziness, and dermatological effects (primarily with the use of the transdermal formulation). Effect may be reduced by the concurrent administration of a tricyclic antidepressant. The abrupt discontinuation of therapy may be followed by a rapid rise in blood pressure; patients should be advised of the importance of complying with the instructions for using the medication and, if therapy is to be discontinued, it should be done so gradually.

Administration: Oral and transdermal.

Preparations: Tablets, 0.1, 0.2, and 0.3 mg. Transdermal system, programmed delivery of 0.1, 0.2, and 0.3 mg clonidine base per day, for 1 week.

CLONOPIN®, former name for Klonopin®—see Clonazepam

CLOPIDOGREL—Plavix®

Description/Actions: An inhibitor of platelet aggregation indicated in the reduction of atherosclerotic events (MI, stroke, and vascular death) in patients with altherosclerosis documented by recent stroke or MI or established peripheral arterial disease. Clopidogrel is also indicated for the treatment of acute coronary syndrome (unstable angina and non-Q-wave MI) including patients who are to be managed medically and those who are to be managed with percutaneous coronary intervention (with or without stent) or CABG.

Warnings: Contraindicated in active pathologic bleeding (e.g., peptic ulcer, intracranial hemorrhage). Use cautiously in the presence of the risk of bleeding (e.g., surgery, ulcers, trauma, concomitant NSAIDS), and severe hepatic disease. Consider discontinu-

76 • CLORAZEPATE DIPOTASSIUM

ing 7 days prior to surgery. Not recommended for use in children. Pregnancy Category C.

Adverse reactions include diarrhea, rash, pruritus, purpura, other GI disturbances, GI ulcers, hemorrhage, neutropenia/agranulocytosis (rare). Instruct patients to report unusual or prolonged bleeding or fever.

Administration: Oral.

Preparations: Tablets, 75 mg.

CLORAZEPATE DIPOTASSIUM—Tranxene®

Benzodiazepine antianxiety agent and anticonvulsant.

Description/Actions: A CNS depressant indicated (1) for the management of anxiety disorders or for the short-term relief of the symptoms of anxiety, (2) for the symptomatic relief of acute alcohol withdrawal, and (3) as adjunctive therapy in the management of partial seizures.

Warnings: Contraindicated in patients with acute narrow-angle glaucoma. Adverse reactions include drowsiness and other CNS effects; patients should be cautioned regarding activities such as driving and operating machinery, as well as interactions with other CNS-acting drugs including alcohol. Can cause dependence and is included in Schedule IV.

Administration: Oral.

Preparations: Tablets, 3.75, 7.5, 11.25, 15, and 22.5 mg. Capsules, 3.75, 7.5, and 15 mg.

CLORPACTIN®, see Oxychlorosene

CLOTRIMAZOLE—Gyne-Lotrimin®, Lotrimin®, Lotrimin AF®, Mycelex®, Mycelex-G®, Trivagizole 3™

Imidazole antifungal agent.

Description/Actions: Indicated for (1) dermal infections—tinea pedis, tinea cruris, tinea corporis, candidiasis, tinea versicolor, (2) vulvovaginal candidiasis, and (3) oropharyngeal candidiasis.

Warnings: Adverse reactions include pruritus, stinging, erythema, vulval irritation.

Administration: Topical and vaginal.

Preparations: Cream, lotion, and solution, 1%. Vaginal cream, 1% and 2%. Vaginal tablets, 100 and 500 mg. Troches, 10 mg.

CLOVE OIL

Description/Actions: Local anesthetic included in some formulations used for the relief of toothache.

Preparations: Drops.

CLOXACILLIN SODIUM—Tegopen®

Description/Actions: Penicillin antibiotic indicated for the treatment of staphylococcal infections.

Preparations: Capsules, 250 and 500 mg. Powder for oral solution, 125 mg/5 ml when reconstituted.

CLOZAPINE—Clozaril®

Antipsychotic agent.

Description/Actions: An atypical antipsychotic drug with effects on dopamine mediated behaviors that differ from those exhibited by the standard antipsychotic agents. Is much less likely than the standard antipsychotic drugs to cause extrapyramidal effects. Indicated for the management of severely ill schizophrenic patients who fail to respond adequately to standard antipsychotic drug treatment, either because of insufficient effectiveness or the inability to achieve an effective dose due to intolerable adverse effects from those drugs. Also indicated in the treatment of patients with schizophrenia or schizoaffective disorder to reduce the risk of recurrent suicidal behavior.

Warnings: Contraindicated in patients with myeloproliferative disorders, or a history of clozapine-induced agranulocytosis or severe granulocytopenia. Should not be used simultaneously with other agents having a well-known potential to suppress bone-marrow function. May cause agranulocytosis and, prior to initiating treatment, a white blood cell (WBC) count should be performed and subsequent WBC counts should be done at least weekly for the duration of therapy, as well as for 4 weeks past discontinuation. If the total WBC count falls below 2000/mm3 or granulocyte count below 1000/mm3 during clozapine therapy, the drug should be discontinued and not resumed because of an even higher risk of agranulocytosis upon rechallenge. Patients should be advised to immediately report the appearance of lethargy, fever, sore throat, flulike symptoms, or any other signs of infection. Use has also been associated with occurrence of seizures as well as other CNS effects (e.g., drowsiness/sedation, dizziness/vertigo). Patients should be cautioned regarding activities such as driving and operating machinery, as well as interactions with other CNS-acting drugs including alcohol. Other adverse reactions include tachycardia, hypotension, constipation, nausea, hypersalivation, sweating, dry mouth, visual disturbances, and fever.

Administration: Oral.

Preparations: Tablets, 25 and 100 mg.

CLOZARIL®, see Clozapine

COAL TAR

Description/Actions: Antipruritic and irritant used in the topical treatment of dermatologic disorders including scalp conditions.

Preparations: Solution, gel, cream, ointment, lotion, soap, and shampoo.

COCAINE

Description/Actions: Local anesthetic applied topically to provide anesthesia for mucous membranes.

Preparations: Powder. Topical solution, 40 mg/ml and 100 mg/ml. Soluble tablets, 135 mg.

CODEINE PHOSPHATE AND SULFATE

Opioid analgesic and antitussive.

Description/Actions: Is a centrally acting analgesic indicated for the relief of pain and the management of cough.

Warnings: Adverse reactions include sedation and other CNS effects; patients should be cautioned regarding activities such as driving and operating machinery, as well as interactions with other CNS-acting drugs including alcohol. Other adverse reactions include constipation, nausea, vomiting, rash, and, in higher doses, respiratory depression. Can cause dependence and formulations are covered under the provisions of the Controlled Substances Act.

Administration: Oral and parenteral.

Preparations: Tablets, 15, 30, and 60 mg. Vials, 30 and 60 mg/ml. Is often used in combination with other agents (e.g., acetaminophen, aspirin) in capsule, tablet, and liquid formulations.

COD LIVER OIL

Description/Actions: Vitamins A and D used to prevent and treat deficiences of these vitamins.

Preparations: Oil, emulsion, capsules.

COGENTIN®, see Benztropine

COGNEX®, see Tacrine hydrochloride

COLACE®, see Docusate sodium

COLAZAL®, see Balsalazide

COLCHICINE

Description/Actions: Agent for gout. Indicated for the relief of pain associated with acute attacks of gout. Has also been used in chronic gouty conditions for the prevention of acute attacks of gout.

Preparations: Tablets, 0.5 and 0.6 mg. Ampules, 1 mg.

COLESEVELAM—Welchol™

Description/Actions: Colesevelam is a nonabsorbable polymer that acts as a bile acid sequestering agent. It is indicated as adjunctive therapy to diet and exercise and used alone or in combination with an HMG-CoA reductase inhibitor for the management of elevated LDL in primary hypercholesterolemia (Fredrickson Type IIa).

Precautions/Adverse Reactions: Usage is contraindicated in patients with hypersensitivity to colesevelam or any component of the formulation and in individuals with bowel obstructions. Because it has not been studied in persons having a triglyceride level greater than 300 mg/dl, caution should be used in treating such patients. Safety and efficacy has not been established in patients with dysphagia, swallowing disorders, severe gastrointestinal motility disorders, or major gastrointestinal tract surgery, and patients susceptible to fat-soluble vitamin deficiencies. Therefore, use in such patients should be with caution. Safety and efficacy have not been established in children. Prior to initiation, secondary causes of hypercholesterolemia should be excluded. Pregnancy Category B. Use only in pregnancy if clearly needed.

Some adverse effects are constipation, dyspepsia, weakness, myalgia, and pharyngitis.

Administration: Oral.

Patient Care Implications: Inform patients to take with a liquid and a meal and to follow dietary guidelines.

Preparations: Tablet: 625 mg.

COLESTID®, see Colestipol

COLESTIPOL HYDROCHLORIDE—Colestid®

Description/Actions: Antihyperlipidemic agent indicated as adjunctive therapy to diet for the reduction of elevated serum cholesterol in patients with primary hypercholesterolemia.

Preparations: Tablets, 1 g. Granules, packets, 5 g.

COLFOSCERIL PALMITATE, CETYL ALCOHOL, AND TYLOXAPOL—Exosurf Neonatal®

Agent for respiratory distress syndrome.

Description/Actions: A synthetic pulmonary surfactant which contains colfosceril palmitate [also known as dipalmitoylphosphatidylcholine (DPPC)], cetyl alcohol, and tyloxapol. Replenishes surfactant and restores surface activity to the lungs. Indicated for the prophylactic treatment of infants with birth weights of less than 1350 g who are at risk of developing (RDS) the prophylactic treatment of infants with birth weights greater than 1350 g who have evidence of pulmonary immaturity; and the rescue treatment of infants who have developed RDS.

Warnings: Adverse reactions include pulmonary bleeding, apnea, and mucous plugging. Suctioning of infant before dosing may lessen the possibility of mucous plugs obstructing the endotracheal tube. May rapidly affect oxygenation and lung compliance.

Administration: Intratracheal. Before administration, the infant should be suctioned. Is administered in the form of a suspension by instillation into the trachea via the side port on a special endotracheal tube adapter without interrupting mechanical ventilation. Each dose is administered in two half doses. The infant is turned from the midline position to the right after the first half-dose, and from the midline position to the left after the second half-dose.

If the suspension appears to separate, the vial should be gently shaken or swirled to resuspend the preparation.

Preparations: Vials, 108 mg colfosceril palmitate, 12 mg cetyl alcohol, 8 mg tyloxapol, and 47 mg sodium chloride.

COLISTIMETHATE SODIUM—Coly-Mycin M®, see Colistin sulfate

COLISTIN SULFATE—Coly-Mycin S®, Polymixin E®

Description/Actions: Antibiotic indicated for the treatment of infections caused by gram-negative bacteria including *Pseudomonas aeruginosa.* Colistimethate is used in the formulation administered parenterally, and colistin is used in the formulations administered orally (for gastro-intestinal infections) and as otic drops.

Preparations: Vials, 150 mg. Oral suspension, 25 mg/5 ml when reconstituted. Otic drops (in combination with other agents), 3 mg/ml.

COLLAGENASE—Santyl®

Description/Actions: Enzyme indicated for debriding chronic dermal ulcers and severely burned areas.

Preparations: Ointment, 250 units/g.

COLLYRIUM®, see Sodium borate

COLY-MYCIN®, see Colistimethate

COLYTE®, see Polyethylene glycol 3350

COMBIVIR®—Combination agent lamivudine and zidovudine

COMBIVENT®—Combination agent ipratopium bromide and albuterol

COMPAZINE®, see Prochlorperazine

COMTAN®, see Entacapone

CONCERTA™, see Methylphenidate hydrochloride

CONDYLOX®, see Podofilox

CONJUGATED ESTROGENS, see Estrogens, conjugated

CORDARONE®, see Amiodarone

CORDRAN®, see Flurandrenolide

COREG®, see Carvedilol

CORGARD®, see Nadolol

CORTEF®, see Hydrocortisone

CORTICOTROPIN— Adrenocorticotropic hormone, ACTH, Acthar®

Description/Actions: Hormone indicated for parenteral use in the diagnostic testing of adrenocortical function. Is of limited value in conditions responsive to corticosteroid therapy.

Preparations: Vials, 25 and 40 units. Vials (gel for repository effect), 40 and 80 units/ml.

CORTISOL, see Hydrocortisone

CORTISONE ACETATE—Cortone acetate®

Description/Actions: Corticosteroid indicated for oral or intramuscular use in a wide range of endocrine, rheumatic, allergic, dermatologic, respiratory, hematologic, neoplastic, and other disorders.

Preparations: Tablets, 5, 10, and 25 mg. Vials, 25 and 50 mg/ml.

CORTISPORIN OTIC®,
Combination of hydrocortisone, neomycin, and polymyxin B

CORTONE®, see Cortisone acetate

CORTROSYN®, see Cosyntropin

CORVERT®, see Ibutilide fumarate

COSMEGEN®, see Dactinomycin

COSOPT®—Combination agent dorzolamide Hcl 2% and timolol maleate 0.5%

COSYNTROPIN—Cortrosyn®

Description/Actions: Synthetic ACTH analogue indicated for parenteral use in the diagnostic testing of adrenocortical function.

Preparations: Vials, 0.25 mg.

COTRIMOXAZOLE, see Trimethoprim-sulfamethoxazole

COUMADIN®, see Warfarin

COVERA-HS®, see Verapamil

COZAAR® see Losartan potassium

CRIXIVAN®, see Indinavir

CROFAB®, see Crotalidae Polyvalent, Immune Fab (Ovine)

CROMOLYN SODIUM—Crolom®, Gastrocrom®, Intal®, Nasalcrom®

Description/Actions: Antiasthmatic agent used by oral inhalation in the prophylactic management of bronchial asthma, and shortly before exposure to factors (e.g., exercise) that precipitate bronchoconstriction. Instruct patients that this agent is not for treatment of acute bronchial asthmatic attacks. Ophthalmic solution is indicated for the treatment of vernal keratoconjunctivitis, vernal conjunctivitis, and vernal keratitis. Nasal solution is indicated for the prevention and treatment of symptoms of allergic rhinitis. Capsules for oral administration are used in the treatment of mastocytosis.

Preparations: Capsules, 100 mg. Oral solution, 100 mg/5 ml. Nebulizer solution (20 mg/2 ml). Metered dose inhalation unit. Nasal solution, 40 mg/ml. Ophthalmic solution, 4%.

CROTALIDAE POLYVALENT IMMUNE FAB (OVINE)— Crofab®

Description/Actions: Indicated for the management of patients with minimal or moderate North American envenomation. Use within 6 hours of a snakebite to prevent coagulation abnormalities.

Precautions/Adverse Reactions: Crotalidae should not be administered to patients with a known history of hypersensitivity to papaya or papain unless the benefits outweigh the risks and appropriate management for anaphylactic reactions is available. Should be used within 6 hours of a snakebite in order to prevent coagulation abnormalities. Recurrent coagulopathy may persist for 1 to 2 weeks or more. Retreatment may be necessary; monitor patient. Patients with allergies to papain, chymopapain, other papaya extracts, or the pineapple enzyme bromelain may also experience a hypersensitivity reaction to crotalidae. Cross sensitivity with dust mites and latex allergens is a possibility due to similar antigenic structures with papain. Contains thimeresal. Anaphylactic reactions are possible due to foreign proteins in the antivenom. Patients should be monitored for the development of delayed hypersensitivity reactions or serum sickness. Caution should be exercised when administering a repeat course of treatment for a second envenomation episode as patients may become sensitized to the foreign protein. Drug interaction studies have not been conducted. Pregnancy Category C. Reproductive studies have not been conducted. Crotalidae contains thimeresal, which has been associated with neurologic and renal toxicities. Developing fetuses and very young children are most at risk. Excretion in human breast milk is unknown. No specific studies have been conducted in children. The absolute venom dose following a snakebite is expected to be the same in children and adults; therefore, no dosage adjustment for age should be made. Adverse reactions observed during therapy with crotalidae include urticaria, rash, pruritis, nausea, coagulation disorders, back pain, chest pain, cellulitis, wound infection, chills, allergic reactions, hypotension, asthma, cough, increased sputum, anorexia, myalgia, ecchymosis, nervousness, and paresthesias.

Administration: Intravenous.

Patient Care Implications: Infusion should proceed slowly during the first 10 minutes. Patient should be monitored for signs and symptoms of an allergic reaction.

Preparations: Injection, 2 vials per box.

CROTAMITON—Eurax®

Description/Actions: Scabicide indicated for the treatment of scabies and for the symptomatic treatment of pruritic skin.

Preparations: Cream and lotion, 10%.

CRYSTICILLIN®, see Procaine Penicillin G

CUPRIMINE®, see Penicillamine

CURARE, see Tubocurarine

CUROSURF®, see Poractant Alfa

CUTIVATE®, see Fluticasone propionate

CYANOCOBALAMIN—Vitamin B_{12}, Nascobal®

Description/Actions: Vitamin indicated in the treatment of pernicious anemia, dietary deficiency of vitamin B_{12}, malabsorption of vitamin B_{12}, and other situations in which there is inadequate utilization of vitamin B_{12}. Also used for the Schilling test. Nascobal® is indicated to maintain therapeutic levels of cyanocobalamin in patients in remission following intramuscular vitamin B_{12} administration and for the maintenance of therapeutic levels of vitamin B_{12} in patients with HIV, AIDS, multiple sclerosis, or Crohn's disease.

Preparations: Tablets, 25, 50, 100, 250, 500, and 1000 ug. Vials, 100 and 1000 urg/ml. Intranasal gel, 500 µg/0.1 ml.

CYCLANDELATE—Cyclospasmol®

Description/Actions: Vasodilator indicated for adjunctive therapy in intermittent claudication, Raynaud's phenomenon, nocturnal leg cramps, and other peripheral vascular disorders. Has also been used in selected cases in ischemic cerebral vascular disease.

Preparations: Tablets, 400 mg. Capsules, 200 and 400 mg.

CYCLESSA™, see Desogestrel/ Ethinyl estradiol

CYCLIZINE—Marezine®

Description/Actions: Antiemetic indicated in the management of nausea and vomiting of motion sickness.

Preparations: Tablets (as the hydrochloride), 50 mg. Ampules (as the lactate), 50 mg.

CYCLOBENZAPRINE HYDROCHLORIDE—Flexeril®

Skeletal muscle relaxant.

Description/Actions: Indicated as an adjunct to rest and physical therapy for relief of muscle spasm associated with acute, painful musculoskeletal conditions.

Warnings: Contraindicated during the acute recovery phase of myocardial infarction, in patients with arrhythmias, heart block or conduction disturbances, congestive heart failure, or hyperthyroidism, and in patients being treated with a monoamine oxidase inhibitor. Adverse reactions include drowsiness and other CNS effects; patients should be cautioned regarding activities such as driving and operating machinery, as well as interactions with other CNS-acting drugs including alcohol. Has an anticholinergic effect and adverse reactions such as dry mouth are common; caution should be exercised in patients with conditions such as angle-closure glaucoma, and in those taking other anticholinergic medications.

Administration: Oral. Use for longer than 2 to 3 weeks is not recommended.

Preparations: Tablets, 5 and 10 mg.

CYCLOCORT®, see Amcinonide

CYCLOGYL®, see Cyclopentolate

CYCLOMEN®, see Danazol

CYCLOPENTOLATE HYDROCHLORIDE—Cyclogyl®

Description/Actions: Anticholinergic agent used to produce mydriasis and cycloplegia in diagnostic procedures.

Preparations: Ophthalmic solution, 0.5% and 1%.

CYCLOPHOSPHAMIDE— Cytoxan®, Neosar®

Description/Actions: Antineoplastic agent indicated in the oral and parenteral treatment of malignant lymphomas, leukemias, multiple myeloma, carcinoma of the breast, neuroblastoma, adenocarcinoma of the ovary, retinoblastoma, and mycosis fungoides.

Preparations: Tablets, 25 and 50 mg. Vials, 100, 200, and 500 mg, 1 and 2 g.

CYCLOSERINE—Seromycin®

Description/Actions: Antibiotic indicated in the treatment of tuberculosis when therapy with the primary medications has not been successful. Has also been used for urinary tract infections in which conventional therapy has failed.

Preparations: Capsules, 250 mg.

CYCLOSPASMOL®, see Cyclandelate

CYCLOSPORINE—Sandimmune®, Neoral®

Description/Actions: Immunosuppressant used orally and intravenously, in conjunction with a corticosteroid, for the prophylaxis of organ rejection in kidney, liver, and heart transplants and severe, active rheumatoid arthritis unresponsive to methotrexate alone.

Preparations: Capsules, 25 and 100 mg. Oral solution, 100 mg/ml. Ampules, 50 mg.

CYCRIN®, see Medroxyprogesterone

CYKLOKAPRON®, see Tranexamic acid

CYLERT®, see Pemoline

CYPROHEPTADINE HYDROCHLORIDE—Periactin®

Description/Actions: Antihistamine indicated for allergic disorders. Also possesses antiserotonin and appetite-stimulating properties.

Preparations: Tablets, 4 mg. Syrup, 2 mg/5 ml.

CYSTAGON®, see Cysteamine bitartrate

CYSTEAMINE BITARTRATE—
Cystagon®

Description/Actions: Cystine-depleting agent indicated in the management of nephropathic cystinosis in children and adults. Contraindicated in patients with known hypersensitivity to this agent or penicillamine. Adverse reactions include vomiting, anorexia, fever, diarrhea, lethargy, and rash. If rash develops, the drug should be withheld until the rash clears. If a severe skin rash (e.g., erythema multiforme) develops, should not be readministered. Has occasionally been associated with reversible leukopenia and abnormal liver function studies; therefore, blood counts and liver function studies should be monitored.

Administration: Oral. Usual maintenance dosage for children through the age of 12 years is 1.3 g/m2/day, given in 4 divided doses. Recommended maintenance dose for patients more than 12 years old and more than 110 pounds is 2 g/day, given in 4 divided doses.

Preparations: Capsules, 50 and 150 mg.

CYTARABINE—Cytosine arabinoside, ARA-C, Cytosar-U®

Description/Actions: Antineoplastic agent indicated for the parenteral treatment of leukemias (primarily acute myelocytic leukemia) and as part of a combination regimen in children with non-Hodgkin's lymphoma.

Preparations: Vials, 100 and 500 mg.

CYTOMEL®, see Liothyronine

CYTOSAR-U®, see Cytarabine

CYTOSINE ARABINOSIDE, see Cytarabine

CYSTOSPAZ®, see Hyoscyamine

CYTOTEC®, see Misoprostol

CYTOVENE®, see Ganciclovir

CYTOXAN®, see Cyclophosphamide

D

DACARBAZINE—DTIC®

Description/Actions: Antineoplastic agent indicated for the parenteral treatment of metastatic malignant melanoma, refractory Hodgkin's disease, various sarcomas, and neuroblastoma.

Preparations: Vials, 100 and 200 mg.

DACTINOMYCIN—Cosmegen®

Description/Actions: Antineoplastic agent indicated for the parenteral treatment of Wilms' tumor, testicular carcinoma, choriocarcinoma, rhabdomyosarcoma, and other neoplasms.

Preparations: Vials, 0.5 mg.

DALFOPRISTIN/QUINUPRISTIN— Synercid®

Description/Actions: Synercid has been approved for vancomycin-resistant *Entercoccus faecium* bacteremia and *Staphylococcus aureus* skin infections.

Precautions/Adverse Reactions: Patients who are known to have a hypersensitivity reaction to dalfopristin, quinupristin, or any other streptogramin should not take Synercid. Synercid has also not been proven to be safe in children under 16, in pregnant women, and or in women who breast-feed. Also Synercid should be used carefully in patients with hepatic disease. Synercid in general has few side effects in patients. The most common reason for discontinuing this drug is nausea, vomiting, pruritus, and a rash. Other possible side effects are arthralgia, myalgia, hepatotoxicity, hyperbilirubinemia, and pseudomembranous colitis.

Administration: Intravenous.

Patient Care Implications: Patients with hepatic impairment may need a reduction in dosage. Monitor liver function enzymes while patient on medicine.

84 • DALGAN®

Not proven to be safe in pregnant women, women who breast-feed, and in children under 16.

Preparations: Vials, 500 mg.

DALGAN®, see Dezocine

DALMANE®, see Flurazepam

DALTEPARIN—Fragmin®

Antithrombotic agent.

Description/Actions: Prevention of deep vein thrombosis and pulmonary embolism following hip replacement and abdominal surgery in high-risk patients (age > 40, obesity, general anesthesia > 30 minutes, history of malignancy or previous thromboembolic phenomena).

Warnings: Contraindicated in active major bleeding and thrombocytopenia associated with positive in vitro tests for antiplatelet antibody in the presence of dalteporin, heparin, or pork allergy. Adverse effects include local hematoma, anaphylaxis, and thrombocytopenia.

Administration: SQ injection.

Preparations: 2500 and 5000 IU/0.2 ml single-dose, prefilled syringe.

DANAPAROID SODIUM—Orgaran®

Description/Actions:

Antithrombic indicated in prevention of post-op DVT.

Warnings: Contraindicated in severe hemorrhagic diathesis, active major bleeding, Type II thrombocytopenia associated with a positive in vitro test for anitiplatelet antibody associated with danaparoid sodium, heparin, or pork allergy.

May cause bleeding or hematomas within the spinal column if used concurrently with spinal or epidural anesthesia analgesia.

Use cautiously in asthma, heparin-induced thrombocytopenia, bleeding disorders, severe renal dysfunction (monitor carefully if serum Cr≥2 mg/dl), severe uncontrolled hypertension, acute bacterial endocarditis, acute ulceration and angiodysplastic GI disease, bleeding diathesis, nonhemorrhagic stroke, invasive procedures, recent brain, spinal, or eye surgery.

Not interchangeable (unit for unit) with heparin or other low molecular weight heparin products. Pregnancy Category C.

Adverse reactions include hemorrhage, thrombocytopenia, local reactions (e.g., hematoma, pain), fever, GI upset, constipation, rash, pruritus, edema, dizziness, insomnia, and anemia.

Administration: SQ injection.

Preparations: 750 units/0.6 ml solution for SC injection, contains sulfites.

DANAZOL—Cyclomen®, Danocrine®

Description/Actions: Androgen indicated for the treatment of endometriosis unresponsive to more conventional treatment, fibrocystic breast disease, and hereditary angioedema.

Preparations: Capsules, 50, 100, and 200 mg.

DANOCRINE®, see Danazol

DANTRIUM®, see Dantrolene

DANTROLENE SODIUM—Dantrium®

Description/Actions: Muscle relaxant and antispastic agent used in controlling the manifestations of spasticity resulting from upper motor neuron disorders (e.g., stroke, cerebral palsy, multiple sclerosis). Also used intravenously in the management of malignant hyperthermia crisis, and orally to prevent or reduce the development of signs of malignant hyperthermia in susceptible patients.

Preparations: Capsules, 25, 50, and 100 mg. Vials, 20 mg.

DAPIPRAZOLE HYDROCHLORIDE—Rev-Eyes™

Antimydriatic agent.

Description/Actions: An alpha-adrenergic blocking agent that reverses the mydriasis caused by agents used in ocular examinations. Indicated in the treatment of iatrogenically induced mydriasis produced by adrenergic (phenylephrine) and parasympatholytic (tropicamide) agents.

Warnings: Contraindicated in patients in whom constriction is undesirable (e.g., acute iritis). Adverse reactions include conjunctival injection, burning on instillation, ptosis, lid erythema, lid edema, chemosis, itching, punctate keratitis, corneal edema, browache, photophobia, and headaches.

Administration: Ophthalmic.

Preparations: Ophthalmic solution, 0.5%.

DAPSONE, Avlosulfan®, DDS®

Description/Actions: Antileprosy agent indicated for the management of all forms of leprosy. Also indicated in the treatment of dermatitis herpetiformis.

Preparations: Tablets, 25 and 100 mg.

DARANIDE®, see Dichlorphenamide

DARAPRIM®, see Pyrimethamine

DARBEPOETIN ALFA—ARANESP™

Description/Actions: Darbepoetin alfa is indicated for the treatment of anemia associated with chronic renal failure, including patients on dialysis and patients not on dialysis. It is also indicated in the treatment of anemia in patients with nonyeloid malignancies where anemia is due to the effect of concomitantly administered chemotherapy.

Precautions/Adverse Reactions: Treatment with darbepoetin has been associated with cardiovascular and neurologic events (including seizures, stroke, and death) in patients with chronic renal failure. Monitor blood pressure and neurologic status during treatment. Supplemental iron therapy is recommended for all patients whose serum ferritin is below 100 mg/l or whose serum transferrin saturation is below 20%. Folic acid and/or vitamin B_{12} deficiencies should be corrected or excluded prior to initiation of therapy with darbepoetin. Infections, inflammatory or malignant processes, osteofibrosis cystica, occult blood loss, hemolysis, severe aluminum toxicity, and bone marrow fibrosis may compromise an erythropoietic response. Pregnancy Category C. There are no adequate and well-controlled studies in pregnant women. Use during pregnancy only if the potential benefit justifies the potential risk to the fetus. Excretion in human breast milk is unknown. Use with caution in nursing women. Safety and efficacy have not been established in pediatric patients. Safety and efficacy have not been established in patients with underlying hematologic diseases such as hemolytic anemia, sickle cell anemia, thalassemia, and porphyria.

Most commonly reported adverse reactions include hypertension, hypotension, infection, headache, myalgia, and diarrhea. The most commonly reported serious side effects associated with darbepoetin therapy are vascular access thrombosis, congestive heart failure, sepsis, and cardiac arrhythmia. The most commonly reported adverse reactions resulting in discontinuation of darbepoetin, dosage adjustment, or the need for concomitant medication to treat an adverse reaction symptom were hypotension, hypertension, fever, myalgia, nausea, and chest pain.

Administration: For intravenous or subcutaneous administration.

Patient Care Implications: Do not exceed a target hemoglobin concentration of 12 g/dl. Do not shake darbepoetin. Shaking will render it inactive. Do not dilute darbepoetin. Monitor blood pressure and neurologic status of patients treated with darbepoetin. Store in refrigerator.

Preparations: Available in 2 solutions for injection: Polysorbate 80 solution (contains 0.05 mg/ml polysorbate/ml) in 1 ml single-dose vials containing 25, 40, 60, 100, and 200 mg/ml.

Albumin solution (contains 2.5 mg/ml human albumin) in 1 ml single-dose vials containing 25, 40, 60, 100, and 200 mg/ml.

DARICON®, see Oxphencyclimine

DARVOCET-N®, Combination of propoxyphene napsylate and acetaminophen

DARVON®, see Propoxyphene hydrochloride

DARVON-N®, see Propoxyphene napsylate

DAUNORUBICIN HYDROCHLORIDE—Cerubidine®

Description/Actions: Antineoplastic agent indicated for the parenteral treatment of acute nonlymphocytic leukemia in adults and in acute lymphocytic leukemia in children.

Preparations: Vials, 20 mg (of the base).

DAYPRO®, see Oxaprozin

DDAVP®, see Desmopressin acetate

DDC, see Zalcitabine

DDI, see Didanosine

DDS®, see Dapsone

DEBRISAN®, see Dextranomer

DEBROX®, see Carbamide peroxide

DECADRON®, see Dexamethasone

DECA-DURABOLIN®, see Nandrolone decanoate

DECHOLIN®, see Dehydrocholic acid

DECLOMYCIN®, see Demeclocycline

DEFEROXAMINE MESYLATE—Desferal®

Description/Actions: Antidote that chelates iron. Indicated for parenteral use to facilitate the removal of iron in the treatment of acute iron intoxication and in chronic iron overload due to transfusion-dependent anemias.

Preparations: Vials, 500 mg.

DEHYDROCHOLIC ACID—Decholin®

Description/Actions: Hydrocholeretic indicated for the relief of constipation. Has also been used as an adjunct in the treatment of various biliary conditions.

Preparations: Tablets, 250 mg.

DELATESTRYL®, see Testosterone enanthate

DELAVIRDINE MESYLATE—Rescriptor®

Description/Actions: Antiretroviral indicated in the treatment of HIV-1 infection in combination with other antiretroviral agents when therapy is warranted. When used as monotherapy viral resistance emerged rapidly.

Warnings: Discontinue if serious rash (or rash with other symptoms) occurs. Use cautiously in patients with impaired liver function or achlorhydria (take with an acidic beverage). Adverse reactions include rash, GI upset.

Administration: Always use in combination with other antiretroviral therapy to minimize the risk of resistance. Potential for cross-resistence between delavirdine and either nucleoside analogues or protease inhibitors is unlikely due to their different mechanisms of action. Take 400 mg 3 times daily. May swallow tabs or disperse them in at least 3 oz of water and drink.

Preparations: Tablets, 100 mg.

DELESTROGEN®, see Estradiol valerate

DELSYM®, see Dextromethorphan

DELTA-CORTEF®, see Prednisolone

DELTASONE®, see Prednisone

DEMADEX®, see Torsemide

DEMECARIUM BROMIDE— Humorsol®

Description/Actions: Cholinesterase inhibitor exhibiting miotic activity. Indicated for ophthalmic use in the treatment of open-angle glaucoma, conditions obstructing aqueous outflow, accommodative esotropia, and following iridectomy.

Preparations: Ophthalmic solution, 0.125% and 0.25%.

DEMEROL®, see Meperidine

DEMECLOCYCLINE HYDROCHLORIDE—Declomycin®

Description/Actions: Tetracycline antibiotic indicated for the treatment of infections caused by susceptible organisms.

Preparations: Tablets, 150 and 300 mg. Capsules, 150 mg.

DEMSER®, see Metyrosine

DENAVIR®, see Penciclovir

DENILEUKIN DIFTITOX—Ontak®

Description/Actions: Denileukin deftitox is used for the treatment of persistent or recurrent cutaneous T-cell lymphoma (CTCL) with CD25 expression of the IL-2 receptor.

Precautions/Adverse Reactions: The drug should be administered in a facility that is equipped for cardiopulmonary resuscitation and where the patient can be monitored for hypersensitivity reactions. Women also should discontinue breast-feeding while receiving the drug. Most patients experience some kind of adverse reaction from the drug. The most common is a flu-like syndrome (91%), then hypersensitivity reaction (69%), infection (48%), vascular leak syndrome (27%), and nervous system disturbances.

Administration: Intravenous.

Patient Care Implications: Should be administered to patients in a facility equipped and staffed for cardiopulmonary resuscitation and where the patient can be closely monitored.

Preparations: Vials, 300 mcg/2 ml.

DEPAKENE®, see Valproic acid

DEPAKOTE®, see Valproic acid

DEPAKOTE® ER, see Divalproex Sodium under Valproic Acid

DEPEN®, see Penicillamine

DEPO-ESTRADIOL®, see Estradiol cypionate

DEPO-MEDROL®, see Methylprednisolone acetate

DEPONIT®, see Nitroglycerin

DEPO-PROVERA®, see Medroxyprogesterone acetate

DEPO-TESTOSTERONE®, see Testosterone cypionate

DERIFIL®, see Chlorophyll

DERMATOP®, see Prednicarbate

DES, see Diethylstilbestrol

DESENEX®, see Undecylenic acid

DESFERAL®, see Deferoxamine mesylate

DESFLURANE—Suprane®
General anesthetic.

Description/Actions: Is a halogenated volatile liquid that is administered via a vaporizer as a general inhalation anesthetic. Indicated as an inhalation agent for induction or maintenance of anesthesia for inpatient and outpatient surgery in adults. Also indicated for maintenance of anesthesia in infants and children after induction of anesthesia with other agents, and for tracheal intubation.

Warnings: Contraindicated in patients with a known or suspected genetic susceptibility to malignant hyperthermia. Adverse reactions include coughing, breathholding, apnea, increased secretions, laryngospasm, pharyngitis, nausea, and vomiting. Because it may increase heart rate, it is recommended that it should not be used as the sole agent for anesthetic induction in patients with coronary artery disease or in any patients in whom increases in heart rate or blood pressure are undesirable. May trigger a skeletal muscle hypermetabolic state that results in malignant hyperthermia. Concurrent use of preanesthetic medications such as an opioid or benzodiazepine may decrease the amount of desflurane required to produce anesthesia. Use will probably reduce the dose of a neuromuscular blocking agent required during anesthesia; however, for endotracheal intubation, it is recommended that the dose of the neuromuscular blocking agent not be reduced.

Administration: Inhalation. Should be administered using a vaporizer (Tec 60) specifically designed for use with the drug.

Preparations: Bottles, 240 ml.

DESIPRAMINE HYDROCHLORIDE—Norpramin®, Pertofrane®
Tricyclic antidepressant.

Description/Actions: Indicated for the relief of depression.

Warnings: Should not be given concomitantly with a monoamine oxidase inhibitor, or following recent myocardial infarction. Adverse reactions include drowsiness and other CNS effects; patients should be cautioned regarding activities such as driving and operating machinery, as well as interactions with other CNS-acting drugs including alcohol. Other adverse reactions include anticholinergic effects (e.g., dry mouth, blurred vision), GI effects (e.g., nausea), and cardiovascular effects (e.g., orthostatic hypotension). Caution should be exercised in patients with cardiovascular disorders.

Administration: Oral.

Preparations: Tablets, 10, 25, 50, 75, 100, and 150 mg. Capsules, 25 and 50 mg.

DESLORATADINE—CLARINEX®, Clarinex® Reditabs

Description/Actions: Desloratadine is indicated for the relief of nasal and nonnasal symptoms of allergic rhinitis (seasonal and perennial) and for symptomatic relief of chronic idiopathic urticaria.

Precautions/Adverse Reactions: Desloratadine is contraindicated in patients who are hypersensitive to desloratadine, loratadine, or any component of the formulation. There are no adequate and well-controlled studies in pregnant women. Pregnancy Category C. Excreted in breast milk/breast-feeding not recommended. Safety and efficacy have not been established for children < 12.

Administration: Oral, adults and children 12 years and older: 5 mg once daily.

Patient Care Implications: May be taken with or without food. Patients should be warned of possible drowsiness and advised not to drive or operate machinery until they see how they react to medication. Dosage should not be increased, because no greater efficacy may be expected and drowsiness might result. No clinically significant changes in the safety profile of desloratadine were observed in clinical studies when combined with erythromycin and ketoconazole. Both of these agents have been associated with potentially dangerous interactions with some other antihistamines.

Preparations: Tablets, 5 mg. Rapidly disintegrating tables, 5 mg.

DESMOPRESSIN ACETATE—DDAVP®, Stimate®

Description/Actions: Antidiuretic hormone indicated for the intranasal or parenteral treatment of diabetes insipidus, intranasal treatment of primary nocturnal enuresis, and parenteral treatment of patients with hemophilia A and von Wille-brand's disease.

Preparations: Nasal solution (DDAVP), 0.1 mg/ml. (available as a nasal tube delivery system and as a nasal spray pump). Nasal solution (Stimate), 1.5 mg/ml. Ampules and vials, 4 µg/ml. Tablets, 0.1 mg, 0.2 mg.

DESOGEN®, see Desogestrel/ethinyl estradiol

DESOGESTREL/ETHINYL ESTRADIOL—Cyclessa™, Desogen®, Ortho-Cept®

Oral contraceptive.

Description/Actions: Is a progestin/estrogen combination that acts primarily by the suppression of gonadotropins and inhibition of ovulation. Desogestrel exhibits a highly selective progestational action and minimal androgenicity. Indicated for the prevention of pregnancy in women who elect to use oral contraceptives as a method of contraception.

Warnings: Contraindicated in women who have thrombophlebitis or a thromboembolic disorder, a past history of such disorders, cerebral vascular or coronary artery disease, known or suspected carcinoma of the breast, carcinoma of the endometrium or other known or suspected estrogen-dependent neoplasia, undiagnosed abnormal genital bleeding, cholestatic jaundice of pregnancy or jaundice with prior oral contraceptive use, hepatic adenomas or carcinomas, or known or suspected pregnancy. Adverse reactions include bleeding irregularities (e.g., breakthrough bleeding, spotting, changes in menstrual flow), gastrointestinal effects e.g., nausea, vomiting, abdominal cramps), fluid retention, melasma, rash, reduced tolerance to carbohydrates, and vaginal candidiasis. Women should be strongly advised not to smoke because of the increased risk of cardiovascular effects.

Administration: Oral. Administered once a day at about the same time each day. Available in packages designed for a 21-day regimen (i.e., one tablet a day for 21 days, followed by 7 days in which medication is not taken) and a 28-day regimen (i.e., one tablet a day for 21 days, followed by one inactive "reminder" tablet a day for 7 days).

Preparations: Tablets, 0.15 mg of desogestrel and 30 µg of ethinyl estradiol in 21-day and 28-day regimens.

DESONIDE—Tridesilon®

Description/Actions: Corticosteroid indicated for the topical treatment of corticosteroid-responsive dermatoses and, in combination with acetic acid in an otic solution, for the management of superficial infections of the external auditory canal.

90 • DESOXIMETASONE

Preparations: Cream and ointment, 0.05%. Otic solution, 0.05% with 2% acetic acid.

DESOXIMETASONE—Topicort®

Description/Actions: Corticosteroid indicated for the topical treatment of corticosteroid-responsive dermatoses.

Preparations: Cream, 0.05% and 0.25%. Ointment, 0.25%. Gel, 0.05%.

DESOXYN®, see Methamphetamine

DESYREL®, see Trazodone

DETROL®, see Tolterodine Tartrate

DETROL® LA, see Tolterodine Tartrate

DEXAMETHASONE—Decadron®, Hexadrol®

Description/Actions: Corticosteroid indicated in a wide range of endocrine, rheumatic, allergic, dermatologic, respiratory, hematologic, neoplastic, and other disorders.

Preparations: Tablets, 0.5, 0.75, 1, 1.5, 2, 3, and 6 mg. Liquid, 0.5 mg/5 ml. Oral concentrate, 0.5 mg/0.5 ml. Vials (as the acetate for intramuscular, intra-articular and intralesional use), 8 mg/ml. Vials and ampules (as the sodium phosphate for parenteral use), 4, 10, 20, and 24 (for IV use only) mg/ml. Topical gel, 0.1%. Topical aerosol, 10 mg/25 g. Cream (as the sodium phosphate), 0.1% Ophthalmic solution (as the sodium phosphate), 0.1%. Ophthalmic ointment (as the sodium phosphate), 0.05%. Aerosols (as the sodium phosphate) for oral inhalation and intranasal administration.

DEXCHLORPHENIRAMINE MALEATE—Polaramine®

Description/Actions: Antihistamine indicated in the treatment of allergic disorders.

Preparations: Tablets, 2 mg. Controlled-release tablets, 4 and 6 mg. Syrup, 2 mg/5 ml.

DEXEDRINE®, see Dextroamphetamine

DEXMEDETOMIDINE HYDROCHLORIDE INJECTION—Precedex®

Description/Actions: Indicated for sedation of initially intubated and mechanically ventilated patients during treatment in an intensive care setting.

Precautions/Adverse Reactions: Precedex should be administered by continuous infusion not to exceed 24 hours. Hypotension and bradycardia have been associated with Precedex infusion. Caution should be used when administering this drug to patients with advanced heart block. Transient hypertension has also been observed, primarily during the loading dose, in association with the initial peripheral vasoconstrictive effects of Precedex. In these cases, reduction of the loading infusion rate may be desirable. Precedex should not be coadministered through the same IV catheter with blood or plasma since physical compatibility has not been established. Withdrawal symptoms including nervousness, agitation, and headaches may occur if Precedex is administered chronically and stopped abruptly. Adverse effects of the drug include hypotension, hypertension, nausea, bradycardia, fever, vomiting, hypoxia, tachycardia, and anemia.

Administration: Intravenous.

Patient Care Implication: Precedex should be administered only by persons skilled in the management of patients in the intensive care setting. Due to known pharmacologic effects of Precedex, patients should be continuously monitored while receiving the drug.

Preparations: Vials and ampules, 2 mL, 100 mcg/mL.

DEXMETHYLPHENIDATE HYDROCHLORIDE— FOCALIN™

Description/Actions: Dexmethylphenidate is indicated for the treatment of ADHD.

Precautions/Adverse Reactions: Contraindicated in patients with marked anxiety, tension, and agitation because the drug may aggravate these symptoms. Contraindicated in patients with motor tics or with a family history or diagnosis of Tourette's syndrome. Contraindicated during treatment with monoamine oxidase inhibitors (MAOIs) and also within a minimum of 14 days following discontinuation of an MAOI (hypertensive crisis may occur). Contraindicated in patients with glaucoma. Should not be used to treat severe depression or for the prevention or treatment of normal fatigue states. Suppression of growth (weight and/or height gain) has been reported with long-term use of stimulants in children. Patients requiring long-term therapy should be monitored carefully. Administration of methylphenidate may exacerbate symptoms of behavior disturbance and thought disorder in psychotic children.

In the presence of seizures, this drug should be discontinued. Use cautiously in patients with hypertension and in patients whose underlying medical conditions might be compromised by increases in blood pressure or heart rate (preexisting hypertension, heart failure, recent myocardial infarction, or hyperthyroidism). Should be given cautiously to patients with a history of drug dependence or alcoholism. Chronic abusive use can lead to marked tolerance and psychological dependence, with varying degrees of abnormal behavior.

Most common adverse reactions were abdominal pain, fever, nausea, and anorexia. Methylphenidate may decrease the effectiveness of drugs used to treat hypertension because of possible effects on blood pressure. Use cautiously with pressor agents. Severe toxic reactions reported when combined with clonidine. Avoid use with linezolid, due to MAO inhibition. Pregancy Category C. Safety and efficacy not established in pregnant women. Use during pregnancy only if the potential benefit to mother outweighs the possible risks to the fetus.

Administration: Oral.

Patient Care Implications: When used for extended periods, physicians should periodically reevaluate the long-term usefulness of the drug for the individual patient. If improvement is not observed after appropriate dosage adjustment over a 1 month period, the drug should be discontinued. Dexmethylphenidate is administered twice a day at least 4 hours apart. It may be given with or without food. Avoid alcohol, caffeine, and other stimulants. Use caution when driving or engaging in tasks requiring alertness until response to drug is known. Do not store medicine in hot, damp, or humid places.

Preparations: Tablets, 2.5, 5, and 10 mg.

DEXPANTHENOL—Ilopan®

Description/Actions: Pantothenic acid derivative used as a GI stimulant. Indicated for parenteral treatment of intestinal atony causing abdominal distention, postoperative and postpartum retention of flatus, or postoperative delay in resumption of intestinal motility, paralytic ileus, and for prophylactic use immediately after major abdominal surgery to minimize the possibility of paralytic ileus.

Preparations: Ampules, vials, and syringes, 250 mg/ml. Has been used orally in combination with choline bitartrate.

DEXRAZOXANE—Zinecard®

Description/Actions: Cardioprotective agent indicated for reducing the incidence and severity of cardiomyopathy associated with doxorubicin administration in women with metastatic breast cancer who have received a cumulative doxorubicin dose of 300 mg/m2 and who would benefit from continuing doxorubicin therapy. Not recommended for use with the initiation of doxorubicin therapy.

Warnings: Contraindicated in chemotherapy regimens which do not contain an anthracycline. Additive myelosuppressive effect of this agent with antineoplastic agents requires careful blood count monitoring.

Administration: Intravenous. Recommended dosage ratio of dexrazoxane: doxorubicin is 10:1 (e.g., 500 mg/m2 dexrazoxane: 50 mg/m2 doxorubicin). After completing the infusion of dexrazoxane, and prior to a total elapsed time of 30 minutes (from the beginning of the dexrazoxane infusion), the intravenous injection of doxorubicin should be given. Doxorubicin should not be given prior to the administration of dexrazoxane.

Preparations: Vials, 250 and 500 mg.

DEXTRAN, LOW MOLECULAR WEIGHT—Dextran 40, Gentran 40®, Rheomacrodex®

DEXTRAN, HIGH MOLECULAR WEIGHT—Dextran 70, Dextran 75, Gentran 75®, Macrodex®

Description/Actions: Synthetic polysaccharide administered parenterally primarily as a plasma expander as adjunctive treatment of shock or impending shock due to hemorrhage, burns, surgery, or other trauma.

Preparations: Injection, 10% low molecular weight dextran and 6% high molecular weight dextran.

DEXTRANOMER—Debrisan®, Envisan®

Description/Actions: Applied topically for use in cleaning wet ulcers and wounds such as venous stasis ulcers, pressure ulcers, infected traumatic and surgical wounds, and infected burns.

Preparations: Beads. Paste.

DEXTROAMPHETAMINE SULFATE—Dexedrine®

Description/Actions: Central nervous system stimulant indicated in the treatment of narcolepsy, attention-deficit disorder with hyperactivity, and in exogenous obesity as a short-term adjunct in a regimen of weight reduction based on caloric restriction.

Preparations: Tablets, 5 mg. Controlled-release capsules, 15 mg.

DEXTROMETHORPHAN—Benylin DM®, Delsym®

Description/Actions: Antitussive indicated for the relief of cough.

Preparations: Syrup (as the hydrobromide) 5, 10, and 15 mg/5 ml.

DEXTROSE—Glucose, Glutose®, Instaglucose®

Description/Actions: Carbohydrate administered parenterally as a source of calories. Oral forms are used to correct hypoglycemia in conscious patients.

Preparations: Solutions, 2.5%, 5%, 10%, 20%, 25%, 30%, 40%, 50%, 60%, and 70%. Oral gel, 40% in 25 g and 30 g tubes and 80 g bottle. Chewable tablets, 5g.

DEXTROTHYROXINE SODIUM—Choloxin®

Description/Actions: Antihyperlipidemic agent used as an adjunct to diet and other measures for the reduction of elevated serum cholesterol levels. May also reduce beta lipoprotein and triglyceride levels.

Preparations: Tablets, 1, 2, and 4 mg.

DEZOCINE—Dalgan®

Analgesic.

Description/Actions: An opioid agonist-antagonist analgesic that exhibits analgesic efficacy, as well as an onset and duration of action, that are comparable to those of morphine. Is most often used in the management of postoperative pain and pain associated with surgery and orthopedic trauma.

Warnings: Adverse reactions include sedation, dizziness/vertigo, and psychotomimetic effects. Patients should be cautioned regarding activities such as driving and operating machinery, as well as interactions with other CNS-acting drugs including alcohol. Other adverse reactions include nausea, vomiting, and injection site reactions. Should not be used in patients who are physically dependent on narcotics because its antagonist action may precipitate withdrawal symptoms.

Administration: Intramuscular and intravenous.

Preparations: Single-dose vials and syringes, 5, 10, and 15 mg. Multiple-dose vials, 10 mg/ml.

DHE 45®, see Dihydroergotamine

DHT®, see Dihydrotachysterol

DIABETA®, see Glyburide

DIABINESE®, see Chlorpropamide

DIACETYLMORPHINE, see Heroin

DIAMOX®, see Acetazolamide

DIASTAT®, see Diazepam

DIAZEPAM—Diastat®, Valium®, Valrelease®

Benzodiazepine antianxiety agent and anticonvulsant.

Description/Actions: A CNS depressant indicated (1) for the management of anxiety disorders or for the short-term relief of the symptoms of anxiety; (2) in acute alcohol withdrawal; (3) as an adjunct for the relief of skeletal muscle spasm due to reflex spasm to local pathology, athetosis, stiff-man syndrome, and tetanus; (4) as an adjunct in convulsive disorders; (5) as an adjunct in status epilepticus and severe recurrent convulsive seizures; (6) as an adjunct prior to endoscopic procedures; and (7) as a premedication in patients who are to undergo surgical procedures.

Warnings: Contraindicated in patients with acute narrow-angle glaucoma. Adverse reactions include drowsiness and other CNS effects; patients should be cautioned regarding activities such as driving and operating machinery, as well as interactions with other CNS-acting drugs including alcohol. Can cause dependence and is included in Schedule IV. Intramuscular injections are painful and erratically absorbed. If IM route is essential for administration, inject deeply into a large muscle mass and rotate sites.

Administration: Oral, intravenous, and intramuscular.

Preparations: Tablets, 2, 5, and 10 mg. Controlled-release capsules, 15 mg. Oral solution, 5 mg/5 ml. Concentrated oral solution, 5 mg/ml. Ampules, vials, and syringes, 5 mg/ml. Rectal gel, 2.5, 5, 10, 15, and 20 mg. Sterile emulsion for injection, 5 mg/ml (contains egg phospholipids, and soybean oil).

DIAZOXIDE—Hyperstat®, Proglycem®

Description/Actions: Antihypertensive agent administered intravenously for short-term use in the emergency reduction of blood pressure in severe hypertension. Also used orally in the management of hypoglycemia due to hyperinsulinism associated with various conditions (e.g., inoperable islet cell carcinoma or adenoma).

Preparations: Ampules, 300 mg. Capsules, 50 mg. Oral suspension, 50 mg/ml.

DIBENT®, see Dicyclomine

DIBENZYLINE®, see Phenoxybenzamine

DIBUCAINE—Nupercainal®

Description/Actions: Local anesthetic used for painful skin conditions and hemorrhoids.

Preparations: Cream, 0.5%. Ointment, 1%.

DICHLORPHENAMIDE— Daranide®, Oratrol®

Description/Actions: Carbonic anhydrase inhibitor indicated for adjunctive treatment of open-angle glaucoma, secondary glaucoma, and preoperatively in acute angle-closure glaucoma.

Preparations: Tablets, 50 mg.

DICLOFENAC POTASSIUM— Cataflam®

DICLOFENAC SODIUM— Voltaren®

Nonsteroidal anti-inflammatory drug.

Description/Actions: Inhibits prostaglandin synthesis. Diclofenac sodium is indicated for the treatment of rheumatoid arthritis, osteoarthritis, and ankylosing spondylitis. Also indicated for ophthalmic use for the treatment of postoperative inflammation following cataract extraction and in photophobia due to incisional refractive surgery. Diclofenac potassium is indicated for the management of pain and primary dysmenorrhea.

Warnings: Should not be given to patients in whom aspirin or another NSAID causes asthma, rhinitis, urticaria, or other allergic-type reactions. May cause GI effects, and use should be avoided in patients with active GI tract disease and closely monitored in patients with a previous history of such disorders. Other adverse reactions include headache, dizziness, rash, pruritus, tinnitus, and fluid retention. Elevations in liver function tests have occurred, and it is recommended that hepatic function tests be performed no later than 8 weeks after starting therapy and periodically thereafter.

Administration: Oral and ophthalmic.

Preparations: Tablets (Cataflam), 25, 50, and 75 mg. Enteric-coated tablets (Voltaren), 25, 50, and 75 mg. Enteric-coated tablets (Cataflam), 75 mg and 100 mg. Ophthalmic solution, 0.1%. Suppositories, 50 and 100 mg, 100 mg extended-release tabs (Voltarum-XR).

DICLOXACILLIN SODIUM— Dycill®, Dynapen®, Pathocil®

Description/Actions: Penicillin antibiotic indicated for the treatment of staphylococcal infections.

Preparations: Capsules, 125, 250, and 500 mg. Powder for oral solution, 62.5 mg/5 ml when reconstituted.

DICUMAROL

Description/Actions: Coumarin anticoagulant indicated for conditions such as prophylaxis and treatment of venous thrombosis and its extension. During period of dosage adjustment, prothrombin activity should be measured daily and dose order obtained.

Preparations: Tablets, 25 and 50 mg.

DICYCLOMINE HYDROCHLORIDE—Antispas®, A-spas®, Bentyl®, Dibent®, Di-Spaz®, Spasmoject®

Anticholinergic agent.

Description/Actions: Relieves smooth muscle spasm of the GI tract and is indicated for the treatment of functional bowel/irritable bowel syndrome (irritable colon, spastic colon, and mucous colitis).

Warnings: Contraindicated in patients with obstructive uropathy, obstructive disease of the GI tract, paralytic ileus, intestinal atony, unstable cardiovascular status in acute hemorrhage, severe ulcerative colitis, myasthenia gravis, and glaucoma. Adverse reactions include dry mouth, blurred vision, and nausea. Anticholinergic psychosis, and heat prostration (in the presence of a high environmental temperature) have been reported in sensitive patients. May cause drowsiness and other CNS effects; patients should be cautioned regarding activities such as driving and operating machinery, as well as interactions with other CNS-acting drugs including alcohol.

Administration: Oral and intramuscular.

Preparations: Tablets, 10 and 20 mg. Extended release tablets, 30 mg. Capsules, 10 and 20 mg. Syrup, 10 mg/5 ml. Solution for injection, 10 mg/ml.

DIDANOSINE—Videx®, Videx® EC

Antiviral agent.

Description/Actions: Also known as dideoxyinosine or ddI. It inhibits the replication of the human immunodeficiency virus (HIV). Is converted by cellular enzymes to the active antiviral metabolite that inhibits viral replication, in part, by interfering with reverse transcriptase. Indicated for adult and pediatric patients (>6 months of age) with advanced HIV infection who are intolerant of zidovudine therapy or who have demonstrated significant clinical or immunologic deterioration during zidovudine therapy. Also indicated for adult patients with advanced HIV infection who have received prolonged prior zidovudine therapy.

Warnings: Fatal lactic acidosis has been reported in pregnant women who receive the combination of didanosine and stavudine with other antiretroviral agents. The combination of didanosine and stavudine should be used with caution during pregnancy and is recommended only if the potential benefits clearly outweigh the potential risks. Redistribution of body fat including central obesity, dorsocervical fat enlargement, peripheral wasting, facial wasting, breast enlargement, and "cushingoid appearance" has been observed in patients receiving antiretroviral therapy. May cause pancreatitis and, if a patient develops abdominal pain and nausea, vomiting, or elevated amylase levels, use of the drug should be interrupted until the possibility of pancreatitis is excluded. Use of didanosine in patients with a history of pancreatitis or alcoholism is best avoided as is the concurrent use with other agents known to be associated with pancreatic toxicity (e.g., intravenous pentamidine). May cause peripheral neuropathy, particularly in patients with a history of neuropathy or neurotoxic drug therapy; patients should be advised to report symptoms such as tingling, burning, pain, or numbness in the hands or feet. Other adverse reactions include headache, diarrhea, insomnia, rash, pruritus, depression, pain, constipation, stomatitis, taste disturbance, myalgia, arthritis, hepatic enzyme elevations, leukopenia, granulocytopenia, and thrombocytopenia. Because two of the three formulations contain (or have added) magnesium and aluminum antacids (to reduce the degradation of the drug by gastric acid), tetracyclines, fluoroquinolones, or other drugs that interact with metals should not be administered within 2 hours of taking didanosine. Ketoconazole should be administered at least 2 hours before dosing with didanosine. Each tablet contains 15.7 mEq of magnesium, 264.5 mg of sodium, as well as a quantity of phenylalanine; caution should be exercised in patients with significant renal impairment, on a sodium-restricted diet, and/or who are phenylketonuric.

Administration: Oral. Food reduces absorption by as much as 50%; therefore, the drug should be administered on an empty stomach (i.e., having nothing to eat or drink, except water, for 1 hour before and 1 to 2 hours after taking the drug). Each dose of the tablet formulation must consist of 2 tablets to achieve adequate acid-neutralizing capacity for maximal absorption. The tablets should be thoroughly chewed, manually crushed, or dispersed in water. The buffered powder for oral solution is provided in packets, the contents of which should be poured into a container with about 4 oz of water. The drug must not be mixed with fruit juice or other acid-containing liquid. The pediatric powder for oral solution is initially constituted with purified water, to which the pharmacist then adds an appropriate quantity of an antacid (Mylanta Double Strength Liquid or Maalox TC Suspension).

Videx® EC capsules should be swallowed whole, the capsules should not be opened.

Preparations: Chewable/dispersible buffered tablets, 25, 50, 100, and 150 mg. Packets of powder for oral solution, 100, 167, 250, and 375 mg. Bottles of pediatric powder for oral solution, 2 and 4 g. Sustained release capsules, 125, 200, 250, and 400 mg.

DIDREX®, see Benzphetamine

DIDRONEL®, see Etidronate

DIENESTROL

Description/Actions: Estrogen indicated for intravaginal use in the treatment of atrophic vaginitis and kraurosis vulvae.

Preparations: Vaginal cream, 0.01%.

DIETHYLPROPION HYDROCHLORIDE—Tenuate®, Tepanil®

Description/Actions: Anorexiant indicated in the management of exogenous obesity as a short-term adjunct in a regimen of weight reduction based on caloric restriction.

Preparations: Tablets, 25 mg. Controlled-release tablets, 75 mg.

DIETHYLSTILBESTROL—DES

DIETHYLSTILBESTROL DIPHOSPHATE—Stilphostrol®

Description/Actions: Estrogen indicated in the treatment of moderate to severe vasomotor symptoms associated with the menopause, atrophic vaginitis, kraurosis vulvae, female hypogonadism, female castration, primary ovarian failure, and breast cancer. Both oral and parenteral (diphosphate) dosage forms are indicated in the treatment of prostatic carcinoma.

Preparations: Tablets, 1 and 5 mg. Enteric-coated tablets, 0.1, 1, and 5 mg. Tablets (diphosphate), 50 mg. Ampules (diphosphate), 250 mg/5 ml.

DIFENOXIN HYDROCHLORIDE/ ATROPINE SULFATE—Motofen®

Antidiarrheal agent.

Description/Actions: Difenoxin is the principal active metabolite of diphenoxylate. A subtherapeutic dose of atropine is included in the formulation to discourage abuse of difenoxin. Indicated as adjunctive therapy in the management of diarrhea.

Warnings: Contraindicated in patients with diarrhea associated with pseudomembranous colitis. Is also contraindicated in children under 2 years of age because of an increased risk of adverse reactions. Adverse reactions include drowsiness and other CNS effects; patients should be cautioned regarding activities such as driving and operating machinery, as well as interactions with other CNS-acting drugs including alcohol. Should not be administered to patients being treated with a monoamine oxidase inhibitor. Is inluded in Schedule IV.

Administration: Oral.

Preparations: Tablets containing 1 mg difenoxin hydrochloride and 0.025 mg atropine sulfate.

DIFFERIN®, see Adaplalene

DIFLORASONE DIACETATE—
Florone®, Maxiflor®

Description/Actions: Corticosteroid used topically in the treatment of corticosteroid-responsive dermatoses.

Preparations: Cream and ointment, 0.05%.

DIFLUCAN®, see Fluconazole

DIFLUNISAL—Dolobid®

Nonsteroidal anti-inflammatory drug.

Description/Actions: A salicylate analogue that exhibits analgesic, antipyretic, and anti-inflammatory effects. Indicated for the treatment of mild to moderate pain, rheumatoid arthritis, and osteoarthritis.

Warnings: Contraindicated in patients in whom acute asthmatic attacks, urticaria, or rhinitis are precipitated by aspirin or other nonsteroidal anti-inflammatory drugs. May cause GI effects and use should be avoided in patients with active GI tract disease and closely supervised in patients with a previous history of such disorders. Other adverse reactions include headache and rash. Effect may be reduced by antacids.

Administration: Oral.

Preparations: Tablets, 250 and 500 mg.

DIGIBIND®, see Digoxin immune FAB

DIGITALIS

Description/Actions: Cardiac glycosides primarily used in the treatment of congestive heart failure.

Preparations: Tablets, 100 mg.

DIGITOXIN

Description/Actions: Cardiac glycoside indicated in the treatment of heart failure, atrial flutter, atrial fibrillation, and supraventricular tachycardia.

Preparations: Tablets, 0.1 and 0.2 mg.

DIGOXIN—Lanoxicaps®, Lanoxin®

Cardiac (digitalis) glycoside.

Actions and Uses: Exhibits a positive inotropic action and also causes a slowing of heart rate and decreased conduction velocity through the AV node. Indicated in the management of heart failure, atrial fibrillation, atrial flutter, and paroxysmal atrial tachycardia.

Warnings: Contraindicated in patients in ventricular fibrillation. May cause serious cardiac toxicity (e.g., arrhythmias), and therapy must be closely supervised. Other adverse reactions include anorexia, nausea, and vomiting, visual disturbances, headache, weakness, apathy, psychosis, and gynecomastia. Certain diuretics and corticosteroids may cause potassium depletion and increase the risk of digoxin toxicity. Simultaneous administration of antacids, cholestyramine, or colestipol may reduce absorption, and as long an interval as possible should separate the administration of digoxin and one of these agents.

Administration: Oral, intravenous, and intramuscular.

Preparations: Tablets, 0.125, 0.25, and 0.5 mg. Liquid in caps, 0.05, 0.1, and 0.2 mg. Elixir (pediatric), 0.05 mg/ml. Ampules, 0.1 mg/ml (pediatric) and 0.25 mg/ml.

DIGOXIN IMMUNE FAB (OVINE)—Digibind®

Antidote for digoxin toxicity.

Description/Actions: Indicated for the treatment of potentially life-threatening digoxin or digitoxin intoxication.

Warnings: A potential for hypersensitivity reactions exists. Low cardiac output states and congestive heart failure may be exacerbated by the withdrawal of the inotropic effects of digoxin. Hypokalemia may result from the rapid reversal of the hyperkalemia associated with digoxin intoxication, and potassium concentrations should be monitored closely.

Administration: Intravenous.

Preparations: Vials, 40 mg.

DIHYDROCODEINE BITARTRATE

Description/Actions: Opioid analgesic indicated for the relief of moderate to moderately severe pain. Used in combination with other analgesics.

DIHYDROERGOTAMINE MESYLATE—DHE 45®

Description/Actions: Vasoconstrictor administered parenterally to abort or prevent vascular headaches (e.g., migraine). In conjunction with low-dose heparin to prevent postoperative deep vein thrombosis and pulmonary embolism.

Preparations: Ampules, 1 mg.

DIHYDROTACHYSTEROL—DHT®, Hytakerol®

Description/Actions: Vitamin D analogue indicated for the treatment of hypoparathyroidism, postoperative tetany, and idiopathic tetany.

Preparations: Capsules, 0.125 mg. Tablets, 0.125, 0.2, and 0.4 mg. Solution, 0.2 mg/5 ml. Concentrated solution, 0.2 mg/ml. Solution in oil, 0.25 mg/ml.

DILACOR XR®, see Diltiazem.

DILANTIN®, see Phenytoin.

DILAUDID®, see Hydromorphone

DILOR®, see Dyphylline

DILTIAZEM HYDROCHLORIDE— Cardizem®, Cardizem SR®, Cardizem CD®, Dilacor XR®, Tiazac®

Antianginal, antiarrhythmic, and antihypertensive agent.

Description/Actions: Is a calcium channel-blocking agent that is indicated in the treatment of (1) angina pectoris due to coronary artery spasm; (2) chronic stable angina in patients who cannot tolerate therapy with beta-blockers and/or nitrates or who remain symptomatic despite adequate doses of these agents; (3) hypertension (Cardizem SR, Cardizem CD, Dilacor XR); (4) atrial fibrillation or flutter (intravenously); and (5) paroxysmal supraventricular tachycardia (intravenously).

Warnings: Contraindicated in patients with sick sinus syndrome (except in the presence of a functioning ventricular pacemaker), second- or third-degree AV block, and hypotension. Adverse reactions include edema, headache, nausea, dizziness, and rash. Although usually well tolerated, concomitant therapy with a beta-adrenergic blocking agent or digitalis glycoside should be monitored closely because there may be additive effects in prolonging AV conduction.

Administration: Oral and intravenous.

Preparations: Tablets, 30, 60, 90, and 120 mg. Sustained-release capsules, 60, 90, and 120 mg (Cardizem SR); 120, 180, 240, and 300 mg and 360 mg (Cardizem CD); 180 and 240 mg (Dilacor XR); 120, 180, 240, 300, 360, and 420 mg (Tiazac). Vials, 25 and 50 mg.

DIMENHYDRINATE—Dramamine®

Description/Actions: Antinauseant/antiemetic indicated for the prevention and treatment of the nausea, vomiting, or vertigo of motion sickness. When used for prophylaxis of motion sickness, administer at least 30 minutes and preferably 1–2 hr before exposure to conditions that may precipitate motion sickness.

Preparations: Tablets and capsules, 50 mg. Extended-release capsules, 25 mg. Chewable tablets, 50 mg. Liquid, 12.5 mg/4 ml. Elixir, 12.5 mg/5 ml and 15 mg/5 ml. Ampules and vials, 50 mg/ml. Suppositories, 50 mg.

DIMERCAPROL—BAL

Description/Actions: Antidote indicated in the parenteral treatment of arsenic, gold, and mercury poisoning. As an adjunct with edetate calcium disodium in the treatment of severe lead poisoning accompanied by encephalopathy.

Preparations: Ampules, 100 mg/ml.

DIMETANE®, see Brompheniramine

DIMETHYL SULFOXIDE—Rimso-50®, DMSO

Description/Actions: Agent for symptomatic relief of *interstitial cystitis* and is instilled directly into the bladder. Is being evaluated for the topical treatment of conditions such as scleroderma and a wide range of musculoskeletal disorders. Also used to protect living cells and tissues during cold storage (cryoprotection).

Preparations: Aqueous solution, 50%.

DINOPROST TROMETHAMINE—Prostaglandin F₂ alpha, Prostin F2 alpha®

Description/Actions: Abortifacient injected into the amniotic sac for the termination of pregnancy during the period from 16 to 20 gestational weeks.

Preparations: Ampules, 5 mg/ml.

DINOPROSTONE—Prostaglandin E₂, Cervidil®, Prepidil®,Prostin E2®

Description/Actions: Abortifacient (Prostin E2) indicated for intravaginal use for the termination of pregnancy during the period from 12 to 20 gestational weeks. Used for the evacuation of the uterine content in the management of missed abortion or intrauterine fetal death up to 28 weeks gestational age. Indicated in the management of nonmetastatic gestational trophoblastic disease (benign hydatiform mole).

Agent for *cervical ripening* (Cervidil®, Prepidil®) used to ripen an unfavorable cervix in pregnant women at or near term with a medical or obstetrical need for labor induction.

Preparations: Vaginal suppositories (Prostin E2), 20 mg. Gel (Prepidil), 0.5 mg. Vaginal insert (Cervidil®), 10 mg.

DIOVAN®, see Valsartan

DIOVAN HCT®—Combination agent valsartan and hydrochlorothiaride (angiotensin II receptor antagonist and diuretic)

DIPENTUM®, see Olsalazine sodium

DIPHENHYDRAMINE HYDROCHLORIDE—Benadryl®, Benylin cough®, Nytol®, Sominex®

Description/Actions: Antihistamine, hypnotic, and antitussive used in the treatment of various allergic disorders, management of cough, treatment of insomnia, prevention of motion sickness, and drug-induced Parkinson's disease or dystonic reactions.

Preparations: Capsules and tablets, 25 and 50 mg. Chewable tablets, 25 mg. Liquid, 12.5 mg/5 ml. Ampules and vials, 10 and 50 mg/ml. Cream and gel, 1%, 2%. Spray, 1%.

DIPHENATOL, see Diphenoxylate hydrochloride with atropine sulfate

DIPHENIDOL—Vontrol®

Description/Actions: Antiemetic indicated in the treatment of peripheral vertigo and associated nausea and vomiting, and in the control of nausea and vomiting as seen in conditions such as postoperative states, malignant neoplasms, and labyrinth disturbances.

Preparations: Tablets, 25 mg.

DIPHENOXYLATE HYDROCHLORIDE WITH ATROPINE SULFATE—
Lomotil®, Diphenatol®, Lofene®, Lomanate®, Lonox®, Lo-Trol®, Low Qual®, Nor-Mil®

Antidiarrheal.

Description/Actions: Diphenoxylate is structurally related to meperidine. Indicated as adjunctive therapy in the management of diarrhea.

Warnings: Contraindicated in patients with obstructive jaundice, and in diarrhea associated with pseudomembranous enterocolitis. Adverse reactions include drowsiness and other CNS effects; patients should be cautioned regarding activities such as driving and operating machinery, as well as interactions with other CNS-acting drugs including alcohol. Effects attributed to the atropine include dry mouth. Use is not recommended for children under 2 years of age because of an increased risk of adverse reactions. Should not be administered to patients being treated with a monoamine oxidase inhibitor. Is included in Schedule V.

Administration: Oral.

Preparations: Tablets and liquid. Each tablet and 5 ml of liquid contains 2.5 mg and 0.025 mg atropine sulfate.

DIPHENYLHYDANTOIN—former name for Phenytoin

DIPIVEFRIN HYDROCHLORIDE— Propine®

Description/Actions: Sympathomimetic agent. A prodrug that is converted to epinephrine following administration. Indicated for ophthalmic use in the treatment of chronic open-angle glaucoma.

Preparations: Ophthalmic solution, 0.1%.

DIPRIVAN®, see Propofol

DIPROLENE®, see Betamethasone dipropionate augmented

DIPROLENE AF®, see Betamethasone dipropionate augmented

DIPROSONE®, see Betamethasone dipropionate

DIPYRIDAMOLE—Persantine®, Persantine IV®

Agent to prevent postoperative thromboembolic complications.

Description/Actions: Indicated as an adjunct to coumarin anticoagulants in the prevention of postoperative thromboembolic complications of cardiac valve replacement. Also indicated for intravenous use as an alternative to exercise in thallium myocardial perfusion imaging for the evaluation of coronary artery disease in patients who cannot exercise regularly.

Warnings: Adverse reactions include dizziness, abdominal distress, headache, and rash.

Administration: Oral and intravenous.

Preparations: Tablets, 25, 50, and 75 mg. Ampules, 10 mg/2 ml.

DIRITHROMYCIN—Dynabac®

Description/Actions: Antiinfective agent. Macrolide antibiotic indicated in the treatment of mild to moderate susceptible infections including acute and chronic bronchitis, secondary bacterial infection of acute bronchitis, community acquired pneumonia, pharyngitis/tonsillitis, uncomplicated skin and skin structure infections. Should not be used in patients with bacteremia.

Warnings: Adverse reactions include abdominal pain, headache, GI upset, dizziness, pain, asthenia, cough, rash, dyspnea, pruritus, insomnia, blood dyscrasias, electrolyte imbalance, and pseudomembranous colitis.
Administration: Oral. Take with food. Do not crush, chew, or cut.
Preparations: Enteric-coated tablets, 250 mg.

DISALCID®, see Salsalate

DISODIUM EDTA®, see Edetate

DISOPYRAMIDE PHOSPHATE—Norpace®, Norpace CR®
Description/Actions: Antiarrhythmic agent indicated for the prevention and suppression of premature ventricular contractions, and episodes of ventricular tachycardia.
Preparations: Capsules and controlled-release capsules, 100 and 150 mg.

DISOTATE, see Edetate

DI-SPAZ®, see Dicyclomine

DISULFIRAM—Antabuse®
Description/Actions: Agent for alcoholism indicated as an aid in the management of selected chronic alcoholic patients who want to remain in a state of enforced sobriety.
Preparations: Tablets, 250 and 500 mg.

DITHRANOL, see Anthralin

DITROPAN® and DITROPAN XL®, see Oxybutynin

DIUCARDIN®, see Hydroflumethiazide

DIURIL®, see Chlorothiazide

DIVALPROEX SODIUM, see Valproic acid

DMSO®, see Dimethyl sulfoxide

DOAN'S PILLS®, see Magnesium salicylate

DOBUTAMINE HYDROCHLORIDE—Dobutrex®
Description/Actions: Inotropic catecholamine indicated in the short-term intravenous treatment of adults with cardiac decompensation due to depressed contractility resulting either from organic heart disease or from cardiac surgical procedures.
Preparations: Vials, 250 mg.

DOBUTREX®, see Dobutamine hydrochloride

DOCETAXEL—Taxotere®
Antineoplastic Agent.
Description/Actions: Antineoplastic agent used in the treatment of patients with locally advanced or metastatic breast cancer who have progressed during anthracycline-based adjuvant therapy. Also indicated as first-line therapy in combination with cisplatin for the treatment of patients with unresectable, locally advanced, or metastatic non-small-cell lung cancer who have not previously received chemotherapy for their condition.
Warnings: Contraindicated in patients with history of severe hypersensitivity reactions to docetaxel or to other drugs formulated with polysorbate 80 or neutrophil counts < 1500 cells/mm3. Toxic deaths have occurred when docetaxel was administered at doses of 100 mg/m2 in patients with and without impaired liver function. Sepsis accounted for the majority of these deaths. Fatal GI bleeds in patients with severe liver impairment has been associated with drug-induced thrombocytopenia. Fluid retention, neutropenia, and cutaneous reactions have also been reported with docetaxel. Careful monitoring of blood

counts, liver, and renal functions is recommended.

Administration: Intravenous. Premedicate patients with oral corticosteroids.

Preparations: Injection, 20 and 80 mg in single dose vials with diluent.

DOCOSANOL 10% CREAM—Abreva®

Description/Actions: Docosanol is indicated in the treatment of herpes labialis of the lips or face.

Precautions/Adverse Reactions: Docosanol is contraindicated in patients with a hypersensitivity to docosanol or to any component of the product. For external use only. Use on lips and face only. Docosanol is not indicated for the treatment of genital herpes. Pregnancy Category B. Excretion in human breast milk is unknown. Adverse effects observed with docosanol were similar to those observed with placebo. Headache and dermatological effects (rash, pruritis, and dry skin) occurred most often.

Administration: Topical.

Patient Care Implications: Use at the first sign of a cold sore or fever blister. Wash hands prior to applying cream. Apply a thin layer, cover entire area and rub until cream completely disappears. Wash hands after applying cream to prevent the spread of the virus.

Preparations: Cream, topical 10% in 2 g tubes.

DOCUSATE CALCIUM—Dioctyl calcium sulfosuccinate, Surfak®

DOCUSATE POTASSIUM—Dioctyl potassium sulfosuccinate

DOCUSATE SODIUM—DSS, Dioctyl sodium sulfosuccinate, Colace®

Description/Actions: Stool softener used in the treatment of constipation due to hard stools.

Preparations: Docusate calcium—Capsules, 50 and 240 mg. Docusate potassium—Capsules, 100 and 240 mg. Docusate sodium—Capsules, 50, 100, and 240 mg. Liquid, 50, 60, and 150 mg/ml and other potencies.

DOFETILIDE—Tikosyn®

Description/Actions: Dofetilide is used for patients in atrial fibrillation/flutter. Used to convert and maintain normal sinus rhythm.

Precautions/Adverse Reactions: Dofetilide can cause a variety of arrhythmias including torsade de pointes and ventricular tachycardia. The drug is contraindicated in patients who already have QT prolongation (QTc > 440 msec), torsade de pointes, renal failure (increases plasma concentration of drug), hypokalemia, and hypomagnesemia because of the increased risk of arrhythmias. Other side effects that can occur are headache, chest pain, and dizziness. Patients taking dofetilide should discontinue breast-feeding and the drug is not proven to be safe in children < 18. Concomitant administration with cimetidine, ketoconazole, megestrol, prochlorperazine, trimethoprim, or verapamil is contraindicated.

Administration: Oral.

Patient Care Implications: Patients starting dofetilide should be kept in a monitored facility where ECG and creatinine clearance can be monitored and cardiac resuscitation can be performed. The dose of dofetilide must be adjusted based on creatinine clearance levels to avoid arrhythmias. Women taking the drug should discontinue breast-feeding and the drug should not be used in children under 18 years of age.

Preparations: Capsule, 125 mcg, 250 mcg, 500 mcg.

DOLASETRON MESYLATE—Anzemet®

Description/Actions: Dolasetron mesylate is indicated in the prevention of nausea and vomiting associated with emetogenic cancer chemotherapy, including initial and repeat courses. Also indicated in the prevention and treatment of post-op nausea and vomiting.

Warnings: Use cautiously in patients at risk of developing prolongation of cardiac conduction intervals, especially Qtc (e.g., congential QT syndrome, hypokalemia, hypomagnesemia). Pregnancy Category B. Not recommended for use in nursing mothers.

Adverse reactions include headache, dizziness, pain, fatigue, diarrhea, tachycardia, and ECG changes.

Administration: Oral and intravenous.

Preparations: Tablets, 50 and 100 mg.

Injection, single use ampules 12.5 mg/ 0.625mL.

Single use vials 100 mg/5 mL.

DOLOBID®, see Diflunisal

DOLOPHINE®, see Methadone

DONEPEZIL HYDROCHLORIDE—Aricept®

Description/Actions: Reversible acetylcholinesterase inhibitor. Indicated in mild to moderate dementia of the Alzheimer's type.

Warnings: Adverse reactions include nausea, diarrhea, insomnia, vomiting, muscle cramps, fatigue and anorexia. Donepezil may have vagotonic effects on the sinoatrial and atrioventricular nodes. This effect may be seen as bradycardia or heart block in patients both with and without known underlying cardiac conduction abnormalities. Syncope and neuroleptic malignant syndrome have also been reported. Monitor for G.I. bleeding, seizures, and asthma.

Administration: Initially 5 mg daily at bedtime; may increase to 10 mg daily at bedtime after 4–6 weeks.

Preparations: Tablets, 5 and 10 mg.

DONNATAL®, Combination of belladonna alkaloids and phenobarbital

DOPAMINE HYDROCHLORIDE— Intropin®

Description/Actions: Inotropic catecholamine indicated for intravenous use in the correction of hemodynamic imbalances present in the shock syndrome due to myocardial infarctions, trauma, endotoxic septicemia, open heart surgery, renal failure, and chronic cardiac decompensation as in congestive failure.

Preparations: Ampules, vials, and syringes, 40, 80, and 160 mg/ml. Bottles (in 5% dextrose), 80, 160, and 320 mg/ 100 ml.

DOPAR®, see Levodopa

DORIGLUTE®, see Glutethimide

DOPRAM®, see Doxapram

DORAL®, see Quazepam

DORNASE ALFA—Pulmozyme®

Agent for cystic fibrosis, mucolytic.

Description/Actions: Is a recombinant form of natural human deoxyribonuclease I (also known as DNase), and contains 260 amino acids in a sequence that is identical to that of the native human enzyme. Is administered by inhalation of an aerosol mist and selectively breaks down extracellular DNA, making the accumulated respiratory secretions less viscous and easier to clear. Indicated for daily use in conjunction with standard therapies, in the management of cystic fibrosis patients to reduce the frequency of respiratory infections requiring parenteral antibiotics, and to improve pulmonary function.

Warnings: Adverse reactions include sore throat, horseness, laryngitis, chest pain, rash, and conjunctivitis.

Administration: Inhalation, using a recommended nebulizer. The drug should not be diluted or mixed with other drugs in the nebulizer.

Preparations: Ampules, 2.5 mg in 2.5 ml of a sterile aqueous solution.

DORYX®, see Doxycycline

DORZOLAMIDE HYDROCHLORIDE—Trusopt®

Antiglaucoma agent.

Description/Actions: Corbonic hydrase inhibitor indicated in the treatment of elevated intraocular pressure in patients with ocular hypertension or open-angle glaucoma.

Warnings: Adverse reactions include ocular burning, stinging, or discomfort and bitter taste following administration. Superficial punctate keratitis, and signs and symptoms of ocular allergic reaction may also occur. Use is not recommended in patients with a creatinine clearance of less than 30 ml/min or concurrently with orally administered carbonic anhydrase inhibitor. Do not administer while wearing soft contact lenses, as the formulation contains benzalkonium chloride as a preservative, which may damage soft contact lenses.

Administration: Ophthalmic. One drop in the affected eye(s) 3 times daily. Administer at least 10 minutes apart from other ophthalmic drugs.

Preparations: Ophthalmic solution, 2%.

DOSTINEX®, see Cabergoline

DOVONEX®, see Calcipotriene

DOXACURIUM CHLORIDE— Nuromax®

Nondepolarizing neuromuscular blocking agent.

Description/Actions: Acts by competing for cholinergic receptors at the motor endplate, resulting in a block of neuromuscular transmission. Has a long duration of action. Indicated as an adjunct to general anesthesia to provide skeletal muscle relaxation during surgery. Also used to provide skeletal muscle relaxation for endotracheal intubation.

Warnings: May cause excessive skeletal muscle weakness resulting in respiratory insufficiency and apnea. Action may be antagonized by neostigmine. Must be used with caution in patients with myasthenia gravis or myasthenic syndrome, and in patients receiving other medications that may increase neuromuscular blockade (e.g., inhalation anesthetics, aminoglycosides, quinidine, magnesium salts).

Administration: Intravenous.

Preparations: Vials, 1 mg/ml.

DOXAPRAM HYDROCHLORIDE—Dopram®

Description/Actions: Respiratory stimulant indicated for intravenous use in the treatment of drug-induced central nervous system depression, chronic pulmonary disease associated with acute hypercapnia, and postanesthesia respiratory depression or apnea other than that due to muscle relaxant drugs.

Precautions/Adverse Reactions: Doxapram should not be used with mechanical ventilation. Pulse oximetry is recommended for assessing oxygenation. Monitor blood pressure, heart rate, and deep tendon reflexes. Doxapram contains the preservative benzyl alcohol, which has been associated with a fatal "gasping syndrome" in neonates; therefore, doxapram is contraindicated in neonates. Anticonvulsants such as intravenous short-acting barbiturates along with oxygen resuscitative equipment should be readily available to manage overdosage.

Preparations: Vials, 20 mg/ml.

DOXAZOSIN MESYLATE— Cardura®

Antihypertensive agent.

Description/Actions: An alpha₁-adrenergic blocking agent that acts on the peripheral vasculature to decrease systemic vascular resistance and lower blood pressure. Indicated for the treatment of hypertension and may be used alone or in combination with a diuretic or beta-adrenergic blocking agent. Also indicated for the treatment of benign prostatic hyperplasia.

Warnings: May cause orthostatic hypotension, resulting in symptoms such as dizziness, lightheadedness, vertigo, and syncope. Orthostatic effects are more common with the first dose (i.e., the "first dose" effect). Treatment should be initiated at a dosage level of 1 mg daily. Patients should be advised of the need to sit or lie down when symptoms of lowered blood pressure occur, and to be careful when rising from a sitting or lying position. Other adverse reactions include edema, fatigue, and somnolence.

Administration: Oral.

Preparations: Tablets, 1, 2, 4, and 8 mg.

DOXEPIN HYDROCHLORIDE—
Sinequan®, Zonalon®

Tricyclic antidepressant and antianxiety agent, and topical antipruritic.

Description/Actions: Indicated in patients with (1) depression and/or anxiety, (2) depression and/or anxiety associated with alcoholism, (3) depression and/or anxiety associated with organic disease, and (4) psychotic depressive disorders with associated anxiety including involutional depression and manic-depressive disorders. Also indicated for the short-term topical management of moderate pruritus in adults with atopic dermatitis and lichen simplex chronicus.

Warnings: Contraindicated in patients with glaucoma or with a tendency to urinary retention. Should not be used in patients being treated with a monoamine oxidase inhibitor. Adverse reactions include CNS effects, and patients should be cautioned regarding activities such as driving and operating machinery, as well as interactions with other CNS-acting drugs including alcohol. Reportedly the most sedating of the tricyclic antidepressants. Other adverse reactions include anticholinergic effects (e.g., dry mouth, blurred vision), GI effects (e.g., nausea, vomiting), and cardiovascular effects (e.g., hypotension).

Administration: Oral and topical.

Preparations: Capsules, 10, 25, 50, 75, 100, and 150 mg. Oral concentrate, 10 mg/ml. Cream, 5%.

DOXERCALCIFEROL—Hectorol®

Description/Actions: Doxercalciferol is a synthetic vitamin D analogue that is used for the treatment of secondary hyperparathyroidism in patients receiving chronic renal dialysis.

Precautions/Adverse Reactions: Doxercalciferol should not be given to patients who are hypercalcemic, hyperphosphatemic, or hypervitaminosis D. Also doxercalciferol's safety has not been determined in children or in breast-feeding women. Patients with hepatic failure should be monitored closely. Some common side effects are edema, headache, malaise, nausea/vomiting, dizziness, dyspnea, confusion, constipation, increase thirst, and sinus bradycardia. Also, long-term use of the drug can lead to hypercalcemia, hyperphosphatemia, and ectopic calcifications.

Administration: Oral.

Patient Care Implications: Patients on the medication should be monitored weekly for PTH levels and calcium-phosphorus product. Also, patients should restrict intake of other vitamin D products while on the medication. Doxercalciferol should not be given to children, breast-feeding women, and pregnant women. Also, hepatic impairment patients should be monitored closely.

Preparations: Tablet, 2.5 mcg.

DOXORUBICIN HYDROCHLORIDE—
Adriamycin PFS®, Adriamycin RDF®, Rubex®

Description/Actions: Antineoplastic agent indicated for intravenous use in the treatment of a number of neoplastic disorders such as acute lymphoblastic leukemia, acute myeloblastic leukemia, Wilms' tumor, neuroblastoma, soft tissue and bone sarcomas, breast carcinoma, ovarian carcinoma, transitional cell bladder carcinoma, thyroid carcinoma, lymphomas of both Hodgkin and non-Hodgkin types, and bronchogenic carcinoma. Serious, irreversible myocardial toxicity with delayed CHF, ventricular arrhythmias and acute left ventricular failure may occur with use of this agent. Follow vesicant precautions for IV administration.

Preparations: Vials, 10, 20, and 50 mg.

DOXYCYCLINE CALCIUM—
Vibramycin®

Preparations: Syrup, 50 mg/5 ml.

DOXYCYCLINE HYCLATE—
Doryx®, Vibramycin®, Vibra-Tabs®, Periostat®

Tetracycline antibiotic.

Description/Actions: Active against many gram-positive and gram-negative bacteria, mycoplasmal, chlamydial, and rickettsial organisms, and certain spirochetes. Indicated in the treatment of respiratory tract infections, urinary tract infections, sexually transmitted infections, and a number of other types of infections. Effective in the treatment of infections caused by *Chlamydia trachomatis* and *Ureaplasma urealyticum.* Also indicated for prophylaxis of malaria due to *Plasmodium falciparum* in short-term travelers (less than 4 months) to areas with chloroquine or pyrimethamine-sulfadoxine resistant strains.

Warnings: Use is best avoided during the last half of pregnancy and in childhood to the age of 8 years because of the risk of discoloration of the teeth. Other adverse reactions include nausea, vomiting, diarrhea, rash, and fungal superinfections. May cause photosensitivity reactions and patients should be cautioned to limit their exposure to sunlight and ultraviolet light. Absorption may be reduced by the simultaneous administration of antacids.

Administration: Oral and intravenous. May be administered orally without regard to meals.

Preparations: Tablets, 20 mg. Capsules and tablets, 50 and 100 mg. Delayed-release capsules, 100 mg. Oral suspension, 25 mg/5 ml., and 50 mg/5 ml. Vials, 100 and 200 mg.

DOXYCYCLINE MONOHYDRATE—Monodox®, Vibramycin®

Preparations: Capsules, 100 mg. Powder for oral suspension, 25 mg/5 ml when reconstituted.

DOXYLAMINE SUCCINATE—
Unisom®

Description/Actions: Antihistamine and hypnotic. Primarily used for the treatment of insomnia.

Preparations: Tablets, 25 mg.

DRAMAMINE®, see Dimenhydrinate

DRISDOL®, see Ergocalciferol

DRONABINOL—Marinol®

Antiemetic and appetite stimulant.

Description/Actions: Is the principal psychoactive substance in marijuana. Indicated for the treatment of nausea and vomiting associated with cancer chemotherapy in patients who have failed to respond adequately to conventional antiemetic treatments. Also indicated for the treatment of anorexia associated with weight loss in patients with AIDS.

Warnings: Can produce physical and psychological dependence and is included in Schedule II of the Controlled Substances Act. CNS adverse reactions include drowsiness, dizziness, impairment of coordination, easy laughing, elation, hallucinations, and brief psychotic reactions.

Administration: Oral.

Preparations: Capsules, 2.5, 5, and 10 mg.

DROPERIDOL—Inapsine®

Description/Actions: Droperidol is indicated to reduce the incidence of nausea and vomiting associated with surgical and diagnostic procedures. It is not recommended for any other use other than for the treatment of perioperative nausea and vomiting in patients for whom other treatments are ineffective or inappropriate.

Precautions/Adverse Reactions: Droperidol is contraindicated in patients with a known hypersensitivity to any component of the formulation. It is contraindicated in patients with a known or suspected QT prolongation (QT$_c$ interval greater than 440 msec for males or 450 msec for females), including patients with congenital long QT syndrome. Cases of QT prolongation and serious arrhythmias (torsades de pointes, ventricular arrhythmias, cardiac arrest, and death) have been reported in patients receiving droperidol at doses at or below recommended doses. Some cases have occurred in patients with no known risk factors for QT prolongation. A dose-dependent prolongation of the QT interval has been observed in clinical trials. Droperidol should be administered with extreme caution to patients who may be at risk for development of prolonged QT syndrome, for example, congestive heart failure, bradycardia, use of a diuretic, cardiac hypertrophy, hypokalemia, hypomagnesemia, or administration of other drugs known to increase the QT interval. Other risk factors may include age > 65, alcohol abuse, and use of agents such as benzodiazepines, volatile anesthetics, and IV opiates. Droperidol should be initiated at a low dose and adjusted upward with caution to achieve the desired effect. All patients should undergo a 12—lead ECG prior to administration of droperidol to determine if a prolonged QT interval is present. If there is a prolonged QT interval, droperidol should not be used. For patients in whom the potential benefit of droperidol treatment outweighs the potential risks of serious arrhythmias, ECG monitoring should be performed prior to treatment and continued for 2–3 hours after completing treatment to monitor for arrhythmias. Droperidol should not be administered with drugs known to prolong the QT interval, such as class I or class III antiarrhythmics, antihistamines that prolong the QT interval, antimalarials, calcium channel blockers, neuroleptics that prolong the QT interval, and antidepressants. Exercise caution when using droperidol with drugs known to induce hypokalemia or hypomagnesemia (diuretics, laxatives, supraphysiological use of steroid hormones with mineralocorticoid potential) as they may precipitate QT prolongation. Concomitant administration of droperidol and central nervous system depressant drugs, such as barbiturates, tranquilizers, opioids, and general anesthetics, requires a reduction in the dose of the CNS depressant drug.

Administration: Adult dose: The maximum recommended initial dose of droperidol is 2.5 mg IM or slow IV. Additional 1.25 mg of droperidol may be administered to achieve the desired effect. Additional doses should be administered with caution. Pediatric dose (children 2–12 years of age): The maximum recommended dose of droperidol is 0.1 mg/kg. Additional doses should be administered with caution only if potential benefit outweighs the potential risk.

Patient Care Implications: ECG monitoring prior to treatment and continued for 2–3 hours after completing treatment to monitor for arrhythmias. Physicians should be alert to palpitations, syncope, or other symptoms suggestive of episodes of irregular cardiac rhythm and promptly evaluate these patients. Monitor vital signs. Fluids and other countermeasures to manage hypotension should be readily available.

Preparations: Ampules and vials 2.5 mg/ml.

DROTRECOGIN ALFA—XIGRIS™

Description/Actions: Drotrecogin alfa (activated) is indicated for the reduction of mortality in adult patients with severe sepsis (sepsis associated with acute organ dysfunction) who have a high risk of death (e.g., APACHE II score ≥ 25).

Precautions/Adverse Reactions: Drotrecogin alfa is contraindicated in anyone with a known hypersensitivity to it or to any component of the formulation. Drotrecogin alfa increases the risk of bleeding; therefore, it is contraindicated in patients with the following clinical situations in which bleeding could be associated with a high risk of death or significant morbidity: active internal bleeding, recent (within 3 months) hemorrhagic stroke, recent (within 2 months) intracranial or intraspinal surgery or severe head trauma, trauma with an increased risk of life-threatening bleeding, presence of an epiduralcatheter, intracranial neoplasm or mass lesion, or evidence of cerebral herniation.

Xigris™ may prolong the activated partial thromboplastin time (aPTT); therefore, its use to access the status of the coagulopathy during drotrecogin alfa infusion is not reliable.

The most common adverse reaction associated with the use of drotrecogin alfa is bleeding. Bleeding may occur from any site. Some common sites include gastrointestinal, intraabdominal, intrathoracic, retroperitoneal, intracranial, genitourinary, and skin/soft tissue (patients requiring the administration of ≥ 3 units of packed red blood cells per day for 2 consecutive days without an identified site of bleeding). There is no known antidote for drotrecogin alfa. In cases of overdose, stop the infusion and monitor closely for hemorrhagic complications.

Administration: Intravenous.

Patient Care Implications: Monitor patient for bleeding. Xigris should be administered via a dedicated line. The only solutions that can be administered through the same line are 0.9% sodium chloride injection lactated Ringer's injection, dextrose, or dextrose and saline mixtures.

Preparations: Powder for injection (preservative-free), 5 and 20 mg.

DTIC®, see Dacarbazine

DULCOLAX® see Bisacodyl

DURABOLIN®, see Nandrolone

DURAGESIC®, see Fentanyl

DURALUTIN®, see Hydroxyprogesterone

DURAMORPH®, see Morphine

DURANEST®, see Etidocaine

DURICEF®, see Cefadroxil

DUTASTERIDE—AVODART™

Description/Actions: Dutasteride is indicated for the treatment of symptomatic benign prostatic hyperplasia in men with enlarged prostates 18 years of age or older.

Precautions/Adverse Reactions: Dutasteride is contraindicated for use in women and children. Pregnancy Category X. Because it is absorbed through the skin, handling of the drug should be avoided by any pregnant woman.

Preclinical data suggest that the suppression of circulating levels of DHT may inhibit the development of the external genital organs in a male fetus carried by a woman exposed to dutasteride. Other urological diseases including cancer should be ruled out before starting therapy. Use caution in hepatic impairment and with the concurrent use of potent chronic CYP3A3/4 inhibitors. Dutasteride is not indicated for use in the pediatric population; safety and efficacy have not been established in this population. Most common adverse reaction was sexual dysfunction. This may include impotence, decreased libido, ejaculation disorders, and gynecomastia.

Administration: Oral.

Patient Care Implications: May be taken with or without food. Capsule should be swallowed whole. Dutasteride is a soft gelatin capsule that may become soft and leak or stick to other capsules if kept at high temperatures. Store at room temperature. If capsules are cracked or leaking, do not use them. Do not donate blood for at least 6 months after last dose to prevent administration of dutasteride to a pregnant transfusion recipient. A new baseline PSA concentration should be established after 3–6 months of treatment. Results may take several months.

Preparations: Capsules, soft gelatin, 0.5 mg.

DYAZIDE®, Combination of triamterene and hydrochlorothiazide

DYCILL®, see Dicloxacillin

DYCLONE®, see Dyclonine

DYCLONINE HYDROCHLORIDE—Dyclone®

Description/Actions: Local anesthetic used primarily for anesthetizing mucous membranes (e.g., mouth, pharynx) prior to endoscopic procedures. Also used to suppress gag reflex, to relieve pain of minor burns or trauma, and to alleviate itching of pruritis ani or vulvae.

Preparations: Topical solution, 0.5% and 1%.

DYFLEX®, see Dyphylline

DYLLINE®, see Dyphylline

DYMELOR®, see Acetohexamide

DYNABAC®, see Dirithromycin

DynaCirc®, see Isradipine

DYNAPEN®, see Dicloxacillin

DYPHYLLINE—Dilor®, Dyflex®, Dylline®, Lufyllin®, Neothylline, Thylline

Description/Actions: Bronchodilator related to theophylline. Indicated for relief of acute bronchial asthma and for reversible bronchospasm associated with chronic bronchitis and emphysema.

Preparations: Tablets, 200 and 400 mg. Elixir, 33.3 mg/5 ml, 53.3 mg/5 ml, and 100 mg/15 ml. Injection, 250 mg/ml.

DYRENIUM®, see Triamterene

E

EASPRIN®, see Aspirin

ECHOTHIOPHATE IODIDE—Phospholine iodide®

Description/Actions: Antiglaucoma agent, Cholinesterase inhibitor indicated for ophthalmic use in the treatment of glaucoma and accommodative esotropia. Use is usually reserved for patients not satisfactorily controlled by less potent miotics.

Preparations: For ophthalmic solution, 1.5 mg (0.03%), 3 mg (0.06%), 6.25 mg (0.125%), and 12.5 mg (0.25%) when reconstituted.

EC-NAPROSYN®, see Naproxen

ECONAZOLE NITRATE—
Spectazole®

Description/Actions: Imidazole antifungal agent indicated for topical use in the treatment of tinea pedis, tinea cruris, tinea corporis, cutaneous candidiasis, and tinea versicolor.

Preparations: Cream, 1%.

ECOTRIN®, see Aspirin

EDECRIN®, see Ethacrynic acid

EDETATE CALCIUM DISODIUM—EDTA, Calcium EDTA, Calcium disodium Versenate®

Description/Actions: Antidote indicated in the parenteral management of acute and chronic lead poisoning and lead encephalopathy.

Preparations: Ampules, 200 mg/ml.

EDETATE DISODIUM—Disotate®, Disodium EDTA®, Endrate®

Description/Actions: Indicated in selected patients for the emergency treatment of hypercalcemia and for the control of ventricular arrhythmias associated with digitalis toxicity.

Preparations: Ampules and vials, 150 mg/ml.

EDEX®, see Alprostadil

EDROPHONIUM CHLORIDE—
Enlon®, Tensilon®, Reversol®

Description/Actions: Cholinesterase inhibitor administered parenterally for the differential diagnosis of myasthenia gravis and as an adjunct in the evaluation of treatment requirements in this disease. Also useful when a curare antagonist is needed to reverse the neuromuscular block produced by tubocurarine and related agents.

Preparations: Ampules and vials, 10 mg/ml.

EDTA, see Edetate calcium disodium

EES®, see Erythromycin ethylsuccinate

EFAVIRENZ—Sustiva®

Description/Actions: Indicated for use in combination with other antiretroviral agents for the treatment of HIV-1 infection. Efavirenz should always be initiated in combination with one other antiretroviral agent to which the patient has not already been exposed.

Precautions/Adverse Reactions: Contraindicated with several other drugs. Prescribers should verify the patient's drug profile before adding this drug. Use cautiously in patients with CNS disturbances and hepatic dysfunction. Monitor liver function and lipid levels in patients with hepatitis. Discontinue the medication if severe rash (with blistering, desquamation, mucosal involvement or fever) occurs. Exclude pregnancy before starting.

Adverse reactions include CNS/psychiatric effects (e.g. insomnia, drowsiness, dizziness, depression, abnormal thinking, impaired concentration, confusion, abnormal dreaming), rash (possibly severe; e.g., Stevens-Johnson, erythema multiforme), GI upset, fever, and cough.

Administration: Oral.

Patient Care Implications: Administer at bedtime for the first 2 weeks to minimize CNS effects. May be taken without regard to food, but avoid taking with a high fat meal. Instruct patients to use appropriate barrier precautions and contraceptives when engaging in sexual intercourse as this medication controls but does not cure HIV.

Preparations: Capsules, 50, 100, and 200 mg. Tablets, 600 mg.

EFEDRON®, see Ephedrine

EFFEXOR®, see Venlafaxine hydrochloride

EFFEXOR® XR, see Venlafaxine hydrochloride

EFIDAC/24®, see Pseudoephedrine hydrochloride

EFLORNITHINE (Topical)—Vaniqa™

Description/Actions: Vaniqa™ is a topical skin product indicated for the reduction of unwanted facial hair and hair in or on adjacent areas under the chin in women.

Precautions/Adverse Reactions: Usage is contraindicated in patients with a hypersensitivity to eflornithine or any component of the formulation. Discontinue if hypersensitivity occurs. For external use only; not for ophthalmic, oral, or intravaginal use. Pregnancy Category C. There are no adequate and well-controlled studies of topical eflornithine cream in pregnant women. The potential risks to the fetus versus the benefit of the medication to the mother should be considered before use. Excretion into breast milk is unknown; exercise caution when administering to nursing women. Safety and efficacy in children < 12 years have not been established.

Some adverse effects (topical): acne, pseudofolliculitis barbe, headache, dizziness, vertigo, pruritus, burning skin, tingling skin, dry skin, skin irritation, and dyspepsia.

Administration: Topical.

Patient Care Implications: Patients should be informed of the following:

1. This medication is not a depilatory, but appears to retard hair growth to improve appearance. Patients will likely need to continue using a hair removal method in conjunction with Vaniqa™.

2. Onset of improvement was seen after as little as 4–8 weeks of treatment; the condition may return to pretreatment levels 8 weeks after cessation of treatment.

3. If skin irritation develops, direct the patient to temporarily reduce the frequency of application (i.e., once daily); if irritation persists, discontinue therapy.

Preparations: Topical cream: 13.9% (30 g) tube.

EFUDEX®, see Fluorouracil

ELAVIL®, see Amitriptyline

ELASE®, see Fibrinolysin

ELDEPRYL®, see Selegiline

ELDOQUIN®, see Hydroquinone

ELIDEL®, see Pimecrolimus

ELIMITE®, see Permethrin

ELIXOPHYLLIN®, see Theophylline

ELLENCE®, see Epirubicin

ELMIRON®, see Pentosan Polysulfate Sodium

ELOCON®, see Mometasone furoate

ELSPAR®, see Asparaginase

ELTROXINE®, see Levothyroxine

EMCYT®, see Estramustine

EMINASE®, see Anistreplase

EMKO®, see Nonoxynol 9

EMLA®

Description/Actions: Eutectic mixture of local anesthetics (lidocaine and prilocaine) that is applied topically.

Warnings: Use on normal intact skin. Contraindicated in methemoglobinemia. Not recommended for use in infants < 37 weeks gestational age.

Administration: Apply thick layer of cream over selected site 1 hour prior to routine procedures and 2 hours prior to painful procedures. Cover with an occlusive dressing. Prior to procedure remove cream and cleanse area with antiseptic.

Preparations: Topical cream and disk.

EMLA CREAM®, see Lidocaine and Prilocaine Cream

E-MYCIN®, see Erythromycin base

E-MYCIN 333®, see Erythromycin base

ENALAPRIL/ HYDROCHLOROTHIAZIDE— Vaseretic®

Description/Actions: Enalapril and hydrochlorothiazide are combined in an oral formulation for the treatment of hypertension. The extent of blood pressure reduction with the combination of these drugs is approximately additive.

Precautions/Adverse Reactions: Thiazide diuretics, such as hydrochlorothiazide, are contraindicated in patients with sulfonamide hypersensitivity or thiazide diuretic hypersensitivity because of the risk of cross-sensitivity. Enalapril is contraindicated in patients with a history of ACE inhibitor-induced, hereditary, or idiopathic angioedema. Enalapril/ hydrochlorothiazide should be used with caution in patients with hypotension, hepatic disease, renal artery stenosis, gout, diabetes mellitus, pregnancy, pancreatitis, SLE, and potassium imbalances. Adverse effects include dizziness, headache, fatigue, cough, muscle cramps, nausea/vomiting, asthenia, impotence, and diarrhea.

Administration: Oral.

Preparations: Tablets, 5/12.5 mg and 10/25 mg.

ENALAPRIL MALEATE—Vasotec®

Antihypertensive agent and agent for treatment of heart failure.

Description/Actions: Is a prodrug that, after oral administration, is hydrolyzed to enalaprilat, a potent angiotensin converting enzyme (ACE) inhibitor. Indicated for the treatment of hypertension and as adjunctive therapy in the management of heart failure, in patients who are not responding adequately to diuretics and digitalis. Also indicated for clinically stable asymptomatic patients with left ventricular dysfunction.

Warnings: Angioedema has occurred infrequently, sometimes after the first dose. Adverse reactions include headache, dizziness, fatigue, cough, proteinuria, and hyperkalemia. Excessive hypotension may occur, particularly in patients with severe salt/ volume depletion (e.g., those being treated vigorously with diuretics). Use during pregnancy should be avoided. Nonsteroidal anti-inflammatory drugs may diminish the antihypertensive effect of ACE inhibitors.

Administration: Oral.

Preparations: Tablets, 2.5, 5, 10, and 20 mg.

ENALAPRILAT—Vasotec IV®, see discussion of enalapril.

Administration: Intravenous.

Preparations: Vials, 1.25 mg/ml.

ENDRATE®, see Edetate disodium

ENDURON®, see Methyclothiazide

ENFLURANE—Ethrane®

Description/Actions: General anesthetic administered by inhalation in the induction and maintenance of general anesthesia.

Preparations: Bottles, 125 and 250 ml.

ENLON®, see Edrophonium

ENOXACIN—Penetrex®

Fluoroquinolone anti-infective agent.

Description/Actions: Inhibits DNA gyrase, an essential bacterial enzyme, and exhibits a bactericidal action against many gram-positive and gram-negative bacteria. Indicated for urinary tract infections caused by susceptible organisms. Also indicated for uncomplicated urethral or cervical gonorrhea.

Warnings: Contraindicated in patients with a known hypersensitivity to any of the fluoroquinolones or the related quinolone antibacterial agents (i.e., nalidixic acid, cinoxacin). Fluoroquinolones have caused erosion of cartilage in weight-bearing joints and other signs of arthropathy in juvenile animals, and use in children under 18, pregnant women, and women who are nursing is best avoided. Adverse reactions include nausea and/or vomiting, abdominal pain, diarrhea, dyspepsia, dizziness, and headache. Because of the possibility of photosensitivity reactions, patients should be advised to avoid excessive sunlight and artificial ultraviolet light during the period of treatment. May cause dizziness, lightheadedness, and other central nervous system effects, and patients should know how they tolerate the drug before they engage in activities that require mental alertness and coordination.

Administration: Oral. Should be administered at least 1 hour before or 2 hours after a meal.

Preparations: Tablets, 200 and 400 mg.

ENOXAPARIN—Lovenox®

Antithrombotic agent.

Description/Actions: Is a low molecular weight heparin fraction that is prepared by the degradation of heparin benzyl ester derived from porcine intestinal mucosa. Does not significantly influence platelet aggregation or the plasma fibrinogen concentration, and does not affect global blood clotting tests [i.e., prothrombin time (PT) or activated partial thromboplastin time (APTT)]. Enoxaparin is indicated for the prophylaxis of deep vein thrombosis, which may lead to pulmonary embolism in patients undergoing abdominal surgery, in patients undergoing hip replacement surgery, and for the prophylaxis of ischemic complications of unstable angina and non-Q-wave myocardial infarction when concurrently administered with aspirin. Enoxaparin is indicated for the inpatient treatment of acute deep vein thrombosis with or without pulmonary embolism when administered with warfarin and for the outpatient treatment of acute deep vein thrombosis without pulmonary embolism when administered with warfarin and for the prevention of deep vein thrombosis in patients at risk due to severely restricted mobility during acute illness.

Warnings: Contraindicated in patients who are hypersensitive to the drug, heparin, or pork products. Also contraindicated in patients with active major bleeding and in patients with thrombocytopenia associated with a positive in vitro test for antiplatelet antibody in the presence of enoxaparin. May cause bleeding episodes although the incidence of such reactions was similar to that with placebo in the clinical studies. Should be used with extreme caution in patients with conditions that are associated with an increased risk of hemorrhage (e.g., congenital or acquired bleeding disorders, active ulceration or a history of recent gastrointestinal ulceration and hemorrhage, uncontrolled arterial hypertension, and hemorrhagic stroke). Cases of epidural or spinal hematomas have been reported with the use of enoxaparin injection and spinal/

epidural anesthesia or spinal puncture resulting in long-term or permanent paralysis. The use of enoxaparin is not recommended for thromboprophylaxis in patients with prosthetic heart valves. Cases of prosthetic heart valve thrombosis have been reported in patients with prosthetic valves who have received enoxaparin for thromboprophylaxis. May cause thrombocytopenia. Periodic complete blood counts, including platelet count, and stool occult blood tests should be conducted during the course of treatment with enoxaparin.

Administration: Subcutaneous injection.

Preparations: Prefilled syringes, 30, 40, 60, 80, 100, 120, and 150 mg.

ENTACAPONE—Comtan®

Descriptions/Actions: Entacapone is used with levodopa/carbidopa in the treatment of Parkinson's disease.

Precautions/Adverse Reactions: Entacapone should be given with caution to patients with hepatic impairment, biliary obstruction, hypotension, and syncope. Also, the safety is questionable in pregnant women, breast-feeding women, and children. Some common adverse effects are dyskinesia, nausea/vomiting, hyperkinesia, diarrhea, brownish-orange urine, hypokinesia, rhabdomyolysis, orthostatic hypotension, and dizziness. Entacapone should not be discontinued abruptly because neuroleptic malignant syndrome could occur.

Administration: Oral.

Patient Care Implications: Patients with hepatic impairment or biliary obstruction may need dosage adjustments. The safety of the drug is not proven in pregnant women, children, or breast-feeding women. The drug should not be discontinued abruptly.

Preparations: Tablet, 200 mg.

ENTEX LA®, Combination of phenylephrine and guaifenesin

ENVISAN®, see Dextranomer

EPHEDRINE HYDROCHLORIDE—Efedron®

Description/Actions: Nasal decongestant often used in combination with other agents. See also pseudoephedrine. Has also been used as a central nervous system stimulant to counteract the depressant effect of certain other agents with which it may be used in combination.

Preparations: Capsules, 25 and 50 mg.

EPHEDRINE SULFATE

Description/Actions: Pressor agent administered parenterally in the management of hypotensive states.

Preparations: Ampules, 25 and 50 mg/ml.

EPI E-Z PEN®, see Epinephrine

EPINEPHRINE—Adrenalin®, Bronkaid mist®, Epinephrine Pediatric®, Epi E-Z Pen®, Epipen AutoInjector®, Primatene Mist Suspension®

Description/Actions: Sympathomimetic agent used to relieve respiratory distress due to bronchospasm, to provide rapid relief of hypersensitivity reactions to drugs and other allergens, to restore cardiac rhythm in cardiac arrest due to various causes, and to prolong the action of infiltration anesthetics. Also used in the treatment of mucosal congestion of hay fever and rhinitis, to relieve bronchial asthmatic paroxysms, for symptomatic relief of serum sickness, urticaria, and angioneurotic edema, for the management of glaucoma and other ocular conditions, and selected other disorders.

Preparations: Ampules and vials (as the hydrochloride), 1:1000, 1:10,000, and 1:100,000. Solution for nebulization (as the hydrochloride), 1.25% and 2.25%. Aerosol, 0.2 and 0.27 mg per spray. Aerosol (as the bitartrate), 0.16 mg per spray. Solution for nasal administration (as the hydrochloride), 0.1%. Ophthalmic solution (as the bitartrate, borate, and hydrochloride), 0.1%, 0.25%, 0.5%, 1%, and 2%. Autoinjector syringes, 0.3 mg and 0.15 mg.

EPIPEN AUTOINJECTOR®—see Epinephrine

EPIRUBICIN—Ellence®

Description/Actions: Epirubicin is used as adjuvant treatment in patients with node positive breast cancer.

Precautions/Adverse Reactions: Epirubicin dosage has to be adjusted in patients with hepatic impairment and renal impairment. Epirubicin should not be administered to patients with neutropenia, thrombocytopenia, pregnant women, and breast-feeding women. The drug should be administered carefully in patients with cardiac disease. Some side effects are bone marrow suppression, cardiotoxicity, alopecia, nausea, vomiting, urine discoloration, skin ulcers, tissue necrosis, and anorexia.

Administration: Intravenous.

Patient Care Implications: Patients with hepatic disease and renal disease need dosage adjustment. CBC with differential, echocardiogram, LFTs, MUGA, bilirubin, and creatinine should be checked before initiation of drug and monitored during therapy.

Preparations: Vials, 50 mg/25 ml, 200 mg/100 ml.

EPIVIR®—see Lamivudine

EPO, see Epoetin alfa

EPOETIN ALFA—EPO, Epogen®, Procrit®

Agent for anemia.

Description/Actions: Also known as recombinant human erythropoietin or EPO. Stimulates red blood cell production in anemic patients decreasing the need for transfusions in these patients. Indicated in the treatment for anemia associated with chronic renal failure, management of anemia secondary to zidovudine therapy (AZT) in HIV-infected patients, and the management of anemia from chemotherapy in patients with nonmyeloid malignancies.

Warnings: Contraindicated in patients with uncontrolled hypertension. Adverse reactions include hypertension, headache, arthralgias, nausea, vomiting, diarrhea, and seizures. For patients who respond to epoetin alfa with a rapid increase in hematocrit (e.g., more than 4 points in any 2-week period), the dose should be decreased to reduce the risk of hypertension. Because of the risk of seizures, patients should be cautioned to avoid potentially hazardous activities such as driving or operating machinery. During hemodialysis, patients treated with epoetin alfa may require increased anticoagulation with heparin to prevent clotting of the artificial kidney.

Administration: Intravenous or subcutaneous. The vials should not be shaken as shaking may denature the glycoprotein, rendering it biologically inactive.

Preparations: Vials, 2000, 3000, 4000, 10,000, and 40,000 units.

EPOGEN®, see Epoetin alfa

EPOPROSTENOL—Flolan®, Prostacyclin®, Prostaglandin 12 (PG 12)®, Prostaglandin X (PGX)®

Prostaglandin, vasodilator.

Description/Actions: Directly dilates pulmonary and systemic arterial vasculature. Also inhibits platelet aggregation. Indicated in the management of primary pulmonary hypertension in selected patients.

116 • EPTIFIBATIDE

Warnings: Side effects include headache, anxiety, dizziness, tachycardia, nausea, vomiting, flushing, myalgia, hypesthesia, hyperesthesia/paresthesia, and flulike symptoms. Dosage adjustments may be necessary in geriatric patients. Unless contraindicated concurrent anticoagulant therapy is usually administered to decrease the risk of pulmonary or systemic embolism.

Administration: Intravenously via continuous infusion.

Preparations: Powder for injection, 0.5 mg and 1.5 mg vials.

EPTIFIBATIDE—Integrilin®

Description/Actions: Platelet aggregation inhibitor indicated in combination with heparin for treating acute coronary syndrome (unstable angina/non Q-wave myocardial infarction) including patients who are to be managed medically and those undergoing percutaneous transluminal angioplasty or artherectomy.

Warnings: Contraindicated in the following conditions within previous 30 days: active internal bleeding, bleeding diathesis, stroke, major surgery, or severe trauma. Contraindicated with a history of intracranial hemorrhage, intracranial neoplasm, arteriovenous malformation, aneurysm, hemorrhagic stroke, thrombocytopenia after previous Integrilin therapy, symptoms or findings suggestive of aortic dissection, severe hypertension, acute pericarditis, and concomitant parenteral GI 11b/111A inhibitor.

Use cautiously in patients with renal failure, platelet count < 150,000/mm³ or hemorrhagic retinopathy. Properly care for femoral artery access site to minimize bleeding. Minimize other arterial and venous punctures, IM injections, catheter use, and other invasive procedures to minimize bleeding risk. Avoid use of noncompressible IV access sites. Do baseline platelet counts, hemoglobin, hematocrit, and monitor during therapy. Discontinue Integrilin if confirmed thrombocytopenia occurs. Adjust heparin to maintain aPTT at 2 times control.

Adverse reactions include bleeding decreased hemoglobin and/or hematocrit, reduced platelet counts, edema, vasovagal reaction, and others.

Administration: Intravenous.

Preparations: Vials, 2 mg/ml (10 ml for bolus dose).

Vials, 0.75 mg/ml (100 ml for infusion).

EQUALACTIN®, see Polycarbophil

EQUANIL®, see Meprobamate

ERGAMISOL®, see Levamisole

ERGOCALCIFEROL—Vitamin D₂, Drisdol®

Description/Actions: A form of vitamin D indicated in the treatment of rickets, familial hypophosphatemia, hypoparathyroidism, osteomalacia, anticonvulsant-induced rickets, osteoporosis, and renal osteodystrophy.

Preparations: Capsules, 25,000 and 50,000 IU. Liquid, 8000 IU/ml. Ampules, 500,000 IU/ml and 500,000 IU/5 ml.

ERGOLOID MESYLATES— Hydergine®

Description/Actions: Ergot derivatives indicated in patients over 60 years of age who manifest signs and symptoms of an idiopathic decline in mental capacity (i.e., cognitive and interpersonal skills, mood).

Preparations: Sublingual tablets, 0.5 and 1 mg. Capsules (liquid) and tablets, 1 mg. Liquid, 1 mg/ml.

ERGOMETRINE, see Ergonovine

ERGONOVINE MALEATE— Ergometrine®, Ergotrate®

Description/Actions: Ergot derivative indicated for the prevention and treatment of postpartum and postabortal hemorrhage due to uterine atony.

Preparations: Tablets, 0.2 mg. Ampules, 0.2 mg/ml.

ERGOSTAT®, see Ergotamine

ERGOTAMINE TARTRATE—
Ergostat®

Description/Actions: Ergot derivative indicated to abort or prevent vascular headache such as migraine and cluster.

Preparations: Sublingual tablets, 2 mg, tablets, 1 mg.

ERGOTRATE®, see Ergonovine

ERTAPENEM—INVANZ™

Description/Actions: Ertapenem is indicated in adults for treatment of moderate to severe infections caused by susceptible strains of gram-positive and gram-negative aerobic and anaerobic organisms.

Precautions/Adverse Reactions: Contraindicated in patients with a known hypersensitivity to lidocaine or other amide-type anesthetics. Serious and fatal anaphylactic reactions noted in patients receiving therapy with betalactams. These reactions are more likely to occur in individuals with a history of sensitivity to multiple allergens. Seizures have occurred most commonly in patients with CNS disorders and/or compromised renal function. Prolonged use of ertapenem may result in pseudomembranous colitis that may range in severity from mild to life threatening. Pregnancy Category B. There are no well-controlled studies in pregnant women. Use only if clearly needed. Ertapenem is excreted in breast milk. Most common adverse reactions were diarrhea, infused vein complication, nausea, headache, constipation, increased platelet count, and elevated hepatic enzymes.

Administration: Intravenous, intramuscular.

Patient Care Implications: Avoid inadvertent injection of intramuscular preparation into intravenous line. The reconstituted solution, after immediately being diluted in NS, may be stored at room temperature (25° C) and used within 6 hours or stored for 24 hours under refrigeration (5° C) and used within 4 hours after removal from refrigeration. Solutions should not be frozen.

Preparations: Sterile lyophilized powder for injection, 1 g ertapenem.

ERYC®, see Erythromycin base

ERYCETTE®, see Erythromycin base (topical)

ERYDERM®, see Erythromycin base (topical)

ERYGEL®, see Erythromycin base (topical)

ERYMAX®, see Erythromycin base (topical)

ERYPED®, see Erythromycin ethylsuccinate

ERY-TAB®, see Erythromycin base

ERYTHRITYL TETRANITRATE—
Cardilate®

Description/Actions: Antianginal agent indicated for the prophylaxis and treatment of patients with frequent or recurrent anginal pain.

Preparations: Oral/sublingual tablets, 10 mg.

ERYTHROMYCIN BASE—E-Mycin®, E-Mycin 333®, Ery-Tab®, Ilotycin®, Robimycin®, ERYC®, PCE®

Macrolide antibiotic.

ERYTHROMYCIN BASE

Description/Actions: Active against most gram-positive and a number of gram-negative bacteria, mycoplasmal and chlamydial organisms, and certain spirochetes. Indicated in the treatment of respiratory tract and a number of other types of infections. Effective in the treatment of primary atypical pneumonia, legionnaires' disease, infections caused by *Chlamydia trachomatis* and *Ureaplasma urealyticum,* and GI infections caused by *Campylobacter jejuni.* Used with neomycin for prophylaxis in colorectal surgery.

Warnings: Adverse reactions include nausea, vomiting, abdominal cramps, and hepatic dysfunction (primarily associated with the use of the estolate). Should not be used concurrently with terfenadine or astemizole.

Administration: Oral. Some formulations may be administered without regard to meals whereas others should be administered apart from meals. Labeling for individual product should be consulted.

Preparations: Enteric-coated tablets, 250, 333, and 500 mg. Capsules with enteric-coated pellets (ERYC), 125 and 250 mg. Tablets with polymer-coated particles (PCE), 333 and 500 mg. Film-coated tablets, 250 and 500 mg.

ERYTHROMYCIN BASE (for topical use)—Akne-mycin®, Erycette®, EryDerm®, Erygel®, Erymax®, Staticin®

Description/Actions: Antibiotic for the topical treatment of acne.

Administration: Topical.

Preparations: Solution, 1.5% and 2%. Gel, 2%.

ERYTHROMYCIN ESTOLATE—Ilosone®

See discussion of erythromycin base.

Administration: Oral. May be administered without regard to meals.

Preparations: Capsules, 250 mg. Tablets, 500 mg. Suspension, 125 and 250 mg/5 ml.

ERYTHROMYCIN ETHYLSUCCINATE—EES®,EryPed®

See discussion of erythromycin base.

Administration: Oral. May be administered without regard to meals.

Preparations: Suspension, 200 and 400 mg/5 ml. Powder for oral suspension, 200 and 400 mg/5 ml when reconstituted. Tablets, 400 mg. Chewable tablets, 200 mg.

ERYTHROMYCIN GLUCEPTATE—Ilotycin gluceptate®

See discussion of erythromycin base.

Administration: Intravenous. Pain, discomfort, and phlebitis may be associated with IV administration.

Preparations: Vials, 250 and 500 mg, 1 g.

ERYTHROMYCIN LACTOBIONATE

See discussion of erythromycin base.

Administration: Intravenous. Pain, discomfort, and phlebitis may be associated with IV administration.

Preparations: Vials, 500 mg, 1 g.

ERYTHROMYCIN STEARATE

See discussion of erythromycin base.

Administration: Oral. Should be administered apart from meals.

Preparations: Tablets, 250 and 500 mg.

ERYTHROPOIETIN, see Epoetin alfa

ESERINE, see Physostigmine

ESGIC-PLUS—Combination barbituate and analgesic. Butalbital, Acetaminophen, and Caffeine.

ESIDRIX®, see Hydrochlorothiazide

ESKALITH®, see Lithium carbonate

ESMOLOL HYDROCHLORIDE— Brevibloc®

Antiarrhythmic agent.

Description/Actions: A beta-adrenergic blocking agent indicated for the rapid control of ventricular rate in patients with atrial fibrillation or atrial flutter in perioperative, postoperative, or other emergent circumstances where short-term control of ventricular rate with a short-acting agent is desirable. Also indicated in noncompensatory sinus tachycardia, where the rapid heart rate requires specific intervention.

Warnings: Contraindicated in patients with sinus bradycardia, heart block greater than first degree, cardiogenic shock, or overt heart failure. Hypotension is the most important adverse reaction, and some patients experience manifestations such as dizziness and diaphoresis. Other adverse reactions include peripheral ischemia, sedation, agitation, nausea, and local reactions at the infusion site; to reduce the incidence of venous irritation and thrombophlebitis, infusion concentrations greater than 10 mg/ml should be avoided. Therapy must be closely monitored in patients with bronchospastic diseases. It must also be used with caution in diabetic patients.

Administration: Intravenous infusion.

Preparations: Ampules, 10 mg/ml, 250 mg/ml.

ESOMEPRAZOLE—Nexium™

Description/Actions: Esomperazole is a proton pump inhibitor indicated for short-term (4–8 weeks) treatment of erosive esophagitis, maintaining symptom resolution and healing of erosive esophagitis, and treatment of symptomatic gastroesophageal reflux disease.

Precautions/Adverse Reactions: Usage is contraindicated in patients with hypersensitivity to esomeprazole, any component of the formulation, or to substituted benzimidazoles. Symptomatic response to therapy does not preclude the presence of gastric malignancy. Atrophic gastritis has been noted by biopsy from patients treated long-term with omeprazole; this may occur with esomeprazole therapy. Safety and efficacy of esomeprazole have not been established in pediatric patients. Pregnancy Category B. This drug should be used during pregnancy only if clearly needed. Excretion in the breast milk is unknown, therefore, breast-feeding is not recommended. Some adverse effects are headache, diarrhea, nausea, flatulence, abdominal pain, constipation, and dry mouth.

Administration: Oral.

Patient Care Implications: Capsule should be swallowed whole and taken at least 1 hour before eating. In patients with swallowing difficulties, open capsule and mix contents with 1 tbsp of applesauce. The mixture should be swallowed immediately and should not be chewed; do not store the mixture for future use.

Preparations: Capsule, delayed release: 20 mg, 40 mg.

ESTAZOLAM—ProSom®

Benzodiazepine hypnotic.

Description/Actions: Usually initiates sleep within 15 to 30 minutes following administration and action continued for an average of 6 to 8 hours. Classified as an intermediate-acting benzodiazepine hypnotic. Indicated for the short-term management of insomnia characterized by difficulty in falling asleep, frequent nocturnal awakenings, and/or early morning awakenings.

Warnings: Contraindicated in pregnancy. Adverse reactions include daytime

120 • ESTINYL®

sedation, hypokinesia, dizziness, and abnormal coordination. Patients should be cautioned regarding activities such as driving and operating machinery, as well as interactions with other CNS-acting drugs including alcohol. Can cause dependence and is included in Schedule IV.

Administration: Oral.

Preparations: Tablets, 1 and 2 mg.

ESTINYL®, see Ethinyl Estradiol

ESTRACE®, see Estradiol

ESTRADERM®, see Estradiol

ESTRADIOL—Alora®, Climara®, Estrace®, Estraderm®, Estring®, Vivelle®

Description/Actions: Estrogen indicated in the treatment of moderate to severe vasomotor symptoms associated with the menopause, atrophic vaginitis, kraurosis vulvae, female hypogonadism, female castration, primary ovarian failure, breast cancer, and prostatic cancer. Transdermal system is also indicated for postmenopausal osteoporosis. Remove vaginal ring when treating vaginal infections and during treatment with other vaginally administered preparations.

Preparations: Tablets, 1 and 2 mg. Transdermal systems 0.025 mg, 0.0375 mg, 0.05 mg, 0.075 mg, 0.1 mg, 4 and 8 mg. Vaginal cream, 0.1 mg/g. Vaginal ring (Estring®) 2 mg Estradiol/90 days.

ESTRADIOL CYPIONATE—Depo-Estradiol cypionate®

See discussion of estradiol.

Preparations: Vials (for intramuscular administration), 1 mg/ml and 5 mg/ml.

ESTRADIOL/ETHINYL ESTRADIOL—Vagifem®

Description/Actions: Estradiol/ethinyl estradiol is a vaginal tablet used to prevent osteoporosis and relieve symptoms associated with menopause.

Precautions/Adverse Reactions: Estradiol/ ethinyl estradiol should not be administered in patients with breast, endometrial, or any estrogen-dependent carcinoma. The drug is also contraindicated in patients with abnormal vaginal bleeding, thromboembolic disorder, and thrombophlebitis. The drug should be avoided in pregnant women and children. Some side effects are gallbladder disease, thromboembolic disorders, spotting, rash, genital pruritis, and endometrial hyperplasia.

Administration: Vaginal tablets.

Patient Care Implication: Estradiol/ ethinyl estradiol should not be given to pregnant women or children. Patients receiving the drug should be checked every 3–6 months to see if the drug is working. Patients on the drug should be monitored for LFTs, lipid profile, and cervical dysplasia.

Preparations: Vaginal tablets, 25 mcg.

ESTRADIOL VALERATE— Delestrogen®

See discussion of estradiol.

Preparations: Vials (for intramuscular administration), 10 mg/ml, 20 mg/ml, and 40 mg/ml.

ESTRAMUSTINE PHOSPHATE SODIUM—Emcyt®

Description/Actions: Antineoplastic agent indicated in the treatment of metastatic and/or progressive carcinoma of the prostate.

Preparations: Capsules, 140 mg.

ESTROGEN—Cenestin®

Description/Actions: Cenestin is a conjugated estrogen product synthesized from soy and yam plants indicated in the treatment of moderate to severe vasomotor spasms associated with menopausal symptoms.

Precautions/Adverse Reactions: Estrogen replacement therapy is contraindicated in breast or estrogen dependent carcinomas (unless palliative), undiagnosed abnormal vaginal bleeding, thromboembolic disorders, thrombophlebitis, and pregnancy. Use cautiously in women with increased risk of endometrial carcinoma or hyperplasia, in women with an intact uterus (consider adding progestin), hepatic or renal dysfunction, gall bladder disease, familial hyperlipoproteinemia, bone disease associated with hypercalcemia, diabetes, depression, uterine leiomyomas and conditions aggravated by fluid retention (e.g., asthma, epilepsy, migraine, cardiac or renal dysfunction). Monitor patients for hypertension. Do an initial complete physical and repeat at 6–12 months. Discontinue if jaundice occurs and during immobilization or at least 4 weeks before surgery associated with thromboembolism.

Adverse reactions include nausea, vomiting, abdominal pain, irregular bleeding, headache, insomnia, edema, weight changes, hypertonia, leg cramps, hypertension, mastodynia, intolerance to contact lenses, and increased size of uterine fibromyomata, chloasma. Long-term continuous use may increase the risk of estrogen dependent cancers.

Use of this medication may increase the incidence of gall bladder disease and thromboembolic disorders.

Administration: Oral.

Patient Care Implications: Instruct the patient in the signs and symptoms of fluid retention, thromboembolic disorders, gall bladder disease, and to report them promptly to the prescriber. Inform patients that exercise has been shown to be of benefit when taking estrogen because of bone loss.

Preparations: Tablets, 0.3, 0.625, 0.9, and 1.25 mg.

ESTROGENS, CONJUGATED—
Premarin®

Estrogen.

Description/Actions: Indicated in the treatment of (1) moderate to severe vasomotor symptoms associated with the menopause and (2) osteoporosis in postmenopausal women. Intravenous dosage form is indicated in the treatment of abnormal uterine bleeding due to hormonal imbalance in the absence of organic pathology. Vaginal cream is indicated in the treatment of atrophic vaginitis and kraurosis vulvae.

Warnings: Contraindicated (1) during pregnancy; (2) in patients with known or suspected cancer of the breast, except in appropriately selected patients being treated for metastatic disease; (3) in patients with known or suspected estrogen-dependent neoplasia; (4) in patients with undiagnosed abnormal genital bleeding; (5) in patients with thrombophlebitis or thromboembolic disorders; and (6) in patients with a past history of thrombophlebitis, thrombosis, or thromboembolic disorders associated with previous estrogen use (except when used in treatment of breast or prostatic malignancy). Estrogens have been reported to increase the risk of endometrial carcinoma. Premarin® alone or in combination with a progestin is not indicated and should not be used to prevent coronary heart disease. Adverse reactions include thromboembolic effects, increased incidence of gallbladder disease, edema, headache, nausea, vomiting, abdominal cramps, tenderness and enlargement of the breasts, and genitourinary effects.

Administration: Oral, intravenous, and vaginal.

Preparations: Tablets, 0.3, 0.625, 0.9, 1.25, and 2.5 mg. Vials, 25 mg. Vaginal cream, 0.625 mg/g.

ESTROGENS, ESTERIFIED—
Menest®

Description/Actions: Estrogen indicated for moderate to severe vasomotor symptoms of menopause, atrophic vaginitis, kraurosis vulvae, female hypogonadism, female castration, pri-

122 • ESTRONE

mary ovarian failure, prostatic carcinoma, and breast cancer.

Preparations: Tablets, 0.3, 0.625, 1.25, and 2.5 mg.

ESTRONE—Theelin®

Description/Actions: Estrogen indicated for intramuscular use for moderate to severe vasomotor symptoms associated with the menopause, atrophic vaginitis, kraurosis vulvae, female hypogonadism, female castration, primary ovarian failure, and prostatic carcinoma.

Preparations: Vials, 2 mg/ml and 5 mg/ml.

ESTROPIPATE—Piperazine estrone sulfate, Ogen®

Description/Actions: Estrogen indicated for moderate to severe vasomotor symptoms of menopause, atrophic vaginitis, kraurosis vulvae, female hypogonadism, female castration, primary ovarian failure, and postmenopausal osteoporosis.

Preparations: Tablets, 0.625, 1.25, 2.5, and 5 mg (equivalent, respectively, to 0.75, 1..5, 3, and 6 mg estropipate). Vaginal cream, 1.5 mg/g.

ESTROSTEP 21®—Oral contraceptive with progestin and estrogen. Also, Estrostep®.

ESTROVIS®, see Quinestrol

ETANERCEPT—Enbrel®

Description/Actions: Indicated in moderately to severely active rheumatoid arthritis (RA) in patients who responded inadequately to one or more disease modifying antirheumatic drugs. Used in the treatment of psoriatic arthritis with or without methotrexate. May be used with methotrexate in patients who have not responded adequately to methotrexate alone.

Precautions/Adverse Reactions: Etanercept is contraindicated in patients with active infection. The needle cover of the diluent syringe contains latex, which should not be handled by persons sensitive to this substance (e.g., nurses, caregivers, patients, etc.) Live vaccines should not be administered during therapy with etanercept.

Use cautiously in patients with recurrent infections and diseases that may predispose to infections (diabetes, CHF). Monitor closely if a new infection does develop and discontinue if a serious infection or sepsis develops. Temporarily suspend therapy if a significant varicella exposure occurs. Attempt to complete childhood immunizations prior to initiating therapy. Pregnancy Category B. Use in nursing mothers not recommended.

Adverse reactions include injection site reactions (may be serious, e.g., sepsis), development of autoantibodies, respiratory disorders, headache, rhinitis, and dyspepsia.

In children, abdominal pain and vomiting has also been reported.

Administration: SQ injection. Inject into the thigh, upper arm, or abdomen.

Patient Care Implications: Instruct patients in correct self administration techniques to ensure safe administration and to reduce the incidence of infection at the injection site. Tell patients to keep vials in the refrigerator and to administer the medication promptly after reconstitution. Corticosteroids, salicylates and NSAIDs, and analgesics may be continued during etanercept therapy. Inform patients that response is generally seen within 1–2 weeks after starting therapy but may not be evident for up to 3 months.

Preparations: Vial, 25 mg powder for reconstitution (diluent contains benzyl alcohol).

ETHACRYNIC ACID—Edecrin®

Description/Actions: Diuretic indicated for the treatment of edema associated with various conditions including the nephrotic syndrome, the short-term management of ascites, the short-term management of hospitalized pediatric patients with congenital heart disease or the nephrotic syndrome, and, intravenously, when a rapid onset of diuresis is desired.

Preparations: Tablets, 25 and 50 mg. Vials (using ethacrynate sodium), 50 mg.

ETHAMBUTOL HYDROCHLORIDE—
Myambutol®

Description/Actions: Antitubercular agent indicated in the treatment of tuberculosis or other mycobacterial diseases in conjunction with at least one other antitubercular drug.

Preparations: Tablets, 100 and 400 mg.

ETHAMOLIN®, see Ethanolamine oleate

ETHANOLAMINE OLEATE—
Ethamolin®

Sclerosing agent.

Description/Actions: Acts primarily by irritation of the intimal endothelium of the vein and produces a sterile inflammatory response which results in fibrosis and occlusion of the vein. Indicated for the treatment of patients with esophageal varices that have recently bled, to prevent rebleeding.

Warnings: Adverse reactions include pleural effusion/infiltration, esophageal ulcer, pyrexia, retrosternal pain, esophageal stricture, and pneumonia. Anaphylactic reactions have occurred infrequently.

Administration: Intravenous (directly into the varix). The maximum total dose per treatment session should not exceed 20 ml or 0.4 ml/kg for a 50 kg patient. To obliterate the varix, injections may be made at the time of the acute bleeding episode and then after 1 week, 6 weeks, 3 months, and 6 months as indicated.

Preparations: Ampules, 5%.

ETHAQUIN®, see Ethautrine

ETHATAB®, see Ethaverine

ETHAVERINE HYDROCHLORIDE—Ethaquin®, Ethatab®, Ethavex-100®, Isovex®

Description/Actions: Peripheral vasodilator indicated in the management of peripheral and cerebral vascular insufficiency associated with arterial spasm. Also used as a smooth muscle spasmolytic in spastic conditions of the gastrointestinal and genitourinary tracts.

Preparations: Tablets, 100 mg.

ETHAVEX-100®, see Ethaverine

ETHCHLORVYNOL—Placidyl®

Description/Actions: Hypnotic indicated for short-term use in the management of insomnia for periods of up to one week.

Preparations: Capsules, 200, 500, and 750 mg.

ETHER

Description/Actions: General anesthetic administered by inhalation to produce anesthesia.

Preparations: Liquid.

ETHINYL ESTRADIOL—Estinyl®

Description/Actions: Estrogen indicated in the treatment of moderate to severe vasomotor symptoms associated with the menopause, female hypogonadism, prostatic carcinoma, and breast cancer in appropriately selected women. Also used as the estrogen component of many oral contraceptive formulations.

Preparations: Tablets, 0.02, 0.05, and 0.5 mg.

ETHINYL ESTRADIOL AND DROSPIRENONE—YASMIN®

Description/Actions: Yasmin® is indicated for the prevention of pregnancy in women who elect to use an oral contraceptive.

Precautions/Adverse Reactions: Yasmin® is contraindicated in women with any of the following conditions: renal insufficiency, hepatic dysfunction, adrenal insufficiency, thrombophlebitis or thromboembolic disorders, a past history of deep vein thrombophlebitis or thromboembolic disorders, cerebrolvascular or coronary artery disease, known or suspected carcinoma of the breast, carcinoma of the endometrium, or other known or suspected estrogen-dependent neoplasia, undiagnosed abnormal genital bleeding, cholestatic jaundice of pregnancy or jaundice with prior pill use, liver tumor (benign or malignant) or active liver disease, known or suspected pregnancy, heavy smoking (≥ 15 cigarettes per day), and over age 35. Cigarette smoking increases the risk of serious cardiovascular side effects from oral contraceptive use.

Oral contraceptive use has been associated with an increased risk of myocardial infarction, thromboembolism, stroke, hepatic neoplasia, gallbladder disease, hypertension, ocular lesions, carbohydrate and lipid metabolic effects, headache, and bleeding irregularities. Women should be advised that this product does not protect against HIV infection and other sexually transmitted diseases.

Concomitant administration of oral contraceptives and rifampin, phenobarbital, phenytoin, griseofulvin, Saint-John's-wort, or phenylbutazone may decrease the effectiveness of the oral contraceptive and lead to menstrual irregularities. Coadministration of oral contraceptives and atorvastatin has resulted in increased plasma concentrations of norethindrone and ethinyl estradiol. Ascorbic acid and acetaminophen may increase plasma concentrations of some synthetic estrogens.

Oral contraceptives may inhibit the metabolism of cyclosporine, prednisolone, and theophylline, resulting in increased plasma concentrations of these drugs. Increased clearance of temazepam, salicylic acid, morphine, and clofibric acid has resulted when these drugs were coadministered with oral contraceptives.

Pregnancy Category X. Known or suspected pregnancy is a contraindication for the use of Yasmin®. Excreted in human breast milk. Nursing is not recommended.

Most common adverse effects associated with Yasmin® therapy and occurring in > 1% of women include headache, menstrual disorders, breast pain, abdominal pain, nausea, leukorrhea, flu syndrome, acne, vaginal moniliasis, depression, diarrhea, asthenia, dysmenorrhea, back pain, infection, sinusitis, cystitis, bronchitis, gastroenteritis, allergic reaction, urinary tract infection, pruritis, emotional lability, surgery, rash, and upper respiratory infection. Most common adverse reactions associated with other oral contraceptives include nausea, vomiting, abdominal cramps, bloating, breakthrough bleeding, spotting, change in menstrual flow, amenorrhea, temporary infertility after discontinuation of treatment, edema, melasma, breast changes (tenderness, enlargement, or secretion), weight changes, changes in cervical erosion and secretion, cholestatic jaundice, migraine, rash, depression, vaginal candidiasis, change in corneal curvature, intolerance to contact lenses, acne, Budd-Chiari syndrome, changes in libido, colitis, cystitis-like syndrome, dizziness, erythema multiforme, erythema nodosum, hemolytic uremic syndrome, hemorrhagic eruption, hirsutism, impaired renal function, loss of scalp hair, nervousness, porphyria, premenstrual syndrome, and vaginitis. Some noncontraceptive benefits of oral contraceptives include: increased menstrual cycle regularity, decreased blood loss and decreased incidence of iron-deficiency anemia, decreased incidence of dysmenorrhea, functional ovarian cysts, ectopic pregnancies, fibroadenomas and fibrocystic disease of the breast, decreased incidence of acute pelvic inflammatory disease, and a decreased incidence of endometrial and ovarian cancer.

Administration: Oral. Missed pills: see package insert.

Patient Care Implications: Instruct patient to take the pills exactly as prescribed. Instruct patient to take the pills at the same time each day either after the evening meal or at bedtime. Monitor serum potassium levels during the first treatment cycle and in high-risk patients. Monitor blood pressure. Advise patients not to smoke.

Preparations: Tablets, ethinyl estradiol, 0.03 mg, and drospirenone, 3 mg (21 active—yellow pills, 7 inactive—white pills).

ETHINYL ESTRADIOL AND ETONOGESTREL— NUVARING®

Description/Actions: NuvaRing® is indicated for the prevention of pregnancy in women who elect to use this product as a method of contraception.

Precautions/Adverse Reactions: NuvaRing® is contraindicated in women with thrombophlebitis or thromboembolic disorders, a past history of deep vein thrombophlebitis or thromboembolic disorders, cerebral vascular or coronary artery disease, valvular heart disease with complications, severe hypertension, diabetes with vascular involvement, headache with focal neurologic symptoms, major surgery with prolonged immobilization, known or suspected carcinoma of the breast or history of breast cancer, carcinoma of the endometrium or other known or suspected estrogen-dependent neoplasia, undiagnosed abnormal genital bleeding, cholestatic jaundice of pregnancy or jaundice with prior hormonal contraceptive use, hepatic tumors, active liver disease, known or suspected pregnancy, heavy smoking (≥ 15 cigarettes/day), and over age 35. Cigarette smoking increases the risk of serious cardiovascular side effects. May lead to increased risk of myocardial infarction, thromboembolism, stroke, hepatic neoplasia, and gallbladder disease. Retinal thrombosis has also been seen in women using oral contraceptives. The risk of morbidity and mortality increases significantly in the presence of hypertension, hyperlipidemias, obesity, and diabetes. There are no data available to determine whether or not safety and efficacy with the vaginal route of administration of combination hormonal contraceptives would be different than the oral route.

Hormonal contraceptives have been shown to cause a decrease in glucose tolerance and hypertriglyceridemia among users. Women with a history of hypertension, hypertension-related disease, or renal disease should be encouraged to use another method of birth control. Breakthrough bleeding and spotting have been reported with NuvaRing®. Fluid retention and depression have also been reported. Patients should be informed that this product does not protect against HIV or other sexually transmitted diseases. Coadministration of herbal products containing Saint-John's-wort may decrease the effectiveness of contraceptive steroids. Coadministration of atorvastatin and certain oral contraceptives containing ethinyl estradiol results in an increase in ethinyl estradiol area under the curve. Ascorbic acid and acetaminophen may increase blood levels of ethinyl estradiol. Coadministration with itraconazole or ketoconazole may increase blood hormone levels. Coadministration of oral contraceptives containing ethinyl estradiol and cyclosporine, prednisolone, and/or theophylline results in increased plasma concentrations of these drugs. Concomitant use of oral contraceptives and acetaminophen results in decreased plasma concentrations of acetaminophen. Coadministration of oral contraceptives and temazepam results in the increased clearance of temazepam. Increased clearance of salicylic acid, morphine, and clofibric acid has been observed when these drugs were administered with oral contraceptives.

Pregnancy Category X. Pregnancy should be ruled out prior to starting NuvaRing®. Effects of NuvaRing® in nursing mothers have not been evaluated. Women who are breast-feeding should be advised not to use NuvaRing®. Safety and efficacy in pediatric patients have not been established. Use before menarche is not indicated.

The most common adverse reactions noted in patients using NuvaRing® were vaginitis, headache, upper respiratory tract infection, leukorrhea, sinusitis, weight gain, and nausea. Most frequently reported adverse reactions leading to discontinuation of NuvaRing® include device-related problems (foreign body sensation, coital problems, device expulsion), vaginal symptoms (discomfort, vaginitis, leukorrhea), headache, emotional lability, and weight gain.

Administration: For vaginal use only—1 ring inserted into the vagina. The ring is to remain in place continuously for 3 weeks. It is then removed for 1 week, during which withdrawal bleeding usually occurs. A new ring is inserted 1 week after the last ring was removed even if menstrual bleeding has not stopped.

Patient Care Implications: Patient should be informed that this product does not protect against HIV or other sexually transmitted diseases. Patient should be advised not to smoke. Patient should be instructed to wash her hands prior to removing the ring from the pouch (save foil pouch for disposal of ring). Ring may be inserted lying down, squatting, or standing with one leg up. Patient should be instructed to hold NuvaRing® between her thumb and index finger and to press the opposite sides of the ring together. Ring should be pushed into the vagina. To remove the ring, hook the index finger under the forward rim or by holding the rim between the index and middle finger and pulling it out. The used ring should be placed in the foil pouch and disposed of in a waste receptacle out of reach of children and pets. It should not be thrown in the toilet.

A new ring should be inseted on the same day of the week as it was inserted in the last cycle and at about the same time.

Patient should be warned that the ring may fall out of the vagina due to incorrect insertion, bowel movements, straining due to severe constipation, or during tampon removal. If the ring accidentally falls out, it may be rinsed with cool or lukewarm water and reinserted as soon as possible within 3 hours of expulsion. Patient should be advised to have an annual health assessment, including blood pressure, laboratory tests, breast exam, Pap test, and abdominal pelvic organ and vaginal examination.

Preparations: Vaginal ring (delivers ethinyl estradiol 0.015 mg/day and etonogestrel 0.12 µg/day).

ETHINYL ESTRADIOL AND NORELGESTROMIN—ORTHO EVRA™

Description/Actions: Ortho Evra™ is a combination contraceptive patch for the prevention of pregnancy.

Precautions/Adverse Reactions: Ortho Evra™ is contraindicated in patients with a known hypersensitivity to ethinyl estradiol, norelgestromin, or any components of the formulation. It should not be used in women who currently have the following conditions: thrombophlebitis or thromboembolic disorders, past history of deep vein thrombophlebitis or thromboembolic disorders, cerebrovascular or coronary disease (past or current), valvular heart disease with complications, severe hypertension, diabetes with vascular involvement, headaches with focal neurologic symptoms, major surgery with prolonged immobilization, known or suspected carcinoma of the breast or personal history of breast cancer, carcinoma of the endometrium or other known or suspected estrogen-dependent neoplasia, undiagnosed abnormal genital bleeding, cholestatic jaundice of pregnancy or jaundice with prior hormonal contraceptive use, acute or chronic hepatocellular disease with abnormal liver function, hepatic adenomas or carcinomas, and known or suspected pregnancy. Cigarette smoking increases the risk of serious cardiovascular side effects from hormonal contraceptive use. Risk increases with age and with heavy smoking (15 or more cigarettes/day). It is quite marked in women over 35 years of age. Women using hormonal contraceptives should be strongly advised not to smoke. Smoking in combination with oral contraceptives has been shown to contribute substantially to the incidence of myocardial infarctions in women in their mid-30s or older. There is an increased risk of thromboembolic and thrombotic disease, myocardial infarction, and both relative and attributable risks of cerebrovascular events (thrombotic and hemorrhagic strokes). A positive association has been observed between the amount of estrogen and progestin in hormonal contraceptives and the risk of vascular disease. Benign hepatic adenomas are associated with hormonal contraceptive use; rupture of benign hepatic adenomas may cause death through intraabdominal hemorrhage. Cases of retinal thrombosis have been reported. Combination hormonal contraceptives may worsen existing gallbladder disease and may accelerate the development of this disease in previously asymptomatic women. Oral contraceptives have been shown to cause a decrease in glucose tolerance in some users. Women being treated for hyperlipidemias should be followed closely; some progestins may elevate LDL levels and may render the control of hyperlipidemias more difficult. If jaundice develops, the medication should be discontinued; the hormones in Ortho Evra™ may be poorly metabolized in patients with impaired liver function. If there is onset or exacerbation of migraine headache or the development of headache with a new pattern that is recurrent, persistent, or severe, Ortho Evra should be discontinued.

Common adverse reactions were abdominal pain, application site reaction, breast symptoms, headache, nausea, upper respiratory infections and emotional lability. Contraceptive effectiveness may be reduced when coadministered with some antibiotics, antifungals, anticonvulsants, and other drugs that increase metabolism of contraceptive steroids. Pregnancy Category X. Enters breast milk; not recommended in nursing mothers.

Administration: Topical. This system uses a 28-day (4 week) cycle. Apply 1 patch each week for 3 weeks (21 days), followed by 1 week that is patch-free. There should be no more than a 7-day patch-free interval. Withdrawal bleeding is expected during this week.

Patient Care Implications: Patients should be counseled that this product does not protect against HIV infection and other sexually transmitted diseases. New patches should be applied on the same day each week. Apply to clean, dry, intact healthy skin on the buttock, abdomen, upper outer arm, or upper torso, or in a place where it will not be rubbed by tight clothing. Should not be placed on skin that is red, irritated, or cut, nor on the breasts. Do not apply makeup, creams, lotions, powders, or any topical products where the patch will be placed. If an uncomfortable irritation should occur, remove patch; a new patch may be applied to a different location until the next change day. Only one patch should be worn at a time. Store patches in their protective pouches. Do not store in refrigerator or freezer. Used patches still contain some active hormones; carefully fold old patch in half so that it sticks to itself before throwing out.

128 • ETHIONAMIDE

Preparations: Patch (transdermal); ethinyl estradiol, 20 μg, and norelgestromin, 150 μg/day.

ETHIONAMIDE—Trecator-SC®

Description/Actions: Antitubercular agent indicated in the treatment of tuberculosis in conjunction with other drugs after failure of treatment with the primary antitubercular agents.

Preparations: Tablets, 250 mg.

ETHMOZINE®, see Moricizine

ETHOPROPAZINE HYDROCHLORIDE—Parsidol®

Description/Actions: Antiparkinson agent indicated in the treatment of parkinsonism and to control extrapyramidal reactions due to drugs such as the phenothiazines.

Preparations: Tablets, 10 and 50 mg.

ETHOSUXIMIDE—Zarontin®

Description/Actions: Anticonvulsant indicated in the treatment of absence (petit mal) epilepsy, myoclonic seizures, and akinetic epilepsy.

Preparations: Capsules, 250 mg. Syrup, 250 mg/5 ml.

ETHOTOIN—Peganone®

Description/Actions: Anticonvulsant indicated for the control of tonic-clonic (grand mal) and complex partial (psychomotor) seizures.

Preparations: Tablets, 250 and 500 mg.

ETHRANE®, see Enflurane

ETHYL ALCOHOL, see Alcohol

ETHYL AMINOBENZOATE, see Benzocaine

ETHYL CHLORIDE

Description/Actions: Local anesthetic used to provide local anesthesia and analgesia when sprayed on the skin.

Preparations: Topical spray.

ETHYLENE

Description/Actions: General anesthetic administered by inhalation to produce anesthesia.

Preparations: Gas.

ETHYLNOREPINEPHRINE HYDROCHLORIDE— Bronkephrine®

Description/Actions: Bronchodilator indicated for parenteral use in the treatment of bronchial asthma and for reversible bronchospasm that may occur in association with bronchitis and emphysema.

Preparations: Ampules, 2 mg/ml.

ETHYNODIOL DIACETATE

Description/Actions: Progestin included in certain oral contraceptive formulations.

ETHYOL®, see Amifostine

ETIDOCAINE HYDROCHLORIDE—Duranest®

Description/Actions: Local anesthetic indicated for infiltration anesthesia, peripheral nerve blocks, and central neural blocks (i.e., lumbar or caudal epidural blocks).

Preparations: Vials, 1% solution. Vials, 1% and 1.5% solutions, both with epinephrine bitartrate, 1:200,000.

ETIDRONATE DISODIUM— Didronel®

Description/Actions: Acts primarily on bone and is indicated for the treatment of symptomatic Paget's disease of bone, and for the prevention and treatment of heterotopic ossification following total hip replacement or due to spinal cord injury. Also used parenterally for the management of hypercalcemia of malignancy inadequately managed by dietary modification or oral hydration, and in the hypercalcemia of malignancy that persists after adequate hydration has been restored.

Preparations: Tablets, 200 and 400 mg. Ampules, 300 mg.

ETODOLAC—Lodine®

Nonsteroidal anti-inflammatory drug.

Description/Actions: Inhibits prostaglandin synthesis and is indicated for the management of osteoarthritis and rheumotoid arthritis. Is also indicated for the management of pain.

Warnings: Should not be given to patients in whom aspirin or another NSAID causes asthma, rhinitis, urticaria, or other allergic-type reactions. May cause GI effects and use should be avoided in patients with active GI tract disease and closely monitored in patients with a previous history of such disorders.

Administration: Oral.

Preparations: Capsules, 200 and 300 mg. Tablets, 400 and 500 mg. Extended-release tablets, 400, 500, and 600 mg.

ETOPOSIDE—VePesid®, VP-16®

Description/Actions: Antineoplastic agent used in treatment of refractory testicular neoplasms in patients who have already received appropriate surgical, chemotherapeutic and radiation therapy. Indicated for the treatment of choriosarcoma in women and small cell carcinoma.

Administration: Oral, intravenous.

Preparations: Capsules, 50 mg. Injection, 50 mg/ml.

ETOMIDATE—Amidate®

Description/Actions: General anesthetic indicated for induction of general anesthesia and for supplementation of subpotent anesthetic agents (e.g., nitrous oxide in oxygen) during maintenance of anesthesia for short surgical procedures.

Preparations: Ampules, 2 mg/ml.

EUGENOL

Description/Actions: Local anesthetic used in some formulations used for the relief of toothache.

Preparations: Drops.

EULEXIN®, see Flutamide

EURAX®, see Crotamiton

EVISTA®, see Raloxifene HCl

EVOXAC®, see Cevimeline hydrochloride

EXCEDRIN®—Combination agent acetaminophen, aspirin, and caffeine (analgesic and salicylate)

EXELDERM®, see Sulconazole nitrate

EXELON®, see Rivastigmine tartrate

EXEMESTANE—Aromasin®

Description/Actions: Exemestane is used as a second-line agent for the treatment of breast cancer in postmenopausal women.

Precautions/Adverse Reactions: Exemestane should not be given to pregnant women, breast-feeding women, or children. Also, the drug should not be given to premenopausal women because exemestane will not be effective. Patients on exemestane should not take any exogenous estrogens. Some common side effects are hot flashes, fever, leg swelling, constipation, weight gain, fatigue, pain, depression, insomnia, anxiety, dyspnea, dizziness, headache, diaphoresis, nausea, and vomiting.

Administration: Oral.

Patient Care Implications: Patients should not take any exogenous estrogens while on the medication. Also, the drug should not be given to pregnant women, breast-feeding women, premenopausal women, and children.

Preparations: Tablets, 25 mg.

EXNA®, see Benzthiazide

EXOSURF NEONATAL®, see Colfosceril palmitate

F

FACTREL®, see Gonadorelin

FAMCICLOVIR—Famvir®

Antiviral agent.

Description/Actions: Is a prodrug that is rapidly converted following administration to the antiviral compound penciclovir. Indicated for the management of acute herpes zoster (shingles), treatment or suppression of recurrent episodes of genital herpes in immunocompetent patients and treatment of recurrent mucocutaneous herpes simplex infections in HIV-infected patients.

Warnings: Adverse reactions include headache, nausea, and fatigue.

Administration: Oral.

Preparations: Tablets, 125, 250, and 500 mg.

FAMOTIDINE—Mylanta AR®, Pepcid®, Pepcid AC®, Pepcid RDP®

Antiulcer agent.

Description/Actions: Indicated in (1) short-term treatment of active duodenal ulcer, (2) maintenance therapy for duodenal ulcer patients at reduced dosage after healing of an active ulcer, (3) short-term treatment of active, benign gastric ulcer, (4) treatment of gastroesophageal reflux disease including erosive esophagitis, and (5) treatment of pathological hypersecretory conditions (e.g., Zollinger-Ellison syndrome, multiple endocrine adenomas). Available without a prescription (Pepcid AC®) to relieve and prevent acid indigestion.

Warnings: Adverse reactions include headache, dizziness, constipation, diarrhea, and transient irritation at the injection site when administered intravenously. Dosage adjustments are required for patients with moderate renal impairment (creatinine clearance < 50 ml/min).

Administration: Oral and intravenous.

Preparations: Tablets, 10 (Pepcid AC®), 20, and 40 mg. Disintegrating tablets (Pepcrd RDP®), 20 and 40 mg. Oral suspension containing 40 mg/5 ml when reconstituted. Vials, 10 mg/ml.

FAMVIR®, see Famciclovir

FANSIDAR®, Combination of sulfadoxine and pyrimethamine

FARESTON®, see Toremifene

FASTIN®, see Phentermine

FELBAMATE—Felbatol®

Antiepileptic agent.

Description/Actions: Because of the risks of aplastic anemia and acute liver failure, should only be used in patients whose epilepsy is so severe that the risk is deemed acceptable in light of the benefits conferred by its use. Indicated as monotherapy and adjunctive therapy in the treatment of partial seizures with and without generalization in adults with epilepsy, and as adjunctive therapy in the treatment of partial and generalized seizures associated with Lennox-Gastaut syndrome in children.

Warnings: Adverse reactions include aplastic anemia, acute liver failure, anorexia, nausea, vomiting, insomnia, somnolence, dizziness, and headache. Do full baseline hematologic evaluation and hepatic function tests before, during, and after therapy. Discontinue if hepatic tests are abnormal or bone marrow depression occurs. Consult hematologist if hematologic abnormalities occur.

Administration: Oral. When felbamate is added to or substituted for existing antiepileptic drugs, it is necessary to reduce the dosage of those drugs in the range of 20–33% to minimize side effects. Avoid abrupt cessation.

Preparations: Tablets, 400 and 600 mg. Oral suspension, 600 mg/5 ml.

FELBATOL®, see Felbamate

FELDENE®, see Piroxicam

FELODIPINE—Plendil®

Antihypertensive agent.

Description/Actions: A calcium channel blocking agent that is indicated in the management of hypertension. May be used alone or concurrently with other antihypertensive agents.

Warnings: Adverse reactions include peripheral edema, headache, flushing, dizziness, asthenia, cough, paresthesia, dyspepsia, chest pain, nausea, muscle cramps, and palpitation. Mild gingival hyperplasia has been reported and may be reduced by good dental hygiene. Caution should be exercised in patients with congestive heart failure, particularly if a beta-blocker is used concurrently. Action may be increased by the concurrent use of cimetidine. Bioavailability of the drug has been reported to be significantly increased when taken with doubly concentrated grapefruit juice. Coadministration of felodipine and cimetidine results in an increase in felodipine plasma levels.

Administration: Oral.

Preparations: Extended-release tablets, 2.5, 5, and 10 mg.

FEMARA®, see Letrozole

FEMSTAT®, see Butoconazole

FENOFIBRATE—Tricor®

Description/Actions: Indicated as an adjunct to diet in treating adults with very high elevations of serum triglyerceride levels (Type IV and V hyperlipidemias) who are at risk of pancreatitis and who do not adequately respond to strict dietary measure of control.

Fenofibrate reduces serum uric acid levels in both hyperuricemic and normal individuals by increasing urinary excretion of uric acid.

Warnings: Contraindicated in hepatic dysfunction (including primary biliary cirrhosis and unexplained persistent liver function abnormality), severe renal dysfunction, and gallbladder disease. Fenofibrate can cause dose related hepatoxicity. Liver function should be monitored at baseline and at regular intervals for the duration of treatment. Pancreatitis has been reported in patients taking fenofibrate, but it is a secondary phenomenon through biliary tract stone or sludge formation and obstruction of the bile duct.

Use cautiously in patients with renal impairment. Monitor CBC for at least a year. Monitor liver function regularly and discontinue if ALT (SGPT) levels are > 3 times upper limit of normal (ULN). Discontinue if myopathy or gallstones occur. Pregnancy Category C. Not recommended in nursing mothers.

Adverse reactions include rash, flulike symptoms, eye irritation, dizziness, eructation, myopathy, rhabdomyolysis, increased serum transaminases, hepatitis, cirrhosis, cholelithiasis, pancreatitis, increased BUN/Cr., transient

132 • FENOPROFEN CALCIUM

moderate hematologic changes, thrombocytopenia, and agranulocytosis (rare).

Administration: Oral. Give with meals. Discontinue if significant improvement is not seen in 2 months.

Preparations: Tablets, 54 and 160 mg.

FENOPROFEN CALCIUM— Nalfon®

Nonsteroidal anti-inflammatory drug.

Description/Actions: Indicated for the relief of mild to moderate pain, rheumatoid arthritis, and osteoarthritis.

Warnings: Should not be used in patients with a history of significantly impaired renal function. Should not be given to patients in whom aspirin or another NSAID causes asthma, rhinitis, urticaria, or other allergic-type reactions. May cause GI effects and use should be avoided in patients with active GI tract disease and closely monitored in patients with a previous history of such disorders. Other adverse reactions include dizziness, pruritus, palpitations, and nervousness.

Administration: Oral.

Preparations: Capsules, 200 and 300 mg. Tablets, 600 mg.

FENTANYL—Duragesic® -25, -50, -75, -100

Description/Actions: Opioid analgesic indicated for the management of chronic pain. Transdermal system provides analgesic activity for up to 72 hours.

Preparations: Transdermal system, 25 µg/hour (2.5 mg), 50 µg/hour (5 mg), 75 µg/hour (7.5 mg), and 100 µg/hour (10 mg).

FENTANYL CITRATE—Actiq®, Sublimaze®, Oralet®

Description/Actions: Opioid analgesic/anesthetic indicated for parenteral use for (1) analgesic action before, during, and following surgery; (2) as an analgesic supplement in general or regional anesthesia; (3) administration with a neuroleptic in conjunction with anesthesia; and (4) as an anesthetic agent with oxygen in selected high risk patients. Also indicated for oral transmucosal use (as a lozenge) for anesthetic premedication in children and adults, and for use in anesthesia or monitored anesthesia care.

Preparations: Ampules, 50 µg/ml. Lozenges, 200, 300, 400, 600, 800, and 1200 µg.

FEOSOL®, see Ferrous sulfate exsiccated

FEOSTAT®, see Ferrous fumarate

FERGON®, see Ferrous gluconate

FER-IN-SOL®, see Ferrous sulfate

FERO-GRADUMET®, see Ferrous sulfate

FERRIC SODIUM GLUCONATE— Ferrlecit®

Description/Actions: Ferric sodium gluconate is used to treat iron deficiency in patients who receive chronic hemodialysis and epoetin alfa.

Precautions/Adverse Reactions: Ferric sodium gluconate should not be administered in neonates, in patients with benzyl alcohol hypersensitivity, and in patients who have an anemia not caused by iron deficiency. The drug may be given to pregnant women but should be administered with caution in breast-feeding patients. One adverse reaction is a hypersensitivity reaction that can cause cardiovascular collapse, cardiac arrest, bronchospasm, angioedema, urticaria, or pruritus. Other side effects are hemosiderosis, flulike syndrome, dizziness, infection, insomnia, upper respiratory infection, hypertension, syncope, tachycardia, bradycardia, pulmonary edema, flatulence, electrolyte disturbance, leg edema, flushing, and hypotension.

Administration: Intravenous.

Patient Care Implications: The drug should not be administered in neonates, in patients with benzyl alcohol hypersensitivity, or in patients who have an anemia not caused by iron deficiency. Ferritin, hemoglobin, hematocrit, iron, and transferrin should be checked before and during therapy.

Preparations: Ampule, 62.5 mg/5 ml.

FERRLECIT®, see Ferric Sodium Gluconate

FERROUS FUMARATE—Feostat®

Description/Actions: Hematinic indicated for the prevention and treatment of iron deficiency anemias.

Preparations: Tablets, 100, 200, and 325 mg. Suspension, 100 mg/5 ml. Drops, 45 mg/0.6 ml.

FERROUS GLUCONATE— Fergon®

Hematinic indicated for the prevention and treatment of iron deficiency anemias.

Preparations: Tablets, 325 mg. Capsules, 325 and 435 mg. Elixir, 300 mg/5 ml.

FERROUS SULFATE—Fero-Gradumet®, Fer-In-Sol®

Description/Actions: Hematinic indicated for the prevention and treatment of iron deficiency anemias.

Preparations: Controlled-release tablets, 525 mg. Syrup, 90 mg/5 ml. Drops, 75 mg/0.6 ml.

FERROUS SULFATE, EXSICCATED—Feosol®, Slow FE®

Description/Actions: Hematinic indicated for the prevention and treatment of iron deficiency anemias.

Preparations: Tablets, 200 mg. Controlled-release capsules and tablets, 160 mg.

FEXOFENADINE HYDROCHLORIDE—Allegra®

Description/Actions: A nonsedating antihistamine with selective peripheral H_1-receptor antagonist activity indicated in the treatment of seasonal allergic rhinitis.

Warnings: Adverse reactions include viral infection, nausea, dysmenorrhea, drowsiness, dyspepsia, and fatigue. Use cautiously in patients with renal impairment. Rash, urticaria, pruritus, and hypersensitivity reactions, with manifestations such as angioedema, chest tightness, dyspnea, flushing, and anaphylaxis, have been reported.

Administration: Oral.

Preparations: Capsules, 60 mg. Tablets, 30, 60, and 180 mg.

FEXOFENADINE/PSEUDO-EPHEDRINE—Allegra-D®

Description/Actions: Fexofenadine and pseudoephedrine are used together in an oral preparation to relieve symptoms of seasonal allergic rhinitis in adults and children 12 years of age and older.

Precautions/Adverse Reactions: Adverse reactions include headache, insomnia, nausea/vomiting, dry mouth, agitation, dizziness, nervousness, anxiety, and palpitations, dyspepsia, throat irritation, upper respiratory infection, back pain, and abdominal pain. Central nervous system stimulation resulting in restlessness, tremor, seizures, and psychological disturbances can be seen. Use cautiously in patients with renal impairment, narrow-angle glaucoma, diabetes mellitus, urinary retention, hyperthyroidism, or prostatic hypertrophy. In addition, since pseudoephedrine is a vasoconstrictor, it should be used cautiously in patients with uncontrolled hypertension or severe coronary artery disease. Due to its pseudoephedrine component, Allegra-D is contraindicated in patients

134 • FIBERCON®

receiving MAOI therapy or within 14 days of stopping such treatment.

Administration: Oral.

Preparations: Extended release tablets, fexofenadine 60 mg/pseudoephedrine 120 mg.

FIBERCON® see Polycarbophil

FIBRINOLYSIN—in Elase®

Description/Actions: Fibrinolytic agent used in combination with desoxyribonuclease for topical use as debriding agents in a variety of inflammatory and infected lesions.

Preparations: Ointment and powder for solution.

FILGRASTIM—Neupogen®

Colony stimulating factor.

Description/Actions: A human granulocyte colony stimulating factor (G-CSF) produced by recombinant DNA technology. Regulates the production of neutrophils within the bone marrow and is indicated to decrease the incidence of infection, as manifested by febrile neutropenia, in patients with nonmyeloid malignancies receiving myelosuppressive anticancer drugs associated with a significant incidence of severe neutropenia with fever may be used to reduce the time of neutrophl recovery and fever duration after induction and consolidation chemotherapy treatment of adults with AML. Also indicated in patients with nonmyeloid malignancies undergoing chemotherapy followed by marrow transplantation. Also indicated to reduce the incidence and duration of sequelae of severe chronic neutropenia.

Warnings: May cause bone pain and leukocytosis. Caution must be exercised in patients with any malignancy with myeloid characteristics because of the possibility that the drug may act as a growth factor for the tumor.

Administration: Intravenous and subcutaneous. Should be administered no earlier than 24 hours after the administration of cytotoxic chemotherapy, and should not be administered in the period 24 hours before the administration of chemotherapy. Vials should not be shaken.

Preparations: Vials, 300 and 480 ug.

FINASTERIDE—Propecia®

Description/Actions: Indicated in the treatment of male pattern hair loss (androgenetic alopecia) in men only.

Warnings: Contraindicated in woman and children. Woman of childbearing potential must not handle crushed or broken tablets. Pregnancy Category X.

Use cautiously in hepatic dysfunction. Consider that the PSA may double in men ≥ 41 years of age without BPH who are undergoing PSA test.

Instruct patients that the benefits may not be seen for 3 months. Must continue to sustain effect. Reversal of effects seen within 12 months of discontinuation.

Adverse reactions include decreased libido, erectile dysfunction, and ejaculation disorder (all rare).

Administration: Oral.

Preparations: Tablets, 1 mg.

FINASTERIDE—Proscar®

Agent for benign prostatic hyperplasia (BPH).

Description/Actions: Inhibits steroid 5-alpha-reductase that converts testosterone into 5-alpha-dihydrotestosterone (DHT), a potent androgen. Indicated for the treatment of symptomatic benign prostatic hyperplasia to improve symptoms and reduce risks of acute urinary retention and the need for prostate surgery.

Warnings: Contraindicated during pregnancy and in nursing mothers. Adverse reactions include impotence, decreased libido, and decreased volume of ejaculate. May cause harm to a male fetus, and women who are pregnant should avoid exposure to the drug—crushed tablets should not be handled by a woman who is pregnant, and, when the patient's sexual partner is or may become pregnant, the patient should avoid exposure of his partner to semen or discontinue the medication. May cause a decrease in serum prostate-specific antigen (PSA).

Administration: Oral. A minimum of 6 months of treatment may be necessary to determine whether an individual will respond to the drug.

Preparations: Tablets, 5 mg.

FIORICET®, Combination of butalbital, acetaminophen, and caffeine

FIORINAL®, Combination of butalbital, aspirin, and caffeine

5 FU®, see Fluorouracil

FLAGYL®, see Metronidazole

FLAVOXATE HYDROCHLORIDE—Urispas®

Description/Actions: Spasmolytic agent indicated for the symptomatic relief of urinary tract problems such as dysuria, urgency, nocturia, suprapubic pain, frequency, and incontinence.

Preparations: Tablets, 100 mg.

FLAXEDIL®, see Gallamine

FLECAINIDE ACETATE—Tambocor®

Antiarrhythmic agent.

Description/Actions: A class IC antiarrhythmic agent. Indicated for the treatment of life-threatening ventricular arrhythmias such as sustained ventricular tachycardia. Also indicated for paroxysmal atrial fibrillation/flutter associated with disabling symptoms and paroxysmal supraventricular tachycardias associated with disabling symptoms in patients without structural heart disease.

Warnings: Contraindicated in patients with second- or third-degree AV block, with right bundle branch block when associated with a left hemiblock (unless a pacemaker is present), or in the presence of cardiogenic shock. Adverse reactions include proarrhythmic events, worsening of congestive heart failure, dizziness, visual disturbances, dyspnea, headache, nausea, fatigue, and palpitation.

Administration: Oral.

Preparations: Tablets, 50, 100, and 150 mg.

FLEXERIL®, see Cyclobenzaprine

FLOLAN®, see Epoprostenol

FLOMAX®, see Tamsulosin Hydrochloride

FLONASE®, see Fluticasone Propionate

FLORINEF®, see Fludrocortisone

FLORONE®, see Diflorasone

FLOROPRYL®, see Isoflurophate

FLOVENT®, see Fluticasone propionate

FLOVENT® DISKUS, see Fluticasone propionate

FLOXIN®, see Ofloxacin

FLOXIN IV®, see Ofloxacin

FLOXURIDINE—FUDR®

Description/Actions: Antineoplastic agent administered by intra-arterial infusion in the management of gastrointestinal adenocarcinoma metastatic to the liver.

Preparations: Vials, 5 mg.

FLUCONAZOLE—Diflucan®

Antifungal agent.

Description/Actions: Indicated for the treatment of cryptococcal meningitis, serious systemic candidal infections including urinary tract infection, peritonitis, and pneumonia, as well as oropharyngeal and esophageal candidiasis. Also indicated as a single-dose treatment for vaginal candidiasis.

Warnings: Adverse reactions include nausea, vomiting, abdominal pain, diarrhea, headache, rash, and hepatic reactions. May increase the plasma concentrations and/or activity of warfarin, phenytoin, cyclosporine, and oral hypoglycemic agents. Rifampin may increase the rate of metabolism, and it may be necessary to increase the dosage of the antifungal agent during the period of concurrent therapy.

Administration: Oral and intravenous.

Preparations: Tablets, 50, 100 and 200 mg. Oral suspension, 10 mg/ml. Glass bottles and plastic containers, 200 mg/100 ml and 400 mg/200 ml.

FLUCYTOSINE—Ancobon®

Description/Actions: Antifungal agent indicated for systemic infections caused by *Candida* and *Cryptococcus*.

Preparations: Capsules, 250 and 500 mg.

FLUDARA®, see Fludarabine

FLUDARABINE PHOSPHATE—Fludara®

Antineoplastic agent.

Description/Actions: Is an analogue of the antiviral agent vidarabine. Indicated for the treatment of patients with B-cell chronic lymphocytic leukemia who have not responded to or have progressed during treatment with at least one standard regimen containing an alkylating agent.

Warnings: May cause fetal harm and should not be used during pregnancy unless safer alternatives are not available. Pulmonary toxicity (e.g., ARDS, respiratory distress, pulmonary hemorrhage, pulmonary fibrosis, and respiratory failure) has occurred in patients treated with fludarabine. Myelosuppression may be severe; several instances of trilineage bone marrow depression or aplastic aplasia resulting in pancytopenia, sometimes death, have been reported. These effects have occurred in both previously treated and untreated patients. Decrease dose of fludarabine by 20% in patients with moderate renal impairment (creatinine clearance 30–70 ml/min/1.73 m^2). Fludarabine should not be administered to patients with severe renal impairment (creatinine clearance < 30 ml/min/1.73 m^2).

Administration: Intravenous.

Preparations: Vials, 50 mg.

FLUDROCORTISONE ACETATE—Florinef®

Description/Actions: Mineralocorticoid indicated for the treatment of Addison's disease and salt-losing adrenogenital syndrome.

Preparations: Tablets, 0.1 mg.

FLUMADINE®, see Rimantadine hydrochloride

FLUMAZENIL—Romazicon®

Benzodiazepine antagonist.

Description/Actions: Reverses the sedating and psychomotor effects of benzodiazepines (e.g., diazepam, midazolam); however, amnesia is less completely and less consistently reversed. Indicated for the complete or partial reversal of the sedative effects of benzodiazepines in cases where general anesthesia has been induced and/or maintained with benzodiazepines, where sedation has been produced with benzodiazepines for diagnostic and therapeutic procedures, and for the management of benzodiazepine overdose.

Warnings: Contraindicated in patients who may be relying on the effects of a benzodiazepine to control potentially life-threatening conditions (e.g., status epilepticus, increased intracranial pressure). Is also contraindicated in cases of serious cyclic antidepressant (e.g., amitriptyline) overdose. May cause seizures including withdrawal seizures in patients who are physically dependent on benzodiazepines. Other adverse reactions include nausea, vomiting, dizziness, agitation, and injection-site pain. In situations in which a patient has received a neuromuscular blocking agent, flumazenil should not be used until the effects of neuromuscular blockade have been fully reversed. Duration of action is shorter than that of the benzodiazepines, and a return of sedation (resedation) may occur following initial reversal; patients should be monitored for resedation, as well as respiratory depression and other residual benzodiazepine effects. Patients should be advised not to engage in any activities requiring complete alertness until at least 18 to 24 hours after discharge and not to take any alcohol or nonprescription drugs for 18 to 24 hours after flumazenil administration or if the effects of the benzodiazepine persist. Because flumazenil does not consistently reverse amnesia, patients cannot be expected to remember information told to them in the postprocedure period, and instructions given to patients should be reinforced in writing or given to a responsible family member.

Administration: Intravenous. Should be administered through a freely running intravenous infusion into a large vein to minimize the likelihood of pain or inflammation at the injection site.

Preparations: Vials, 0.1 mg/ml.

FLUMETHIAZIDE

Description/Actions: Thiazide diuretic used in combination with other agents in the treatment of hypertension.

FLUNISOLIDE—Aerobid®, Aerobid-M® (menthol flavor), Nasalide®, Nasarel®

Corticosteroid.

Description/Actions: Nasalide: Indicated for the topical treatment of the symptoms of seasonal or perennial rhinitis when effectiveness of or tolerance of conventional treatment is unsatisfactory. Nasarel: Treatment of seasonal or perennial rhinitis. Aerobid®: Maintenance treatment of asthma as prophylactic therapy or to reduce the need for systemic corticosteroids in individuals requiring systemic steroid therapy.

Warnings: Adverse reactions include transient nasal burning and stinging and nasal congestion. Caution must be exercised when transferring a patient from systemic corticosteroid therapy to flunisolide therapy. Contraindicated as primary treatment of an acute attack, in varicella and vaccinia.

Administration: Nasal spray.

Preparations: Nasal solution spray bottle, 6.25 mg, metered dose inhaler 250 µg/inh.

FLUOCINOLONE ACETONIDE— Synalar®

Description/Actions: Corticosteroid applied topically for relief of inflammatory and pruritic manifestations of corticosteroid-responsive dermatoses.

Preparations: Cream, 0.01%, 0.025%, and 0.2%. Ointment, 0.025%. Topical solution, 0.01%.

FLUOCINONIDE—Lidex®, Lidex-E®

Topical corticosteroid.

Description/Actions: Indicated for the relief of the inflammatory and pruritic manifestations of corticosteroid-responsive dermatoses.

Warnings: Adverse reactions include burning, itching, dryness, irritation, and a potential for systemic effects.

Administration: Topical.

Preparations: Cream, gel, ointment, and solution, 0.05%. Lidex-E cream utilizes water-washable aqueous base.

FLUORESCEIN SODIUM

Description/Actions: Diagnostic aid used in various ocular conditions.

Preparations: Solution, 2%. Strips, 0.6 and 1 mg. Ampules, 10% and 25%.

FLUOROMETHOLONE—FML®

Description/Actions: Corticosteroid indicated for ophthalmic use in the treatment of inflammatory conditions of the eye.

Preparations: Ophthalmic suspension and ointment, 0.1%.

FLUOROPLEX®, see Fluorouracil

FLUOROURACIL—Adrucil®, Carac™, Efudex®, 5 FU®, Fluoroplex®

Description/Actions: Antineoplastic agent indicated for intravenous use in the management of carcinoma of the colon, rectum, breast, stomach, and pancreas, and for the topical treatment of active or solar keratoses, and superficial basal cell carcinomas.

Preparations: Ampules, 500 mg. Cream, 05%, 1% and 5%. Topical solution, 1%, 2%, and 5%.

FLUOTHANE®, see Halothane

FLUOXETINE HYDROCHLORIDE— Prozac®, Prozac® Weekly™, Sarafem™

Antidepressant.

Description/Actions: Fluoxetine is a selective serotonin reuptake inhibitor. It is indicated for the treatment of depression, obsessive-compulsive disorder (OCD), bulimia nervosa, and panic disorder and for the treatment of premenstrual dysphoric disorder (PMDD). It is also indicated for the treatment of depression and OCD in pediatric patients.

Warnings: Adverse reactions include anxiety, nervousness, insomnia, nausea, diarrhea, and rash and/or urticaria. Dizziness and other CNS effects may develop and patients should be cautioned regarding activities such as driving and operating machinery, as well as interactions with other CNS-acting drugs including alcohol. Concurrent use with tryptophan has resulted in the development of agitation and restlessness in some patients. Use in combination with a monoamine oxidase inhibitor should be avoided and at least 14 days should elapse between discontinuation of a MAO inhibitor and initiation of treatment with fluoxetine. At least 5 weeks should elapse between discontinuation of fluoxetine and initiation of therapy with an MAOI.

Administration: Oral.

Preparations: Tablets, 10 mg. Capsules, 10 and 20 mg. Liquid, 20 mg/5 ml.

Sustained release capsule, 90 mg.

FLUOXYMESTERONE— Halotestin®

Description/Actions: Androgen indicated in male patients for replacement therapy in conditions associated with symptoms of deficiency or absence of endogenous testosterone (e.g., primary hypogonadism—testicular failure), and delayed puberty. Also indicated in the treatment of recurrent mammary cancer in selected female patients.

Preparations: Tablets, 2, 5, and 10 mg.

FLUPHENAZINE DECANOATE—Prolixin decanoate®

FLUPHENAZINE ENANTHATE—Prolixin enanthate®

Description/Actions: Phenothiazine antipsychotic agent indicated for the parenteral treatment of patients requiring prolonged parenteral neuroleptic therapy (e.g., chronic schizophrenics).

Preparations: Vials and syringes, 25 mg/ml.

FLUPHENAZINE HYDROCHLORIDE—Permitil®, Prolixin®

Description/Actions: Phenothiazine antipsychotic agent indicated for the management of manifestations of psychotic disorders.

Preparations: Tablets, 1, 2.5, 5, and 10 mg. Elixir, 2.5 mg/5 ml. Concentrate, 5 mg/ml. Vials, 2.5 mg/ml.

FLURANDRENOLIDE—Cordran®

Description/Actions: Corticosteroid applied topically for the relief of inflammatory and pruritic manifestations of corticosteroid-responsive dermatoses.

Preparations: Cream and ointment, 0.025% and 0.05%. Lotion, 0.05%. Tape, 4 µg/sq. cm. Patch, 2 3 inches.

FLURAZEPAM HYDROCHLORIDE—Dalmane®

Benzodiazepine hypnotic.

Description/Actions: A CNS depressant indicated for the management of insomnia.

Warnings: Contraindicated during pregnancy. Adverse reactions include residual sedation and other CNS effects upon awakening; patients should be cautioned regarding activities such as driving and operating machinery, as well as interactions with other CNS-acting drugs, including alcohol. Can cause dependence and is included in Schedule IV.

Administration: Oral.

Preparations: Capsules, 15 and 30 mg.

FLURBIPROFEN—Ansaid®

Nonsteroidal anti-inflammatory drug.

Description/Actions: Inhibits prostaglandin synthesis and is indicated for the treatment of rheumatoid arthritis and osteoarthritis.

Warnings: Should not be given to patients in whom aspirin or another NSAID causes asthma, rhinitis, urticaria, or other allergic-type reactions. May cause GI effects and use should be avoided in patients with active GI tract disease and closely monitored in patients with a previous history of such disorders.

Administration: Oral.

Preparations: Tablets, 50 and 100 mg.

FLURBIPROFEN SODIUM—Ocufen®

Nonsteroidal anti-inflammatory drug for ophthalmic use.

Description/Actions: Indicated for the inhibition of intraoperative miosis to reduce the risk of complications associated with procedures such as cataract surgery.

Warnings: Contraindicated in epithelial herpes simplex keratitis. Adverse reactions include transient burning and stinging upon instillation; the drug may also delay wound healing. Caution should be exercised in the treatment of patients having a history of sensitivity to aspirin or another nonsteroidal anti-inflammatory drug.

Administration: Ophthalmic.

Preparations: Ophthalmic solution, 0.03%.

FLUTAMIDE—Eulexin®

Antineoplastic agent.

Description/Actions: An antiandrogen that inhibits the uptake and binding of androgen. Is rapidly converted to hydroxyflutamide which is the major active metabolite. Indicated in the treatment of locally confined stage A_2–C or metastatic prostatic carcinoma (stage D_2) in combination with an analogue of luteinizing hormone-releasing hormone (LH-RH) such as leuprolide.

Warnings: Adverse reactions include diarrhea, nausea, vomiting, hot flashes, loss of libido, impotence, and gynecomastia. Has caused elevations of hepatic enzyme levels, as well as clinically evident hepatitis, and periodic liver function tests should be considered in patients on long-term therapy.

Administration: Oral. It is recommended that treatment be started simultaneously with both flutamide and leuprolide. Patients should be informed that the two drugs are to be administered concurrently and that they should not discontinue taking either medication without consulting their physician.

Preparations: Capsules, 125 mg.

FLUTICASONE PROPIONATE—
Cutivate®, Flonase®, Flovent®, Flovent® Diskus™

Corticosteroid.

Description/Actions: Indicated (Cutivate®) for the relief of the inflammatory and pruritic manifestations of corticosteroid-responsive dermatoses. Also administered (Zlonase®) by nasal inhalation for the managment of seasonal and perennial allergic rhinitis.

Warnings: Adverse reactions include pruritus, dryness, burning, increased erythema, hypertrichosis, and numbness of fingers.

Administration: Topical, nasal, and inhalation.

Preparations: Cream, 0.05%; ointment, 0.005%. Nasal spray, 44 µg, 50 µg, 110 µg, 220 µg per actuation. Metered dose inhaler, 44, 110, and 220 µg/inh. Rotadisk, 50, 100, and 250 µg/inh. via dry powder.

FLUVASTATIN SODIUM—Lescol®, Lescol® XL

Agent for hypercholesterolemia.

Description/Actions: Produces a significant reduction in total and low-density lipoprotein (LDL) cholesterol concentrations, a modest reduction in triglyceride concentrations, and an increase in high-density lipoprotein (HDL) cholesterol concentrations. Indicated as an adjunct to diet in the treatment of elevated total cholesterol and low-density lipoprotein cholesterol in patients with primary hypercholesterolemia whose response to dietary restriction of saturated fat and cholesterol and other nonpharmacological measures has not been adequate. Also indicated to slow the progression of coronary atherasclerosis in patients with coronary heart disease.

Warnings: Contraindicated in patients with active liver disease or unexplained, persistent elevations of serum transaminases. Is also contraindicated in pregnant women and nursing mothers. Increases in serum transaminases may occur and it is recommended that liver function tests be performed before the initiation of treatment, at 6 and 12 weeks after initiation of therapy or elevation in dose, and periodically thereafter (e.g., every 6 months). Should be used with caution in patients with a history of liver disease or heavy alcohol ingestion. Adverse reactions include dyspepsia, abdominal pain, arthropathy, and exercise-related muscle pain. Patients should be advised to promptly report unexplained muscle pain, tenderness or weakness. The concurrent use of clofibrate or gemfibrozil is best avoided, and caution should be exercised if cyclosporine or erythromycin is used concurrently. When used concomitantly with a bile acid-binding resin, it should be administered at least 4 hours after the resin.

Administration: Oral. Should be administered at bedtime.

Preparations: Capsules, 20 and 40 mg, extended release tablet, 80 mg.

FLUVOXAMINE MALEATE—Luvox®

Description/Actions: Selective serotonin reuptake inhibitor indicated for the treatment of obsessive compulsive disorder.

Warnings: Concurrent administration of terfenadine or astemizole is contraindicated. Adverse reactions include somnolence, insomnia, nervousness, dizziness, and tremor. Advise patients to avoid driving or operating machinery until response is ascertained. Alcohol should be avoided. It is recommended that fluvoxamine not be used in combination with MAOIs or within 14 days of discontinuing an MAOI.

Administration: Oral.

Preparations: Tablets, 50 and 100 mg.

FML®, see Fluorometholone

FOCALIN™, see Dexmethylphenidate Hydrochloride

FOLIC ACID—Folvite®

Description/Actions: Agent for anemias that is indicated in the prevention and treatment of megaloblastic anemias due to a deficiency of folic acid as may be seen in sprue, anemias of nutritional origin, pregnancy, infancy, or childhood.

Preparations: Tablets, 0.1, 0.4, 0.8, and 1 mg. Vials 5 mg/ml and 10 mg/ml.

FOLINIC ACID, see Leucovorin

FOLLUTEIN®, see Chorionic gonadotropin

FOLVITE®, see Folic Acid

FOMIVIRSEN NA—Vitravene®

Description/Actions: Indicated for the local treatment of human cytomegalovirus (CMV) retinitis in patients with AIDs who are intolerant of or have a contraindication to other treatment for CMV retinitis or who are insufficiently responsive to previous treatment for CMV retinitis.

Precautions/Adverse Reactions: Fomivirsen is contraindicated in patients who have recently (within 2–4 weeks) been treated with either intravenous or intravitreal cidofovir because of the risk of exaggerated ocular inflammation. CMV retinitis may be associated with CMV disease elsewhere in the body. Fomivirsen provides localized therapy limited to the treated eye. The use of fomivirsen does not provide treatment for systemic CMV disease. Patients should be monitored for extraocular CMV disease or disease of the contralateral eye.

Adverse reactions include ocular inflammation, uveitis, including iritis and vitreitis. Inflammation is more commonly reported during the induction dosing.

Administration: Intravitreal injection. Treatment with fomivirsen involves an induction and an maintenance phase. Dosing for both phases is 330 mcg (0.05 mL).

Patient Care Implications: If inflammatory reactions are severe, delaying additional treatment and using topical corticosteroids have been shown to be useful in medical management of these reactions.

For patients whose disease progresses while on fomivirsen, an attempt at reinduction at the same dose may result in resumed disease control. Instruct patients that fomivirsen is not a cure for their opthalmic CMV and that adherence to consistent follow-up appointments is necessary. Warn patients that their disease may still progress despite treatment with fomivirsen.

Preparations: Single-use vial, 0.25 ml (6.6 mg/ml).

FONDAPARINUX—ARIXTRA®

Description/Actions: Fondaparinux is indicated for the prophylaxis of deep vein thrombosis, which may lead to pulmonary embolism in patients undergoing hip fracture surgery, hip replacement surgery, and knee replacement surgery.

Precautions/Adverse Reactions: Fondaparinux cannot be used interchangeably (unit for unit) with heparin, low molecular weight heparins (LMWHs) or heparinoids. Each of these medicines has their own instructions for use. Use with extreme caution in conditions with increased risk of hemorrhage, such as congenital or acquired bleeding disorders, active ulcerative and angiodysplastic disease, and hemorrhagic stroke; shortly after brain, spinal, or opthalmological surgery, or in patients treated concomitantly with platelet inhibitors. Discontinue agents that may increase the risk of hemorrhage before starting fondaparinux. Should be used with caution in elderly ptients and in patients with a history of heparin-induced thrombocytopenia.

Warning: When neuraxial anesthesia or spinal puncture is used, patients anticoagulated or scheduled to be anticoagulated with LMWH, heparinoids, or fondaparinux for prevention of thromboembolic complications are at risk of developing an epidural or spinal hematoma, which can result in long-term or permanent paralysis.

Pregnancy Category B. No adequate or well-controlled studies in pregnant women; use only if clearly needed. Excretion in breast milk unknown; use caution.

The most common adverse reactions were bleeding complications. Other adverse reactions were mild local irritation, edema, fever, nausea, constipation, vomiting, and insomnia. Antiplatelet agents (anagrelide, clopidogrel, dipyridamole, abciximab), NSAIDs, and salicylates may increase its anticoagulant effect.

Administration: SQ Injection.

Patient Care Implications: Inform patients they may have tendency to bleed easily while on fondaparinux; brush teeth with soft brush, floss with waxed floss, use electric razor, and avoid potentially harmful activities.

Preparations: Injection: 2.5 mg in 0.5 ml single-dose prefilled syringe, affixed with a 27 gauge X ½ inch needle with an automatic needle protection system.

FORADIL®—see Formoterol Fumarate

FORMOTEROL FUMARATE—FORADIL®

Description/Actions: Formoterol fumarate is indicated for long-term twice daily (morning and evening) administration in the maintenance treatment of asthma and in the prevention of bronchopasm in adults and children > 5 years of age with reversible obstructive airway disease including patients with symptoms of nocturnal asthma who require regular treatment with inhaled, short-acting beta-2-agonists. Formoterol is also indicated for the acute prevention of exercise-induced bronchospasm in adults and children 12 years of age when administered on an occasional, as needed basis. Formoterol is indicated for the long-term, twice daily (morning and evening) administration in the maintenance treatment of bronchoconstriction in patients with chronic obstructive pulmonary disease, including chronic bronchitis and emphysema.

Precautions/Adverse Reactions: Therapy with formoterol should not be initiated in patients with worsening or acutely deteriorating asthma that may be a life-threatening condition. Formoterol is not a substitute for inhaled or oral corticosteroids. Corticosteroid therapy should not be stopped or reduced at the time formoterol is initiated. When initiating therapy with formoterol in patients who have been taking inhaled, short-acting beta-2-agonists on a regular basis, patients should be instructed to discontinue the regular use of the short-acting beta-2-agonist and to use them only on an as needed basis for symptomatic relief of acute asthma symptoms. Formoterol can produce paradoxical bronchospasms that may be life-threatening. If it occurs, discontinue formoterol immediately. Formoterol should not be used more frequently than twice daily at the recommended dose. Worsening asthma may warrant a reevaluation of the patient and treatment regimen.

Formoterol can produce clinically significant cardiovascular effects in some patients, such as increased heart rate, increased blood pressure, and/or symptoms. Use with caution in patients with cardiovascular disorders such as coronary insufficiency, cardiac arrhythmias, and hypertension. Use with caution in patients with seizure disorders and thyrotoxicosis and in patients who are unusually sensitive to sympathomimetic amines. Beta-2-agonists have been reported to produce ECG changes such as flattening of the T wave, prolongation of the QT_c interval, and ST segment depression. Immediate hypersensitivity reactions (anaphylactic reactions, urticaria, angioedema, rash, and bronchospasm) may occur following the administration of formoterol.

Concurrent use of formoterol with xanthine derivatives, steroids, or diuretics may potentiate the hypokalemic effects of adrenergic agonists. Concomitant administration of formoterol with monoamine oxidase inhibitors, tricyclic antidepressants, or drugs known to prolong the QT_c interval may potentiate cardiovascular side effects. Coadministration of beta-blockers and formoterol may inhibit the effects of each other. Beta-blockers not only block the therapeutic effects of beta agonists, but may produce severe bronchospasms in asthmatic patients. Use a cardioselective beta-blocker if therapy with a beta-blocker is necessary.

Concurrent administration of formoterol and adrenergic drugs may potentiate the sympathetic effects of formoterol. Pregnancy Category C. Formoterol has been shown to cause stillbirth and neonatal mortality in rats. No adequate and well-controlled studies in pregnant women. Use during pregnancy only if the potential benefit justifies the potential risk to the fetus. Excretion in human breast milk is unknown. Beta-2-agonists may potentially interfere with uterine contractility. Use during labor only if the potential benefit justifies the potential risk. Safety and efficacy in children < 5 years of age have not been established.

Most common adverse effects noted in patients treated with formoterol include angina, hypertension or hypotension, tachycardia, arrhythmias, nervousness, headache, tremor, dry mouth, palpitation, muscle cramps, nausea, dizziness, fatigue, malaise, dysphonia, hypokalemia, hyperglycemia, metabolic acidosis, and insomnia. Most common adverse events seen in children include viral infection, inflammation, abdominal pain, nausea, and dyspepsia.

Administration: Foradil® capsules should be administered by the oral inhalation route and only using the Aerolizer inhaler.

Patient Care Implications: Patients should be advised not to increase the dose or frequency of formoterol without consulting their physician. Patients should be informed that formoterol is not intended to relieve acute asthma symptoms. When formoterol is used for the prevention of exercise-induced bronchospasms, the contents of 1 capsule should be taken at least 15 minutes prior to exercise.

Formoterol should not be used as a substitute for oral or inhaled corticosteroids. The dosage of these medications should not be changed, and they should not be stopped without consulting a physician.

Patients should be informed that treatment with beta-2-agonists may cause palpitations, chest pain, rapid heart rate, tremor, or nervousness. Patients should be advised never to use formoterol with a spacer and never to exhale into the device.

Patient should be instructed to avoid exposing formoterol capsules to moisture and should be instructed to handle the capsule with dry hands.

The Aerolizer inhaler should never be washed and should be kept dry. Patients should be informed that in rare cases the gelatin capsule may break into small pieces. These pieces should be retained by the screen built into the Aerolizer inhaler. However, tiny pieces of gelatin may reach the mouth or throat after inhalation.

Patients should be informed that formoterol capsules should always be stored in the blister and only removed immediately before use. Formoterol capsules should only be administered by oral inhalation. Formoterol capsules should not be ingested.

Preparations: Gelatin capsules containing 12 mg of formoterol fumarate for oral inhalation, and one Aerolizer inhaler.

FORTAZ®, see Ceftazidime

FORTOVASE®, see Saquinavir

FOSAMAX®, see Alendronate

FOSCARNET SODIUM—Foscavir®

Antiviral agent.

Description/Actions: Inhibits replication of herpes viruses including cytomegalovirus (CMV). Indicated for the treatment of cytomegalovirus retinitis in patients with AIDS. Also indicated for the treatment of acyclovir-resistant mucocutaneous herpes simplex virus infections in immunocompromised patients.

Warnings: May cause renal impairment and creatinine clearance should be determined at baseline, 2–3 times per week during induction therapy, and at least once every 1 or 2 weeks during maintenance therapy. Concurrent use with other potentially nephrotoxic drugs (e.g., aminoglycosides) should be avoided when possible.

Has the potential to chelate divalent metal ions such as calcium and has been associated with changes in serum electrolytes including hypocalcemia and hypomagnesemia, as well as hypokalemia, hypophosphatemia, and hyperphosphatemia. Serum calcium, magnesium, potassium, and phosphorus should be monitored on a schedule similar to that recommended for serum creatinine. Patients should be advised to report symptoms such as perioral tingling, numbness in the extremities, and paresthesias which may be associated with electrolyte abnormalities. The concomitant use with intravenous pentamidine may increase the risk of severe hypocalcemia. Other adverse reactions include seizures, anemia, granulocytopenia, fever, nausea, vomiting, diarrhea, and headache.

Administration: Intravenous infusion. Must not be administered by rapid or bolus injection because of the increased risk of toxicity.

Preparations: Bottles, 250 and 500 ml containing the drug in a concentration of 24 mg/ml.

FOSCAVIR®, see Foscarnet

FOSFOMYCIN—Monurol®

Description/Actions: Synthetic, broad-spectrum antibiotic that has bactericidal activity in the urine at therapeutic doses. Indicated in the treatment of uncomplicated susceptible UTIs in women.

Warnings: Adverse reactions include diarrhea, vaginitis, nausea, headache, dizziness, asthenia, and dyspepsia.

Usual adult dose (oral) for UTIs: Female: single dose of 3 g in 4 oz. of water; male: 3 g once daily for 2–3 days for complicated UTIs. Dissolve granules in 3–4 oz of water (not hot), stir to dissolve, and drink immediately. Follow manufacturer's guidelines for dosing for each episode of acute cystitis, since repeated daily doses do not improve clinical success but increase the incidence of adverse events. If bacteria persist or reappear after treatment with fosfomycin, other therapeutic agents should be selected. Urine specimen should be obtained for culture and sensitivity testing before and after completion of therapy.

Preparations: Single-dose sachet packets of 3 g.

FOSINOPRIL SODIUM—Monopril®

Antihypertensive agent.

Description/Actions: An angiotensin converting enzyme (ACE) inhibitor that is a prodrug. Following oral administration, is converted to its active metabolite, fosinoprilat. Indicated for the treatment of hypertension and may be used alone or in combination with a thiazide diuretic. Also indicated in the management of congestive heart failure.

Warnings: Adverse reactions include headache, dizziness, fatigue, cough, diarrhea, and nausea/vomiting. May cause an elevation in serum potassium levels; the risk of hyperkalemia is increased in patients also taking a potassium-sparing diuretic, a potassium supplement, and/or a potassium-containing salt substitute. May cause symptomatic postural hypotension. There have been infrequent reports of angioedema of the face, extremities, lips, tongue, glottis, and larynx, especially following the first dose. Patients should be told to report immediately any symptoms suggesting angioedema and to stop taking the drug. When used during the second and third trimesters of pregnancy, ACE inhibitors have been reported to be associated with the development of neonatal hypertension, renal failure, and skull hypoplasia; use during pregnancy should be avoided. May increase serum lithium levels and concurrent therapy should be closely monitored.

Administration: Oral.

Preparations: Tablets, 10 and 20 mg.

FOSPHENYTOIN SODIUM—Cerebyx®

Description/Actions: For short-term (up to 5 days) IV/IM administration when other forms of phenytoin administration are unavailable or deemed less advantageous. See phenytoin.

FRAGMIN®, see Dalteparin

FROVA™, see Frovatriptan

FROVATRIPTAN—FROVA™

Description/Actions: Frovatriptan is indicated for acute treatment of migraine with or without aura in adult patients.

Precautions/Adverse Reactions: Because of the potential of this class of compound (5-HT1 agonists) to cause coronary vasospasm, frovatriptan should not be given to patients with documented ischemic or vasospastic coronary artery disease (CAD). Not intended for the prophylactic therapy of migraine or for use in the management of hemiplegic or basilar migraine. Frovatriptan is contraindicated in the following conditions: cerebrovascular syndromes, peripheral vascular disease, and uncontrolled hypertension. It is strongly recommended that frovatriptan not be given to patients in whom unrecognized CAD is predicted by the presence of risk factors (e.g., hypertension, hypercholesterolemia, smoker, obesity, diabetes, strong family history of CAD, female with surgical or physiological menopause, or male over 40 years of age) unless a cardiovascular evaluation provides satisfactory clinical evidence that the patient is reasonably free of coronary artery and ischemic myocardial disease or other significant underlying cardiovascular disease. It should not be used within 24 hours of treatment with another 5-HT1 agonist, an ergotamine-containing or ergot-type medication or methysergide. Ergot-containing drugs have been reported to cause prolonged vasospastic reactions. The most common adverse events were dizziness, paresthesia, headache, dry mouth, fatigue, flushing, hot or cold sensation, and chest pain. Serious cardiac events, including some that have been fatal, have occurred following the use of a 5-HT1 agonist. These events are extremely rare, and most have been reported in patients with risk factors predictive of CAD. There are no adequate and well-controlled studies in pregnant women. Pregnancy Category C. Use only if potential benefit to mother outweighs the potential risk to fetus. Excretion in breast milk is unknown; use caution. Safety and effectiveness in pediatrics have not been established.

Administration: Oral, adult migraine: 2.5 mg. If headache recurs, a second dose of 2.5 mg may be given if the first dose provided some relief. Two hours must elapse between doses. Maximum daily dose: 7.5 mg.

Patient Care Implications: Take with fluids. Take at first sign of migraine attack. It does not prevent migraine. For patients with risk factors predictive of CAD who have been determined to have a satisfactory cardiovascular evaluation, it is strongly recommended that administration of the first dose be given in a physician's office.

Preparations: Tablets, 2.5 mg.

FRUCTOSE—Levulose

Description/Actions: Carbohydrate administered parenterally as a source of calories.

Preparations: Solution, 10%.

FUDR®, see Floxuridine

FULVICIN®, see Griseofulvin

FUNGIZONE®, see Amphotericin B

FURACIN®, see Nitrofurazone

FURADANTIN®, see Nitrofurantoin

FURAZOLIDONE—Furoxone®

Description/Actions: Anti-infective agent indicated in the treatment of bacterial or protozoal diarrhea and enteritis caused by susceptible organisms.

Preparations: Tablets, 100 mg. Liquid, 50 mg/15 ml.

FUROSEMIDE—Lasix®

Diuretic and antihypertensive agent.

Description/Actions: Is a loop diuretic indicated (1) for the treatment of edema associated with congestive heart failure, cirrhosis of the liver, and renal diseases and (2) hypertension. Is also indicated via intravenous use as adjunctive therapy in acute pulmonary edema.

Warnings: Is contraindicated in anuria. May cause volume and electrolyte depletion. Potential for hypokalemia warrants periodic measurement of serum potassium levels. Reduction in potassium levels may increase the action and toxicity of digoxin and related glycosides. Parenteral therapy is best avoided in patients receiving aminoglycoside antibiotics because of an increased risk of ototoxicity.

Administration: Oral, intravenous, and intramuscular.

Preparations: Tablets, 20, 40, and 80 mg. Oral solution, 10 mg/ml. Ampules, vials, and syringes, 10 mg/ml.

FUROXONE®, see Furazolidone

G

GABAPENTIN—Neurontin®

Antiepileptic agent.

Description/Actions: Gabapentin is indicated as adjunctive therapy in the treatment of partial seizures with and without secondary generalizations in patients over 12 years of age with epilepsy. Gabapentin is also indicated as adjunctive therapy in the treatment of partial seizures in pediatric patients age 3–12 years and for the management of postherpetic neuralgia in adults.

Warnings: Adverse reactions include somnolence, dizziness, ataxia, nystagmus, and tremor. Patients should be cautioned not to drive or operate machinery until they have gained sufficient experience with the use of the drug to determine whether it affects their mental and/or motor performance adversely. Bioavailability is reduced by the administration of aluminum/magnesiun-containing antacids and it should be administered at least 2 hours following the antacid.

Administration: Oral. If treatment is to be discontinued and/or an alternative anticonvulsant is added to the therapy, this should be done gradually over a minimum of 1 week.

Preparations: Capsules, 100, 300, and 400 mg tablets, 600 and 800 mg. Oral solution, 250 mg/ 5 mL.

GABITRIL®, see Tiagabine Hydrochloride

GALLAMINE TRIETHIODIDE— Flaxedil®

Description/Actions: Neuromuscular blocking agent indicated as an adjunct to anesthesia to induce skeletal muscle relaxation. Also used to manage patients undergoing mechanical ventilation.

Preparations: Vials, 20 mg/ml.

GALLIUM NITRATE—Ganite®

Agent for hypercalcemia.

Description/Actions: Exerts a hypocalcemic effect by inhibiting calcium resorption from bone. Indicated for the treatment of symptomatic cancer-related hypercalcemia that has not responded to adequate hydration.

Warnings: Contraindicated in patients with severe renal impairment. May cause renal effects and serum creatinine levels should be monitored. Concurrent use with other potentially nephrotoxic drugs (e.g., aminoglycosides, amphotericin B) may increase the risk of developing severe renal insufficiency. Other adverse reactions include hypocalcemia, transient hypophosphatemia, decreased sodium bicarbonate, anemia, decreased blood pressure, and nausea and/or vomiting.

Administration: Intravenous. The daily dose must be administered as an IV infusion over 24 hours. Adequate hydration must be maintained throughout the treatment period.

Preparations: Vials, 500 mg.

GAMMA BENZENE HEXACHLORIDE, see Lindane

GANCICLOVIR SODIUM— Cytovene®

Antiviral agent.

Description/Actions: Inhibits replication of herpes viruses including cytomegalovirus (CMV). Indicated for the treatment of cytomegalovirus retinitis in immunocompromised individuals, including patients with AIDS. Also indicated in transplant patients at risk for CMV disease.

Warnings: May cause granulocytopenia and thrombocytopenia and it is recommended that neutrophil counts and platelet counts be performed every 2 days during the period in which ganciclovir is dosed twice daily and at least weekly thereafter. Other adverse reactions include anemia, fever, rash, and abnormal liver function values. Has been reported to be teratogenic in animals and it should be used during pregnancy only if the benefits outweigh the risks. Because of the mutagenic potential of ganciclovir, women of childbearing potential should be advised to use effective contraception during treatment, and male patients should be advised to practice barrier contraception during and for at least 90 days following treatment with the drug. The concurrent use of ganciclovir and zidovudine is associated with an increased risk of granulocytopenia. Seizures have been reported in some patients receiving ganciclovir and imipenem-cilastatin concurrently and the use of these agents in combination should be avoided if possible. Probenecid may reduce the renal clearance and increase the action of ganciclovir.

Administration: Intravenous infusion (at a constant rate over a period of 1 hour) and oral, which should be taken with food.

Preparations: Vials, containing ganciclovir sodium equivalent to 500 mg ganciclovir. Capsules, 250 mg.

GANIRELIX—Antagon®

Description/Actions: Ganirelix is a gonadotropin-releasing hormone antagonist (GnRH) that is used in women receiving assisted insemination or reproductive technology (ART) procedures.

Precautions/Adverse Reactions: Ganirelix should not be given to patients who have a hypersensitivity to mannitol or ganirelix, have primary ovarian failure, or have an ovarian cyst. The drug should be given carefully to patients with either kidney or hepatic impairment. Also, ganirelix should be avoided in pregnant women, breast-feeding women, and children. Ganirelix is usually well tolerated but some common adverse reactions are abdominal pain, headache, ovarian hyperstimulation syndrome, vaginal bleeding, menstrual irregularity, nausea, vomiting, and hot flashes.

Administration: SQ injection.

Patient Care Implications: Patients should avoid excessive alcohol or tobacco consumption during therapy. Patients with renal or hepatic impairment should be monitored carefully. A pregnancy test should be done before therapy is started. Monitor the patient by getting serum estradiol and gonadotropin levels and also conducting pelvic exams and pelvic ultrasounds.

Preparations: Syringe, 250 mcg.

GANITE®, see Gallium nitrate

GANTANOL®, see Sulfamethoxazole

GANTRISIN®, see Sulfisoxazole

GANTRISIN ACETYL®, see Sulfisoxazole acetyl

GARAMYCIN®, see Gentamicin

GASTROCROM®, see Cromolyn

GATIFLOXACIN—Tequin®

Description/Actions: Indicated for the treatment of infections in the following conditions: acute bacterial exacerbation of chronic bronchitis, acute sinusitis, community-acquired pneumonia, uncomplicated urinary tract infections, pyelonephritis, uncomplicated urethral and cervical gonorrhea, and acute, uncomplicated rectal infections in women. Uncomplicated skin and skin structure infections.

Precautions/Adverse Reactions: Tequin is contraindicated in persons with a history of hypersensitivity to gatifloxacin or any member of the quinolone class of antimicrobial agents. The safety and effectiveness of gatifloxacin in pediatric patients, adolescents, and pregnant or lactating women have not been established. Gatifloxacin may have the potential to prolong the QTc interval of the electrocardiogram of some patients. Due to the lack of clinical experience, Gatifloxacin should be avoided in patients with known prolongation of the QTc interval, patients with uncorrected hypokalemia, and patients receiving class IA or class III antiarrhythmic agents. Quinolones may cause CNS events including nervousness, agitation, insomnia, anxiety, nightmares, or paranoia. Caution should be used in patients with renal insufficiency..

Administration: Oral, intravenous.

Preparations: Tablets, 200 and 400 mg.

IV solution, 20- and 40-ml vials, 10 mg/ml; 100- and 200-ml flexible containers, 2 mg/ml.

G-CSF, see Filgrastim

GEMCITABINE HYDRO-CHLORIDE—Gemzar®

Antineoplastic.

Description/Actions: Antineoplastic agent used in the treatment of adenocarcinoma of the pancreas and as a first-line treatment for patients with locally advanced (nonresectable stage II or III) or metastatic (stage IV) disease in patients previously treated with 5-FU.

Warnings: Prolongation of infusion time beyond 30 minutes and more frequent administration than weekly dosing have been shown to increase toxicity. Side effects include myelosuppression, fever, rash, pruritis, transient elevations in serum transaminases, mild hematuria, and proteinuria. Monitor patients prior to each dose with a CBC including differential and platelet count.

Administration: Intravenous.

Preparations: Powder for injection 20 mg/ml (10 ml/50 ml)

GEMFIBROZIL—Lopid®

Description/Actions: Antihyperlipidemic agent indicated as adjunctive therapy to diet for (1) the treatment of patients with very high serum triglyceride levels (Type IV or Type V hyperlipoproteinemia) who present a risk of abdominal pain and pancreatitis and who do not respond adequately to dietary measures and (2) reducing the risk of coronary heart disease.

Precautions/Adverse Reactions: Concomitant therapy with gemfibrozil and an HMG-CoA reductase inhibitor (simvastatin, fluvastatin, lovastatin, atorvastatin, pravastatin) is associated with an increased risk of skeletal muscle toxicity manifested as rhabdomyolysis, markedly elevated creatine kinase (CPK) levels, and myoglobinuria, leading to acute renal failure and death.

Preparations: Capsules, 300 mg. Tablets 600 mg.

GEMTUZUMAB OZOGAMICIN—Mylotarg®

Description/Actions: Gemtuzumab is a chemotherapeutic agent that is indicated for the treatment of patients with CD33 positive acute myeloid leukemia in first relapse who are 60 years of age or older and who are not considered candidates for other cytotoxic chemotherapy.

Precautions/Adverse Reactions: Gemtuzumab is contraindicated in patients with a known hypersensitivity to gemtuzumab ozogamicin or any of it components, anti-CD33 antibody, calicheamicin derivatives, or inactive ingredients. Gemtuzumab should be administered under the supervision of physicians experienced in the treatment of acute leukemia. Since there is no data to support using gemtuzumab in combination with other chemotherapeutic agents, it should only be used as single-agent therapy. Severe myelosuppression will occur in all patients. Severe hypersensitivity reactions including anaphylaxis, infusion reactions, and pulmonary events can occur during the infusion or within 24 hours of the start of the infusion. Postinfusion reactions characterized by fever, chills, hypotension, or dyspnea may occur during the first 24 hours after administration. Vital signs should be monitored during the infusion and for 4 hours following the infusion. Hepatotoxicity has been reported with gemtuzumab therapy. Caution should be exercised when administering to patients with hepatic impairment. Tumor lysis syndrome may occur as a consequence of leukemic treatment. Prophylactic hydration and allopurinol should be started to prevent hyperuricemia. Leukoreduction with hydroxyurea and leukapheresis to decrease the peripheral white blood cell count to < 30,000 cells/ml prior to the administration of gemtuzumab. Do not administer as an intravenous push or bolus. No formal drug interaction studies have been performed. Pregnancy Category D. There are no adequate and well-controlled studies in pregnant women. May cause fetal harm if administered to pregnant women. Excretion in human breast milk is unknown. The most common side effects observed in patients on gemtuzumab were infusion related effects such as chills, fever, nausea, vomiting, headache, hypotension, hypertension, hypoxia, dyspnea, and hyperglycemia. Severe myelosuppression is the major toxicity associated with gemtuzumab. In clinical trials, neutropenia was observed in 98% of patients, thrombocytopenia (99%), anemia (47%), infection (28%), herpes simplex infections (22%), and 15% of patients experienced bleeding. Mucositis was observed in 35% of patients. Increased bilirubin, AST, and ALT were also observed during gemtuzumab therapy.

Administration: For intravenous infusion only.

Patient Care Implications: Vital signs should be monitored during the infusion and for 4 hours after the infusion. The solution must not be given as an intravenous push or bolus. Administer diphenhydramine and acetaminophen 1 hour prior to the start of the infusion. Gemtuzumab is light sensitive; use an UV protective bag over the IV bag during infusion. A separate IV line equipped with a low protein-binding 1.2–micron filter must be used for administration of the drug. Chemotherapeutic agent should be handled and disposed of properly.

Preparations: Powder for injection, 5 mg of lyophilized powder in 20 ml amber glass vial.

GEMZAR®—see Gemcitabine

GENOTROPIN®—see Somatropin

GENTAMICIN SULFATE—
   Garamycin®

Aminoglycoside antibiotic.

Description/Actions: Indicated for the parenteral treatment of serious infections caused by gram-negative bacteria including *Pseudomonas aeruginosa*. Is also effective in the treatment of staphylococcal infections. Has also been used topically in the treatment of dermatologic and ocular infections.

Warnings: May cause nephrotoxicity, ototoxicity and neurotoxicity, and the concurrent or serial use of other nephrotoxic or ototoxic agents should be avoided.

Administration: Intravenous, intramuscular, intrathecal, topical, and ophthalmic.

Preparations: Vials, 40 mg/ml. Vials, syringes, and piggyback units, 60, 70, 80, 90, 100, 120, 160, and 180 mg. Vials (for intrathecal use), 2 mg/ml. Cream and ointment, 0.1%. Ophthalmic solution and ointment, 0.3%.

GENTIAN VIOLET—
   Methylrosaniline chloride

Description/Actions: Anti-infective agent used topically in the treatment of dermatologic and vaginal infections.

Preparations: Solutions, 1% and 2%.

GENTRAN®, see Dextran

GEOCILLIN®, see Carbenicillin indanyl sodium

GEODON™, see Ziprasidone

GLEEVEC™, see Imatinib Mesylate

GLIMEPIRIDE—Amaryl®

Oral antidiabetic sulfonylurea.

Description/Actions: Used as an adjunct to diet and exercise in noninsulin dependent diabetes mellitus (NIDDM) in individuals who are unable to maintain glycemic control by diet and exercise alone. Also indicated for secondary failure in combination with insulin.

Warnings: Contraindicated in ketoacidosis as this condition should be treated with insulin. Administration of oral hypoglycemic drugs has been reported to be associated with increased cardiovascular mortality as compared to treatment with diet alone or diet plus insulin. May cause hypoglycemia, dizziness, asthenia, headache, nausea, allergic skin reactions, and blood dyscrasias.

Administration: Oral once daily with breakfast or first main meal.

Preparations: Scored tablets, 1, 2, and 4 mg.

GLIPIZIDE—Glucotrol®, Glucotrol XL

Sulfonylurea hypoglycemic agent.

Description/Actions: Indicated as an adjunct to diet for the control of hyperglycemia and its associated symptomatology in patients with noninsulin-dependent diabetes mellitus, after an adequate trial of dietary therapy has proved unsatisfactory.

Warnings: May cause hypoglycemia and patients should be advised to contact their physician if symptoms of hypoglycemia develop. Adverse reactions include nausea, diarrhea, pruritus, and erythema. Oral hypoglycemic agents have been suggested to be associated with increased cardiovascular mortality as compared to treatment with diet alone or diet plus insulin. Corticosteroids and thiazide and other diuretics may increase blood glucose levels and necessitate an increase in dosage of glipizide. Therapy in patients also receiving a beta-adrenergic blocking agent should be monitored closely.

Administration: Oral.

Preparations: Tablets, 5 and 10 mg. Controlled-release tablet (Glucotrol XL), 5 and 10 mg.

GLUCAGON

Description/Actions: Agent to increase blood glucose levels. Indicated for parenteral use in counteracting severe hypoglycemic reactions in diabetic patients or during insulin shock therapy in psychiatric patients. Used to facilitate radiographic examination of the GI tract.

Warnings: Contraindicated in pheochromocytoma. Adverse reactions include GI upset and hypersensitivity reaction (urticaria, respiratory distress, hypotension).

Preparations: Vials, 1 and 10 mg.

GLUCOPHAGE® see Metformin hydrochloride

GLUCOPHAGE® XR see Metformin hydrochloride

GLUCOSE, see Dextrose

GLUCOTROL®, see Glipizide

GLUCOTROL XL®, see Glipizide

GLUCOVANCE™, Combination of Glyburide and metformin hydrochloride

GLUTAMIC ACID HYDROCHLORIDE

Description/Actions: Gastric acidifier used in the treatment of conditions associated with a deficiency of hydrochloric acid in the gastric juice.

Preparations: Capsules, 340 mg.

GLUTETHIMIDE—Doriglute®

Description/Actions: Hypnotic indicated for the short-term treatment of insomnia, sedative effect preoperatively and during the first stage of labor.

Preparations: Tablets, 250 mg.

GLYBURIDE—DiaBeta®, Micronase®, Glynase®

Sulfonylurea hypoglycemic agent.

Description/Actions: Indicated as an adjunct to diet to lower the blood glucose in patients with non–insulin-dependent diabetes mellitus whose hyperglycemia cannot be controlled by diet alone.

Warnings: May cause hypoglycemia and patients should be advised to contact their physician if symptoms of hypoglycemia develop. Adverse reactions include nausea, heartburn, epigastric fullness, pruritus, erythema, urticaria, and rash. Oral hypoglycemic agents have been suggested to be associated with increased cardiovascular mortality as compared to treatment with diet alone or diet plus insulin. Corticosteroids and thiazide and other diuretics may increase blood glucose levels and necessitate an increase in dosage of glyburide. Therapy in patients also receiving a beta-adrenergic blocking agent should be monitored closely.

Administration: Oral.

Preparations: Tablets, 1.25, 2.5, and 5 mg. Tablets, micronized, 1.5, 3, and 6 mg (Glynase PresTab).

GLYCERYL TRIACETATE, see Triacetin

GLYCERYL TRINITRATE—Former name for Nitroglycerin

GLYCINE, see Aminoacetic Acid

GLYCOPYRROLATE—Robinul®

Description/Actions: Anticholinergic agent used as adjunctive therapy in the treatment of peptic ulcer. Is also used parenterally as a preoperative antimuscarinic, intraoperatively to counteract drug induced or vagal traction reflexes with the associated arrhythmias, or to protect against the peripheral muscarinic effects of cholinergic agents given to reverse the neuromuscular blockade due to nondepolarizing muscle relaxants.

Preparations: Tablets, 1 and 2 mg. Vials, 0.2 mg/ml.

GLYNASE®, see Glyburide

GLY-OXIDE®, see Carbamide peroxide

GM-CSF, see Sargramostim

GOLD SODIUM THIOMALATE—Myochrysine®

Description/Actions: Gold formulation indicated for the intramuscular treatment of rheumatoid arthritis.

Preparations: Ampules, 10, 25, and 50 mg.

GoLYTELY®, see Polyethylene glycol 3350

GONADORELIN HYDROCHLORIDE—Factrel®

Description/Actions: Synthetic luteinizing hormone–releasing hormone indicated for diagnostic use in evaluating the functional capacity and response of the gonadotropes of the anterior pituitary.

Preparations: Vials, 100 mg.

GONADOTROPIN, CHORIONIC
see Chorionic gonadotropin

GOSERELIN ACETATE—Zoladex®

Antineoplastic agent.

Description/Actions: Is a synthetic analogue of gonadotropin-releasing hormone. Chronic administration leads to a sustained suppression of pituitary gonadotropins, resulting in a fall in serum testosterone levels. Indicated in the palliative treatment of advanced carcinoma of the prostate, treatment of endometriosis, and palliative treatment of advanced breast cancer in peri- and postmenopausal women. May be used in combination with Flutamide and radiation therapy for locally confined stage T2B–T4 (stage B2-C) prostatic carcinoma.

Warnings: Is contraindicated during pregnancy. Adverse reactions include hot flashes, sexual dysfunction, decreased erections, lower urinary tract symptoms, pain, lethargy, dizziness, insomnia, anorexia, nausea, upper respiratory infection, chronic obstructive pulmonary disease, edema, congestive heart failure, rash, and sweating. When treatment is initiated, there is a transient increase in serum testosterone levels, which may cause a temporary worsening of signs and symptoms during the first few weeks of therapy.

Administration: Subcutaneous. The formulation is implanted into the upper abdominal wall and provides a continuous release of the drug over a 28-day period.

Preparations: Implant, 3.6 mg.

GRANISETRON HYDROCHLORIDE—Kytril®

Antiemetic.

Description/Actions: Is a selective blocking agent of the serotonin 5-HT$_3$ receptor type. Indicated for the prevention of nausea and vomiting associated with initial and repeat courses of emetogenic cancer therapy, including high-dose cisplatin, radiation therapy—induced nausea and vomiting, and for the prophylaxis and treatment of postoperative nausea and vomiting.

Warnings: Adverse reactions include headache, asthenia, somnolence, diarrhea, and constipation.

Administration: Oral and intravenous. Oral doses are administered up to 1 hour before chemotherapy and second dose 12 hours after the first. Postoperative nausea and vomiting: 1 mg.

Preparations: Tablets, 1 mg. Vials, 1 mg.

GRANULOCYTE COLONY STIMULATING FACTOR, see Filgrastim

GRANULOCYTE-MACROPHAGE COLONY STIMULATING FACTOR, see Sargramostim

GRIFULVIN®, see Griseofulvin

GRISACTIN®, see Griseofulvin

GRISEOFULVIN MICROSIZE—
Fulvicin-U/F®, Grifulvin V®, Grisactin®

GRISEOFULVIN ULTRAMICROSIZE—Fulvicin P/G®, Grisactin Ultra®, Gris-PEG®.

Description/Actions: Antifungal agent administered orally for tinea (ringworm) infections of the skin, hair, and nails.

Should not be used for superficial infection that may respond to topical antifungals.

Preparations: Microsize—Capsules and tablets, 125, 250, and 500 mg. Suspension, 125 mg/5 ml. Ultramicrosize—Tablets, 125, 165, 250, and 330 mg.

GRIS-PEG®, see Griseofulvin

GUAIFENESIN—Humabid LA®, Humabid Sprinkle®, Robitussin®, Sinumist SR Caplets®

Description/Actions: Expectorant indicated for the symptomatic relief of respiratory conditions characterized by dry, nonproductive cough and in the presence of mucus in the respiratory tract.

Preparations: Capsules and tablets, 100 and 200 mg. Syrup, 67 mg/5 ml, 100 mg/5 ml, and 200 mg/5 ml. Extended release capsules/tablets, 300 and 600 mg.

GUANABENZ ACETATE— Wytensin®

Description/Actions: Antihypertensive agent that exhibits a central alpha-2 adrenergic agonist action.

Preparations: Tablets, 4 and 8 mg.

GUANADREL SULFATE—Hylorel®

Description/Actions: Antihypertensive agent indicated in the treatment of hypertension in patients who have not responded adequately to a thiazide-type diuretic.

Preparations: Tablets, 10 and 25 mg.

GUANETHIDINE MONOSULFATE—Ismelin®

Description/Actions: Antihypertensive agent indicated for the treatment of moderate and severe hypertension, and for the management of renal hypertension.

Preparations: Tablets, 10 and 25 mg.

GUANFACINE HYDROCHLORIDE—Tenex®

Antihypertensive agent.

Description/Actions: Is a centrally acting alpha-2 adrenergic receptor agonist. Indicated in the management of hypertension.

Warnings: Adverse reactions include sedation, weakness, dizziness, dry mouth, constipation, and impotence. Patients should be advised to exercise caution when operating machinery or driving motor vehicles until it is determined that they do not become drowsy or dizzy from the medication. A potential exists for interactions with other drugs that have a central nervous system depressant action, and patients should be warned that their tolerance for alcohol and other CNS depressants may be decreased. The abrupt discontinuation of therapy may be associated with symptoms of nervousness and anxiety as well as increases in blood pressure (rebound hypertension).

Administration: Oral.

Preparations: Tablets, 1 mg.

GYNE-LOTRIMIN®, see Clotrimazole

H

HABITROL®, see Nicotine

HALAZEPAM—Paxipam®

Description/Actions: Benzodiazepine antianxiety agent indicated for the management of anxiety disorders or the short-term relief of the symptoms of anxiety.

Preparations: Tablets, 20 and 40 mg.

HALCINONIDE—Halog®

Description/Actions: Corticosteroid applied topically for the relief of the inflammatory and pruritic manifestations of corticosteroid-responsive dermatoses.

Preparations: Cream, 0.025% and 0.1%. Ointment and solution, 0.1%.

HALCION®, see Triazolam

HALDOL®, see Haloperidol

HALOBETASOL PROPIONATE—Ultravate®

Topical corticosteroid.

Description/Actions: A high- to super-high potency topical corticosteroid indicated for the relief of the inflammatory and pruritic manifestations of corticosteroid-responsive dermatoses.

Warnings: Adverse reactions include stinging, burning, itching, dry skin, erythema, and skin atrophy. May cause suppression of the hypothalamic-pituitary-adrenal (HPA) axis and appropriate precautions should be taken (e.g., regarding the extent and duration of treatment).

Administration: Topical. Should not be used with occlusive dressings. Because of its high potency, treatment should be limited to 2 weeks, and amounts greater than 50 g/week should not be used.

Preparations: Cream and ointment, 0.05%.

HALOG®, see Halcinonide

HALOPERIDOL—Haldol®

Antipsychotic agent.

Description/Actions: A butyrophenone derivative indicated for (1) the management of manifestations of psychotic disorders; (2) the control of tics and vocal utterances of Tourette's disorder; and, in children who have not responded to psychotherapy or medications other than neuroleptics, (3) the treatment of severe behavior problems in children of combative, explosive hyperexcitability, and (4) the short-term treatment of hyperactive children who show excessive motor activity with accompanying conduct disorders.

Warnings: Contraindicated in patients with parkinsonism or severe CNS depression. Adverse reactions include drowsiness and other CNS effects; patients should be cautioned regarding activities such as driving and operating machinery, as well as interactions with other CNS-acting drugs including alcohol. Other adverse reactions include extrapyramidal reactions, tardive dyskinesia, neuroleptic malignant syndrome, and hypotension. Concomitant therapy with lithium must be closely monitored because there have been reports of an encephalopathic syndrome in some patients receiving both medications.

Administration: Oral and intramuscular.

Preparations: Tablets, 0.5, 1, 2, 5, 10, and 20 mg. Solution concentrate (as the lactate), 2 mg/ml. Ampules and vials (as the lactate), 5 mg/ml.

HALOPERIDOL DECANOATE—Haldol decanoate®

Antipsychotic agent.

Description/Actions: Is a long-acting parenterally administered form of haloperidol indicated in the management of patients requiring prolonged parenteral neuroleptic therapy.

Warnings: See discussion of haloperidol.

Administration: Intramuscular. The recommended interval between doses is 4 weeks.

Preparations: Ampules, 50 and 100 mg per ml.

HALOPROGIN—Halotex®

Description/Actions: Antifungal agent indicated for the topical treatment of superficial tinea (ringworm) infections and tinea versicolor.

Preparations: Cream and solution, 1%.

HALOTESTIN®, see Fluoxymesterone

HALOTEX®, see Haloprogin

HALOTHANE—Fluothane®

Description/Actions: Inhalation general anesthetic indicated for the induction and maintenance of general anesthesia.

Preparations: Liquid, 125 and 250 ml.

HECTOROL®, see Doxercalciferol

HELIDAC®

Description/Actions: Combination agent used in treatment of active duodenal ulcer associated with *H. pylori*. Bismuth subsalicylate, metronidazole, tetracyline.

HEMABATE®, see Carboprost tromethamine

HEPARIN SODIUM—Liquaemin sodium®

Anticoagulant.

Description/Actions: Exhibits an anticoagulant action, in part, by inhibiting the conversion of fibrinogen to fibrin. Indicated in the prophylaxis and treatment of venous thrombosis and its extension, pulmonary embolism, peripheral arterial embolism, and atrial fibrillation with embolization. Also used in the diagnosis and treatment of acute and chronic consumptive coagulopathies, in a low-dose regimen for prevention of postoperative deep vein thrombosis and pulmonary embolism in patients undergoing major surgery, as an adjunct in the treatment of coronary occlusion with acute myocardial infarction, in the prevention of clotting in arterial and heart surgery, and in blood transfusions, extracorporeal circulation, and dialysis procedures. Used in very low doses to maintain patency of IV catheters (heparin flush).

Warnings: May cause hemorrhage and therapy must be closely monitored. Action may be increased by agents such as aspirin and nonsteroidal anti-inflammatory drugs.

Administration: Intravenous or deep subcutaneous. Intramuscular use should be avoided because of the danger of hematoma formation.

Preparations: Ampules and vials, 10, 100, 1000, 5000, 10,000, 20,000, and 40,000 units/ml.

HEPSERA™, see Adefovir Dipivoxil

HEROIN—Diacetylmorphine

Description/Actions: Narcotic analgesic not legally available in the United States.

HERPLEX®, see Idoxuridine

HESPAN®, see Hetastarch

HETASTARCH—Hespan®

Description/Actions: Plasma expander with colloidal properties approximating those of human albumin. Indicated for intravenous infusion when plasma volume expansion is desired as an adjunct in the treatment of shock due to hemorrhage, burns, surgery, sepsis, or other trauma.

Preparations: Solution, 6% in 250 and 500 cc bottles.

HEXACHLOROPHENE— pHisoHex®

Description/Actions: Anti-infective agent indicated for topical use as a surgical scrub and a bacteriostatic skin cleanser.

Preparations: Emulsion, 3%.

HEXADROL®, see Dexamethasone

HEXALEN®, see Altretamine

HEXAVITAMIN

Description/Actions: Vitamin mixture that includes Vitamins A, D, B_1, B_2, and C, and nicotinic acid. Used in the prevention and treatment of deficiencies of these vitamins.

Preparations: Capsules and Tablets.

HIBICLENS®, see Chlorhexidine gluconate

HIBISTAT®, see Chlorhexidine gluconate.

HIPREX®, see Methenamine hippurate

HISTAMINE PHOSPHATE

Description/Actions: Diagnostic agent used to test the ability of the gastric mucosa to produce hydrochloric acid, and in the diagnosis of pheochromocytoma.

Preparations: Ampules containing the equivalent of 0.1 and 0.2 mg histamine base/ml.

HISTRELIN ACETATE—Supprelin®

Agent for precocious puberty.

Description/Actions: Is an analogue of naturally occurring gonadotropin-releasing hormone (GnRH), and is a potent inhibitor of gonadotropin secretion when administered daily in therapeutic doses. Chronic daily administration inhibits the secretion of pituitary gonadotropin, which, in turn, causes a reduction in ovarian and testicular steroid production. Indicated for the control of the manifestations of centrally mediated precocious puberty occurring before the age of 8 years in girls or 9.5 years in boys.

Warnings: Also contraindicated in women who are or may become pregnant while receiving the drug and in nursing mothers. Adverse reactions include skin reactions at the injection site (e.g., redness, swelling, itching), vaginal bleeding, and hypersensitivity reactions.

Administration: Subcutaneous. Daily injection should be rotated through different body sites (upper arms, thighs, abdomen). Patients and their families should be informed of the need to give injections at approximately the same time each day; otherwise, the pubertal process may be reactivated. Treatment should be discontinued when the onset of puberty is desired.

Preparations: Vials (and syringes with needles) that deliver 0.6 ml of a solution containing 200 µg/ml (120 µg/vial), 500 µg/ml (300 µg/vial), or 1000 µg/ml (600 µg/vial).

HIVID®, see Zalcitabine

HOMATROPINE HYDROBROMIDE

Description/Actions: Anticholinergic agent for ophthalmic use. Indicated for use as a mydriatic and cycloplegic for refraction, and in the management of certain ocular inflammatory conditions. Also used orally for anticholinergic action in combination with other agents.

Preparations: Ophthalmic solutions, 2% and 5%.

HUMABID LA®, see Guaifenesin

HUMABID SPRINKLE®, see Guaifenesin

HUMALOG®, see Insulin

HUMATIN®, see Paromomycin

HUMATROPE®, see Somatropin

HUMIRA™, see Adalimunab

HUMORSOL®, see Demecarium

HUMULIN®, see Insulin

HYALURONIDASE—Wydase®

Description/Actions: Enzyme indicated as an adjuvant to increase the absorption and dispersion of other injected drugs, for hypodermoclysis, and as an adjunct in subcutaneous urography for improving resorption of radiopaque agents.

Preparations: Vials, 150 and 1500 units.

HYCAMTIN®, see Topotecan Hydrochloride

HYCODAN®, Combination of hydrocodone and homatropine

HYDELTRA®, see Prednisolone tebutate

HYDELTRASOL®, see Prednisolone sodium phosphate

HYDERGINE®, see Ergoloid mesylates

HYDRALAZINE HYDROCHLORIDE—Apresoline®

Antihypertensive agent.

Preparations: Tablets, 10, 25, 50, and 100 mg. Injection, 20 mg/ml.

HYDREA®, see Hydroxyurea

HYDROCHLOROTHIAZIDE— Esidrix®, HydroDIURIL®, MIcrozide®, Oretic®

Thiazide diuretic.

Description/Actions: Indicated in the management of hypertension, and as adjunctive therapy in edema associated with congestive heart failure, hepatic cirrhosis, and corticosteroid and estrogen therapy. Is also useful in edema due to various forms of renal dysfunction such as nephrotic syndrome.

Warnings: May cause hypokalemia, and serum potassium levels should be determined periodically. Reduction in potassium levels may increase the action and toxicity of digoxin and related glycosides. Concurrent use with lithium is best avoided because of an increased risk of lithium toxicity. May cause hyperglycemia and hyperuricemia, and therapy in patients having diabetes or gout should be closely monitored. Excreted in breast milk. If drug therapy with hydrochlorothiazide is essential, patient should be instructed to stop nursing.

Administration: Oral.

Preparations: Tablets, 25, 50, and 100 mg. Capsules, 12.5 mg. Oral solution, 50 mg/5 ml. Concentrated oral solution, 100 mg/ml.

HYDROCODONE BITARTRATE— Hycodan®

Description/Actions: Opioid analgesic and antitussive indicated for the relief of moderate to moderately severe pain and for the relief of cough. Used in combination with other agents.

HYDROCODONE BITARTRATE WITH ACETAMINOPHEN— Norco®

HYDROCORTISONE—Cortisol, Cortef®, Hydrocortone®, Pandel®

Description/Actions: Corticosteroid indicated in a wide range of endocrine, rheumatic, allergic, dermatologic, respiratory, hematologic, neoplastic, and other disorders.

Preparations: Tablets, 5, 10, and 20 mg. Oral suspension (as the cypionate), 10 mg/5 ml. Vials, (as the sodium phosphate), 50 mg/ml. Vials (as the sodium succinate), 100, 250, 500, and 1000 mg. Vials (as the acetate for intralesional, intraarticular, or soft tissue injection), 25 mg/ml and 50 mg/ml. Retention enema, 100 mg. Cream, ointment, lotion, gel, aerosol for topical use (some for mulations contain the acetate salt), 0.25%, 0.5%, 1%, and 2.5%. Cream and ointment (as the butyrate), 0.1%. Cream (as buteprate) and ointment (as the valerate), 0.2%.

HYDROCORTONE®, see Hydrocortisone

HYDRODIURIL®, see Hydrochlorothiazide

HYDROFLUMETHIAZIDE—Diucardin®, Saluron®

Description/Actions: Thiazide diuretic indicated as adjunctive therapy in the treatment of edema. Is also indicated in the management of hypertension.

Preparations: Tablets, 50 mg.

HYDROGEN PEROXIDE

Description/Actions: Antiseptic/cleansing *agent* applied to the skin and certain mucous membranes.

Preparations: Solution, 3%.

HYDROMORPHONE HYDROCHLORIDE—Dilaudid®

Description/Actions: Opioid analgesic indicated for the relief of moderate to severe pain. Has also been used to suppress cough.

Preparations: Tablets, 1, 2, 4, and 8 mg. Suppositories, 3 mg. Ampules, vials, and syringes, 1 mg/ml, 2 mg/ml, 3 mg/ml, 4 mg/ml, and 10 mg/ml.

HYDROMOX®, see Quinethazone

HYDROPHILIC OINTMENT

Description/Actions: Ointment base that is "water removable" and into which medications are often incorporated and applied.

HYDROPHILIC PETROLATUM

Description/Actions: Ointment base capable of absorbing quantities of water or aqueous solutions containing medications.

HYDROQUINONE—Eldoquin®, Lustra®

Description/Actions: A depigmenting agent indicated in ultraviolet-induced dyschromia and discoloration of the skin due to pregnancy, oral contraceptives, hormone replacement therapy or skin trauma.

Warnings: Do skin sensitivity test before use. If itching, vesicle formation, or excessive inflammation occurs, avoid further treatment. Avoid sun and UV light. Avoid contact with eyes. Pregnancy Category C.

Adverse reactions include localized contact dermatitis (discontinue if occurs).

Administration: Topical.

Discontinue if lightening effect does not occur after 2 months.

Preparations: 4% cream in 2 oz jar.

HYDROXOCOBALAMIN

Description/Actions: Vitamin B_{12} analogue indicated in the parenteral treatment of pernicious anemia, dietary deficiency of vitamin B_{12}, malabsorption of vitamin B_{12}, and other situations in which there is inadequate utilization of vitamin B_{12}. Also used for the Schilling test.

Preparations: Vials, 1000 µg/ml.

HYDROXYAMPHETAMINE HYDROBROMIDE

Description/Actions: Sympathomimetic *amine* indicated for ophthalmic use to dilate the pupil.

Preparations: Ophthalmic solution, in combination with other agents.

HYDROXYCHLOROQUINE SULFATE—Plaquenil®

Description/Actions: Antimalarial agent indicated for the treatment of acute attacks and suppression of malaria. Also used in the management of rheumatoid arthritis and lupus erythematosus in patients who have not responded satisfactorily to drugs having a lesser potential to cause serious adverse effects.

Preparations: Tablets, 200 mg.

HYDROXYPROGESTERONE CAPROATE—Duralutin®

Description/Actions: Progestin administered intramuscularly in the management of amenorrhea, abnormal uterine bleeding due to hormonal imbalance, production of secretory endometrium and desquamation, and adenocarcinoma of uterine corpus in advanced stage.

Preparations: Vials, 125 mg/ml and 250 mg/ml.

HYDROXYUREA—Hydrea®

Description/Actions: Antineoplastic agent indicated in the treatment of melanoma, chronic myelocytic leukemia, and carcinoma of the ovary. Has also been of benefit in reducing the frequency and severity of painful sickle cell crises.

Preparations: Capsules, 500 mg.

HYDROXYZINE—Atarax®, Vistaril

Antianxiety agent.

Description/Actions: Exhibits sedative and antihistaminic actions. Indicated (1) for symptomatic relief of anxiety and tension associated with psychoneurosis and as an adjunct in organic disease states in which anxiety is manifested; (2) in the management of pruritus due to allergic conditions such as chronic urticaria and atopic and contact dermatoses, and in histamine-mediated pruritus; and (3) as a sedative when used as premedication and following general anesthesia.

Warnings: Contraindicated in early pregnancy. Adverse reactions include drowsiness and other CNS effects; patients should be cautioned regarding activities such as driving and operating machinery, as well as interactions with other CNS-acting drugs including alcohol. When other CNS-depressant drugs are administered concurrently, their dosage should be appropriately reduced.

Administration: Oral and intramuscular.

Preparations: Tablets and capsules, 10, 25, 50, and 100 mg. Syrup, 10 mg/5 ml, oral suspension, 25 mg/5 ml. Vials, 25 and 50 mg/ml.

HYGROTON®, see Chlorthalidone

HYLOREL®, see Guanadrel

HYOSCINE, see Scopolamine

HYOSCYAMINE SULFATE— Anaspaz, Cystospaz®, Levbid®, Levsin®, Levsinex®

Description/Actions: Anticholinergic agent used as adjunctive therapy in the treatment of peptic ulcer. Also used in other gastrointestinal disorders, biliary and renal conditions, as a drying agent in acute rhinitis, and in the management of parkinsonism.

Preparations: Tablets, 0.125 and 0.15 mg. Controlled-release capsules, 0.375 mg. Elixir, 0.125 mg/5 ml. Drops, 0.125 mg/ml. Vials, 0.5 mg/ml.

HYPERSTAT®, see Diazoxide

HYTAKEROL®, see Dihydrotachysterol

HYTRIN®, see Terazosin

HYZAAR®, Combination drug containing Lorsartan potassium 50 mg and Hydrochlorothiazide 12.5 mg

I

IBRITUMOMAB TIUXETAN— ZEVALIN™

Description/Actions: Zevalin™ is indicated for the treatment of patients with relapsed or refractory low-grade, follicular, or transformed B-cell non-

Hodgkin's lymphoma, including patients with rituximab refractory follicular non-Hodgkin's lymphoma.

Precautions/Adverse Reactions: Zevalin™ is contraindicated in patients with known Type I hypersensitivity or anaphylactic reactions to murine proteins or to any component of this product, including rituximab, yttrium chloride, and indium chloride. Because rituximab is part of the regimen, consult warnings for rituximab. Fatal infusion reactions have occurred; deaths have occurred within 24 hours of rituximab infusion. Fatalities associated with an infusion reaction symptom complex that included hypoxia, pulmonary infiltrates, acute respiratory distress, myocardial infarction, ventricular fibrillation, or cardiogenic shock. These severe reactions typically occur during the first rituximab infusion, with time to onset of 30 to 120 minutes. These signs and symptoms may require interruption of rituximab, In 111 Zevalin™, or y 90 Zevalin administration.

Y 90 Zevalin™ administration results in severe and prolonged cytopenias in most patients. It should not be given to patients with ≥25% lymphoma marrow involvement and/or impaired bone marrow reserve. Y 90 Zevalin™ should not be administered to patients with altered biodistribution of In 111 Zevalin™.

The therapeutic regimen is intended as a single-course treatment and is to be used in combination with rituximab. The contents of the kit are not radioactive.

Pregnancy Category D. There is a potential risk that the Zevalin™ regimen could cause toxic effects on the male and female gonads. Effective contraceptive methods should be used during treatment and for up to 12 months following the regimen.

The most serious adverse reactions include infections, allergic reactions (bronchospasm and angioedema), and hemorrhage while thrombocytopenic (resulting in death). Patients who have received Zevalin™ regimen have developed myeloid malignancies and dysplasias. Most common toxicities were neutropenia, thrombocytopenia, anemia, nausea, vomiting, abdominal pain, increased cough, dyspnea, dizziness, asthenia, chills, fever, and headache. No formal drug interaction studies have been performed. Because of the frequent occurrence of severe thrombocytopenia, agents that interfere with platelet function and/or anticoagulation should be weighed against the potential increased risks of bleeding and hemorrhage. Safety and effectiveness in children have not been established.

Administration: Intravenous.

Patient Care Implications: Do not give y 90 Zevalin to patients with a platelet count <100,000/mm^3. Y 90 dose should not exceed the absolute maximum allowable dose of 32.0 mCi (1184 MEq), regardless of the patient's weight. Patient should be measured by a suitable radioactivity calibration system immediately prior to administration. Proper aseptic technique and precautions for handling radioactive materials should be employed. Radiolabeling of ibritumomab with y 90 and In 111 (not included in kit) must be performed by appropriate personnel in a specialized facility. Human antimurine antibody should be done prior to treatment. If positive, the patient may have an allergic or hypersensitivity reaction when treated. Monitor for infusion-related allergic reactions. Obtain complete blood counts and platelet counts at least weekly. Platelet count must be done prior to step 2. Biodistribution of In 111 Zevalin should be assessed by imaging at 2–24 hours and at 48–72 hours postinjection, and a third image may be necessary at 90–120 hours. If biodistribution is not acceptable, the patient should not proceed to step 2. Kit is not radioactive. Do not freeze. To prepare radiolabeled injection, follow manufacturer's guidelines. Should be prepared only by individuals trained in the prep-

162 • IBUPROFEN

aration of radiopharmaceuticals in a facility that is designated for this purpose.

Preparations: Each kit contains 4 vials for preparation of either In 111 or y 90. In 111 Zevalin kit provides for the radiolabeling of ibritumomab tiuxetan with In-111. Has 4 vials; 1 Zevalin vial containing 3.2 mg of ibritumomab tiuxetan in 2 ml of 0.9% sodium chloride solution, 1 vial containing 50 mM of sodium acetate, 1 formulation buffer vial, 1 empty reaction vial, and 4 identification labels. Y 90 Zevalin kit provides for radiolabeling of ibritumomab tiuxetan with y 90. Kit has 4 vials: 1 Zevalin vial containing 3.2 mg of ibritumomab tiuxetan in 2 ml 0.9% sodium chloride, 1 vial containing 50 mM of sodium acetate, 1 formulation buffer vial, 1 empty reaction vial, and 4 identification labels.

IBUPROFEN—Advil®, Children's Advil®, Motrin®, Children's Motrin®, Nuprin®, Pediacare Fever Liquid®, Rufen®

Nonsteroidal anti-inflammatory drug.

Description/Actions: Inhibits prostaglandin synthesis and is indicated for the relief of mild to moderate pain, primary dysmenorrhea, rheumatoid arthritis, osteoarthritis, and reduction of fever.

Warnings: Should not be given to patients in whom aspirin or another NSAID causes asthma, rhinitis, urticaria, or other allergic-type reactions. May cause GI effects, and use should be avoided in patients with active GI tract disease and closely monitored in patients with a previous history of such disorders. Other adverse reactions include dizziness and rash.

Administration: Oral.

Preparations: Caplets and tablets, 100, 200, 300, 400, 600, and 800 mg. Gelcaps, 200 mg. Chewable tablets, 50 and 100 mg. Suspension, 100 mg/5 ml, oral drops 40 mg/ml and 50 mg/1.25 ml (dropperful).

IBUTILIDE FUMARATE—Corvert®

Antiarrhythmic.

Description/Actions: Predominantly class III antiarrhythmic used in the Rapid Conversion of atrial fibrillation or atrial flutter of recent onset to sinus rhythm. Patients with atrial arrhythmias of longer duration are less likely to respond to ibutilide. The effectiveness of ibutilide has not been determined in patients with arrhythmias of > 90 days duration.

Warnings: Administer in appropriate treatment environment as this drug may cause life-threatening arrhythmias such as sustained polymorphic ventricular tachycardia, usually in association with QT prolongation (torsades de pointes) but sometimes without QT prolongation. These arrhythmias can be reversed if treated promptly with cardioversion. An appropriate environment should include continuous ECG monitoring, personnel skilled in arrhythmia recognition, and life-support equipment. Reports of reversible heart block have been associated with ibutilide administration.

Administration: Intravenous with an initial dose over 10 minutes with a second 10-minute infusion if arrhythmia does not terminate within 10 minutes after the end of the initial infusion. Maintain continuous ECG monitoring for 4 hours following the infusion or until QT has returned to baseline.

Preparations: Solution, 0.1mg/ml in 10 ml vials.

ICHTHAMMOL

Description/Actions: Antibacterial agent and astringent applied topically in certain dermatologic disorders.

Preparations: Ointment, 10% and 20%.

IDAMYCIN®, see Idarubicin hydrochloride

IDARUBICIN HYDROCHLORIDE—Idamycin®

Antineoplastic agent.

Description/Actions: Is an anthracycline derivative that is indicated for use in combination with other antileukemic drugs (usually cytarabine) for the treatment of acute myeloid leukemia in adults.

Warnings: May cause severe myelosuppression and should not be given to patients with preexisting bone marrow suppression induced by previous drug therapy or radiotherapy unless the benefit warrants the risk. Other adverse reactions include myocardial toxicity (e.g., congestive heart failure, arrhythmias), GI effects (e.g., nausea, vomiting, mucositis, abdominal pain, diarrhea), alopecia, dermatologic effects (e.g., rash, urticaria), pulmonary effects, mental status effects, fever, headache, neurologic effects, hyperuricemia secondary to rapid lysis of leukemic cells, and extravasation. Should not be used in pregnant women unless the benefit outweighs the risk. In patients with hepatic or renal impairment, a reduction in dosage should be considered and treatment should be closely monitored.

Administration. Intravenous. Follow vesicant procedures.

Preparations: Vials, 5 and 10 mg.

IDOXURIDINE—IDU, Herplex®, Stoxil®

Description/Actions: Antiviral agent indicated for ophthalmic use in the treatment of herpes simplex keratitis.

Preparations: Ophthalmic solution, 0.1%. Ophthalmic ointment, 0.5%

IDU, see Idoxuridine

IFEX® see Ifosfamide

IFOSFAMIDE—Ifex®

Antineoplastic agent.

Description/Actions: Is an analogue of cyclophosphamide and requires metabolic activation by liver microsomal enzymes to produce biologically active metabolites. Indicated for use in combination with other antineoplastic agents, for third line chemotherapy of germ cell testicular cancer. Should be used in combination with mesna to reduce the risk of hemorrhagic cystitis.

Warnings: May cause leukopenia, thrombocytopenia, and urotoxic effects, especially hemorrhagic cystitis. Other adverse reactions include sedation confusion, hallucinations, alopecia, nausea, and vomiting.

Administration: Intravenous infusion (lasting a minimum of 30 minutes). Should be given with extensive hydration consisting of at least 2 liters of oral or intravenous fluid per day, and with the uroprotective agent, mesna.

Preparations: Vials, 1 and 3 g.

ILETIN®, see Insulin

ILOPAN®, see Dexpanthenol

ILOSONE®, see Erythromycin estolate.

ILOTYCIN®, see Erythromycin base and gluceptate

IMATINIB MESYLATE— GLEEVEC™

Description/Actions: Imatinib is indicated as first-line treatment of patients with chronic myeloid leukemia; for the treatment of patients with Philadelphia chromosome–positive chronic myeloid leukemia in blast crisis, accelerated phase; or for chronic phase after failure of interferon–alpha therapy. Imatinib is also indicated for the treatment of patients with kit-positive unresectable and or metastatic gastrointestinal stromal tumors.

Precautions/Adverse Reactions: Imatinib is contraindicated in patients with a known hypersensitivity to it or to any component of the formulation. Women of childbearing age should be advised not to become pregnant while on imatinib therapy. Therapy with imatinib is often associated with edema and occasionally serious fluid retention. Probability of edema was increased with higher imatinib doses and age > 65 years. Severe fluid retention (pleural effusion, pericardial effusion, pulmonary edema, and ascites) has been reported. Severe superficial edema has also been reported. Imatinib may cause gastrointestinal irritation. To minimize this effect, Gleevec should be taken with food and with a large glass of water.

Hemorrhage is possible with imatinib therapy. Treatment with imatinib is associated with hematologic toxicity, namely, neutropenia or thrombocytopenia. Complete blood counts should be performed weekly for the first month, biweekly for the second month, and periodically thereafter as clinically indicated.

Hepatotoxicity may occur with imatinib therapy. It may be severe. Liver function tests (transaminases, bilirubin, and alkaline phosphatase) should be monitored before initiation of therapy and monthly or as clinically indicated. Long-term safety data on treatment with imatinib are unknown; however, potential long-term toxicities include liver toxicity, renal toxicity, and immunosuppression.

Imatinib is metabolized primarily by the cytochrome P450 enzyme system 3A4. Coadministration of imatinib and CYP3A4 inhibitors such as ketoconazole, itraconazole, erythromycin, and clarithromycin resulted in decreased metabolism and increased plasma levels of imatinib. Coadministration of imatinib and CYP3A4 inducers such as dexamethasone, phenytoin, carbamazepine, rifampin, phenobarbital, and Saint-John's-wort may reduce plasma levels of imatinib. Coadministration of imatinib and simvastatin resulted in increased plasma concentrations of simvastatin. Use caution when coadministering imatinib and drugs with a narrow therapeutic index such as cyclosporine and pimozide. Imatinib will increase serum concentrations of other drugs metabolized by CYP3A4 such as triazole-benzodiazepines, dihydropyridine calcium channel blockers, and certain HMG-CoA reductase inhibitors. Coadministration of imatinib and warfarin resulted in decreased metabolism of warfarin. It is recommended that patients requiring anticoagulation should receive low molecular weight or standard heparin. In vitro imatinib inhibits cytochrome P450 2D6 activity at similar concentrations that affect CYP3A4 activity. Plasma concentrations of substrates of CYP2D6 are expected to increase when coadministered with imatinib.

Pregnancy Category D. Women of childbearing potential are advised to avoid becoming pregnant while receiving imatinib therapy. Excretion in human breast milk is unknown. Women should be advised against breastfeeding while taking imatinib. Safety and efficacy in pediatric patients have not been established.

The most frequently reported drug-related adverse events were nausea, vomiting, diarrhea, edema, and muscle cramps. Edema was mostly periorbital or in the lower limbs and was managed with diuretics or by reducing the dose of imatinib. Peripheral effusions, ascites, pulmonary edema and rapid weight gain with or without superficial edema have been reported. These events appear to be dose related and were more common in the blast crisis and accelerated phase studies and are more common in the elderly. Neutropenia and thrombocytopenia has been associated with imatinib therapy, occurring with a higher frequency at doses ≥ 750 mg.

Administration: Oral.

Patient Care Implications: Imatinib should be taken with a meal and a large glass of water. Patients should be weighed and monitored regularly for signs and symptoms of fluid retention. Complete blood counts should be performed weekly for the first month, biweekly for the second month, and periodically thereafter as clinically indicated. Liver function tests should be monitored before initiation of treatment and monthly or as clinically indicated. Patients should be monitored for potential renal toxicity and immunosuppression. Female patiets should be advised to avoid becoming pregnant.

Preparations: Capsules, 100 mg.

IMDUR®, see Isosorbide mononitrate

IMIGLUCERASE—Cerezyme®

Agent for Gaucher's disease.

Description/Actions: Is an analogue of the human enzyme, beta-glucocerebrosidase produced by recombinant technology. Indicated for long-term enzyme replacement therapy for patients with a confirmed diagnoses of Type I Gaucher's disease that results in one or more of the following conditions: anemia, thrombocytopenia, bone disease, hepatomegaly, or splenomegaly.

Warnings: Adverse reactions include headache, nausea, abdominal discomfort, dizziness, pruritus, and rash. Caution should be exercised in patients previously treated with alglucerase and who have developed antibody to alglucerase or who have exhibited symptoms of hypersensitivity to alglucerase. Anaphylactoid reactions have been reported during treatment with imiglucerase. Use caution with further treatments. Most patients have successfully completed therapy after a reduction in the rate of infusion and pretreatment with antihistamines and/or corticosteroids. Pulmonary hypertension has also been reported with the use of imiglucerase.

Administration: Intravenous. Is administered by IV infusion over 1–2 hours.

Preparations: Vials, 200 units.

IMIPENEM-CILASTATIN SODIUM—Primaxin IV®, Primaxin IM®

Carbapenem antibiotic.

Description/Actions: Imipenem has a very broad spectrum of action that includes almost all gram-positive and gram-negative bacteria. Cilastatin is an enzyme inhibitor that significantly reduces the renal metabolism of imipenem, resulting in a much greater urinary recovery of the antibiotic. Indicated for intravenous use for the treatment of lower respiratory tract infections, urinary tract infections, intraabdominal infections, gynecologic infections, bacterial septicemia, bone and joint infections, skin and skin-structure infections, endocarditis, and polymicrobic infections caused by susceptible organisms. Indicated for intramuscular use in the treatment of serious infections of mild to moderate severity for which IM therapy is appropriate.

Warnings: Must be used cautiously, if at all, in patients who have experienced hypersensitivity reactions to a penicillin or cephalosporin. Seizures have been reported although infrequently, and therapy must be closely supervised in patients with predisposing factors such as a history of seizures.

Administration: Intravenous and intramuscular.

Preparations: Vials and infusion bottles for intravenous use, 250 mg imipenem equivalent with 250 mg cilastatin equivalent, and 500 mg of each agent. Vials for intramuscular use, 500 mg imipenem equivalent with 500 mg cilastatin equivalent, and 750 mg of each agent.

IMIPRAMINE HYDROCHLORIDE—Tofranil®

IMIPRAMINE PAMOATE—Tofranil-PM®

Description/Actions: Tricyclic antidepressant indicated for the relief of symptoms of depression. Oral formulation of imipramine hydrochloride is also used in the management of childhood enuresis.

Preparations: Tablets, 10, 25, and 50 mg. Capsules (pamoate), 75, 100, 125, and 150 mg. Ampules, 25 mg.

IMIQUIMOD—Aldara®

Description/Actions: Immune response modifier indicated for the treatment of external genital and perianal warts (condyloma acuminata) in individuals 12 years of age and older. Imiquimod induces mRNA encoding cytokines including interferon-alpha at the treatment site. In addition, HPLV1 mRNA and HPV DNA are significantly decreased following treatment. Other therapies used to treat genital warts can cause damage to tissue and surrounding areas and imiquimod should not be applied until these areas have healed.

Warnings: Not for use in treating urethral, intravaginal, cervical, rectal, or intraanal human papilloma viral disease. Not for use on lesions that have not healed from other therapies (drug or surgical). Avoid sexual contact while cream is applied to skin. Avoid eyes. Do not occlude. May exacerbate inflammatory skin conditions. Concomitant use of diaphragms or condoms not recommended. Adverse reactions include local and remote reactions (e.g., erythema, erosion, itching, burning, soreness), headache, flulike symptoms, and myalgia. Safety and efficacy in patients below the age of 12 have not been established.

Administration: Apply a thin layer to warts and rub in 3 times per week at bedtime (e.g., Mon-Wed-Fri or Tues-Thurs-Sat). Maximum usage not to exceed 16 weeks. Remove with soap and water after 6–10 hours. If local reactions occur, suspend therapy until reaction subsides. When treating warts under foreskin of uncircumcised males, the foreskin should be retracted and cleansed daily. New warts may develop during therapy. Wash hands before and after application. Notify prescriber of severe skin reactions. Instruct female patients to avoid using the product in the vagina.

Preparations: Single-use packets of 5% cream (250 mg each).

IMITREX®, see Sumatriptan succinate

IMODIUM®, see Loperamide

IMODIUM ADVANCED®—
Combination agent loperamide and simethicone (opiod and antiflatulent)

IMODIUM A-D®, see Loperamide

IMURAN®, see Azathioprine

INAMRINONE—Inocor® Inotropic agent.

Description/Actions: Increases myocardial contractility and decreases preload and afterload by a direct dilating effect on vascular smooth muscle. Indicated for short-term treatment of congestive heart failure unresponsive to glycosides, diuretics, and vasodilators.

Warnings: Contraindicated in idiopathic hypertrophic subaortic stenosis (IHSS). Correct fluid and electrolytes associated with previous aggressive diuretic therapy prior to initiating amrinone. Adverse reactions include arrhythmias, hypotension, thrombocytopenia, and tachyphylaxis. Initiate in monitored environment.

Administration: Intravenous.

Preparations: Injection, 5 mg/ml.

INAPSINE®, see Droperidol

INDAPAMIDE—Lozol®

Description/Actions: Diuretic indicated for the treatment of hypertension and for the treatment of salt and fluid retention associated with congestive heart failure.

Preparations: Tablets, 1.25 and 2.5 mg.

INDERAL®, see Propranolol

INDINAVIR—Crixivan®

Antiviral, protease inhibitor.

Description/Actions: Used in treatment of HIV infection.

Warnings: Contraindicated with concurrent use of terfenadine, astemizole, cisapride, triazolam, and midazolam. Adverse reactions include nephrolithiasis, aymptomatic hyperbilirubinemia, GI upset, abdominal pain, kidney stones, headache, fatigue, insomnia, flank pain, and dysguesia. Maintain adequate hydration (1.5 L/day). Discontinue or suspend therapy (e.g., 1–3 days) during acute nephrolithiasis or impaired hepatic function.

Administration: Oral with water on an empty stomach or with a light meal. Usual dose is 800 mg every 8 hours. Reduce dose of indinavir sulfate to 600 mg every 8 hours in hepatic insufficiency or with concomitant use of Ketoconazole.

Preparations: Capsules, 200, 333, and 400 mg.

INDOCIN®, see Indomethacin

INDOMETHACIN—Indocin®, Indocin SR®

Nonsteroidal anti-inflammatory drug.

Description/Actions: Inhibits prostaglandin synthesis and is indicated in the treatment of rheumatoid arthritis, osteoarthritis, ankylosing spondylitis, acute painful shoulder, and acute gouty arthritis. Used as an alternative to surgery in the management of patent ductus arteriosus in premature neonates.

Warnings: Should not be given to patients in whom aspirin or another NSAID causes asthma, rhinitis, urticaria, or other allergic-type reactions. Suppositories are contraindicated in patients with a history of proctitis or recent rectal bleeding. May cause GI effects and use should be avoided in patients with active GI tract disease and closely monitored in patients with a previous history of such disorders. Other reactions include headache and dizziness.

Administration: Oral, rectal, and intravenous. Should be administered with food or antacids, or immediately after meals, to reduce GI effects.

Preparations: Capsules, 25 and 50 mg. Sustained-release capsules, 75 mg. Oral suspension, 25 mg/5 ml. Suppositories, 50 mg. Injection, 1 mg vials.

InFeD®, see Iron dextran

INFLIXIMAB—Remicade®

Description/Actions: Anti-inflammatory agent indicated for reducing signs and symptoms and inducing and maintaining clinical remission in patients with moderately to severely active Crohn's disease who have had an inadequate response to conventional therapy. Useful in reducing the number of draining enterocutaneous fistula(s) in fistulizing Crohn's disease.

Precautions/Adverse Reactions: Contraindicated in patients with allergy to murine protein. Discontinue if lupus-like syndrome with antibody formation occurs. Use cautiously in elderly. Pregnancy Category C. Use in children and nursing mothers not recommended. Tuberculosis (frequently disseminated or extrapulmonary at clinical presentation), invasive fungal infections, and other opportunistic infections have been observed in patients receiving infliximab. Some have been fatal. Patients should be evaluated for latent tuberculosis infection. Cases of histoplasmosis, listeriosis, pneumocystosis, and worsening heart failure have been reported in patients treated with infliximab. Do not initiate therapy in patients with congestive heart failure.

Adverse reactions include infection, infusion reactions, nausea, vomiting, fatigue, fever, pain, dizziness, bronchitis, sinusitis, rhinitis, rash, antibody formation, lupus-like syndrome, and anaphylaxis.

Administration: Intravenous.

Reconstitute vial with 10 ml of sterile water for injection. The total dose of reconstituted product should be further diluted in 250 ml of normal saline.

Patient Care Implications: Administration of infliximab has been associated with hypersensitivity reactions. Discontinue the medication for severe reactions. Instruct patients in the signs and symptoms of infection and to promptly report onset to the prescriber.

Preparations: Powder for injection, 100 mg.

INH, see Isoniazid

INNOHEP®, see Tinzaparin

INOCOR®, see Inamrinone

INOMAX®, see Nitric oxide

INSULATARD®, see Insulin

INSULIN ASPART—Novolog®

Description/Actions: Indicated in the treatment of hyperglycemia in adult patients with diabetes mellitus. It should be used together with intermediate-acting or long-acting insulin. Insulin aspart may also be infused subcutaneously by external insulin pump.

Precautions/Adverse Reactions: Insulin aspart is contraindicated in patients with a known hypersensitivity to insulin aspart or to any component of the product. It is also contraindicated during episodes of hypoglycemia. Injection of insulin aspart should be immediately followed by a meal. It should be used in conjunction with a longer acting insulin in Type I diabetics. Hypoglycemia and hypokalemia are common adverse effects during insulin therapy. Changes in insulin therapy should be made cautiously and under medical supervision. Monitoring of blood glucose levels is recommended for all diabetics. Lipodystrophy and hypersensitivity reactions may occur at the injection site. Decreased doses of insulin aspart may be required in patients with renal or hepatic impairment. Oral antidiabetic agents, ACE inhibitors, disopyramide, fibrates, fluoxetine, monoamine oxidase inhibitors, propoxyphene, salicylates, octreotide, and sulfonamide antibiotics may increase the blood glucose-lowering effects of insulin aspart. Corticosteroids, niacin, danazol, diuretics, sympathomimetic agents, isoniazid, phenothiazine derivatives, somatropin, thyroid hormones, estrogens, and progestins may decrease the blood glucose–lowering effects of insulin aspart. Beta-blockers, clonidine, lithium salts, and alcohol may either increase or decrease the blood glucose–lowering effects of insulin aspart. Pentamidine has the potential for causing both hyperglycemia and hypoglycemia. Beta blockers, clonidine, guanethidine, and reserpine may mask the signs of hypoglycemia. Pregnancy Category C. There are no well-controlled clinical studies on the use of insulin aspart during pregnancy. Excretion in human breast milk is unknown. Safety and efficacy in children have not been studied. The most common adverse effect observed in patients on insulin therapy is hypoglycemia. Other side effects include lipodystrophy, injection site pain, pruritus, rash, and allergic reactions.

Administration: SQ injection.

Patient Care Implications: For subcutaneous administration. Injection should immediately be followed by a meal. Insulin aspart may be mixed with NPH human insulin. When insulin aspart is mixed with NPH human insulin, the insulin aspart should be drawn up first, and the mixture should be used immediately. Insulin aspart should not be mixed with crystalline zinc insulins. Monitor patient for signs and symptoms of hypoglycemia. Rotate injection sites. Instruct patient on the proper injection technique. Insulin aspart should be stored in the refrigerator—do not freeze. Do not use insulin aspart if it has been frozen. Cartridges or vials may be kept at ambient temperature away from excessive heat or sunlight for up to 28 days. Patients should be educated on the importance of self-monitoring of blood glucose levels.

Preparations: Injection, 100 units/ml, 10 ml vials.

Cartridges, 3 ml PenFill® cartridges for use with NovoPen® 3 Insulin delivery devices and Norofine® disposable needles.

INSULIN GLARGINE—Lantus®

Description/Actions: Indicated in the treatment of adult and pediatric patients with Type I diabetes mellitus or adults with Type II diabetes mellitus who require basal (long-acting) insulin therapy.

Precautions/Adverse Effects: Insulin glargine is contraindicated in patients with a known hypersensitivity to insulin glargine or to any component of the product. Prolonged hypoglycemia and recovery from hypoglycemia may occur with insulin glargine. Glucose monitoring is recommended for all patients. Any changes in insulin dosage should be made cautiously and under medical supervision. Insulin glargine is not intended for intravenous administration. Lantus® must not be diluted or mixed with any other insulin or solution, as this may alter the pH and therefore the onset or duration of the insulin glargine. Lantus® requirements may be decreased in patients with renal or hepatic impairment. Lipodystrophy may occur at the injection site. Injection sites should be rotated. Insulin requirements may be altered during periods of illness, stress, or emotional disturbances. Do not use in the treatment of diabetic ketoacidosis. Oral antidiabetic agents, ACE inhibitors, disopyramide, fibrates, fluoxetine, monoamine oxidase inhibitors, propoxyphene, salicylates, octreotide, and sulfonamide antibiotics may increase the blood glucose–lowering effects of insulin glargine. Corticosteroids, niacin, danazol, diuretics, sympathomimetic agents, isoniazid, phenothiazine derivatives, somatropin, thyroid hormones, estrogens, and progestins may decrease the blood glucose–lowering effects of insulin glargine. Beta–blockers, clonidine, lithium salts, and alcohol may either increase or decrease the blood glucose–lowering effects of insulin glargine. Pentamidine has the potential for causing both hyperglycemia and hypoglycemia. Beta blockers, clonidine, guanethidine, and reserpine may mask the signs of hypoglycemia. Pregnancy Category C. There are no well-controlled clinical studies in pregnant women. Excretion in human breast milk is unknown. Studies have shown Lantus® to be safe and effective in children 6–15 years of age with Type I diabetes mellitus. The most common adverse effect observed in patients on insulin therapy is hypoglycemia. Other adverse effects include injection site pain, lipodystrophy, pruritis and rash.

Administration: SQ injection.

Patient Care Implications: Do not mix or dilute with any other insulin or solution. Monitor patients for signs and symptoms of hypoglycemia. Store unopened vials in the refrigerator. Opened 10 ml vials may be kept at room temperature for up to 28 days away from excessive heat and direct sunlight. Opened 5 ml vials may be kept at room temperature for up to 14 days away from excessive heat and direct sunlight. Use only if the solution is clear and colorless with no particles visible. Rotate injection sites. Instruct patient on the proper injection technique. Educate patients on the importance of self-monitoring blood glucose levels.

Preparations: Injection, 100 units/ml, 10 ml vials.

INSULIN INJECTION—Regular
Iletin I and II®, Humalog®, Humulin R®, Novolin R®, Velosulin®

INSULIN ZINC SUSPENSION, PROMPT (Semilente)

ISOPHANE INSULIN SUSPENSION (NPH)—NPH
Iletin I and II®, Insulatard NPH®, Humulin N®, Novolin N®

INSULIN ZINC SUSPENSION (LENTE)—Lente Iletin I and II®, Humulin L®, Novolin L®

PROTAMINE ZINC INSULIN SUSPENSION (PZI)

INSULIN ZINC SUSPENSION, EXTENDED (Ultralente)

Hypoglycemic agent.

Description/Actions: Is the principal hormone required for proper glucose use in normal metabolic processes. Indicated in the treatment of diabetes mellitus that cannot be properly controlled by diet alone. Also used in severe ketoacidosis or diabetic coma.

Warnings: Hypoglycemia may result from excessive dosage. Adverse reactions include allergic responses and lipodystrophy. Corticosteroids and thiazide and other diuretics may increase blood glucose levels and necessitate an increase in insulin dosage.

Administration: Subcutaneous. Insulin injection (regular insulin) has been administered intravenously or intramuscularly in certain situations (e.g., severe ketoacidosis, diabetic coma).

Preparations: Preparations are classified as rapid-acting (Regular, Semilente), intermediate-acting (NPH, Lente), and long-acting (PZI, Ultralente), based on the promptness, duration, and intensity of action following subcutaneous administration. Some preparations contain human insulin prepared using recombinant DNA technology (Humulin) or semisynthetically (Novolin, Insulatard, Velosulin); other preparations are derived from beef and pork sources. Vials, 100 units/ml. A concentrated solution of regular insulin containing 500 units per ml is available for the treatment of patients with insulin resistance.

INTAL®, see Cromolyn

INTEGRILIN®, see Eptifibatide

INTERFERON ALFACON-1—Intergen®

Description/Actions: Indicated in treatment of chronic hepatitis C virus (HCV) infection in patients with compensated liver disease who have anti-HCV serum antibodies and/or presence of HCV-RNA.

Warnings: Contraindicated in hypersensitivity to *E. coli* derived products. Use only under the supervision of qualified MDs. Do not interchange brands. Exclude other causes of hepatitis (e.g., hepatitis B, autoimmune hepatitis). Use cautiously in cardiac disease, endocrine disorders, autoimmune disorders, leukopenia (esp. granulocytopenia), thrombocytopenia, and other myelosuppressive conditions. Withhold treatment if absolute neutrophil count $< 500 \times 10^6/L$ or if platelet count is $< 50 \times 10^9/L$.

Not recommended for use in severe psychiatric disorders or decompensated liver disease. Discontinue if either occurs. Not for use in pregnancy (Category C) or nursing mothers. Do pretreatment eye exams in diabetics and hypertensives. Refer to opthalmologist if visual disturbances occur.

Monitor lab values (blood counts, TSH, and T_4 creatinine, albumin, triglycerides, bilirubin) before, 2 weeks after starting, and periodically thereafter.

Adverse reactions include flulike symptoms, pain, edema, psychiatric/CNS effects (e.g., depression, insomnia, dizziness), local reactions, GI upset, cardiac or upper respiratory effects, rash, alopecia, pruritis, and visual or lab abnormalities.

Instruct patients in effective contraception (both males and females).

Administration: SQ injection.

If tolerated and unresponsive or relapsed, may give 15 μg SC 3 times per week for 6 months.

Preparations: 9 and 15 μg vials for SC inj., preservative free.

INTERFERON ALFA-2a RECOMBINANT—Roferon-A®

INTERFERON ALFA-2b RECOMBINANT—Intron A®

Antineoplastic agent/antiviral agent.

Description/Actions: Prepared using recombinant DNA technology. Indicated for the treatment of hairy-cell leukemia in patients 18 years of age or older and in the treatment of AIDS-related Kaposi's sarcoma in patients 18 years of age or older. Interferon alfa-2b is also indicated for the treatment of chronic hepatitis non-A, non-B/C, chronic hepatitis B, and for the intralesional treatment of condylomata acuminata (venereal or genital warts). Interferon alfa-2a is indicated in the treatment of chronic hepatitis C in patients with compensated liver disease.

Warnings: Most patients experience flulike symptoms (e.g., fever, headache, myalgia, chills) at the beginning of therapy; these effects can often be effectively managed with an analgesic-antipyretic such as acetaminophen. Fatigue, dizziness, and other CNS effects may occur, and patients should be cautioned about the risks of engaging in activities in which full mental and physical alertness and coordination are required.

INTERFERON BETA-1A • 171

Administration: Intramuscular and subcutaneous for hairy-cell leukemia, AIDS-related Kaposi's sarcoma, and chronic hepatitis non-A, non-B/C. Intralesional for condylomata acuminata.

Preparations: Interferon alfa-2a: Vials 3, 9, 18, and 36 million IU, and a powder formulation in vials containing 18 million IU. Interferon alfa-2b: Vials containing 3, 5, 10, 18, 25, and 50 million IU of lyophilized powder.

INTERFERON ALFA-N3 (HUMAN LEUKOCYTE DERIVED)— Alferon N®

Antiviral agent.

Description/Actions: Is manufactured from pooled units of human leukocytes and is designated as a natural interferon. Indicated for the intralesional treatment of refractory or recurring external condylomata acuminata (genital warts) in patients 18 years of age or older.

Warnings: Adverse reactions include flulike symptoms (e.g., fever, headache, myalgia, chills, back pain, and insomnia).

Administration: Intralesional. The drug should be injected into the base of each wart.

Preparations: Vials, 5 million IU.

INTERFERON BETA-1A—Avonex®

Description/Actions: For the treatment of relapsing forms of multiple sclerosis to slow the accumulation of physical disability and decrease the frequency of clinical exacerbations. Interferon Beta-1A is also approved for the treatment of patients with a first multiple sclerosis (MS) attack if magnetic resonance imaging (MRI) of the brain shows abnormalities characteristic of MS.

Preparations: Powder for injection, 33 mg (6.6 million units).

INTERFERON BETA-1B—
Betaseron®

Agent for multiple sclerosis.

Description/Actions: Produced by recombinant DNA technology and exhibits antiviral and immunoregulatory activities. Indicated for use in ambulatory patients with relapsing-remitting multiple sclerosis to reduce the frequency of clinical exacerbations and slow the accumulation of physical disability.

Warnings: Adverse reactions include injection site reactions, flulike symptoms, menstrual disorders, reduction in neutrophil and white blood cell counts, and elevation in SGPT levels. Use has been associated with depression and suicide attempts, and patients should be advised to immediately report symptoms of depression. Has been reported in animal studies to have abortifacient activity.

Administration: Subcutaneous, administered every other day. Sites for self-injection include arms, abdomen, hips, and thighs.

Preparations: Room temperature formulation—injectible. Vials, 0.3 mg Betaseron (9.6 million IU), plus a separate vial containing diluent.

INTERFERON GAMMA-1B - Actimmune®

Biologic response modifier.

Description/Actions: Prepared by recombinant DNA technology. Exhibits immunomodulatory properties and a phagocyte-activating effect, which mediates the killing of microorganisms. Indicated for reducing the frequency and severity of serious infections associated with chronic granulomatous disease.

Warnings: Adverse reactions include flulike symptoms (e.g., fever, headache, chills, myalgia, fatigue), which may decrease in severity as treatment continues. Some symptoms may be minimized by bedtime administration. Acetaminophen may be useful in alleviating fever and headache. May cause CNS effects (e.g., dizziness, decreased mental status) and caution should be exercised in patients with known seizure disorders and/or compromised CNS function. May cause hematologic effects (e.g., neutropenia) and caution should be exercised when used in patients with myelosuppression or when used in combination with other potentially myelosuppressive agents.

Administration: Subcutaneous. Optimum sites of injection are the right deltoid and anterior thigh. Vials should not be shaken.

Preparations: Vials, 100 µg (3 million units).

INTERGEN, see Interferon Alfacon-1

INTERLEUKIN-2, see Aldesleukin

INTRON A®, see Interferon alfa-2b recombinant

INTROPIN®, see Dopamine

INVERSINE®, see Mecamylamine

INVERT SUGAR—Travert®

Description/Actions: Mixture of *dextrose* and *fructose* used intravenously for fluid and caloric replacement.

Preparations: Solution, 10%.

INVIRASE®, see Saquinavir

IODINATED GLYCEROL

Description/Actions: Mucolytic/expectorant indicated as adjunctive treatment in respiratory conditions such as bronchitis and asthma.

Preparations: Tablets, 30 mg. Elixir, 1.2%. Solution, 5%.

IODINE

Description/Actions: Antiseptic applied

topically to prevent or treat dermatologic infections. Also used to disinfect the skin preoperatively. Has also been used (often as sodium iodide or potassium iodide) orally and parenterally in the management of certain thyroid conditions.

Preparations: Solution (with sodium or potassium iodide), 2% and 5% (Lugol's solution). Tincture (with sodium or potassium iodide), 2% and 5%.

IODOCHLORHYDROXYQUIN— former name of Clioquinol

IODOQUINOL— Diiodohydroxyquin, Yodoxin®

Description/Actions: Amebicide indicated in the treatment of intestinal amebiasis.

Preparations: Tablets, 210 and 650 mg.

IOPIDINE®, see Apraclonidine

IPECAC

Emetic used in the management of drug overdose and in certain other poisonings.

Preparations: Syrup.

IPRATROPIUM BROMIDE— Atrovent®

Bronchodilator, anticholinergic.

Description/Actions: Is an anticholinergic agent administered by inhalation for the maintenance treatment of bronchospasm associated with chronic obstructive pulmonary disease, including chronic bronchitis and emphysema. Nasal spray is used for rhinorrhea associated with allergic and nonallergic perennial rhinitis and rhinorrhea associated with the common cold.

Warnings: Adverse reactions include cough, exacerbation of symptoms, nervousness, dizziness, headache, nausea, gastrointestinal distress, and palpitations. Nasal spray may cause epistaxis, pharyngitis, nasal dryness or irritation. Systemic anticholinergic effects are uncommon, but caution should be exercised in patients with narrow-angle glaucoma, prostatic hypertrophy, or bladder-neck obstruction. Teach patients to avoid use during acute bronchospasm. Patients should be warned against spraying the aerosol into their eyes, because temporary blurring of vision may result.

Administration: Oral inhalation, nasal spray.

Preparations: Metered-dose inhaler. Inhalation solution, 0.02%. Nasal spray, 0.03% aqueous solution.

IRBESARTAN—Avapro®

Description/Actions: Angiotensin II receptor antagonist indicated in the treatment of hypertension and for use in patients with type 2 diabetes for the treatment of nephropathy with an elevated serum creatinine and proteinuria (> 300 mg/day) in patients with type 2 diabetes and hypertension.

Warnings: Correct salt/volume depletion (e.g., patients vigorously treated with diuretics or those on dialysis) before beginning therapy, or use a low initial dose. Use cautiously in renal impairment, severe CHF, renal artery stenosis. Pregnancy Category C in first trimester. Pregnancy Category D in second and third trimesters.

Adverse reactions include diarrhea, dyspepsia, and fatigue.

Administration: Oral.

Preparations: Tablets, 75, 150, and 300 mg.

IRON DEXTRAN—InFeD®

Description/Actions: Iron formulation indicated for the parenteral treatment of iron deficiency anemia.

Preparations: Ampules and vials, 50 mg iron/ml.

ISMELIN®, see Guanethidine

ISMO®, see Isosorbide mononitrate

ISOETHARINE—Bronkometer®, Bronkosol®

Description/Actions: Bronchodilator administered by inhalation and indicated for bronchial asthma and for reversible bronchospasm that may occur in association with bronchitis and emphysema.

Preparations: Solution for nebulization (as the hydrochloride), numerous concentrations ranging from 0.062% to 1%. Metered dose inhaler (as the mesylate), 340 μg/metered dose.

ISOFLUROPHATE—Floropryl®

Description/Actions: Cholinesterase inhibitor indicated for ophthalmic use in the treatment of open-angle glaucoma, conditions obstructing aqueous outflow, following iridectomy, and accommodative esotropia.

Preparations: Ophthalmic ointment, 0.025%

ISOMETHEPTENE MUCATE

Description/Actions: Sympathomimetic agent used in combination with other agents in the treatment of tension and vascular headaches.

ISONIAZID—INH, Nydrazid®

Description/Actions: Antitubercular agent used in the treatment of tuberculosis and as preventive therapy in selected patients who are at risk of tubercular infection.

Preparations: Tablets, 50, 100, and 300 mg. Syrup, 50 mg/ml. Vials, 100 mg/ml.

ISOPROPYL ALCOHOL

Description/Actions: Antiseptic that is applied to the skin as isopropyl rubbing alcohol and in other formulations.

Preparations: Solutions, 70%, 91%, and 100%.

ISOPROTERENOL HYDROCHLORIDE—Isuprel®

Description/Actions: Bronchodilator indicated for the treatment of bronchospasm associated with bronchial asthma, pulmonary emphysema, bronchitis, and bronchiectasis. Also used as an adjunct in the management of shock and in the treatment of cardiac standstill or arrest, in the management of certain ventricular arrhythmias and other serious cardiac complications. May also be used in the management of bronchospasm during anesthesia.

Preparations: Solution for nebulization, 0.25% (1:400), 0.5% (1:200), and 1% (1:100). Aerosol solution and metered-dose inhalers. Sublingual tablets, 10 and 15 mg. Ampules, vials, and syringes, 0.2 mg/ml. (1:5000).

ISOPTIN®, see Verapamil

ISOPTIN SR®, see Verapamil

ISOPTO-CARBACHOL®, see Carbachol

ISORDIL®, see Isosorbide dinitrate

ISOSORBIDE DINITRATE—Isordil®, Sorbitrate®

Antianginal agent.

Description/Actions: An organic nitrate indicated for the treatment and prevention of angina pectoris.

Warnings: Adverse reactions include headache, dizziness, hypotension, and cutaneous vasodilation with flushing.

Administration: Oral and sublingual.

Preparations: Sublingual tablets, 2.5, 5, and 10 mg. Tablets, 2.5, 5, 10, 20, 30, and 40 mg. Controlled-release tablets, 40 mg. Chewable tablets, 5 and 10 mg.

ISOSORBIDE MONONITRATE—Imdur®, Ismo®, Monoket®

Antianginal agent.

Description/Actions: An organic nitrate that has a primary action of relaxation of vascular smooth muscle. Is the major active metabolite of isosorbide dinitrate. Indicated for the prevention of angina pectoris due to coronary artery disease.

Warnings: Adverse reactions include headache, dizziness, and nausea/vomiting. May cause hypotension and should be used with caution in patients who are volume depleted or who are already hypotensive.

Symptomatic hypotension may occur when used concurrently with a calcium channel-blocking agent and dosage adjustments may be necessary.

Administration: Oral. When administered twice a day, is given in an "asymmetric" dosing schedule (2 doses per day given 7 hours apart), which has been designed to avoid tolerance. The controlled-release formulation is administered once a day.

Preparations: Tablets, 10 and 20 mg. Controlled-release tablets (Imdur®), 30, 60, 120 mg.

ISOTRETINOIN—Accutane®

Description/Actions: Retinoid (vitamin A analogue) indicated for the treatment of severe recalcitrant cystic acne. Isotretinoin should be reserved for patients with severe nodular acne who are unresponsive to conventional therapy, including systemic antibiotics. Only indicated for those female patients who are not pregnant because isotretinoin can cause severe birth defects. The Accutane® Pregnancy Prevention and Risk Management Programs, consisting of the System to Manage Accutane® Related Teratogenicity (S.M.A.R.T.) and the Accutane® Pregnancy Prevention Program (PPP), should be followed for prescribing Accutane® with the goal of preventing fetal exposure to isotretinoin.

Warnings: May cause fetal abnormalities and must not be taken during pregnancy. Pregnancy category X. Exercise caution when prescribing to patients with a genetic predisposition for age related osteoporosis, a history of childhood osteoporosis, osteomalacia, or other disorders of bone metabolism including patients diagnosed with anorexia nervosa and those on chronic drug therapy that cause drug induced osteoporosis/osteomalacia and or affects vitamin D metabolism such as systemic corticosteroids and any anticonvulsant. Accutane® may cause depression, psychosis and rarely suicidal ideation, suicide attempts, suicide and aggressive and or violent behaviors. Discontinuation of Accutane® may be insufficient, further evaluation may be necessary.

Preparations: Capsules, 10, 20, and 40 mg.

ISOVEX®, see Ethaverine

ISOXSUPRINE HYDROCHLORIDE—Vasodilan®

Description/Actions: Peripheral vasodilator used for relief of symptoms associated with cerebral vascular insufficiency, in peripheral vascular disease of arteriosclerosis obliterans, thromboangiitis obliterans, and Raynaud's disease. Has been utilized investigationally in threatened premature labor.

Preparations: Tablets, 10 and 20 mg.

ISRADIPINE—DynaCirc®

Antihypertensive agent.

Description/Actions: A calcium channel-blocking agent that is indicated in the management of hypertension. May be used alone or concurrently with a thiazide-type diuretic.

Warnings: Adverse reactions include dizziness, edema, palpitations, flushing, tachycardia, fatigue, and headache. Caution should be exercised when the drug is used in patients with congestive heart failure. Concurrent use with a beta-adrenergic blocking agent may be employed advantageously in some patients but may be associated with risks such as an excessive reduction in blood pressure.

Administration: Oral.

Preparations: Capsules, 2.5 and 5 mg. Controlled-release tablets, 5 and 10 mg.

ISUPREL®, see Isoproterenol

ITRACONAZOLE—Sporanox®

Triazole antifungal agent.

Description/Actions: Inhibits the cytochrome P-450-dependent synthesis of ergosterol, which is a vital component of fungal cell membranes. Indicated for the treatment of blastomycosis (pulmonary and extrapulmonary) and histoplasmosis, including chronic cavitary pulmonary disease and disseminated, nonmeningeal histoplasmosis. Is indicated for these infections in both immunocompromised and non-immunocompromised patients. Also indicated for the treatment of pulmonary aspergillosis in patients who are intolerant of or who are refractory to amphotericin B therapy. Indicated the onchomycosis of the toenail with or without fingernail involvement and in onchomycosis of the fingernail.

Warnings: Caution must be exercised in patients who are hypersensitive to other azole antifungal agents. Concurrent use with terfenadine astemizole or cisapride, is contraindicated. Adverse reactions include nausea, vomiting, diarrhea, edema, fatigue, fever, rash, headache, and hypertension. Abnormal hepatic function, including rare reports of reversible idiosyncratic hepatitis, has been experienced, and patients should be advised to report any signs or symptoms that may suggest liver dysfunction. Rare cases of serious hepatotoxicity including liver failure and death have been reported with itraconazole; some of the events developed within the first week of treatment. Treatment should be stopped immediately and liver function testing should be conducted in patients who develop signs and symptoms suggestive of liver disease, such as unusual fatigue, anorexia, nausea, vomiting, jaundice, dark urine,. or palor stools.

Administration: Oral. Should be administered with food.

Preparations: Capsules, 100 mg. Oral solution, 10 mg/ml.

Injection kit, 10 mg/ml–25 ml ampule with one 50 ml bag of 0.9% Sodium Chloride and filtered infusion set.

K

KADIAN®, see Morphine Sulfate

KALETRA™, see Lopinavir and Ritonavir

KANAMYCIN SULFATE—Kantrex®

Description/Actions: Aminoglycoside antibiotic primarily used in the parenteral treatment of infections caused by gram-negative bacteria. Has been used orally for the suppression of intestinal bacteria in the management of hepatic coma and in combination with other drugs to treat tuberculosis in patients resistant to conventional therapy.

Administration: IV, IM, intraperitoneal, inhalation, and irrigation.

Preparations: Vials and syringes, 75 and 500 mg and 1 g. Capsules, 500 mg.

KANTREX®, see Kanamycin

KAOLIN

Description/Actions: Adsorbent used in combination with other agents in the management of diarrhea.

KAON®, see Potassium gluconate

KAY CIEL®, see Potassium chloride

KAYEXALATE®, see Sodium polystyrene sulfonate

KEFLEX®, see Cephalexin

KEFLIN®, see Cephalothin

KEFTAB®, see Cephalexin hydrochloride

KEFUROX®, see Cefuroxime sodium

KEFZOL®, see Cefazolin

KEPPRA®, see Levetiracetam

KEMADRIN®, see Procyclidine

KENACORT®, see Triamcinolone

KENALOG®, see Triamcinolone

KERLONE®, see Betaxolol

KETALAR®, see Ketamine

KETAMINE HYDROCHLORIDE— Ketalar®

Description/Actions: General anesthetic administered parenterally as the sole anesthetic in certain procedures, for the induction of anesthesia prior to the administration of other general anesthetic agents, and to supplement low-potency agents such as nitrous oxide.

Preparations: Vials, 10 mg/ml, 50 mg/ml, and 100 mg/ml.

KETOCONAZOLE—Nizoral®

Antifungal agent.

Description/Actions: Indicated for oral use in the treatment of systemic fungal infections and for the treatment of severe recalcitrant cutaneous dermatophytic infections that have not responded to topical therapy or oral griseofulvin, or in patients who are unable to take griseofulvin. Also used topically in the treatment of tinea corporis, tinea cruris, and tinea versicolor, cutaneous candidiasis, and seborrheic dermatitis. Used as a shampoo in the reduction of scaling due to dandruff.

Warnings: Should not be used concurrently with terfenadine, astemizole, or cisapride.

Administration: Oral and topical.

Preparations: Tablets, 200 mg. Cream, 2%. Shampoo, 2%.

KETOPROFEN—Actron®,Orudis®, Oruvail®

Nonsteroidal anti-inflammatory drug.

Description/Actions: Inhibits prostaglandin synthesis and is indicated for the treatment of rheumatoid arthritis and osteoarthritis, mild to moderate pain, and dysmenorrhea.

Warnings: Should not be given to patients in whom aspirin or another NSAID causes asthma, rhinitis, urticaria, or other allergic-type reactions. May cause GI effects and use should be avoided in patients with active GI tract disease and closely supervised in patients with a previous history of such disorders. Other adverse reactions include headache, malaise, nervousness, and edema.

Administration: Oral.

Preparations: Tablets, 12.5 mg. Capsules, 25, 50, and 75 mg. Controlled-release capsules (Oruvail®), 200 mg.

KETOROLAC TROMETHAMINE— Acular®, Acular PF®, Toradol®

Analgesic.

Description/Actions: A nonsteroidal anti-inflammatory drug (NSAID) that inhibits prostaglandin synthesis. Indicated for intramuscular or intravenous use for the short-term (up to 5 days) management of moderately severe, acute pain, usually in a postoperative setting. Therapy should be initiated by the IM or IV route and is to be used orally only as a continuation treatment. Treatment by any route (or combination of routes) of administration should not exceed 5

178 • KETOTIFEN

days. Indicated for ophthalmic use for the relief of itching due to seasonal allergic conjunctivitis and post-op inflammation after cataract extraction.

Warnings: Should not be given to patients in whom aspirin or another NSAID causes asthma, rhinitis, urticaria, or other allergic-type reactions. Use is contraindicated in patients at risk of GI bleeding or other bleeding reactions, and in patients with advanced renal impairment. Adverse reactions include nausea, dyspepsia, gastrointestinal pain, and drowsiness.

Administration: Oral, intravenous, intramuscular, and ophthalmic.

Preparations: Tablets, 10 mg. Single-dose syringes, 15, 30, and 60 mg. Ophthalmic solution, 0.5% and as persative free.

KETOTIFEN—Zaditor®

Description/Actions: Ketotifen is used to provide temporary relief of itching due to allergic conjunctivitis.

Precautions/Adverse Reactions: Ketotifen should be administered to a contact lens wearer 10 minutes before they insert their lenses. The drug has not been established in pregnant women, breast-feeding women, and children under the age of 3. Ketotifen is usually well tolerated. Some side effects are conjuctival hyperemia, headache, rhinitis, conjunctivitis, eyelid swelling, flu syndrome, keratitis, lacrimation disorder, mydriasis, ocular pain, photophobia, and xerophthalmia.

Administration: Adults, adolescents, and children ≥ 3 years: One drop in affected eye twice daily every 8–12 hours.

Patient Care Implications: Ketotifen should be used 10 minutes before patient inserts contact lens. Drug safety not established in pregnant women, breast-feeding women, and children under age 3. Do not share drops between patients, and wash hands before and after use.

Preparations: Eye drops, 5 ml bottle.

KINERET™, see Anakinra

KLARON®, see Sulfacetamide sodium

KLONOPIN®, see Clonazepam

K-LOR®, see Potassium chloride

KLORVESS®, see Potassium chloride

KLOTRIX®, see Potassium chloride

KONAKION®, see Phytonadione

K-TAB®, see Potassium chloride

KWELL®, see Lindane

KYTRIL®, see Granisetron hydrochloride

L

LABETALOL HYDROCHLORIDE—
Normodyne®, Trandate®

Antihypertensive agent.

Description/Actions: Exhibits nonselective beta-adrenergic and selective alpha 1-adrenergic-blocking actions. Indicated in the management of hypertension and, when administered intravenously, is also indicated for the treatment of severe hypertension.

Warnings: Contraindicated in patients with bronchial asthma, overt cardiac failure, greater than first-degree heart block, cardiogenic shock, or severe bradycardia. Adverse reactions include fatigue, dizziness, nausea, and nasal stuffiness. Use is best avoided in patients with bronchospastic diseases, and therapy in diabetic patients must be closely monitored.

Administration: Oral and intravenous. Patients should be cautioned about the interruption or discontinuation of therapy; exacerbation of angina pectoris may occur following the abrupt cessation of therapy, and, when therapy is to be discontinued, the dosage should be gradually reduced over a period of 1 to 2 weeks.

Preparations: Tablets, 100, 200, and 300 mg. Ampules and vials, 5 mg/ml.

LAC-HYDRIN®, see Ammonium lactate

LACTATED RINGER'S INJECTION

Description/Actions: Intravenous electrolyte replenishment solution containing sodium, potassium, calium, chloride, and lactate.

Preparations: Solutions, 250, 500, and 1000 ml.

LACTULOSE—Cephulac®, Chronulac®

Description/Actions: Disaccharide used orally in the treatment of constipation, and orally or rectally in the prevention and treatment of portal-systemic encephalopathy, including the states of hepatic precoma and coma.

Preparations: Syrup, 10 g/15 ml.

LAMICTAL®, see Lamotrigine

LAMISIL®, see Terbinafine hydrochloride

LAMIVUDINE—Epivir®, HBV 3TC®

Description/Actions: Antiretroviral indicated in the management of HIV infection (AIDS) in combination with zidovudine.

Warnings: Use cautiously in patients with renal dysfunction and children with a history of, or other risk factors for, pancreatitis. Adverse reactions in adults include headache, malaise, fever, GI upset, neuropathy, dizziness, sleep or depressive disorders, rash, respiratory effects, and musculoskeletal pain. Adverse reactions in children include pancreatitis, paresthesias, and peripheral neuropathy.

Administration: Oral without regard to food.

Preparations: Tablets, 100 mg and 150 mg. Oral solution, 10 mg/ml.

LAMOTRIGINE—Lamictal®

Description/Actions: Antiepileptic drug indicated as an adjunctive therapy in the treatment of partial seizures in patients with epilepsy, as adjunct in Lennox-Gastaut Syndrome in adults, and for the treatment of inadequately controlled partial seizures in children 2 years of age or older.

Warnings: Use cautiously in patients with reduced renal function, impaired cardiac or hepatic function. Adverse reactions include ataxia, dizziness, headache, somnolence, nausea, vomiting, rash, and photosensitivity.

Administration: Oral without regard to meals. Abrupt discontinuation may result in an increase in seizure activity so gradual withdrawal over 2 weeks is recommended unless safety concerns require more rapid withdrawal.

Preparations: Tablets, 25, 100, 150, and 200 mg. Chewable/dispersible tablets, 5 and 25 mg.

LAMPRENE®, see Clofazimine

LANOLIN—Wool fat

Description/Actions: Ointment base used topically in the management of certain dermatological conditions associated with dry skin and as a vehicle into which other medications are incorporated.

LANOXICAPS®, see Digoxin

LANOXIN®, see Digoxin

LANSOPRAZOLE—Prevacid®, Prevacid® Solutab

Description/Actions: Indicated for short-term treatment (up to 4 weeks) of active duodenal ulcer, short-term treatment (up to 8 weeks) of erosive esophagitis, and long-term treatment of pathological hypersecretory states (e.g., Zollinger-Ellison syndrome). In combination with clarithromgcin and/or amoxilillin for *H. pylori* eradication in duoderal ulcer disease, to reduce the risk of duodenal ulcer recurrence. Also indicated for the short-term treatment of symptomatic gastroesophageal reflux disease and for the short-term treatment of esophagitis in children ages 1 to 11.

Warnings: Adverse reactions include diarrhea, abdominal pain, and nausea. Because it is a potent acid inhibitor, those drugs that require an acidic environment may not be as well absorbed.

Administration: Oral or may open capsules and mix intact granule with 40 ml of apple juice and inject via nasogastric tube.

Preparations: Delayed release capsules, 15 and 30 mg. Delayed release oral suspension packets, 15 and 30 mg. Delayed release orally disintegrating tablets, 15 and 30 mg.

LARGON®, see Propiomazine

LARIAM®, see Mefloquine

LARODOPA®, see Levodopa

LASIX®, see Furosemide

LATANOPROST—Xalatan®

Description/Actions: Latanoprost is indicated for the initial treatment of elevated intraocular pressure associated with open-angle glaucoma or ocular hypertension and for the reduction of elevated intraocular pressure in patients with open-angle glaucoma and ocular hypertension who are intolerant of other intraocular pressure-lowering medications or are insufficiently responsive to other intraocular pressure-lowering medications.

Warnings: Use cautiously in renal or hepatic impairment. Adverse reactions include blurred vision, burning, stinging, increased pigmentation of the iris, punctate epithelial keratopathy, photophobia, upper respiratory tract infection, pain, angina, and rash. Latanoprost may gradually change eyelashes and vellus hair. These changes include increased length, thickness, pigmentation, and number of lashes or hairs and misdirected growth of eyelashes.

Administration: 1 drop once daily in the PM. Do not exceed the once daily dosage because it has been shown that more frequent administration may decrease the IOP lowering effect. Remove contact lenses before use, and do not reinsert for 15 minutes afterwards. Allow at least 5 minutes between application of other topical ophthalmic agents.

Preparations: 0.005% ophthalmic solution containing benzalkonium chloride.

LEDERCILLIN VK®, see Penicillin V potassium

LEFLUNOMIDE—Arava®

Description/Actions: Disease-modifying antirheumatic drug indicated to reduce the signs and symptoms of active rheumatoid arthritis (RA) and to retard structural damage as evidenced by X-ray erosions and joint space narrowing. Leflunomide has antiproliferative and anti-inflammatory activity.

Precautions/Adverse Reactions: Leflunomide is contraindicated in women of childbearing potential who are not using reliable contraception and in patients with significant hepatic impairment and hepatitis.

Pregnancy Category X. Use in nursing mothers not recommended.

Monitor liver function tests at the start of therapy to establish baseline values, and then monthly until stable, then do periodic testing. Obtain a negative pregnancy test before starting therapy. Use cautiously in patients with renal impairment, severe immunodifficiency, bone marrow dysplasia, and severe uncontrolled infections. Delay giving live vaccines.

Adverse reactions include diarrhea, elevated liver enzymes, alopecia, rash, respiratory infections, hypertension, headaches, and GI upset. Leflunomide may cause immunosuppression.

Administration: Oral.

Patient Care Implications: Instruct patients that leflunomide can remain within the body for up to 2 years unless an elimination procedure is followed. Contraception must be practiced while on this medication. Both men and women who wish to engage in pregnancy should be warned that they should seek the advice of their prescriber and undergo an elimination procedure before attempting to become pregnant. Simply stopping the drug and then attempting to become pregnant may result in serious birth defects or fetal death.

Aspirin, NSAIDs, and low-dose corticosteroids may be used concurrently.

Preparations: Tablets, 10, 20, and 100 mg.

LENTE INSULIN, see Insulin

LEPIRUDAN—Refludan®

Description/Actions: Indicated to treat heparin-induced thrombocytopenin and associated thromboembolic disease in order to prevent further thromboembolic complications.

Warnings: Carefully assess risk in patients with increased risk of bleeding (e.g., recent puncture of large vessels or organ biopsy, anomaly of vessels or organs, recent cerebrovascular accident, stroke, intercerebral surgery or other neuraxial procedures, severe uncontrolled hypertension, bacterial endocarditis, advanced renal impairment, hemorrhagic diathesis, recent major surgery, recent major bleeding). Obtain baseline aPTT ratio and continue to monitor closely during therapy. Use cautiously in renal insufficiency, liver injury, and reexposure.

Adverse reactions include hemorrhagic events, abnormal liver function, allergic skin reactions, infections, multiorgan failure, and ventricular fibrillation.

Administration: Intravenous.

Preparations: Vials, 50 mg.

LESCOL®, see Fluvastatin sodium

LESCOL® XL, see Fluvastatin sodium

LETROZOLE—Femara®

Description/Actions: Letrozole is a non-steroid aromatase inhibitor indicated in advanced breast cancer in postmenopausal woman with disease progression following antiestrogen therapy. Letrozole is also indicated as first-line treatment of postmenopausal women with hormone receptor positive or hormone receptor unknown locally advanced metastatic breast cancer.

Warnings: Adverse reactions include pain, nausea, headache, fatigue, arthralgia, GI upset, edema, hot flashes, hypercalcemia, alopecia, depression, elevated liver enzymes, thrombocytopenia (rare), and others.

Pregnancy Category D. Use cautiously in severe hepatic impairment.

Administration: Oral.

Preparations: Tablets, 2.5 mg.

LEUCOVORIN CALCIUM—Citrovorum factor, folinic acid, Wellcovorin®

Description/Actions: Folic acid analogue indicated to prevent and treat the hematologic and other undesired ef-

LEUKERAN

fects of folic acid antagonists (e.g., methotrexate) and to counteract the effect of overdosage of these agents. Has also been used in the treatment of certain megaloblastic anemias. Is also indicated for parenteral use in combination with 5-fluorouracil to prolong survival in the palliative treatment of patients with advanced colorectal cancer.

Preparations: Tablets, 5, 10, 15, and 25 mg. Ampules, 3 mg/ml and 5 mg/ml. Vials, 50, 100, and 350 mg. Implant, 72 mg, 65 mg free base.

LEUKERAN®, see Chlorambucil

LEUKINE®, see Sargramostim

LEUPROLIDE ACETATE—Lupron®, Lupron Depot-3 month®, Lupron Depot-Ped®, Viadur™

Description/Actions: Gonadotropin-releasing hormone analogue administered parenterally in the treatment of advanced prostatic cancer, endometriosis, and central precocious puberty. Also indicated for the treatment of uterine leimyomata in women who fail iron therapy. Leuprolide acetate solution is injected daily via the subcutaneous route. The depot formulation is injected via the intramuscular route once a month (Lupron Depot® 3.75 mg and 7.5 mg), once every 3 months (Lupon Depot® - 3 month (11.25 and 22.5 mg) or once every 4 months (Lupron Depot® - 4 month (30 mg).

Viadur™ (implant formulation): One subcutaneous implant for 12 months. Must be removed after 12 months of hormonal therapy; another implant may be inserted to continue therapy.

Patient Care Implications: Patient should be counseled on the possibility of the development or worsening of depression and the occurrence of memory disorders during treatment.

Preparations: Powder for injection, 3.75 mg, 7.5 mg, 11.25 mg, and 15 mg., 22.5 mg and 30 mg. Solution for injection, 5 mg/ml. Implant, 72 mg, 65 mg free base.

LEUSTATIN®, see Cladribine

LEVALBUTEROL—Xopenex®

Description/Actions: Indicated in the prevention and treatment of bronchospasm in reversible obstructive airway disease.

Precautions/Adverse Reactions: Use cautiously in patients with cardiovascular disease (esp. coronary insufficiency, arrhythmias, hypertension), seizure disorders, diabetes, and hyperthyroidism. Pregnancy Category C. Use not recommended in nursing mothers.

Adverse reactions include nervousness, tremor, infection, tachycardia, migraine, anxiety, dypepsia, leg cramps, dizziness, cough, turbinate edema, hypokalemia, and paradoxical bronchospasm.

Administration: Inhaled via nebulizer.

Patient Care Implications: Instruct patients to seek medical attention if the drug becomes less effective, if they do not experience significant improvement within 60 minutes of treatment, if symptoms worsen, or if more drug is needed to control symptoms. Use appropriate nebulizer. Do not mix other drugs in the nebulizer with the levalbuterol. Teach patients not to exceed dosing limits and to contact the prescriber if they feel this is necessary.

Preparations: Preservative-free inhalation solution, 0.31 mg/3 ml, 0.63 mg/3 ml, and 1.25 mg/3 ml per vial.

LEVAMISOLE—Ergamisol®

Antineoplastic agent.

Description/Actions: An immunomodulator that appears to restore depressed immune function. Indicated as adjunct treatment in combination with fluorouracil after surgical resection in patients with Dukes' stage C colon cancer.

Warnings: May cause agranulocytosis. Use in combination with fluorouracil has been associated with neutropenia, anemia, and thrombocytopenia. Adverse reactions include nausea, vomiting, diarrhea, stomatitis, anorexia, rash and/or pruritus, flulike symptoms, dizziness, ataxia, depression, and confusion. Disulfiram-like reactions may occur following the consumption of alcoholic beverages.

Administration: Oral. Treatment should be initiated no earlier than 7 days and no later than 30 days after surgery.

Preparations: Tablets, 50 mg.

LEVAQUIN®, see Levofloxacin

LEVARTERENOL, see Norepinephrine

LEVATOL®, see Penbutolol

LEVBID®, see Hyoscyamine sulfate

LEVETIRACETAM—Keppra®

Description/Actions: Levetiracetam is used as adjunctive therapy for the treatment of partial seizures.

Precautions/Adverse Reactions: Levetiracetam dosage should be adjusted in patients with renal impairment and the drug should not be stopped abruptly. The drug should also be given with caution to patients who are pregnant or breast-feeding and children under 16. Levetiracetam may affect patient's mental or motor performance, so caution should be used in operating machinery until patient knows how drug affects him or her. Some side effects are drowsiness, fatigue, difficulty breathing, ataxia, lack of coordination, agitation, anxiety, apathy, depression, hallucinations, and nervousness.

Administration: Oral.

Patient Care Implication: Levetiracetam dosage must be adjusted in patients with renal impairment, and creatinine and BUN must be monitored in all patients receiving the drug. Levetiracetam should be given cautiously to patients who are pregnant or breast-feeding and children under 16. Patients should avoid operating machinery after taking the medication.

Preparations: Tablet, 250, 500, and 750 mg.

LEVOBETAXOLOL HCL OPHTHALMIC SUSPENSION 0.5%—Betaxon®

Description/Actions: Indicated for lowering intraocular pressure in patients with chronic open-angle glaucoma or ocular hypertension.

Precautions/Adverse Reactions: Levobetaxolol is contraindicated in patients with sinus bradycardia greater than a first-degree atrioventricular block, cardiogenic shock, patients with overt cardiac failure, or in patients with a hypersensitivity to levobetaxolol or to any component of the product. Some systemic absorption may occur with topically applied beta-adrenergic-blocking agents. Severe respiratory and cardiac reactions including death due to bronchospasm can occur in patients with asthma. Use caution when using in patients with a history of cardiac failure or heart block. Discontinue therapy with levobetaxolol at the first sign of heart failure. Use cautiously in patients with diabetes mellitus, patients suspected of developing thyrotoxicosis, patients with myasthenic symptoms, and patients with restriction of pulmonary function. Gradually withdraw beta-adrenergic-blocking agents prior to general anesthesia. Potential additive effect with concomitant administration of an orally active beta-adrenergic blocking agent. Additive hypotension and or bradycardia may occur in patients receiving concomitant therapy with catecholamine-depleting drugs such as reserpine. Use cautiously in patients using concomitant adrenergic psychotropic drugs. Pregnancy Category C. There are no adequate and well-controlled studies in pregnant women. Use during pregnancy only if the potential benefit justifies the potential risk to the fetus. Excretion in human breast milk is unknown. Safety and efficacy in pediatric patients have not been established. Most common adverse effects observed during therapy with levobetaxolol include transient ocular discomfort upon instillation (11%) and transient blurred vision (2%). Cataracts and vitreous disorders have been reported in less than 2% of patients.

Administration: Adults: 1 drop in the affected eye twice a day.

Patient Care Implications: Do not use with contact lenses in the eyes. Protect from light. Shake well before using.

Preparations: Ophthalmic suspension, 5 ml, 10 ml, and 15 ml Drop-Tainer® dispenser.

LEVOBUNOLOL HYDROCHLORIDE—Betagan®

Agent for glaucoma.

Description/Actions: A noncardioselective beta-adrenergic-blocking agent indicated for ophthalmic use in the treatment of chronic open-angle glaucoma and ocular hypertension.

Warnings: Contraindicated in patients with bronchial asthma or severe chronic obstructive pulmonaryy disease, sinus bradycardia, second- and third-degree AV block, overt cardiac failure, or cardiogenic shock. Adverse reactions include transient ocular burning and stinging and systemic effects such as decrease in heart rate and blood pressure. Caution must be exercised in patients who are also taking another beta-blocker orally for another indication.

Administration: Ophthalmic.

Preparations: Ophthalmic solution, 0.25% and 0.5%.

LEVOCABASTINE HYDROCHLORIDE—Livostin®

Antihistamine.

Description/Actions: Indicated for topical ophthalmic use for the temporary relief of the signs and symptoms of seasonal allergic conjunctivitis.

Warnings: Adverse reactions include mild, transient stinging and burning, and headache. Contains benzalkonium chloride and patients should be instructed not to wear soft contact lenses during treatment.

Administration: Ophthalmic.

Preparations: Ophthalmic suspension, 0.05%.

LEVOCARNITINE—Carnitor®

Description/Actions: Amino acid derivative used as replacement therapy in primary and secondary carnitine deficiency.

Precautions/Adverse Reactions: Adverse reactions include nausea, vomiting, abdominal cramps, diarrhea, and patient body odor. Reducing the dosage often decreases or eliminates the GI effects of drug-related odor.

Administration: Oral, intravenous.

Preparations: Tablets, 330 mg.

Enteral liquid, 100 mg/ml.

Injection, 200 mg/ml in 2.5 and 5 ml ampules.

LEVODOPA—Dopar®, Larodopa®

Antiparkinson agent.

Description/Actions: Is converted to dopamine, which is the active pharmacologic agent. Indicated in the treatment of parkinsonism.

Warnings: Should not be given concomitantly with a monoamine oxidase inhibitor or in patients with narrow-angle glaucoma. Should be administered cautiously in patients with severe cardiovascular or pulmonary disease, bronchial asthma, renal, hepatic, or endocrine disease. Adverse reactions include choreiform and/or dystonic movements, palpitations, orthostatic hypotension, mental changes, headache, dizziness, nausea, and vomiting. Effect may be reduced by pyridoxine, and preparations containing this vitamin should be avoided unless carbidopa is being given concomitantly with levodopa (i.e., in the combination product, Sinemet® and Sinemet CR®). Not useful for treatment of drug-induced extrapyramidal reactions.

Administration: Oral.

Preparations: Capsules and tablets, 100, 250, and 500 mg. Sinemet tablets, 10 mg/100 mg, 25 mg/100 mg, and 25 mg/250 mg carbidopa/levodopa. Sinemet CR (controlled release) tablets, 50 mg/200 mg carbidopa/levodopa.

LEVO-DROMORAN®, see Levorphanol

LEVOFLOXACIN—Levaquin®, Quixin™

Fluoroquinolone

Description/Actions: Anti-infective agent indicated in the treatment of susceptible infections including respiratory tract infections, urinary tract infections, pyelonephritis, and nosocomial pneumonia.

Precautions/Adverse Reactions: Maintain adequate hydration. Use cautiously in patients with renal impairment, severe cerebral arterioslcerosis, epilepsy, and other seizure risks. Discontinue if rash, other signs of hypersensitivity, hypoglycemic reactions, phototoxicity, or tendon pain with inflammation or rupture, occurs. Risk of tendon rupture may be increased in patients receiving concomitant corticosteroids, especially in the elderly. Has been associated with QT interval prolongation and torsades de pointes in patients with concurrent medical conditions or concomitant medications that may prolong the QT interval (e.g., class Ia or class III antiarrhythmic agents). Use of levofloxacin in the presence of risk factors for torsades de pointes, such as hypokalemia,

significant bradycardia, and cardiomyopathy, should be avoided. Monitor blood, renal, hepatic, and hematopoetic function in prolonged use. Adverse reactions include nausea and diarrhea. Not recommended for children < 18 years of age.

Administration: Oral, intravenous and opththalmic. Take tabs with full glass of water. Infuse IV over 60 minutes. Ophthalmic (children ≥ 1 year and adults).

Preparations: Tablets, 250 mg, 500 mg, and 750 mg. Solution for IV infusion, 25 mg/ml.

Opthalmic solution, 0.5%.

LEVOMETHADYL ACETATE HYDROCHLORIDE—ORLAAM®

Agent for opiate dependence.

Description/Actions: Is an opiate agonist indicated for the management of opiate dependence as part of a comprehensive treatment plan that also includes appropriate medical evaluation, treatment planning, and counseling. Is approved for use only when dispensed by a licensed facility.

Warnings: Cases of QT interval prolongation and serious arrhythmias (torsades de pointes) have been observed during treatment with levomethadyl. ORLAAM should be reserved for use in the treatment of opiate-addicted patients who fail to show an acceptable response to other treatments for opiate addiction. All patients should undergo a 12—lead ECG prior to administration. If QT interval prolongation is present, ORLAAM should not be used. Administer with caution to patients at risk for developing QT interval prolongation. May cause CNS effects and impair the mental and physical abilities required for such potentially hazardous tasks as driving a car. May cause dependence and is classified in Schedule II. Other adverse reactions include abdominal pain, constipation, diarrhea, dry mouth, nausea, vomiting, cough, rhinitis, rash, sweating, difficult ejaculation, impotence, bradycardia, arthralgia, blurred vision, flu syndrome, and malaise. Withdrawal symptoms are likely to occur if a narcotic antagonist (e.g., naloxone) or a mixed agonist/ antagonist analgesic (e.g., pentozocine) is used concurrently. Should not be used concurrently with meperidine or propoxyphene. Is not recommended for use during pregnancy, and monthly pregnancy tests are required in patients of childbearing potential.

Administration: Oral. Is usually administered 3 times per week. Doses must not be given on consecutive days.

Preparations: Oral solution, 10 mg/ml. Should always be diluted before administration.

LEVONORGESTREL

Progestin component in certain oral contraceptive formulations.

LEVONORGESTREL AND ETHYL ESTRADIOL—Preven®

Description/Actions: This product is a hormonal contraceptive kit containing 4 tablets of a combination oral contraceptive, one hCG pregnancy test, and detailed patient information and product labeling. The tablets are indicated for the prevention of pregnancy in women after known or suspected contraceptive failure or unprotected intercourse.

Precautions/Adverse Reactions: Contraindicated in known or suspected pregnancy, pulmonary embolism, ischemic heart disease, history of cerebrovascular accident, valvular heart disease with complications, severe hypertension, diabetes with vascular involvement, headaches with focal neurological symptoms, major surgery with prolonged immobilization, breast cancer, liver tumors, active liver disease, and over 35 y/o if a heavy smoker (more than 15 cigarettes/day).

Use cautiously in patients during postpartum, in smokers, patients with cardiovascular disease, hypertension, diabetes, liver disease, ectopic pregnancy, unexplained vaginal bleeding, migraine, and conditions that may decrease GI transit time (may decrease ethinyl estradiol levels).

Adverse reactions include nausea, vomiting, menstrual irregularities, breast tenderness, headache, abdominal pain/cramps, and dizziness. Contact the prescriber if vomiting occurs within 1 hour of taking the medication.

Administration: Rule out pregnancy first by using the enclosed pregnancy test kit. Take 2 tablets as soon as possible (but no longer than 72 hours after unprotected intercourse) then take the remaining 2 tablets 12 hours later.

Patient Care Implications: Instruct patients that this is not a substitute for regular contraception. The effect of repeated use (more than once in a menstrual cycle or in multiple cycles) of emergency contraception is not known. Emergency contraceptives are not as effective as some other methods of contraception. Warn patients if the pregnancy test is positive not to take the tablets. Inform patients that this medication does not prevent transmission of sexually transmitted diseases.

Preparations: Levonorgesterel 0.25 mg + Ethinyl Estradiol 0.05 mg—4 tablets and 1 urine hCG test.

LEVONORGESTREL IMPLANT— Norplant®

Description/Actions: Progestin implant system used as a contraceptive and which is effective for up to 5 years.

Preparations: Kit containing 6 capsules (each containing 36 mg) and the equipment needed to implant all 6 capsules subdermally in the mid-portion of the upper arm.

LEVOPHED®, see Norepinephrine

LEVOPROME®, see Methotrimeprazine

LEVORPHANOL TARTRATE—Levo-Dromoran®

Opioid analgesic indicated for the relief of moderate to severe pain.

Preparations: Tablets, 2 mg. Ampules and vials, 2 mg/ml.

LEVOTHYROXINE SODIUM—Eltroxin®, Levoxyl®, Synthroid®

Agent for thyroid replacement.

Description/Actions: Is the principal hormone secreted by the normal thyroid gland. Indicated as replacement therapy for reduced or absent thyroid function.

Warnings: Use is best avoided in patients with acute myocardial infarction, uncorrected adrenal insufficiency, and thyrotoxicosis. Must be used cautiously in patients with cardiovascular disorders and endocrine disorders such as diabetes. Adverse reactions include headache, nervousness, palpitations, tachycardia, and nausea. May increase the action of anticoagulants.

Administration: Oral, intravenous, and intramuscular.

Preparations: Tablets, 0.025, 0.05, 0.075, 0.088, 0.1, 0.112, 0.125, 0.137, 0.15, 0.175, 0.2, and 0.3 mg. Vials, 0.2 and 0.5 mg.

LEVOXYL®, see Levothyroxine sodium

LEVSIN®, see Hyoscyamine

LEVSINEX®, see Hyoscyamine

LEVULAN KERASTICK®, see Aminolevulinic Acid Hydrochloride

LEVULOSE, see Fructose

LEXXEL®—Combination of Enalapril maleate extended release tablets, 5 mg and felodipine, 5 mg.

LIBRAX®, Combination of chlordiazepoxide and clindinium

LIBRITABS®, see Chlordiazepoxide

LIBRIUM®, see Chlordiazepoxide

LIDEX®, see Fluocinonide

LIDOCAINE AND PRILOCAINE CREAM—EMLA Cream®

Description/Actions: An emulsion of lidocaine and prilocaine indicated for use on normal intact skin for local analgesia and on genital mucous membranes as pretreatment for infiltration anesthesia.

Precautions/Adverse Reactions: EMLA is contraindicated in patients with a known history of sensitivity to local anesthetics of the amide type or to any other component of the product. EMLA should be used with caution in patients who may be more sensitive to the systemic effects of lidocaine and prilocaine including acutely ill, debilitated, or elderly patients as well as those with severe hepatic disease. Application to larger areas or for longer times than those recommended could result in serious adverse effects. Adverse reactions most commonly involve application site reactions (e.g. erythema, edema, hyperpigmentation, itching, rash). Dose-related systemic reactions occur more rarely and include CNS excitation and/or depression as well as cardiovascular effects such as bradycardia, hypotension, and cardiovascular collapse.

Administrations: Topical.

Preparations: Tubes, 5 and 30 g with or without Tegaderm™ dressing.

LIDOCAINE HYDROCHLORIDE—Xylocaine®

Description/Actions: Local anesthetic and antiarrhythmic agent. Used by the intravenous and intramuscular routes in the management of ventricular arrhythmias. Also administered parenterally as a local anesthetic for infiltration and nerve block, and by transtracheal and retrobulbar injection. Is also used topically during certain procedures (e.g., urological) and for dermatologic conditions. Several formulations are intended for application to the mucous membranes of the mouth and pharynx.

Preparations: Vials (for IV infusion), 0.2%, 0.4%, and 0.8%. Vials and syringes (for IV admixtures), 4%, 10%, and 20%. Ampules, vials, and syringes (for direct IV administration), 1%, and 2%. Ampules and automatic injection device (for IM administration), 10%. Ampules, vials, and syringes (for infiltration and nerve block), 0.5%, 1%, 1.5%, 2%, 4%, and in combination with epinephrine. Premixed IV solutions for infusion, 2 mg/ml (0.2%), 4 mg/ml (0.4%), and 8 mg/ml (0.8%) in 250 and 500 ml containers. Ointment, 2.5% and 5%. Solution (for topical application to mucous membranes), 2%, 4%, and 10%. Jelly, 2% and ointment, 5%, both for topical application to mucous membranes.

LIME SULFUR SOLUTION, see Sulfurated lime

LINCOCIN®, see Lincomycin

LINCOMYCIN HYDROCHLORIDE—Lincocin®

Description/Actions: Antibiotic indicated for the treatment of infections caused by susceptible gram-positive bacteria. Infrequently used drug as it has been replaced by safer, more effective agents.

Preparations: Capsules, 250 and 500 mg. Vials and syringes, 300 mg/ml.

LINDANE—Gamma benzene hexachloride, Kwell®

Description/Actions: Parasiticide indicated in the treatment of patients with scabies and lice infestations. Contraindicated in neonates. Adverse reactions include seizures. Children are at increased risk of systemic absorption and CNS side effects. Instruct parents and/or patients to follow application instructions carefully to minimize systemic absorption and toxic effects.

Preparations: Cream, lotion, and shampoo, 1%.

LINEZOLID—Zyvox®

Description/Actions: Indicated for the treatment of vancomycin-resistant enterococcus faecium infections. It is also indicated for the treatment of nosocomial pneumonia, complicated skin and skin-structure infections, uncomplicated skin and skin-structure infections, and community-acquired pneumonia.

Precautions/Adverse Reactions: Linezolid should not be taken with tyramine foods and should be used with caution in pregnant women, breast-feeding women, and hypertensive patients. Linezolid should not be given to children. The most common adverse events are diarrhea, headache, nausea, constipation, dizziness, insomnia, and rash. Other adverse events reported include pseudomembranous colitis, hypertension, dyspepsia, localized abdominal pain, pruritis, and tongue discoloration. Myelosupression including anemia, leukopenia, pancytopenia and thrombocytopenia have been reported in patients receiving linezolid.

Administration: Oral, intravenous.

Patient Care Implications: Patients who are pregnant, breast-feeding, or hypertensive should be careful using the drug. Linezolid should not be given to children. Platelets should be monitored in patients receiving the medication.

Monitor weekly complete blood counts for patients receiving linezoid especially, those patients receiving linezoid for longer than 2 weeks, patients with preexising myelosuppression, patients receiving concomitant therapy with other myelosuppressive agents, and patients with a chronic infection who have received previous or concomitant antibiotic therapy.

Preparations: Tablets, 400 and 600 mg.

Injection, 200 mg/100 ml, 400 mg/200 ml, 600 mg/300 ml.

Oral Suspension, 100 mg/5 ml, 150 ml bottle.

LIORESAL®, see Baclofen

LIOTHYRONINE SODIUM—Triiodothyronine, T$_3$, Cytomel®, Triostat®

Description/Actions: A thyroid hormone indicated as replacement or supplemental therapy in patients with hypothyroidism, as a pituitary/ thyroid–stimulating hormone suppressant in the treatment or prevention of various goiters, as a diagnostic agent, and, via parenteral use, for myxedema coma and precoma.

Preparations: Tablets, 5, 25, and 50 µg. Vials, 10 µg/ml (Triostat®).

LIPITOR®, see Atorvastatin

LIQUAEMIN®, see Heparin

LIQUEFIED PHENOL, see Phenol

LIQUID PETROLATUM, see Mineral oil

LISINOPRIL—Prinivil®, Zestril®

Antihypertensive agent.

LITHIUM CARBONATE • 189

Description/Actions: An angiotensin converting enzyme (ACE) inhibitor that is a derivative of enalaprilat, the active form of enalapril. Indicated for the treatment of hypertension and may be used alone or concomitantly with other antihypertensive agents. Also indicated as adjunctive therapy in the management of congestive heart failure in patients not responding adequately to diuretics and digitalis. Used as an adjunct to other therapies within 24 hours post MI in hemodynamically stable patients, to reduce mortality.

Warnings: Lisinopril is contraindicated in patients with a known hypersensitivity to any component of the product, in patients with a history of angioedema related to previous treatment with an ACE inhibitor, and in patients with hereditary or idiopathic angioedema. Lisinopril should be given with caution to patients with obstruction in the outflow tract of the left ventricle. Adverse reactions include dizziness, headache, fatigue, diarrhea, upper respiratory symptoms, cough, and hyperkalemia. An excessive reduction in blood pressure may occur, particularly in patients with severe salt/ volume depletion (e.g., those treated vigorously with diuretics). Angioedema has occurred infrequently, sometimes after the first dose. Coadministration of lisinopril and nonsteroidal anti-inflammatory drugs in patients with compromised renal function may result in a further deterioration of renal function. These effects are usually reversible.

Administration: Oral.

Preparations: Tablets, 2.5, 5, 10, 20, and 40 mg.

LITHANE®, see Lithium carbonate

LITHIUM CARBONATE—Eskalith®, Lithane®, Lithium citrate, Lithonate®

Description/Actions: Psychotherapeutic agent indicated in the acute treatment of manic episodes of manic-depressive illnesses, and as prophylaxis against their recurrence.

Preparations: Capsules and tablets, 150, 300 and 600 mg. Controlled-release tablets, 300 and 450 mg. Syrup, 300 mg/5ml.

LITHONATE®, see Lithium carbonate

LITHOSTAT®, see Acetohydroxamic acid

LIVER

Description/Actions: Antianemic agent used as a source of vitamin B_{12}.

Preparations: Tablets. Vials, 2, 10, and 20 μg vitamin B_{12}/ml.

LOBELINE

Description/Actions: Smoking deterrent used as a temporary aid to break the habit of smoking cigarettes.

Preparations: Tablets, 2 mg.

LODINE®, see Etodolac

LODOSYN®, see Carbidopa

LODOXAMIDE TROMETHAMINE—Alomide®

Agent for ocular disorders.

Description/Actions: Indicated for the topical treatment of vernal keratoconjunctivitis, vernal conjunctivitis, and vernal keratitis.

Warnings: Adverse reactions include transient burning, stinging, or discomfort upon instillation. Contains benzalkonium chloride and patients should be instructed not to wear soft contact lenses during treatment.

Administration: Ophthalmic.

Preparations: Ophthalmic solution, 0.1%.

LOESTRIN®—Oral contraceptive combination of ethinyl estradiol and norethindrone acetate

LOFENE®, see Diphenoxylate

LOMANATE®, see Diphenoxylate

LOMEFLOXACIN HYDROCHLORIDE— Maxaquin®

Fluoroquinolone anti-infective agent.

Description/Actions: Inhibits DNA gyrase and exhibits a bactericidal action against many gram-positive and gram-negative bacteria. Indicated for lower respiratory tract infections and urinary tract infections caused by susceptible organisms. Also indicated for prophylaxis (preoperatively) to reduce the incidence of urinary tract infections in the early postoperative period (3–5 days postsurgery) in patients undergoing transurethral surgical procedures.

Warnings: Contraindicated in patients with a known hypersensitivity to any of the fluoroquinolones or the related quinolone antibacterial agents (i.e., nalidixic acid, cinoxacin). Fluoroquinolones have caused erosion of cartilage in weight-bearing joints and other signs of arthropathy in juvenile animals, and use in children under 18, pregnant women, and women who are nursing is best avoided. Adverse reactions include nausea, diarrhea, headache, dizziness, and photosensitivity reactions. Patients should be advised to avoid excessive sunlight and artificial ultraviolet light during the period of treatment. May cause dizziness, lightheadedness, and other central nervous system effects, and patients should know how they tolerate the drug before they engage in activities that require mental alertness and coordination. Convulsions have been reported in patients receiving lomefloxacin.

Administration: Oral.

Preparations: Tablets, 400 mg.

LOMOTIL®, see Diphenoxylate

LOMUSTINE—CCNU®, CeeNU®

Description/Actions: Antineoplastic agent indicated in the treatment of brain tumors and Hodgkin's disease.

Preparations: Capsules, 10, 40, and 100 mg.

LONITEN®, see Minoxidil

LONOX®, see Diphenoxylate

LO/OVRAL®, Oral contraceptive combination of ethinyl estradiol and norgestrel

LOPERAMIDE HYDROCHLORIDE—Imodium®, Imodium A-D®, Imodium Advanced®

Antidiarrheal.

Description/Actions: Indicated for the control and symptomatic relief of acute nonspecific diarrhea and of chronic diarrhea associated with inflammatory bowel disease. Also indicated for reducing the volume of discharge from ileostomies.

Warnings: Adverse reactions include abdominal pain, nausea, vomiting, constipation, and tiredness.

Administration: Oral.

Preparations: Capsules and caplets, 2 mg. Liquid, 1 mg/5 ml. Also as a combination agent containing loperamide HCl 2 mg and Simethicone 125 mg in a chewable tablet (Imodium Advanced®).

LOPID®, see Gemfibrozil

LOPINAVIR AND RITONAVIR— Kaletra™

Description/Actions: Kaletra™ is a coformulation of lopinavir and ritonavir. It is used in the treatment of HIV in combination with other antiretroviral agents.

Precautions/Adverse Reactions: Kaletra™ is contraindicated in patients with known hypersensitivity to any of its ingredients, including ritonavir. Breastfeeding is contraindicated while receiving Kaletra™. Certain drugs that are metabolized via the cytochrome P450 isoform CYP3A or CYP2D6 are associated with increased levels and possible serious and/or life-threatening events when administered with Kaletra™. The following drugs should *not* be used in combination with Kaletra™: flecainide, propafenone, astemizole, terfenadine, dihydroergotamine, ergotamine, methylergonovine, cisapride, pimozide, midazolam, and triazolam. Avoid concurrent use with Saint-John's-wort, lovastatin, and simvastatin. Pancreatitis has been observed in patients on Kaletra™; use caution in patients with a history of pancreatitis. Patients with signs or symptoms of pancreatitis should be evaluated and therapy should be suspended as clinically appropriate. New onset diabetes mellitus and exacerbation of preexisting diabetes have been reported in patients receiving protease inhibitors. Use caution in patients with hepatic dysfunction; patients with underlying hepatic disease or marked elevations in transaminase prior to treatment may be at increased risk for further increases in transaminase levels. The potential of resistance/cross-resistance with other protease inhibitors is currently being evaluated. Increased bleeding has been reported in hemophilia Type A and B patients treated with Kaletra™. Redistribution/accumulation of body fat has been observed in patients on antiretroviral therapy. Large increases in the concentration of total cholesterol and triglycerides have occurred in patients on Kaletra™; Lipid testing should be performed prior to initiating therapy and periodically throughout treatment. Pregnancy Category C. No adequate and well-controlled studies in pregnant women. Kaletra™ should be used during

192 • LOPRESSOR®

pregnancy only if the potential benefit justifies the potential risk to the fetus. Safety and efficacy in pediatric patients < 6 months have not been established. Kaletra™ is an inhibitor of CYP3A and CYP2D6; coadministration of Kaletra™ and drugs primarily metabolized by these isoenzyme systems may result in increased plasma concentrations that could increase their therapeutic and/or adverse effects. Some adverse effects are nausea, abdominal pain, hypercholesterolemia, increased triglycerides, increased amylase, increased liver function tests, headache, insomnia, rash, and hyperglycemia.

Administration: Oral.

Preparations: Capsule: lopinavir 133.3 mg and ritonavir 33.3 mg. Solution, oral: Lopinavir 80 mg and ritonavir 20 mg per ml. Oral solution and gelatin capsules should be refrigerated (stored) at 2° C to 8° C (36°–46° F). If stored at room temperature (25° C or 77° F), use within 2 months.

LOPRESSOR®, see Metroprolol

LOPROX®, see Ciclopirox olamine

LOPURIN®, see Allopurinol

LORABID®, see Loracarbef

LORACARBEF—Lorabid®

Carbacephem antibiotic.

Description/Actions: Inhibits bacterial cell wall synthesis and exhibits a bactericidal action against many gram-positive and gram-negative bacteria. Indicated for upper respiratory tract infections, lower respiratory tract infections, acute maxillary sinusitis, uncomplicated skin and skin structure infections, and urinary tract infections caused by susceptible organisms.

Warnings: Contraindicated in patients with a known hypersensitivity to loracarbef or any of the cephalosporins. Must be used cautiously, if at all, in penicillin-sensitive patients and use should be avoided in patients with a history of immediate and/or severe reactions to penicillins. Adverse reactions include diarrhea, nausea, vomiting, abdominal pain, rash, headache, and vaginitis.

Administration: Oral. Should be administered at least one hour before or 2 hours after a meal. The rate of absorption from the suspension is faster than from the capsule; capsules should not be substituted for the oral suspension in the treatment of otitis media.

Preparations: Capsules, 200 mg. Powder for oral suspension, 100 mg/5 ml and 200 mg/5 ml.

LORATADINE—Claritin®

Antihistamine.

Description/Actions: Selectively antagonizes peripheral histamine H_1-receptors and is designated as a nonsedating antihistamine. Indicated for the relief of symptoms of seasonal allergic rhinitis and idiopathic chronic urticaria.

Warnings: Adverse reactions include headache, somnolence, fatigue, and dry mouth although the incidence of these effects was similar in patients receiving placebo.

Administration: Oral. Should be administered on an empty stomach.

Preparations: Tablets, 10 mg. Reditabs, 10 mg. Syrup, 1 mg/ml.

LORAZEPAM—Ativan®

Benzodiazepine antianxiety agent.

Description/Actions: A CNS depressant indicated for the management of anxiety disorders or for the short-term relief of the symptoms of anxiety and insomnia. Also indicated for parenteral use as a preanesthetic medication and in status epilepticus.

Warnings: Contraindicated in patients with acute narrow-angle glaucoma. Adverse reactions include drowsiness and other CNS effects; patients should be cautioned regarding activities such as driving and operating machinery, as well as interactions with other CNS-acting drugs including alcohol. Can cause dependence and is included in Schedule IV.

Administration: Oral, intravenous, and intramuscular.

Preparations: Tablets, 0.5, 1, and 2 mg. Vials, 2 and 4 mg/ml. Concentrated solution, 2 mg/ml.

LORTAB®, Combination opioid and analgesic.

Hydrocodone bitartrate and acetaminophen

LOSARTAN POTASSIUM— Cozaar®, Hyzaar®

Description/Actions: Angiotensin II receptor antagonist indicated in the treatment of hypertension and for use in patients with type 2 diabetes for the treatment of nephropathy with an elevated serum creatinine and proteinuria (> 300 mg/day) in patients with type 2 diabetes and hypertension.

Precautions: Adverse reactions include hypotension and dizziness. Contraindicated in pregnancy. May increase serum potassium levels. The antihypertensive effect of losartan may be diminished by concomitant administration of indomethacin.

Administration: Oral.

Preparations: Tablets, 25 and 50 mg. Available in combination formulation (Hyzaar) that contains 50 mg of losartan potassium and 12.5 mg of hydrochlorothiazide and 100 mg of losartan and 25 mg of hydrochlorothiazide.

LOTEMEX®, see Loteprednol etabonate

Description/Actions: Anti-inflammatry agent indicated in the treatment of seasonal allergic conjunctives (Alrex®) steroid responsive ocular disease, and postop inflammation after ocular surgery (Lotemax®).

Warnings: Contraindicated in ocular fungal, viral, or mycobacterial infections. Revaluate if no improvement after 2 days. Prescribe initially and renew after 14 days only after appropriate exam. use cautiously in corneal or scleral thinning, glaucoma, or a history of herpes simplex. Monitor IOP and for secondary infections in prolonged therapy (> 10 days). Avoid abrupt cessation. Remove soft contact lenses for installation and wait 10 minutes before reinserting. Included local reactions (e.g., blurred vision, burning, itching eyes, dry eye), photophobia, headache, rhinitis, and pharyngitis. May mask or exacerbate ocular infections. Prolonged use may result in increased IOP, optic nerve damage, visual acuity and field defects, cataract formation, and corneal perforation.

Administrations: Opthalmic.

Preparations: 2% opthalmic suspension (contains benzakonium chloride).

LOTENSIN®, see Benazepril hydrochloride

LOTEPREDNOL ETABONATE— Alrex®, Lotemax®

LOTREL®, Combination of Amlodipine and benazepril

LOTRIMIN®, see Clotrimazole

LOTRIMIN AF®, see Clotrimazole.

LOTRISONE®, Combination of clotrimazole and betamethasone dipropionate

LO-TROL®, see Diphenoxylate

LOVASTATIN—Mevacor®

Antihyperlipidemic agent.

Description/Actions: Results in a reduction of low-density lipoprotein (LDL) cholesterol and total plasma cholesterol, while high-density lipoprotein (HDL) concentrations increase. Indicated as an adjunct to diet for the reduction of elevated total and LDL cholesterol levels in patients with primary hypercholesterolemia (Types IIa and IIb), when the response to diet and other nonpharmacologic measures alone has been inadequate. Also indicated to slow the progression of coronary atherosclerosis in patients with coronary heart disease.

Warnings: Contraindicated during pregnancy and lactation because lovastatin has been reported to exhibit teratogenic effects in some animal studies. It is also contraindicated in patients with active liver disease or unexplained persistent elevations of serum transaminases. Marked persistent increases in serum transaminases may occur and it is recommended that liver function tests be performed every 4 to 6 weeks during the first 15 months of therapy and periodically thereafter. Adverse reactions include headache, rash, pruritus, nausea, diarrhea, constipation, abdominal pain, and myalgia. Some individuals experience myositis and patients should be advised to report unexplained muscle pain or tenderness. Although it is not known whether lovastatin causes ocular problems, it is recommended that ophthalmologic exams be conducted before or shortly after starting therapy, and annually thereafter.

Administration: Oral.

Preparations: Tablets, 10, 20, and 40 mg.

LOVENOX®, see Enoxaparin

LOXAPINE—Loxitane®

Description/Actions: Antipsychotic agent indicated for the management of the manifestations of psychotic disorders.

Preparations: Capsules (as the succinate), 5, 10, 25, and 50 mg. Oral concentrate (as the hydrochloride), 25 mg/ml. Ampules and vials (as the hydrochloride and for IM use), 50 mg/ml.

LOW-QUEL®, see Diphenoxylate

LOXITANE®, see Loxapine

LOZOL®, see Indapamide

LUDIOMIL®, see Maprotiline

LUFYLLIN®, see Dyphylline

LUGOL'S SOLUTION, see Iodine

LUMIGAN®, see Bimatoprost

LUMINAL®, see Phenobarbital

LUNELLE™, Combination of Medroxyprogesterone acetate and estradiol cypionate

LUPRON®, see Leuprolide

LUPRON DEPOT®, see Leuprolide

LUPRON DEPOT-PED®, see Leuprolide

LURIDE®, see Sodium fluoride

LUSTRA®, see Hydroquinone

LUTREPULSE®, see Gonadorelin acetate

LUXIOL®, see Betamethasome Valerate

LUVOX®, see Fluvoxamine maleate

LYPHOCIN®, see Vancomycin

LYSODREN®, see Mitotane

M

MAALOX®, see Aluminum and magnesium hydroxide

MACROBID®, see Nitrofurantoin

MACRODANTIN®, see Nitrofurantoin macrocrystals

MACRODEX®, see Dextran

MAFENIDE ACETATE— Sulfamylon®

Description/Actions: Sulfonamide anti-infective agent indicated for topical use as adjunctive therapy of patients with second- and third-degree burns.

Preparations: Cream, 8.5%.

MAGALDRATE—Riopan®

Description/Actions: Antacid indicated for the relief of hyperacidity and related symptoms.

Preparations: Tablets and chewable tablets, 480 mg. Suspension, 540 mg/5 ml.

MAGAN®, see Magnesium salicylate

MAGNESIUM CARBONATE

Description/Actions: Antacid used in combination with other agents.

MAGNESIUM CHLORIDE—Slow-Mag®

Magnesium supplement.

Preparations: Controlled-release tablets, 64 mg magnesium (as chloride).

MAGNESIUM CITRATE—Citrate of magnesia

Description/Actions: Laxative used in the treatment of constipation and with other agents as a bowel evacuant in the preparation of the colon for radiologic examinations.

Preparations: Solution.

MAGNESIUM HYDROXIDE—Milk of magnesia

Description/Actions: Antacid and laxative used alone or in combination with other agents.

Preparations: Tablets, 325 mg. Suspension.

MAGNESIUM OXIDE

Description/Actions: Used for the replacement of magnesium in various magnesium deficiencies.

Preparations: Capsules 140 mg, Tablets, 400 mg, 420 mg, and 500 mg.

MAGNESIUM SALICYLATE— Doan's Pills®, Magan®

Description/Actions: Salicylate analgesic/anti-inflammatory agent indicated for the relief of pain and the signs and symptoms of arthritic disorders.

Preparations: Tablets, 325, 545, and 600 mg.

MAGNESIUM SULFATE

Description/Actions: Laxative, anticonvulsant, and electrolyte. Used orally in the treatment of constipation, and parenterally to prevent or control convulsions. Also used parenterally as replacement therapy in the treatment of hypomagnesemia.

Preparations: Granules (to prepare solution for oral administration). Ampules and vials, 10%, 12.5%, 25%, and 50%.

MAGNESIUM TRISILICATE

Description/Actions: Antacid used in combination with other agents.

MALARONE™, see Atovaquone and proguanil hydrochloride

MANDELAMINE®, see Methenamine mandelate

MANDOL®, see Cefamandole

MANNITOL—Osmitrol®

MAOLATE®

Description/Actions: Osmotic diuretic indicated in the prevention and treatment of the oliguric phase of acute renal failure following cardiovascular surgery, severe traumatic injury, surgery in the presence of severe jaundice, hemolytic transfusion reaction, to reduce intraocular pressure (IOP) and intracranial pressure (ICP). Most common adverse reaction is electrolyte imbalance, especially hyponatremia.

Administration: Intravenous, GU irrigant.

Preparations: IV injection, 5, 10, 15, and 20%. GU irrigant, 5%. Also in combination with sorbitol for GU irrigation.

MAOLATE®, see Chlorphenesin carbamate

MAPROTILINE HYDROCHLORIDE—Ludiomil®

Description/Actions: Tetracyclic antidepressant indicated in the treatment of depression and for the relief of anxiety associated with depression.

Preparations: Tablets, 25, 50, and 75 mg.

MARCAINE®, see Bupivacaine

MAREZINE®, see Cyclizine

MARIJUANA, see Dronabinol

MARINOL®, see Dronabinol

MASOPROCOL—Actinex®

Agent for actinic keratoses.

Description/Actions: Indicated for the topical treatment of actinic (solar) keratoses.

Warnings: Adverse reactions include erythema, flaking, itching, dryness, edema, burning, and soreness. May induce sensitization (allergic contact dermatitis) and, if such reactions occur, the drug should be discontinued.

Administration: Topical. Patients may experience a transient local burning sensation after applying the cream. May stain clothing or fabrics.

Preparations: Cream, 10%.

MATULANE®, see Procarbazine

MAVIK®, see Trandolapril

MAXAIR®, see Pirbuterol

MAXAQUIN®, see Lomefloxacin

MAXIFLOR®, see Diflorasone

MAXIPIME®, see Cefepime

MAXIVATE®, see Betamethasone dipropionate

MAXZIDE®, Combination of triamterene and hydrochlorothiazide

MAZANOR®, see Mazindol

MAZINDOL—Mazanor®, Sanorex®

Description/Actions: Anorexiant indicated in the management of exogenous obesity as a short-term adjunct in a regimen of weight reduction based on caloric restriction.

Preparations: Tablets, 1 and 2 mg.

MEBARAL®, see Mephobarbital

MEBENDAZOLE—Vermox®

Description/Actions: Anthelmintic indicated for the treatment of pinworm, whipworm, roundworm, and hookworm infections.

Preparations: Chewable tablets, 100 mg.

MECAMYLAMINE HYDROCHLORIDE—Inversine®

Description/Actions: Antihypertensive agent indicated in the management of moderately severe to severe hypertension.

Preparations: Tablets, 2.5 mg.

MECHLORETHAMINE HYDROCHLORIDE—
Mustargen®, Nitrogen Mustard

Description/Actions: Antineoplastic agent indicated for the parenteral treatment of Hodgkin's disease, lymphosarcoma, chronic myelocytic or chronic lymphocytic leukemia, polycythemia vera, mycosis fungoides, and bronchogenic carcinoma. Also administered intrapleurally, intraperitoneally, or intrapericardially for the palliative treatment of metastatic carcinoma resulting in effusion.

Preparations: Vials, 10 mg.

MECLAN®, see Meclocycline

MECLIZINE HYDROCHLORIDE—
Antivert®, Bonine®

Antihistamine.

Description/Actions: Exhibits antihistaminic and anticholinergic activity. Indicated for the management of nausea, vomiting, and dizziness associated with motion sickness, and in vertigo associated with diseases affecting the vestibular system.

Warnings: Must be used with caution in patients with asthma, glaucoma, or enlargement of the prostate. Adverse reactions include drowsiness, and patients should be cautioned regarding activities such as driving and operating machinery, as well as interactions with other CNS-acting drugs including alcohol. Other adverse reactions include dry mouth.

Administration: Oral.

Preparations: Tablets, 12.5, 25, and 50 mg. Chewable tablets, 25 mg. Capsules, 15, 25, and 30 mg.

MECLOCYCLINE SULFOSALICYLATE—Meclan®

Description/Actions: Tetracycline antibiotic indicated for topical use in the treatment of inflammatory acne vulgaris.

Preparations: Cream, 1%

MEDROL®, see Methylprednisolone

MEDROXYPROGESTERONE ACETATE—Cycrin®, Depo-Provera®, Provera®

Progestational agent.

Description/Actions: Is a derivative of progesterone and is indicated in the treatment of secondary amenorrhea, and abnormal uterine bleeding due to hormonal imbalance in the absence of organic pathology, such as fibroids or uterine cancer. Also indicated for intramuscular use as adjunctive therapy and palliative treatment of inoperable, recurrent, and metastatic endometrial carcinoma or renal carcinoma. Also indicated for intramuscular use as a long-term injectable contraceptive when administered at 3-month intervals.

Warnings: Contraindicated in patients with hepatic dysfunction, undiagnosed vaginal bleeding, and known or suspected malignancy of breast or genital organs. May cause thromboembolic phenomena including thrombophlebitis and pulmonary embolism, and use is contraindicated in patients with a history of such disorders. May cause adverse effects in the fetus, and use during the first 4 months of pregnancy is not recommended. Other adverse reactions include rash, pruritus, edema, nausea, insomnia, depression, somnolence, and breakthrough bleeding.

Administration: Oral and intramuscular.

Preparations: Tablets, 2.5, 5, and 10 mg. Vials (Depo-Provera), 100 mg/ml, 150 mg/ml, and 400 mg/ml. Prefilled syringe, 150 mg/ml.

MEFENAMIC ACID—Ponstel®

Description/Actions: Nonsteroidal anti-inflammatory drug indicated for the relief of moderate pain and the treatment of primary dysmenorrhea.

MEFLOQUINE HYDROCHLORIDE

Preparations: Capsules, 250 mg.

MEFLOQUINE HYDROCHLORIDE—Lariam®

Antimalarial agent

Description/Actions: Acts as a blood schizonticide, but does not eliminate exoerythrocytic (hepatic phase) parasites. Indicated for the treatment of moderate acute malaria caused by susceptible strains of *Plasmodium falciparum* or *Plasmodium vivax*. Is also indicated for the prophylaxis of *Plasmodium falciparum* and *Plasmodium vivax* malaria infections.

Warnings: The drug should not be used during pregnancy and women of childbearing potential should use reliable contraceptive measures for the duration of mefloquine use and for 2 months after the last dose. Adverse reactions include CNS effects and patients should be cautioned regarding activities such as driving and operating machinery, as well as interactions with other CNS-acting drugs including alcohol. Rare cases of suicidal ideation and suicide have been reported. Other adverse reactions include nausea, vomiting, diarrhea, abdominal pain, loss of appetite, headache, tinnitus, fever, chills, myalgia, and rash. Concomitant use with chloroquine may increase the risk of convulsions.

Administration: Oral. For malaria prophylaxis, therapy should be initiated one week prior to departure to an endemic area and the drug should be administered on the same day of the week. Prophylaxis should be continued for 4 additional weeks following return. Doses of mefloquine should not be taken on an empty stomach and should be administered with at least 8 oz of water.

Preparations: Tablets, 250 mg.

MEFOXIN®, see Cefoxitin

MEGACE®, see Megestrol

MEGESTROL ACETATE— Megace®

Description/Actions: Antineoplastic agent indicated for the treatment of advanced carcinoma of the breast or endometrium. Also indicated for the treatment of anorexia, cachexia, or significant weight loss in patients with AIDS.

Preparations: Tablets, 20 and 40 mg. Suspension, 40 mg/ml.

MELLARIL®, see Thioridazine

MELOXICAM—Mobic®

Description/Actions: Indicated to relieve the signs and symptoms of osteoarthritis and also has been used as an analgesic to treat mild to moderate acute pain.

Precautions/Adverse Reaction: Meloxicam should not be given to patients who have experienced asthma, urticaria, or allergic-type reactions after taking aspirin or other NSAIDs. Severe, rarely fatal, anaphylactic-like reactions have been reported in such patients. Serious gastrointestinal toxicity such as bleeding, ulceration, and perforation of the stomach, and small or large intestine, can occur at any time. The most common adverse events reported are gastrointestinal including abdominal pain, diarrhea, dyspepsia, flatulence, constipation, and nausea and vomiting. Less common GI effects reported are colitis, xerostomia, peptic ulcer disease, eructation, esophagitis, gastritis, and GERD. In general, anorexia may also occur. Other adverse events are allergic or respiratory reactions including ingioedema, asthma, bronchospasm, dyspnea, dizziness, flu-like symptoms, headache, rash, edema, and upper respiratory tract infections.

Administrations: Oral.

Patient Care Implications: As with other NSAIDs, higher doses were associated with an increased risk of serious GI events. Therefore, the daily dose should not exceed 15 mg. Monitor signs and symptoms of GI perforation, ulceration, and bleeding. Experience with chronic NSAID therapy in elderly and debilitated patients suggests greater potential for serious GI adverse events. Monitor liver function tests. Use of meloxicam is not recommended in patients with severe hepatic insufficiency. If clinical signs and symptoms consistent with liver disease develop, or if systemic manifestations occur (i.e., eosinophilia, rash, etc.), meloxicam should be discontinued.

Preparations: Tablets, 7.5 and 15 mg.

MELPHALAN—Alkeran®

Description/Actions: Antineoplastic agent indicated for the treatment of multiple myeloma and for the palliation of nonresectable carcinoma of the ovary. Administered by intravenous infusion for the palliative treatment of multiple myeloma when oral therapy is not appropriate.

Preparations: Tablets, 2 mg. Vials, 50 mg.

MENEST®, see Estrogens, esterified

MENOTROPINS—Pergonal®

Gonadotropins [follicle-stimulating hormone (FSH) and luteinizing hormone (LH)] administered intramuscularly for the induction of ovulation and pregnancy in anovulatory women, and to stimulate spermatogenesis in men with infertility.

Preparations: Ampules, 75 IU each of FSH and LH and 150 IU each of FSH and LH.

MENTAX®, see Butenafine Hydrochloride

MENTHOL

Description/Actions: Analgesic/cooling agent included with other agents in formulations that are applied topically to the skin or throat (e.g., lozenges).

MEPERIDINE HYDROCHLORIDE—Demerol®

Opioid analgesic.

Description/Actions: Indicated for the relief of moderate to severe pain, for preoperative medication, for support of anesthesia, and for obstetrical analgesia.

Warnings: Adverse reactions include sedation and other CNS effects; patients should be cautioned regarding activities such as driving and operating machinery, as well as interactions with other CNS-acting drugs including alcohol. Other adverse reactions include flushing of the face, hypotension, and pain at the injection site. Is contraindicated in patients receiving a monoamine oxidase inhibitor. Can cause dependence, and formulations are covered under the provisions of the Controlled Substances Act.

Administration: Oral, intramuscular, intravenous, and subcutaneous.

Preparations: Tablets, 50 and 100 mg. Syrup, 50 mg/5 ml. Ampules, vials, and syringes, 10 mg/ml, 25 mg/ml, 50 mg/ml, 75 mg/ml, and 100 mg/ml.

MEPHENTERMINE SULFATE— Wyamine®

Description/Actions: Sympathomimetic agent indicated for the parenteral treatment of hypotension secondary to ganglionic blockade and that occurring with spinal anesthesia.

Preparations: Ampules and vials, 15 mg/ml and 30 mg/ml.

MEPHENYTOIN—Mesantoin®

Description/Actions: Anticonvulsant indicated for the control of grand mal, focal, Jacksonian, and psychomotor seizures in those patients who are refractory to less toxic anticonvulsants.

Preparations: Tablets, 100 mg.

MEPHOBARBITAL—Mebaral®

Description/Actions: Barbiturate indicated as a sedative for the relief of anxiety and tension, and as an anticonvulsant for the treatment of grand mal and petit mal epilepsy.

Preparations: Tablets 32, 50, and 100 mg.

MEPHYTON®, see Phytonadione

MEPIVACAINE HYDROCHLORIDE—Carbocaine®

Description/Actions: Local anesthetic used to produce local anesthesia by infiltration injection, peripheral nerve block, and central neural blocks by the lumbar or caudal epidural route. Also indicated for use in dental procedures.

Preparations: Vials, 1%, 1.5%, and 2%. Dental cartridges, 3%.

MEPROBAMATE—Equanil®, Meprospan®, Miltown®

Description/Actions: Antianxiety agent indicated for the management of anxiety disorders or for the short-term relief of the symptoms of anxiety.

Preparations: Tablets, 200, 400, and 600 mg. Controlled-release capsules, 200 and 400 mg.

MEPRON®, see Atovaquone

MEPROSPAN®, see Meprobamate

MEQUINOL/TRETINOIN TOPICAL SOLUTION—Solag®

Description/Actions: A solution containing 2% mequinol and 0.01% tretinoin indicated for the treatment of solar lentigines.

Preparations/Adverse Reactions: The combination of mequinol and tretinoin may cause fetal harm when administered to pregnant women. Solag Topical Solution should therefore not be used in women of childbearing potential. Solag is also contraindicated in individuals with a history of sensitivity reactions to any of its ingredients. Solag should not be administered if the patient is also taking drugs known to be photosensitizers because of the possibility of augmented phototoxicity. Caution should be used in patients with eczematous skin or a history of vitiligo. During the use of Solag, exposure of the treated area to sunlight should be avoided or minimized. Adverse reactions include erythema, burning, stinging or tingling, desquamation, pruritus, and skin irritation. Some patients experience temporary hypopigmentation of treated lesions or of the skin surrounding treated lesions.

Administration: Apply Solag to solar lentigines using the applicator top while avoiding application to the surrounding skin. The usual application schedule is twice daily, morning and evening, at least 8 hours apart. Patients should not shower or bathe the treatment areas for at least 6 hours after application. When applying, avoid the eyes, mouth, paranasal sinuses, and mucous membranes. With discontinuation of Solag therapy, a majority of patients will experience some repigmentation of their lesions over time.

Patient Care Implications: Solag should only be used as an adjunct to a comprehensive skin care and sun avoidance program. If a drug sensitivity, chemical irritation, or systemic adverse reaction develops, use of Solag should be discontinued. Patients require detailed instruction to obtain maximal benefits and to understand all the precautions necessary to use this drug with greatest safety.

Preparations: Topical solution, 30 ml bottle.

MERBROMIN—Mercurochrome

Description/Actions: Antiseptic that is applied topically.

Preparations: Solution, 2%.

MERCAPTOPURINE—Purinethol®

Description/Actions: Antineoplastic agent indicated in the management of leukemias.

Preparations: Tablets, 50 mg.

MERCUROCHROME®, see Merbromin

MERCURY, AMMONIATED, see Ammoniated mercury

MERREM®, see Meropenem

MEROPENEM—Merrem®

Description/Actions: Synthetic, broad-spectrum carbapenem antibiotic. Bactericidal activity results from the inhibition of cell wall synthesis.

Warnings: Contraindicated in patients who have experienced anaphylactic reactions to other carbopenems (imipenem) or to beta-lactam antibiotics. Use cautiously in patients with CNS disorders, history of seizures or renal impairment. Monitor renal, hepatic, and hematopoietic function in long-term use. Adverse reactions include local reactions, GI upset, headache, rash, pruritis, apnea, seizures, constipation, superinfection, and pseudomembraneous colitis. Meropenem may decrease serum levels of valproic acid to subtherapeutic.

Administration: IV infusion or bolus with dosages adjusted to renal function (see manufacturer's guidelines).

Preparations: Powder for reconstitution, 500 mg and 1 g.

MERTHIOLATE®, see Thimerosal

MESALAMINE—Asacol®, Pentasa®, Rowasa®

Agent for ulcerative colitis.

Description/Actions: Also known as 5-aminosalicylic acid (5-ASA) and is a metabolite of sulfasalazine. Indicated in the treatment of active mild to moderate distal ulcerative colitis.

Warnings: Contraindicated in patients who are hypersensitive to the drug or to any component (e.g., sulfite) of the formulation. Adverse reactions include an acute intolerance syndrome characterized by cramping, acute abdominal pain, bloody diarrhea, and sometimes fever, headache, and a rash. Some patients experience mild hair loss.

Administration: Oral and rectal.

Preparations: Tablets, delayed release, 400 mg (Asacol®). Capsules, controlled release, 250 mg (Pentasa®). Suspension enema, 4 g/60 ml (Rowasa). Suppositories, 500 mg (Rowasa).

MESANTOIN®, see Mephenytoin

MESNA—Mesnex®

Uroprotective agent.

Description/Actions: Reacts with the urotoxic metabolites (e.g., acrolein) of ifosfamide. Indicated as a prophylactic agent in reducing the incidence of hemorrhagic cystitis caused by ifosfamide.

Warnings: Adverse reactions include nausea, vomiting, and diarrhea.

Administration: Oral and intraveneous. Intravenous bolus injection. The total daily dose of mesna is 60% of the ifosfamide dose. It is given as intravenous bolus injections in a dosage equal to 20% of the ifosfamide dosage at the time of ifosfamide administration and 4 and 8 hours after each dose of ifosfamide.

Preparations: Ampules, 200 and 400 mg; 1 g. Tablets, 400 mg.

MESNEX®, see Mesna

MESORIDAZINE BESYLATE— Serentil®

Description/Actions: Phenothiazine antipsychotic agent indicated in the treatment of schizophrenia, behavioral problems in mental deficiency and chronic brain syndrome, alcoholism, and psychoneurotic manifestations.

Preparations: Tablets, 10, 25, 50, and 100 mg. Oral concentrate, 25 mg/ml. Ampules, 25 mg.

MESTINON®, see Pyridostigmine

MESTRANOL

Description/Actions: Estrogen included in combination with a progestin in various oral contraceptive formulations.

METAHYDRIN®, see Trichlormethiazide

METAMUCIL®, see Psyllium

METAPROTERENOL SULFATE— Alupent®, Metaprel®

Bronchodilator.

Description/Actions: Stimulates beta-adrenergic receptors. Indicated for bronchial asthma and for reversible bronchospasm that may occur in association with bronchitis and emphysema.

Warnings: Contraindicated in patients with cardiac arrhythmias associated with tachycardia, and should be used with caution in patients with other cardiovascular disorders. Adverse reactions include nervousness, tremor, tachycardia, palpitations, hypertension, nausea, and vomiting. Other sympathomimetic agents should not be used concurrently. Beta-adrenergic blocking agents and metaproterenol may inhibit the effect of each other.

Administration: Oral and oral inhalation.

Preparations: Tablets, 10 and 20 mg. Syrup, 10 mg/5 ml. Metered dose inhaler. Inhalant solution, 0.4%, 0.6%, and 5%.

METARAMINOL BITARTRATE— Aramine®

Description/Actions: Sympathomimetic agent indicated for parenteral administration in the prevention and treatment of the acute hypotensive state occurring with spinal anesthesia. Also used for the adjunctive treatment of hypotension due to other causes.

Preparations: Vials, 1%.

METASTRON®, see Strontium-89 chloride

METAXALONE—Skelaxin®

Description/Actions: Skeletal muscle relaxant indicated as an adjunct to rest, physical therapy, and other measures for the relief of discomfort associated with acute, painful musculoskeletal conditions.

Preparations: Tablets, 400 mg, and 800 mg.

METFORMIN HYDROCHLORIDE— Glucophage®, Glucophape® XR

Antihyperglycemic agent.

Description/Actions: Indicated as monotherapy or as an adjunct to sulfonylureas or insulin in combination with diet to lower blood glucose in patients with non-insulin-dependent diabetes mellitus (NIDDM) whose diet or sulfonylurea does not result in adequate glycemic control.

Warnings: Contraindicated in patients with renal disease and acute or chronic metabolic acidosis, CHF requiring drug treatment and concomitant intravascular iodinated radiocontrast agent. Withhold the drug in patients undergoing radiologic studies involving iodinated contrast materials as such products may result in an acute alteration of renal function. Adverse reactions include lactic acidosis, diarrhea, nausea, vomiting, abdominal bloating, flatulence, anorexia, metallic taste, and asymptotic subnormal serum vitamin B_{12} concentrations.

Administration: Oral with meals to reduce the incidence of GI effects.

Preparations: Tablets, 500 and 850 mg, 1000 mg. Extended-release tablets, 500 mg.

METHADONE HYDROCHLORIDE— Dolophine®

Description/Actions: Opioid analgesic indicated for relief of severe pain, for detoxification treatment of narcotic addiction, and for temporary maintenance treatment of narcotic addiction.

Preparations: Tablets, 5, 10, and 40 mg. Oral solution, 5 mg/5 ml, and 10 mg/5 ml. Ampules and vials, 10 mg/ml.

METHAMPHETAMINE HYDROCHLORIDE—Desoxyn®

Description/Actions: Anorexiant indicated as a short-term adjunct in a regimen of weight reduction based on caloric restriction. Also used in attention deficit disorder with hyperactivity, narcolepsy, epilepsy, postencephalitic parkinsonism and in treatment of certain depressive reactions.

Preparations: Tablets, 5 mg. Long-acting tablets, 5, 10, and 15 mg.

METHAZOLAMIDE—Neptazane®

Description/Actions: Carbonic anhydrase inhibitor indicated for adjunctive treatment of open-angle glaucoma, secondary glaucoma, and preoperatively in acute angle-closure glaucoma where delay of surgery is desired in order to lower intraocular pressure.

Preparations: Tablets, 25 and 50 mg.

METHENAMINE HIPPURATE— Hiprex®

METHENAMINE MANDELATE— Mandelamine®

Description/Actions: Urinary tract antibacterial indicated for prophylactic or suppressive treatment of frequently recurring urinary tract infections.

Preparations: Tablets, 500 mg and 1 g.

METHERGINE®, see Methylergonovine

METHICILLIN SODIUM— Staphcillin®

Description/Actions: Penicillin antibiotic indicated for the parenteral treatment of staphylococcal infections.

Preparations: Vials, 1, 4, 6, and 10 g.

METHIMAZOLE—Tapazole®

Description/Actions: Antithyroid agent indicated for the treatment of hyperthyroidism.

Preparations: Tablets, 5 and 10 mg.

METHIONINE—Pedameth®

Description/Actions: Indicated for the treatment of diaper rash in infants, and for control of odor, dermatitis and ulceration caused by ammoniacal urine in incontinent adults.

Preparations: Capsules, 200 mg. Liquid, 75 mg/5 ml.

METHOCARBAMOL—Robaxin®

Description/Actions: Skeletal muscle relaxant indicated as an adjunct to rest, physical therapy, and other measures for the relief of discomfort associated with acute, painful musculoskeletal conditions.

Preparations: Tablets, 500 and 750 mg. Vials, 100 mg/ml.

METHOHEXITAL SODIUM— Brevital sodium®

Description/Actions: Barbiturate general anesthetic indicated for intravenous use for induction of anesthesia, for supplementing other anesthetic agents, as anesthesia for short surgical procedures with minimum painful stimuli, or as an agent for inducing a hypnotic state.

Preparations: Vials, 500 mg, 2.5 and 5 g.

METHOTREXATE—Rheumatrex®

Description/Actions: Antineoplastic agent

indicated for the treatment of gestational choriocarcinoma, in patients with chorioadenoma destruens and hydatiform mole, acute lymphocytic leukemia, meningeal leukemia, breast cancer, epidermoid cancers of the head and neck, lung cancer, lymphosarcoma, and mycosis fungoides. Also used in the symptomatic control of severe, recalcitrant disabling psoriasis, and in the treatment of severe, active, classical or definite rheumatoid arthritis in selected adults who have had an insufficient therapeutic response to, or are intolerant of an adequate trial of first line therapy, including full dose NSAIDs.

Preparations: Tablets, 2.5 mg. Dose pack, 2.5 mg tablets (Rheumatrex). Vials, 20, 50, 100, and 250 mg. Vials, 2.5 mg/ml and 25 mg/ml.

METHOTRIMEPRAZINE— Levoprome®

Description/Actions: Analgesic administered parenterally for the treatment of moderate to severe pain in nonambulatory patients.

Preparations: Vials, 20 mg/ml.

METHOXAMINE HYDROCHLORIDE—Vasoxyl®

Description/Actions: Sympathomimetic amine indicated for parenteral use for restoring or maintaining blood pressure during anesthesia. Also used to terminate some episodes of supraventricular tachycardia.

Preparations: Ampules, 20 mg.

METHOXSALEN—Oxsoralen®, Oxsoralen-Ultra®

Description/Actions: Photoactive agent indicated for topical use with long wave ultraviolet radiation for the repigmentation of vitiligo, and for oral use with long-wave UVA radiation for the symptomatic control of severe, recalcitrant disabling psoriasis.

Preparations: Capsules (Oxsoralen-Ultra), 10 mg. Lotion (to be applied by a physician and not to be dispensed to patients), 1%.

METHOXYFLURANE—Penthrane®

Description/Actions: Inhalation general anesthetic usually indicated in combination with oxygen and nitrous oxide. Also used to provide analgesia in obstetrics and in minor surgical procedures.

Preparations: Bottles, 15 and 125 ml.

METHSUXIMIDE—Celontin®

Description/Actions: Anticonvulsant indicated for the control of absence (petit mal) seizures that are refractory to other drugs.

Preparations: Capsules, 150 and 300 mg.

METHYL SALICYLATE—Oil of wintergreen

Description/Actions: Salicylate analgesic used in combination with other agents and applied topically in the management of certain dermatologic and muscular conditions.

Preparations: Lotion, liniment, and cream formulations.

METHYLCELLULOSE—Citrucel®

Description/Actions: Laxative used in the treatment of constipation.

Preparations: Powder and liquid.

METHYCLOTHIAZIDE—Enduron®

Description/Actions: Thiazide diuretic indicated as adjunctive therapy in edema, and in the management of hypertension.

Preparations: Tablets, 2.5 and 5 mg.

METHYLDOPA, METHYLDOPATE HYDROCHLORIDE—Aldomet®

Antihypertensive agent.

Description/Actions: Indicated in the treatment of hypertension.

Warnings: Contraindicated in patients with active hepatic disease because liver disorders have been associated with therapy. Other adverse reactions include sedation, headache, orthostatic hypotension, edema, bradycardia, nausea, vomiting, positive Coombs' test, and hemolytic anemia.

Administration: Oral and intravenous.

Preparations: Tablets, 125, 250, and 500 mg. Suspension, 250 mg/5 ml. Vials, 250 mg/5 ml.

METHYLENE BLUE

Description/Actions: Antiseptic and antidote. Has been used as a genitourinary antiseptic and in the management of patients with oxalate urinary tract calculi. Has also been used in the management of methemoglobinemia and as an antidote for cyanide poisoning.

Preparations: Tablets, 65 mg. Ampules, 10 mg/ml.

METHYLERGONOVINE MALEATE—Methergine®

Description/Actions: Oxytocic indicated for routine management after delivery of the placenta; postpartum atony and hemorrhage; subinvolution. Under full obstetric supervision, may be given in the second stage of labor following delivery of the anterior shoulder.

Preparations: Tablets, 0.2 mg. Ampules, 0.2 mg/ml.

METHYLPHENIDATE HYDROCHLORIDE— Concerta™, Ritalin®, Ritalin-SR®

Description/Actions: Central nervous system stimulant indicated in the management of attention-deficit disorder and narcolepsy.

Preparations: Tablets, 5, 10, and 20 mg. Controlled-release tablets, 20 mg, Osmotic controlled-release tablets, 18, 36, and 54 mg. Extended-release tablets, 27 mg.

METHYLPREDNISOLONE— Medrol®

Corticosteroid.

Description/Actions: Indicated in a wide range of endocrine, rheumatic, allergic, dermatologic, respiratory, hematologic, neoplastic, and other disorders. Use has been reported to improve neurologic recovery in patients with acute spinal cord injury when the medication (as methylprednisolone sodium succinate) is given in the first 8 hours.

Warnings: Contraindicated in patients with systemic fungal infections. Adverse reactions include sodium and fluid retention, potassium depletion, muscle weakness, osteoporosis, peptic ulcer, thin fragile skin, development of cushingoid state, glaucoma, cataracts, and negative nitrogen balance. May mask signs of infection and new infections may appear during use. May increase requirements for hypoglycemic agents in diabetic patients.

Administration: Oral.

Preparations: Tablets, 2, 4, 8, 16, 24, and 32 mg.

METHYLPREDNISOLONE ACETATE—Depo-Medrol®, Medrol acetate topical®

See discussion of methylprednisolone.

Administration: Intramuscular, intra-articular, intralesional, and soft tissue administration. Topical.

Preparations: Vials, 20, 40, and 80 mg/ml. Ointment, 0.25% and 1%.

METHYLPREDNISOLONE SODIUM SUCCINATE—Solu-Medrol®. See discussion of methylprednisolone.

Administration: Intravenous and intramuscular.

Preparations: Vials, 40, 125, and 500 mg, 1 and 2 g.

METHYLROSANILINE CHLORIDE, see Gentian violet

METHYLTESTOSTERONE— Oreton methyl®

Description/Actions: Androgen indicated for replacement therapy in conditions associated with a deficiency or absence of endogenous testosterone including primary hypogonadism (e.g., testicular failure due to cryptorchidism) and hypogonadotropic hypogonadism.

May be used to stimulate puberty in carefully selected males with clearly delayed puberty, and for the treatment of impotence and male climacteric symptoms when these are secondary to androgen deficiency. May also be used in women with advanced inoperable metastatic mammary cancer who are 1 to 5 years postmenopausal, and for the management of postpartum breast pain and engorgement.

Preparations: Tablets, 10 and 25 mg. Buccal tablets, 5 and 10 mg.

METHYSERGIDE MALEATE— Sansert®

Description/Actions: Indicated for the prevention or reduction of intensity and frequency of vascular headaches in patients who experience frequent and/or severe headaches. Observe for development of retroperitoneal fibrosis during long-term therapy.

Preparations: Tablets, 2 mg.

METICORTEN®, see Prednisone

METIPRANOLOL HYDROCHLORIDE— OptiPranolol®

Agent for glaucoma.

Description/Actions: A nonselective beta-adrenergic-blocking agent indicated for ophthalmic use in the treatment of ocular conditions like chronic open-angle glaucoma and ocular hypertension.

Warnings: Contraindicated in patients with a history of bronchial asthma, severe chronic obstructive pulmonary disease, symptomatic sinus bradycardia, greater than a first degree atrioventricular block, cardiogenic shock, or overt cardiac failure. Adverse reactions include transient local discomfort, conjunctivitis, abnormal vision, and occasional systemic effects. Caution must be exercised in patients taking another beta-blocker orally for another indication.

Administration: Ophthalmic.

Preparations: Ophthalmic solution, 0.3%.

METOCLOPRAMIDE HYDROCHLORIDE—Reglan®

Agent to increase GI tract motility.

Description/Actions: Stimulates motility of the upper GI tract. Indicated (1) as short-term therapy for patients with symptomatic, gastroesophageal reflux who fail to respond to conventional therapy; (2) for the relief of symptoms associated with diabetic gastric stasis; (3) for the prophylaxis of vomiting associated with cancer chemotherapy; (4) to facilitate small bowel intubation; and (5) to stimulate gastric emptying and intestinal transit of barium in radiological examinations.

Warnings: Contraindicated in patients in whom the stimulation of GI motility may be dangerous (e.g., in the presence of GI hemorrhage), and in patients with epilepsy or pheochromocytoma. May cause extrapyramidal reactions and should not be used in patients receiving other drugs likely to cause such reactions. Metoclopramide produces a transient increase in plasma aldosterone, certain patients (patients with cirrhosis or congestive heart failure) may be at risk for developing fluid retention and volume overload.

If this occurs, the drug should be discontinued. Adverse reactions include drowsiness and other CNS effects; patients should be cautioned regarding activities such as driving and operating machinery, as well as interactions with other CNS-acting drugs including alcohol. Other adverse reactions include nausea, diarrhea, visual disturbances, fluid retention, amenorrhea, gynecomastia, and impotence.

Administration: Oral, intravenous, and intramuscular. Oral administration should be 30 minutes before meals and at bedtime.

Preparations: Tablets, 5 and 10 mg. Syrup, 5 mg/5 ml. Ampules and vials, 5 mg/ml.

METOCURINE IODIDE—Metubine iodide®

Description/Actions: Muscle relaxant administered intravenously as an adjunct to anesthesia to induce skeletal muscle relaxation.

Preparations: Vials, 2 mg/ml.

METOLAZONE—Zaroxolyn®

METOLAZONE (rapidly available formulation)—Mykrox®

Description/Actions: Diuretic indicated in the management of hypertension and in the treatment of edema.

Preparations: Tablets, 0.5 (Mykrox®), 2.5, 5, and 10 mg.

METOPROLOL TARTRATE— Lopressor®

METOPROLOL SUCCINATE— Toprol XL®

Antihypertensive and antianginal agent.

Description/Actions: A cardioselective beta-adrenergic-blocking agent indicated in the management of hypertension, angina pectoris, and hemodynamically stable patients with definite or suspected acute myocardial infarction to reduce cardiovascular mortality. Metoprolol succinate is also indicated in the treatment of stable, symptomatic NYHA class II or III heart failure of ischemic, hypertensive, or cardiomyopathic origin.

Warnings: Contraindicated in patients with sinus bradycardia, heart block greater than first degree, cardiogenic shock, and overt cardiac failure. Adverse reactions include tiredness, dizziness, depression, bradycardia, shortness of breath, diarrhea, pruritus, and rash. Use is best avoided in patients with bronchospastic diseases and therapy in diabetic patients must be closely monitored.

Administration: Oral and intravenous. When administered orally should be taken with or immediately following meals. Patients should be cautioned about the interruption or discontinuation of therapy; exacerbation of angina pectoris has occurred following the abrupt cessation of therapy and, when therapy is to be discontinued, the dosage should be gradually reduced over a period of 1 to 2 weeks. Adult dose: Hypertension: Initially, 50–100 mg once daily. Dosage may be increased at weekly intervals up to a maximum of 400 mg/day. Angina: Initially, 100 mg/day. Dosage may be gradually increased at weekly intervals up to a maximum of 400 mg/day. Heart failure: Initially, 25 mg once daily for 2 weeks in patients with NYHA class II heart failure and 12.5 mg once daily in patients with more severe heart failure. The dose should then be doubled every 2 weeks to the highest dosage level tolerated by the patient or up to 200 mg/day.

Preparations: Tablets 50 and 100 mg. Controlled-release tablets (Toprol XL), 25 mg, 50 mg, 100 mg, and 200 mg. Ampules and syringes, 5 mg/5 ml.

METRODIN®, see Urofollitropin

METROGEL®, see Metronidazole

METROGEL-VAGINAL®, see Metronidazole

METRONIDAZOLE—Flagyl®, MetroGel®, MetroGel-Vaginal®, Noritate®

Description/Actions: Anti-infective agent indicated in the treatment of trichomoniasis, amebiasis, and anaerobic bacterial infections, and in the topical treatment of rosacea. Vaginal gel is indicated in the treatment of bacterial vaginosis.

Preparations: Tablets, 250 and 500 mg. Capsules, 375 mg. Extended release tablets, 750 mg. Vials (for intravenous administration), 500 mg and 500 mg/100 ml. Gel, 0.75%. Vaginal gel, 0.75%. Cream, 1%.

METUBINE®, see Metocurine

METYRAPONE

Description/Actions: Diagnostic test of pituitary adrenocorticotropic function.

Preparations: Tablets, 250 mg.

METYROSINE—Demser®

Description/Actions: Agent for pheochromocytoma. Indicated in the treatment of patients with pheochromocytoma for preoperative preparation of patients for surgery, management of patients when surgery is contraindicated, and the chronic treatment of patients with malignant pheochromocytoma.

Preparations: Tablets, 250 mg.

MEVACOR®, see Lovastatin

MEXILETINE HYDROCHLORIDE—Mexitil®

Antiarrhythmic agent.

Description/Actions: A class IB antiarrhythmic agent that is similar to lidocaine in its electrophysiologic properties. Indicated for the suppression of symptomatic ventricular arrhythmias, including frequent premature ventricular contractions (unifocal or multifocal), couplets, and ventricular tachycardia.

Warnings: Contraindicated in patients with cardiogenic shock or second- or third-degree AV block (unless a pacemaker is present). Adverse reactions include proarrhythmic events, GI distress, lightheadedness, tremor, and coordination difficulties.

Administration: Oral.

Preparations: Capsules, 150, 200, and 250 mg.

MEXITIL®, see Mexiletine

MEZLIN®, see Mezlocillin

MEZLOCILLIN SODIUM—Mezlin®

Penicillin antibiotic.

Description/Actions: Is bactericidal and is active against many gram-positive and gram-negative bacteria, including *Pseudomonas aeruginosa*. Is usually used in conjunction with an aminoglycoside antibiotic in the treatment of *Pseudomonas* infections.

Warnings: Contraindicated in patients with a history of allergic reaction to any of the penicillins. Adverse reactions include hypersensitivity reactions, GI disturbances, and local reactions at the injection site.

Administration: Intravenous and intramuscular.

Preparations: Vials and infusion bottles, 1, 2, 3, 4, and 20 g.

MIACALCIN®, see Calcitonin-salmon

MICARDIS®, see Telmisartan

MICARDIS® HCT, Combination of telmisartan and hydrochlorothiazide

MICATIN®, see Miconazole

MICONAZOLE—Monistat IV®

MICONAZOLE NITRATE—
Monistat 3®, Monistat 7®,
Monistat-Derm®, Micatin®

Imidazole antifungal agent.

Description/Actions: Indicated for (1) topical application in the treatment of tinea pedis, tinea cruris, tinea corporis, candidiasis, and tinea versicolor; (2) vaginal administration for vulvovaginal candidiasis; and (3) intravenous administration for systemic fungal infections.

Warnings: Adverse reactions associated with topical and vaginal use include local irritation and itching. Adverse reactions associated with intravenous use include phlebitis, pruritus, rash, fever, nausea, and vomiting. Base contained in the vaginal suppository formulation may interact with certain rubber or latex products, such as those used in vaginal contraceptive diaphragms; therefore, concurrent use is not recommended.

Administration: Topical, vaginal, intravenous, intrathecal, and bladder instillation.

Preparations: Cream, lotion, powder, and spray, 2%. Vaginal cream, 1%. Vaginal suppositories, 100 and 200 mg. Ampules, 10 mg/ml.

MICRO-K®, see Potassium chloride

MICRONASE®, see Glyburide

MICRONOR®, see Norethindrone

MICROZIDE®, see Hydrochlorothiazide

MIDAMOR®, see Amiloride

MIDAZOLAM HYDROCHLORIDE—Versed®

Sedative/anesthetic.

Description/Actions: A short-acting benzodiazepine CNS depressant. Indicated (1) intramuscularly for preoperative sedation and to impair memory of perioperative events; (2) intravenously as an agent for conscious sedation prior to short diagnostic or endoscopic procedures, and in therapeutic procedures; and (3) intravenously for induction of general anesthesia, before administration of other anesthetic agents. Can also be used as a component of intravenous supplementation of nitrous oxide and oxygen (balanced anesthesia) for short surgical procedures.

Warnings: Contraindicated in patients with acute narrow-angle glaucoma. Adverse reactions include apnea, decreased tidal volume and/or respiratory rate decrease, hypotension, and oversedation. Effects may be increased by the concurrent administration of other agents having CNS depressant, respiratory depressant and/or hypotensive effects, and the dosage of one or both agents should be appropriately reduced. Lower dosages should be used in elderly, debilitated, and other high-risk patients.

Administration: Intravenous and intramuscular.

Preparations: Vials, 1 mg/ml and 5 mg/ml.

MIDODRINE HYDROCHLORIDE—
ProAmatine®

Description/Actions: Alpha-adrenergic agonist, indicated in the treatment of orthostatic hypotension. Also used (investigational) in managing urinary incontinence.

Warnings: Contraindicated in patients with severe heart disease, acute renal disease, urinary retention, thyrotoxicosis, pheochromocytoma, supine hypertension. Caution must be exercised in patients with diabetes. Adverse reactions include supine hypertension, bradycardia, paresthesia, pruritus (primarily of the scalp), piloerection (goose bumps), chills, dysuria, urinary frequency and urgency, and urinary retention. Use cautiously with other medications which may reduce the heart rate. Discontinue and reevaluate if the patient develops signs or symptoms of bradycardia (e.g., pulse slowing, increased dizziness, or syncope).

Administration: 10 mg 3 times a day, during daytime hours when patient is upright. Maximum dose is 40 mg/day.

Preparations: Tablets, 2.5 and 5 mg.

MIFEPREX®, see Mifepristone

MIFEPRISTONE—Mifeprex®

Description/Actions: Indicated for the medical termination of intrauterine pregnancy through the first 49 days of pregnancy.

Precautions/Adverse Reactions: Mifepristone is contraindicated in women with a known hypersensitivity to mifepristone, misoprostol, other prostaglandins, or to any component of the product. It is also contraindicated in ectopic pregnancy, intrauterine device (IUD) in place, chronic adrenal failure, porphyrias, pregnancy greater than 49 days, hemorrhagic disorders, concurrent anticoagulant therapy, concurrent long-term corticosteroid therapy, undiagnosed adnexal mass, and inadequate or lack of access to medical facilities equipped to provide emergency medical care of incomplete abortion, blood transfusions, and emergency resuscitation from the first visit until discharged by the physician. In addition, mifepristone should not be used in patients unable to fully understand and comply with the treatment regimen. Women should be instructed to review the Medication Guide and Patient Agreement. Signed informed consent is required prior to treatment initiation, and a copy must be kept in the patient's file. There is no safety or efficacy data on the use of mifepristone in women with chronic medical conditions such as cardiovascular, hypertensive, hepatic, or renal disease, insulin-dependent diabetes mellitus; severe anemia; or history of heavy smoking. Women greater than 35 years of age who also smoke more than 10 cigarettes per day were not included in clinical trials; therefore, treat with caution. Pregnancy termination must be confirmed by ultrasound or clinical exam. Treatment failures must be managed with surgical abortions. Vaginal bleeding is expected to last 9–16 days, but as long as 69 days has been reported. Vaginal bleeding may be severe and may require treatment with vasoconstrictors, curettage, saline infusions and or blood transfusions. Use with caution in patients with severe anemia. The effectiveness of mifepristone may be decreased if misoprostol is administered more than 2 days after mifepristone. May only be administered by qualified physicians able to assess the duration of pregnancy accurately, diagnose ectopic pregnancies, and provide surgical intervention in the event of an incomplete abortion or severe bleeding. The physician has agreed to provide these services or has made plans to provide these services through others and can assure patient access to emergency medical services. The physician must report to the manufacturer any hospitalization, transfusion, or other serious event encountered during treatment of a patient with mifepristone. No drug interaction studies have been done; however, mifepristone is metabolized by the cytochrome p450 system 3A4 and is expected to interact with drugs metabolized via the same enzyme system. Ketoconazole, itraconazole, erythromycin, and grapefruit juice may increase serum levels of mifepristone by inhibiting its metabolism. Rifampin, dexamethasone, phenytoin, phenobarbital, carbamazepine, and Saint-John's-Wort may decrease mifepristone levels by inducing its metabolism. Mifepristone may inhibit the metabolism of drugs that are cytochrome p450 3A4 substrates. Exercise caution when coadministering with mifepristone. Pregnancy Category X. Mifepristone is used to terminate pregnancy. Excretion in human breast milk is unknown. Safety and efficacy in pediatric patients have not been established. Major adverse effects associated with mifepristone include bleeding more heavily than during a normal menstrual period (80–90%), abdominal pain/cramping (96%), nausea, vomiting, diarrhea, headache, back pain, dizziness, and fatigue.

Administration: Oral. Treatment with mifepristone requires three office visits. Signed informed consent is required by the patient prior to initiation of therapy.

Patient Care Implications: Serum human chorionic gonadotropin (HCG) levels will not adequately confirm termination of pregnancy until at least 10 days after the administration of mifepristone. Pregnancy termination must be confirmed by ultrasound and/or clinical exam. Vaginal bleeding may be heavy and require medical treatment with curettage, transfusions, vasoconstrictors, and saline infusions. Hemoglobin and hematocrit levels should be monitored. Patients should be advised to review the Medication Guide and Patient Agreement. Patients must understand the importance of completing the entire treatment schedule and returning for follow-up visits. Patients should be aware that bleeding and cramping will occur. Patients should be aware that bleeding is not proof of a complete abortion and that surgical intervention will be required for incomplete abortions. Fetal harm may occur if pregnancy is not terminated after a failed abortion with mifepristone. Physician must give the patient a phone number to call for questions or for emergencies. Patients may become pregnant again before their next menstrual period. Contraception may be resumed once termination of pregnancy is confirmed.

Preparations: Tablets, 200 mg supplied in single-dose blister packets containing 3 tablets.

MIGLITOL—Glyset®

Description/Actions: Miglitol is an antidiabetic drug indicated as an adjunct to diet in Type II diabetes, alone or with a sulfonylurea.

Precautions/Adverse Reactions: Miglitol is contraindicated in ketoacidosis, inflammatory bowel disease, colonic ulceration, partial intestinal obstruction (or predisposition to such), chronic intestinal diseases associated with marked disorders of digestion, or absorption or conditions that may deteriorate from increased intestinal gas formation.

Use not recommended in patients with significant renal dysfunction (serum cr > 2 mg/dl), in pregnancy (Category B) and nursing mothers.

Adverse reactions include flatulence, diarrhea, and abdominal pain.

Administration: Oral. Take with the first bite of each main meal.

Patient Care Implications: While miglitol does not cause hypoglycemia when used alone, it can contribute to hypoglycemia when used in conjunction with sulfonylurea agents. If treatable hypoglycemia develops because of the mechanism of action of miglitol, treat with glucose instead of fructose.

Preparations: Tablets, 25, 50, and 100 mg.

MILK OF MAGNESIA, see Magnesium hydroxide

MILONTIN®, see Phensuximide

MILRINONE LACTATE— Primacor®

Agent for congestive heart failure.

Description/Actions: Is a phosphodiesterase inhibitor and increases cardiac output by inhibiting the enzymatic hydrolysis of cAMP, resulting in both positive inotropic and vasodilating ef-

212 • MILTOWN®

fects. Indicated for the short-term intravenous treatment of congestive heart failure.

Warnings: Adverse reactions include ventricular arrhythmias, supraventricular arrhythmias, hypotension, angina or chest pain, and headache. Should not be used in patients with severe obstructive aortic or pulmonic valvular disease in lieu of surgical relief of the obstruction. It is recommended that it not be used in patients in the acute phase after myocardial infarction. May aggravate outflow tract obstruction in hypertrophic subaortic stenosis. If hypokalemia exists, should be corrected with a potassium supplement before or during the use of milrinone.

Administration: Intravenous. Administered in a loading dose (administered slowly over 10 minutes), followed by a continuous IV infusion (as the maintenance dose).

Preparations: Vials, milrinone lactate equivalent to 1 mg of milrinone per ml. Carpuject sterile cartridge-needle unit with Interlink System Cannula (1 mg/ml).

MILTOWN®, see Meprobamate

MINERAL OIL—Liquid petrolatum

Description/Actions: Laxative used in the form of oil or in emulsion formulations.

MINIPRESS®, see Prazosin

MINITRAN®, see Nitroglycerin

MINOCIN®, see Minocycline

MINOCYCLINE HYDROCHLORIDE—Minocin®

Tetracycline antibiotic.

Description/Actions: Active against many gram-positive and gram-negative bacteria, mycoplasmal, chlamydial, and rickettsial organisms, and certain spirochetes. Indicated in the treatment of respiratory and urinary tract infections and a number of other types of infections. Effective in the treatment of infections caused by *Chlamydia trachomatis* and *Ureaplasma urealyticum*. Is useful as adjunctive therapy in the management of severe acne. Is also indicated in the treatment of asymptomatic carriers of *Neisseria meningitidis*.

Warnings: Use is best avoided during the last half of pregnancy and in childhood to the age of 8 years because of the risk of discoloration of the teeth. May cause lightheadedness, dizziness, and vertigo, and patients should be cautioned about activities such as driving or operating machinery. Other adverse reactions include nausea, vomiting, diarrhea, rash, photosensitivity reactions, and fungal superinfections. Must be used with caution in patients with impaired renal function. Absorption may be reduced by the simultaneous administration of antacids.

Administration: Oral and intravenous. May be administered orally without regard to meals.

Preparations: Capsules and tablets, 50 and 100 mg. Suspension, 50 mg/5 ml. Vials, 100 mg.

MINOXIDIL—Loniten®, Rogaine®

Description/Actions: Indicated for the treatment of hypertension that is symptomatic or associated with target organ damage and is not manageable with conventional antihypertensive regimens. Also indicated for the topical treatment of male pattern baldness of the vertex of the scalp, and female androgenetic alopecia (i.e., diffuse hair loss or thinning of the frontoparietal areas).

Preparations: Tablets, 2.5 and 10 mg (Loniten). Topical solution, 2% and 5% (Rogaine).

MINTEZOL®, see Thiabendazole

MIOSTAT®, see Carbachol

MIRADON®, see Anisindione

MIRTAZAPINE—Remeron®

Description/Actions: Antidepressant of tetracylic chemical structure indicated in the treatment of depression. Patients may begin to see improvements in one to four weeks.

Warnings: Do not administer concurrently with or within 14 days of MAO-Is. Use cautiously in patients with hepatic or renal dysfunction, conditions that may be exacerbated by hypotension, disease that affects hemodynamic response, history of mania or hypomania, seizure disorders, suicidal ideation, immunocompromised patients, and elderly. Adverse reactions include somnolence, increased appetite, weight gain, dizziness, nausa, dry mouth, constipation, asthenia, flu syndrome, edema, and CNS effects.

Administrations: Initially 15 mg once daily at bedtime. Increase at intervals of at least 1–2 weeks. Usual range is 15–45 mg daily.

Preparations: Tablets, 15 and 30 mg.

MISOPROSTOL—Cytotec®

Prostaglandin.

Description/Actions: An analogue of prostaglandin E_1 that exhibits actions which protect the gastroduodenal mucosa. Indicated for the prevention of NSAID-induced gastric ulcers in patients at high risk of complications from a gastric ulcer (e.g., patients over age 60, individuals with a history of ulcer, patients taking corticosteroids).

Warnings: Contraindicated during pregnancy because the drug exhibits an abortifacient action. Adverse reactions include diarrhea, abdominal pain, nausea, flatulence, dyspepsia, and headache. Should not be used in women of childbearing potential unless the patient requires NSAID therapy and is at high risk of developing gastric ulcers and/or associated complications.

Administration: Oral. Should be taken with a meal and the last dose of the day should be at bedtime.

Preparations: Tablets, 100 and 200 µg.

MITHRACIN®, see Plicamycin

MITHRAMYCIN, see Plicamycin

MITOMYCIN—Mutamycin®

Description/Actions: Antineoplastic agent indicated for the parenteral treatment of disseminated adenocarcinoma of the stomach or pancreas, in combination with other agents.

Preparations: Vials, 5, 20, and 40 mg.

MITOTANE—Lysodren®

Description/Actions: Antineoplastic agent indicated in the treatment of inoperable adrenal cortical carcinoma.

Preparations: Tablets, 500 mg.

MITOXANTRONE HYDROCHLORIDE—Novantrone®

Antineoplastic agent.

Description/Actions: Indicated in combination with other approved drug(s) (e.g., cytosine arabinoside) in the initial therapy of acute nonlymphocytic leukemia in adults. Mitoxantrone is also indicated in the treatment of patients with secondary progressive multiple sclerosis, including progressive relapsing disease.

Warnings: Severe myelosuppression occurs and complete blood counts are necessary for appropriate dose adjustments. Other adverse reactions include bleeding, infection, nausea, vomiting, diarrhea, abdominal pain, stomatitis, fever, headache, alopecia, cough, dyspnea, conjunctivitis, tachycardia, and congestive heart failure. The drug may cause fetal harm when administered during pregnancy. The drug may impart a blue-green color to the urine for 24 hours after administration, and patients should be advised to expect this during the therapy.

Administration: Intravenous infusion.

Preparations: Vials, 2 mg mitoxantrone free base per ml [10 ml (20 mg), 12.5 ml (25 mg), 15 ml (30 mg)].

MITROLAN®, see Polycarbophil

MIVACRON®, see Mivacurium

MIVACURIUM CHLORIDE— Mivacron®

Nondepolarizing neuromuscular blocking agent.

Description/Actions: Indicated as an adjunct to general anesthesia, to facilitate tracheal intubation and to provide skeletal muscle relaxation during surgery or mechanical ventilation.

Warnings: Use from multidose vials is contraindicated in patients with a known allergy to benzyl alcohol. Adverse reactions include transient cutaneous flushing of the face, neck and/or chest. Must be used with caution in patients with neuromuscular disease (e.g., myasthenia gravis, myasthenic syndrome), and in patients receiving other medications that may increase and/or prolong neuromuscular block (e.g., inhalation anesthetics, aminoglycosides, quinidine, magnesium salts). May cause histamine release, and caution should be exercised in patients with clinically significant cardiovascular disease and patients with any history (e.g., asthma) suggesting a greater sensitivity to the release of histamine. Is metabolized by plasma cholinesterase, and duration of action may be markedly prolonged in the presence of genetic abnormalities of plasma cholinesterase.

Administration: Intravenous.

Preparations: Vials, 2 mg/ml. Premixed infusion in 5% Dextrose Injection, 0.5 mg/ml. Solutions are acidic and may not be compatible with alkaline solutions having a pH greater than 8.5 (e.g., barbiturate solutions).

MOBAN®, see Molindone

MOBIC®, see Meloxicam

MOCTANIN®, see Monooctanoin

MODAFINIL—Provigil®

Description/Actions: An antinarcoleptic drug indicated to improve wakefulness in patients with excessive daytime sleepiness (EDS) associated with narcolepsy.

Precautions/Adverse Reactions: Use is not recommended in patients with a history of LV hypertrophy, ischemic EKG changes, chest pain, arrhythmias, or other significant manifestations of mitral valve prolapse. Use cautiously in patients with a history of recent MI, unstable angina, hypertension, cardiovascular disease, psychosis, severe hepatic or renal impairment, and the elderly. Pregnancy Category C. Monitor patients periodically as abuse potential exists. May antagonize hormonal contraceptives. Reduce dose in the elderly.

Adverse reactions include headache, infection, nausea, anxiety, depression, insomnia, and other CNS effects.

Administration: Oral.

Patient Care Implications: Instruct patients of childbearing potential who employ oral contraceptives for birth control to use alternate means of contraception. Instruct patients to avoid alcohol.

Preparations: Tablets, 100 mg and 200 (scored) mg.

MODANE®, see Bisacodyl

MODERIL®, see Rescinnamine

MODURETIC®, Combination of amiloride and hydrochlorothiazide

MOEXIPRIL HYDROCHLORIDE— Univasc®

MOLINDONE HYDROCHLORIDE—Moban®

Description/Actions: Antipsychotic agent indicated for the management of the manifestations of psychotic disorders.

Preparations: Tablets, 5, 10, 25, 50, and 100 mg. Oral concentrate, 20 mg/ml.

MOMETASONE FUROATE— Elocon®

Topical corticosteroid.

Description/Actions: Indicated for the relief of the inflammatory and pruritic manifestations of corticosteroid-responsive dermatoses.

Warnings: Adverse reactions include burning, tingling/stinging, pruritus, and signs of skin atrophy.

Administration: Topical.

Preparations: Cream, ointment, and lotion, 0.1%

MOMETASONE FUROATE— Nasonex®

Description/Actions: Corticosteroid indicated in prophylaxis and treatment of seasonal allergic rhinitis symptoms and treatment of perennial allergic rhinitis symptoms.

Warnings: Use not recommended in tuberculosis, varicella, vaccinia, unhealed nasal wounds, untreated fungal, bacterial, and viral infections, or ocular herpes simplex. Discontinue if nasopharyngeal candida infection occurs. If adrenal insufficiency exists following systemic corticosteroid therapy, replacement with topical corticosteroids may exacerbate symptoms of adrenal insufficiency (e.g., depression). Monitor for vision changes or if there is a history of glaucoma or cataracts. Pregnancy Category C. Cautious use in nursing mothers.

Adverse reactions include headache, viral infection, pharyngitis, epistaxis, cough, upper respiratory tract infections, pain, sinusitis, and others. Instruct patients to adhere to dosing and interval recommendations. Advise patients to seek medical advice if exposed to chicken pox or measles.

Administration: Two sprays in each nostril once daily.

Preparations: 50 μg/spray in 17 g (120 sprays) metered dose, manual pump spray, and dosage counter spray.

MONISTAT®, see Miconazole nitrate

MONOBENZONE—Benoquin®

Description/Actions: Depigmenting agent indicated for final depigmentation in extensive vitiligo.

Preparations: Cream, 20%.

MONODOX®, see Doxycycline monohydrate

MONOOCTANOIN—Moctanin®

Agent for gallstones.

Description/Actions: A solubilizing agent for treatment of cholesterol gallstones retained in the biliary tract after cholecystectomy, when other means of removing cholesterol stones in the common bile duct have failed or cannot be undertaken.

Warnings: Contraindicated in patients with clinical jaundice, significant biliary tract infection, or with a history of recent duodenal ulcer or jejunitis. Adverse reactions include GI pain, nausea, vomiting, and diarrhea. Patients should have periodic liver function tests.

Administration: As a continuous perfusion through a catheter inserted directly into the common bile duct, or through a nasobiliary tube placed by endoscopy.

Preparations: Bottles containing 120 ml.

MONOPRIL®, see Fosinopril sodium

MONTELUKAST—Singulair®

Description/Actions: A leukotriene antagonist indicated in prophylaxis and chronic treatment of asthma.

Warnings: Not for primary treatment of acute attack. Not for monotherapy in treatment and management of exercise-induced bronchospasm. Monitor patients closely when withdrawing from oral steroids. Safety and efficacy in pediatric patients < 12 months of age have not been established.

Adverse reactions include headache, asthenia/fatigue, fever, GI disturbances, laryngitis, and pharyngitis.

Instruct patients to report increased need for short acting bronchodilators. Have appropriate rescue meds available. Continue usual regimen for exercise-induced bronchospasm prophylaxis.

Pregnancy Category B.

Administration: Oral.

Preparations: Chewable tablets in cherry flavor, 4 and 5 mg.

Tablets, 10 mg.

4 mg granule packets.

MONUROL®, see Fosfomycin

MORICIZINE HYDROCHLORIDE—Ethmozine®

Antiarrhythmic agent.

Description/Actions: A class I antiarrhythmic agent. Indicated for the treatment of documented life-threatening arrhythmias.

Warnings: Contraindicated in the presence of cardiogenic shock, and in patients with preexisting second or third-degree atrioventricular block, and in patients with right bundle branch block when associated with left hemiblock unless a pacemaker is present. Adverse reactions include proarrhythmic effects, congestive heart failure, conduction abnormalities, chest pain, palpitations, dizziness, fatigue, sleep disorders, nervousness, headache, nausea, vomiting, dyspepsia, abdominal pain, paresthesias, musculoskeletal pain, blurred vision, and dyspnea.

Administration: Oral.

Preparations: Tablets, 200, 250, and 300 mg.

MORPHINE SULFATE—Astramorph PF®, Duramorph®, Kadian®, MS Contin®, MSIR®, Oramorph SR®, RMS®, Roxanol®, Roxanol SR®

Opiate analgesic.

Description/Actions: Indicated for the relief of moderate to severe pain, for preoperative medication, to facilitate induction of anesthesia, and as an anesthetic or adjunct to anesthesia.

Warnings: Adverse reactions include sedation and other CNS effects; patients should be cautioned regarding activities such as driving and operating machinery, as well as interactions with other CNS-acting drugs including alcohol. Other adverse reactions include constipation and hypotension. Cases of anaphylaxis; intestinal obstruction, and death have also been reported. Can cause dependence and formulations are covered under the provisions of the Controlled Substances Act.

Administration: Oral, rectal, intravenous, intramuscular, subcutaneous, epidural, intrathecal.

Preparations: Tablets, 10, 15, and 30 mg. Controlled-release tablet, 15, 30, 60, and 100 mg. (MS Contin, Oramorph SR, Roxanol SR). Sustained-release pellets in capsules, 20, 50, and 100 mg. Oral solution, 4 mg/ml, 20 mg/ml, 10 mg/5 ml, 20 mg/5 ml, and 100 mg/5 ml. Suppositories, 5, 10, 20, and

30 mg (RMS). Ampules, vials, and syringes, 2, 4, 5, 8, 10, 15, 25, and 50 mg/ml. Ampules and vials (preservative-free and can be used via epidural and intrathecal routes), 0.5 and 1 mg/ml. (Astramorph PF, Duramorph). Solution for IV injection (PCA device), 1 mg/ml, 2 mg/ml, 3 mg/ml, and 5 mg/ml.

MOTOFEN®, see Difenoxin hydrochloride/atropine sulfate

MOTRIN®, see Ibuprofen

MOXIFLOXACIN HYDROCHLODIDE—Avelox®

Description/Actions: A synthetic broad-spectrum fluoroquinolone antibiotic indicated for the treatment of adults with acute bacterial sinusitis, acute bacterial exacerbation of chronic bronchitis, and community-acquired pneumonia.

Precautions/Adverse Reactions: Contraindicated in patients with a history of hypersensitivity to moxifloxacin or any member of the quinolone class of antimicrobial agents. The safety and effectiveness of moxifloxacin in patients less than 18 years of age and pregnant or lactating women has not been established. The drug should be avoided in patients with known prolongation of the QT interval, patients with uncorrected hypokalemia, and patients receiving class IA or class III antiarrhythmic agents due to lack of clinical experience with the drug in these patient populations. Adverse reactions include nausea, diarrhea, dizziness, headache, abdominal pain, vomiting, taste perversion, abnormal liver function tests, and dyspepsia.

Administration: Intravenous and oral.

Preparations: Tablets, 400 mg. Injection, 400 mg/250 mL.

MS CONTIN®, see Morphine

MSIR®, see Morphine

MUCOMYST®, see Acetylcysteine

MUPIROCIN—Bactroban®

Topical and intranasal antibiotic.

Description/Actions: Indicated for the topical treatment of impetigo due to *Staphylococcus aureus*, beta hemolytic *Streptococcus*, and *Streptococcus pyogenes*. Eradication of nasal colonization of methicillin-resistant *S. aureus* (MRSA) in adult patients and healthcare workers in certain institutional settings during outbreaks MRSA.

Warnings: Topical adverse reactions include burning, stinging, pain, and itching. Reactions to nasal applications include headache, rhinitis, respiratory disorder, pharyngitis, taste perversion, cough, and pruritus.

Administration: Topical, nasal. Nasal application is performed twice daily by applying approximately 0.25 g to the inside of each nostril for 5 days. Spread ointment by repeatedly closing and releasing nostrils for 1 minute after application.

Preparations: Ointment, 2%. (15 g and 30 g). Cream, 2% (15 g and 30 g).

MUROMONAB-CD3—Orthoclone OKT3®

Immunosuppressant.

Description/Actions: Indicated for the treatment of acute allograft rejection in renal, heart, and liver transplant patients.

Warnings: Contraindicated in patients who are in fluid overload. The most severe reaction is potentially fatal pulmonary edema, which has occurred in some patients with fluid overload prior to treatment. Patients should be evaluated for fluid overload by chest X-ray or according to the criterion of weight gain. Most patients experience fever and chills during the first 2 days of therapy. Other adverse reactions commonly encountered during the first 2 days of therapy include dyspnea, chest pain, nausea, vomiting, wheezing, diarrhea, and tremor. Therapy can result in increased susceptibility to infection. The dosage of other immunosuppresants (e.g., prednisone, azathioprine) used concomitantly should be reduced. The use of cyclosporine should be reduced or discontinued to reduce the risk of nephrotoxicity.

Administration: Intravenous as an IV bolus (in less than 1 minute).

Preparations: Ampules, 5 mg.

MUSTARGEN®, see Mechlorethamine

MUTAMYCIN®, see Mitomycin

MYAMBUTOL®, see Ethambutol

MYCELEX®, see Clotrimazole

MYCIFRADIN®, see Neomycin

MYCOBUTIN®, see Rifabutin

MYCOPHENOLATE MOFETIL— CellCept®

Description/Actions: Immunosuppressant indicated in prophylaxis of organ rejection in patients receiving allogeneic renal transplants as an adjunct to cyclosporine and corticosteroids.

Warnings: May cause neutropenia so complete blood counts should be performed weekly for the first month, twice monthly for the second and third months, and then monthly for the first year. If neutropenia develops (absolute neutrophil count of less than 1300/mm_2), treatment should be interrupted or dosage reduced. Adverse reactions include sepsis, diarrhea, vomiting, and GI tract hemorrhage. Caution must be exercised in patients with active digestive system disease. Counseling of appropriate, contraception to prevent pregnancy is recommended as the drug is contraindicated in pregnancy.

Administration: Oral on an empty stomach. Initiate within 72 hours following transplantation. Administer IV if unable to take orally.

Preparations: Capsules, 250 mg. Tablets 500 mg. Powder for oral suspension 200 mg/ml. Powder for injection, lyophylized 500 mg.

MYCOSTATIN®, see Nystatin

MYDRIACYL®, see Tropicamide

MYKROX®, see Metolazone

MYLANTA®, see Aluminum hydroxide 200 mg, magnesium hydroxide 200 mg, simethicone 20 mg/5 ml.

MYLANTA AR®, see Famotidine

MYLANTA—Children's tablets and liquid, tablets, calcium carbonate 400 mg, liquid, calcium carbonate 400 mg/5 ml

MYLANTA GELCAPS®—Calcium carbonate 550 mg, magnesium 125 mg.

MYLANTA DS TABLETS®— Calcium carbonate 700 mg, magnesium 300 mg

MYLANTA TABLETS®—Calcium carbonate 350 mg, magnesium hydroxide 150 mg

MYLANTA SUPREME®— Combination drug containing calcium carbonate 400 mg and magnesium hydroxide 135 mg/5 ml

MYLERAN®, see Busulfan

MYLICON®, see Simethicone

MYLOTARG®, see Gemtuzumab Oogamicin

MYOFLEX®, see Trolamine salicylate

MYSOLINE®, see Primidone

MYTELASE®, see Ambenonium

N

NABUMETONE—Relafen®
Nonsteroidal anti-inflammatory drug.

Description/Actions: Exhibits analgesic, anti-inflammatory, and antipyretic actions indicated for the treatment of signs and symptoms of rheumatoid arthritis and osteoarthritis.

Warnings: Contraindicated in patients in whom aspirin or another nonsteroidal anti-inflammatory drug induces asthma, urticaria, or other allergic-type reactionss. May cause gastrointestinal effects including diarrhea, dyspepsia, abdominal pain, constipation, flatulence, nausea, vomiting, gastritis, dry mouth, and stomatitis. Use should be avoided in patients with active gastrointestinal tract disease and closely monitored in patients with a previous history of such disorders. Other adverse reactions include fluid retention, edema, dizziness, headache, pruritus, rash, tinnitus, fatigue, increased sweating, insomnia, nervousness, somnolence, and photosensitivity reactions. Use is not recommended during the third trimester of pregnancy or in nursing mothers.

Administration: Oral.

Preparations: Tablets, 500 and 750 mg.

NADOLOL—Corgard®
Antihypertensive and antianginal agent.

Description/Actions: A nonselective beta-adrenergic-blocking agent indicated in the management of hypertension and angina pectoris.

Warnings: Contraindicated in patients with bronchial asthma, sinus bradycardia and greater than first degree conduction block, cardiogenic shock, and overt cardiac failure. Adverse reactions include sedation, dizziness, fatigue, bradycardia, and symptoms of peripheral vascular insufficiency. Use is best avoided in patients with bronchospastic diseases, and therapy in diabetic patients must be closely monitored.

Administration: Oral. Patients should be cautioned about the interruption or discontinuation of therapy; exacerbation of angina pectoris has occurred following the abrupt cessation of therapy, and, when therapy is to be discontinued, the dosage should be gradually reduced over a period of 1 to 2 weeks.

Preparations: Tablets, 20, 40, 80, 120, and 160 mg.

NAFARELIN ACETATE—Synarel®
Agent for endometriosis.

Description/Actions: A synthetic agonistic analogue of gonadotropin-releasing hormone. With repeated dosing, it causes a decrease in sex hormone levels. Indicated for the management of endometriosis in women 18 years of age and older, and for the treatment of central precocious puberty in children.

Warnings: Contraindicated in pregnancy, in women who are breast-feeding, and in women with undiagnosed abnormal vaginal bleeding. Adverse reactions include hot flashes, decreased libido, vaginal dryness, headaches, and emotional lability. Although the drug usually inhibits ovulation and stops menstruation, contraception is not insured, particularly if patients miss successive doses and experience breakthrough bleeding or ovulation. Patients should use a nonhormonal method of contraception.

Administration: Nasal. Treatment of endometriosis should be started between days 2 and 4 of the menstrual cycle. Patients should be advised of the importance of having their prescription refilled in a timely manner so that they do not miss a dose. The duration of treatment should be limited to 6 months, primarily because of a concern about a loss in bone density. However, if symptoms of endometriosis recur following a 6-month course of therapy and further treatment is being considered, it is recommended that bone density be assessed before retreatment begins.

Preparations: Nasal solution, 2 mg/ml.

NAFCIL®, see Nafcillin sodium

NAFCILLIN SODIUM—Nafcil®, Nallpen®, Unipen®

Description/Actions: Penicillin antibiotic indicated in the treatment of staphylococcal infections.

Preparations: Capsules, 250 mg. Tablets, 500 mg. Vials, 500 mg, 1, 2, and 10 g.

NAFTIFINE HYDROCHLORIDE— Naftin®

Antifungal agent.

Description/Actions: Indicated for the topical treatment of tinea pedis, tinea cruris, and tinea corporis.

Warnings: Adverse reactions include burning/stinging, dryness, erythema, itching, and local irritation.

Administration: Topical.

Preparations: Cream and gel, 1%.

NAFTIN®, see Naftifine

NALBUPHINE HYDROCHLORIDE—Nubain®

Description/Actions: Opioid agonist-antagonist analgesic indicated for parenteral use for the relief of moderate to severe pain. Also used as a supplement to balanced anesthesia, for preoperative and postoperative analgesia, and for obstetrical analgesia during labor and delivery.

Preparations: Ampules, vials, and syringes, 10 mg/ml and 20 mg/ml.

NALFON®, see Fenoprofen

NALIDIXIC ACID—NegGram®

Description/Actions: Anti-infective agent indicated for the treatment of urinary tract infections caused by susceptible gram-negative bacteria.

Preparations: Tablets, 250 and 500 mg., 1 g. Suspension, 250 mg/5 ml.

NALLPEN®, see Nafcillin sodium

NALMEFENE HYDROCHLORIDE—Revex®

Description/Actions: Opioid antagonist indicated in the complete or partial reversal of effects induced by opioids and in the management of known or suspected opioid overdose. Is longer acting than naloxone.

Warnings: Adverse reactions include nausea, vomiting, tachycardia, and hypertension. Can produce acute withdrawal symptoms in patients with physical dependence on opioids or following surgery involving high doses of opioids.

Administration: Intravenous bolus, but may be given intramuscularly or subcutaneously if venous access cannot be established.

Preparations: Ampules, 100 μg/ml and 1 mg/ml.

NALOXONE HYDROCHLORIDE—Narcan®

Description/Actions: Opioid antagonist indicated for parenteral use for the reversal of narcotic depression induced by opioids. Is also used for the diagnosis of suspected acute opioid overdosage. Is also included in tablet formulations of pentazocine to prevent the effect of the analgesic if the product is misused by injection. Can produce acute withdrawal symptoms in patients with physical dependence on opioids or following surgery involving high doses of opioids.

Preparations: Ampules, vials, and syringes, 0.02 mg/ml and 0.4 mg/ml.

NALTREXONE HYDROCHLORIDE—ReVia®

Description/Actions: Opioid antagonist indicated to provide blockade of the pharmacologic effects of exogenously administered opioids as an adjunct to the maintenance of the opioid-free state in detoxified formerly opioid-dependent individuals. Also indicated for the treatment of alcohol dependence.

Precaution/Adverse Reactions: Naltrexone is contraindicated in patients currently dependent on opioids, including those currently maintained on opiate agonists [(e.g., methadone or LAAM (levo-alpha-acetyl-methadol)].

Preparations: Tablets, 50 mg.

NANDROLONE DECANOATE— Deca-Durabolin®

Description/Actions: Anabolic steroid indicated for the parenteral management of the anemia of renal insufficiency. Adequate iron intake is required for optimal response. Should be administered deep into gluteal muscle.

Preparations: Ampules, vials, and syringes, 50 mg/ml, 100 mg/ml, and 200 mg/ml.

NANDROLONE PHENPROPIONATE— Durabolin®

Description/Actions: Anabolic steroid indicated for the parenteral treatment of metastatic breast cancer. Administer deep into gluteal muscle.

Preparations: Vials, 25 mg/ml and 50 mg/ml.

NAPHAZOLINE HYDROCHLORIDE—Privine®

Description/Actions: Decongestant indicated for nasal and ophthalmic use in the relief of congestion and related symptoms associated with various nasal and ocular conditions.

Preparations: Nasal drops and spray, 0.05%. Ophthalmic solution, 0.012%, 0.02%, 0.03%, 0.05%, 0.1%.

NAPRELAN, see Naproxen sodium

NAPROSYN®, see Naproxen

NAPROXEN—Naprosyn®, EC-Naprosyn®

NAPROXEN SODIUM—Aleve®, Anaprox®, Anaprox DS®, Naprelan®

Nonsteroidal anti-inflammatory drug.

Description/Actions: Inhibits prostaglandin synthesis and is indicated for the relief of mild to moderate pain, primary dysmenorrhea, rheumatoid arthritis, osteoarthritis, juvenile arthritis, ankylosing spondylitis, tendinitis and bursitis, and acute gout. Also used in the treatment of fever.

Warnings: Should not be given to patients in whom aspirin or another NSAID causes asthma, rhinitis, urticaria, or other allergic-type reactions. May cause GI effects, and use should be avoided in patients with active GI tract disease and closely monitored in patients with a previous history of such disorders. Other adverse reactions include headache, dizziness, drowsiness, itching, skin eruptions, tinnitus, edema, and dyspnea.

222 • NARATRIPTAN

Administration: Oral.

Preparations: Naproxen—Tablets, 250, 375, and 500 mg. Enteric-coated tablets, 375 and 500 mg. Suspension, 125 mg/5 ml. Naproxen sodium—Tablets, 220 (Aleve), 275 and 550 mg. Controlled-release tablets (Naprelan), 375 and 500 mg.

NARATRIPTAN—Amerge®

Description/Actions: Selective 5HT Ib/Id receptor agonist indicated in acute treatment of migraine with or without aura, in adults. Effective in relieving the pain and other symptoms associated with migraine (e.g., nausea, photophobia). Due to its long half-life relative to other "triptans" it may be an appropriate choice for patients who have longer lasting migraines.

Warnings: Confirm diagnosis. Exclude underlying cardiovascular disease, supervise first dose, and consider ECG monitoring in patients with likelihood of unrecognized coronary disease. Monitor cardiovascular function in long-term intermittent use. Use cautiously in hepatic or renal dysfunction. Not recommended for use in the elderly.

Contraindicated in ischemic cardiac disease, cerebrovascular disease, peripheral vascular disease, uncontrolled hypertension, severe renal or hepatic impairment, basilar or hemoplegic migraine, and within 24 hours of other 5-HT, agonist, or ergot-type drugs. Pregnancy Category C.

Adverse reactions include paresthesia, dizziness, drowsiness, malaise/fatigue, and throat/neck symptoms.

Administration: Oral.

Preparations: Tablets, 1 and 2.5 mg.

NAROPIN®, see Ropivicaine Hydrochloride

NAQUA®, see Trichlormethiazide

NARCAN®, see Naloxone

NASACORT®, NASACORT AQ®, see Triamcinolone acetonide

NASALCROM®, see Cromolyn

NASALIDE®, see Flunisolide

NASAREL®, see Flunisolide

NASCOBAL®, see Cyanocobalamin

NASONEX®, see Mometasone Furoate

NATACYN®, see Natamycin

NATAMYCIN—Natacyn®

Description/Actions: Antifungal agent indicated for ophthalmic use in the treatment of fungal blepharitis, conjunctivitis, and keratitis.

Preparations: Ophthalmic suspension, 5%.

NATEGLINIDE—Starlix®

Description/Actions: Indicated for the management of patients with Type II diabetes mellitus either as monotherapy in patients whose hyperglycemia cannot be adequately controlled by diet and exercise alone or in combination with metformin in patients whose hyperglycemia in not adequately controlled by metformin, diet, and exercise alone. Nateglinide should not be added to or substituted for regimens containing glyburide or other insulin secretagogues.

Precautions/Adverse Reactions: Nateglinide is contraindicated in patients with a known hypersensitivity to the drug, Type I diabetes mellitus, and diabetic ketoacidosis. Hypoglycemia is a possibility with nateglinide therapy. Risk of hypoglycemia may be increased by strenuous exercise, alcohol, insufficient caloric intake or combining with other antidiabetic agents. Use caution in patients with moderate to severe hepatic insufficiency. Glycemic control may be lost with infection, fever, trauma, or surgery, necessitating insulin therapy. Nateglinide is metabolized by the cytochrome P450 isoenzyme CYP2C9 and CYP3A4. It is an inhibitor of CYP2C9. No significant interactions were observed with the concomitant administration of glyburide, metformin, digoxin, warfarin or diclofenac. Thiazide diuretics, corticosteroids, thyroid products, and sympathomimetic agents may decrease the hypoglycemic effect of nateglinide. Nonsteroidal anti-inflammatory agents, salicylates, monoamine oxidase inhibitors, and nonselective beta-adrenergic agents may increase the hypoglycemic effect of nateglinide. Pregnancy Category C. There are no adequate and well-controlled studies in pregnant women. Nateglinide should not be used during pregnancy. Excretion in human breast milk is unknown; therefore, nateglinide should not be administered to nursing women. Safety and efficacy in pediatric patients have not been studied. Adverse reactions observed in ≥ 2% of patients treated with nateglinide alone include upper respiratory infections, back pain, flu symptoms, dizziness, weight gain, arthropathy, diarrhea, accidental trauma, bronchitis, coughing, and hypoglycemia. Hyperuricemia was observed in patients treated with nateglinide alone and in combination with metformin. Hypersensitivity reactions such as rash, itching, and urticaria have been reported.

Administration: Oral.

Preparations: Tablets, 60 mg and 120 mg.

NATRECOR®, see Nesiritide Citrate

NATURETIN®, see Bendroflumethiazide

NAVANE®, see Thiothixene

NAVELBINE®, see Vinorelbine tartrate

NEBCIN®, see Tobramycin

NEBUPENT®, see Pentamidine

NEDOCROMIL SODIUM—Tilade®
Antiasthmatic agent.

Description/Actions: Is an anti-inflammatory agent that appears to inhibit the activation of, and release of mediators (e.g., histamine) from, various inflammatory cell types associated with asthma. Indicated for maintenance therapy in the management of patients with mild to moderate bronchial asthma. Should not be used for the reversal of acute bronchospasm.

Warnings: Adverse reactions include unpleasant taste, cough, pharyngitis, headache, upper respiratory tract infection, nausea, and vomiting.

Administration: Oral inhalation. Should be added to the patient's existing treatment regimen (e.g., bronchodilator).

Preparations: Metered-dose inhaler, at least 112 metered inhalations with each actuation delivering 1.75 mg of the drug from the mouthpiece. Nebulizer solution, 0.5%.

NEDOCROMIL SODIUM OPHTHALMIC SODIUM— Alocril®

Description/Actions: Indicated for the treatment of itching associated with allergic conjunctivitis.

Precautions/Adverse Reactions: The most frequently reported adverse effect is headache. Ocular burning, irritation and stinging, unpleasant taste, and nasal congestion can also occur. More rarely, asthma, conjunctivitis, eye redness, photophobia, and rhinitis are seen.

Administration: One or two drops in each eye BID.

Preparations: Solution, 2% in 5 ml.

NEFAZODONE HYDROCHLORIDE—Serzone®

Description/Actions: Inhibits neuronal reuptake of serotonin and norepinephrine and indicated in the treatment of depression.

Warnings: Nefazodone therapy has been associated with liver abnormalities ranging from asymptomatic reversible serum transaminase increases to cases of necrosis and liver failure resulting in transplant and/or death. Treatment should not be initiated in individuals with active liver disease or with elevated baseline serum transaminases. Patients should be alert for signs and symptoms of developing liver failure (jaundice, anorexia, gastrointestinal complaints, malaise, etc.) and to report them to their physician immediately. Nefazodone should be discontinued in patients with signs or symptoms suggestive of hepatocellular injury such as increased serum AST or serum ALT levels greater than 3 times the upper limit of normal. Nefazodone is contraindicated in patients who were withdrawn from therapy because of evidence of liver injury. Nefazodone is also contraindicated in patients with a known hypersensitivity to any component of the formulation or to other phenylpiperazine antidepressants. Concurrent administration of terfenadine or astemizole is contraindicated. Adverse reactions include somnolence, dizziness, lightheadedness, confusion, nausea, constipation, dry mouth, asthenia, blurred vision, abnormal vision, headache, sinus bradycardia, and orthostatic hypotension. Patients should be advised to avoid the consumption of alcoholic beverages, and cautioned about operating machinery until response is ascertained.

Administration: Oral.

Preparations: Tablets, 100, 150, 200, and 250 mg.

NEGGRAM®, see Nalidixic acid

NELFINAVIR—Viracept®

Description/Actions: Protease inhibitor indicated in the treatment of HIV infection when antiretroviral therapy is warranted, preferably in combination with other antiretroviral agents.

Warnings: Contraindicated with concurrent use of terfenadine, astemisole, cisapride, triazolam, or midazolam. Prescribers should review patient's drug profile and adjust accordingly prior to prescribing. Use cautiously in patients with hepatic impairment and hemophilia. Avoid use of powder in patients with phenylketonuria, since it contains phenylalanine. Adverse reactions include diarrhea, nausea, flatulence, abdominal pain, and rash.

Administration: Take with meals or light snack. Powder may be mixed in a small amount of nonacidic food or beverage (e.g., water, milk, formula) with meals. Once mixed with food or a beverage, must be used immediately or may be refrigerated for up to 6 hours. Antiviral activity is enhanced when administered with nucleoside analogues.

Preparations: Tablets, 250 mg. Oral powder, 50 mg/g (contains 11.2 mg phenylalanine).

NELOVA®

Description/Actions: Oral contraceptive combination of mestranol and norethindrone.

NEMBUTAL®, see Pentobarbital

NEOMYCIN SULFATE— Mycifradin®

Description/Actions: Aminoglycoside antibiotic most often used topically, alone or in combination with other anti-infective agents, in the treatment of dermatologic, ocular, and otic infections. Has also been used orally for preoperative suppression of intestinal bacteria, for GI infections, in hepatic coma, and to reduce elevated blood cholesterol levels. Has been used as a bladder irrigant (usually with polymyxin B to prevent urinary tract infections).

Preparations: Cream and ointment, 0.5%. Tablets, 500 mg. Oral solution, 125 mg/5 ml.

NEORAL®, see Cyclosporine

NEOSAR®, see Cyclophosphamide

NEOSTIGMINE METHYLSULFATE—
Prostigmin®

Description/Actions: Anticholinesterase indicated for the symptomatic control of myasthenia gravis. Methylsulfate derivative is administered parenterally and is also indicated for the prevention and treatment of postoperative distention and urinary retention, and to reverse the effects of nondepolarizing neuromuscular blocking agents (e.g., tubocurarine).

Preparations: Tablets, 15 mg. Ampules and vials, 1:4000, 1:2000, and 1:1000.

NEO-SYNEPHRINE®, see Phenylephrine

NEOTHYLLINE®, see Dyphylline

NEPTAZANE®, see Methazolamide

NESACAINE®, see Chloroprocaine

NESIRITIDE CITRATE—
NATRECOR®

Description/Actions: Natrecor® is indicated for the intravenous treatment of patients with acutely decompensated congestive heart failure who have dyspnea at rest or with minimal activity.

Precautions/Adverse Reactions: Nesiritide should not be used as primary therapy for patients with cardiogenic shock or in patients with a systolic blood pressure < 90 mmHg. Avoid using nesiritide in patients suspected of having, or known to have low cardiac filling pressures. Not recommended for use in patients with significant valvular stenosis, restrictive or obstructive cardiomyopathy, constrictive pericarditis, pericardial tamponade, or other conditions in which cardiac output is dependent upon venous return, or for patients suspected to have low cardiac filling pressures. There is an increased incidence of symptomatic hypotension in patients receiving oral angiotensin converting enzyme (ACE) inhibitors and nesiritide.

Pregnancy Category C. No adequate and well-controlled studies in pregnant women. Use in pregnancy only if the potential benefit justifies the potential risk to the fetus. Excretion in human breast milk is unknown. Safety and efficacy in pediatric patients have not been established.

Adverse reactions noted in at least 3% of the patients treated with nesiritide include hypotension, ventricular tachycardia, nonsustained ventricular tachycardia, ventricular extra systoles, headache, back pain, dizziness, anxiety, and nausea. The dose-limiting effect of nesiritide is hypotension. Use cautiously in patients with systolic blood pressure < 100 mmHg at baseline, as the rate of symptomatic hypotension may be increased in this patient population. Hypotension may be prolonged. Administer only in settings where blood pressure can be monitored closely. Dosage reductions and/or discontinuation of the drug may be warranted in patients who develop hypotension.

Administration: Intravenous.

Patient Care Implications: Monitor blood pressure closely during nesiritide administration.

Preparations: Powder for injection, 1.5 mg, single-use vials.

NETILMICIN SULFATE—
Netromycin®

Description/Actions: Aminoglycoside antibiotic indicated for parenteral use, primarily in the treatment of infections caused by gram-negative bacteria.

Preparations: Vials, 100 mg/ml.

NETROMYCIN®, see Netilmicin

NEUPOGEN®, see Filgrastim

NEURONTIN®, see Gabapentin

NEUTRA-PHOS K®, see Potassium phosphate

NEUTREXIN®, see Trimetrexate glucuronate

NEVIRAPINE—Viramune®

Description/Actions: Indicated in combination with nucleoside analogues in the treatment of HIV-1 infected adults who have experienced clinical and/or immunologic deterioration.

Warnings: Suspend therapy if severe rash or any rash accompanied by fever, blistering, oral lesions, conjunctivitis, swellling, muscle or joint aches, or general malaise occurs. Discontinue if rash reoccurs on rechallenge. Use cautiously in patients with hepatic dsyfunction. Monitor and discontinue if moderate or severe liver dysfunction occurs. Advere reactions include rash (may be life threatening), fever, nausea, headache, and liver dysfunction.

Administration: 200 mg once daily for 14 days and if no rash appears then 200 mg twice daily.

Preparations: Tablets, 200 mg (scored). Oral suspension, 50 mg/5 ml.

NEXIUM™, see Esomeprazole

NIACIN, see Nicotinic acid

NIACIN AND LOVASTATIN— ADVICOR™

Description/Actions: Advicor™ is indicated for the treatment of primary hypercholesterolemia (heterozygous familial and nonfamilial) and mixed lipidemia (Frederickson Types IIa and IIb).

Precautions/Adverse Reactions: Advicor™ is contraindicated in patients with active liver disease or unexplained persistent elevations of serum transaminases; active peptic ulcer disease; arterial bleeding; or pregnancy. It should not be substituted for equivalent doses of immediate-release (crystalline) niacin. Cases of severe hepatic toxicity, including fulminant hepatic necrosis, have occurred in patients who have substituted sustained-release niacin products for immediate-release niacin. It should be used with caution in patients who consume substantial quantities of alcohol and/or have a past history of liver disease. Niacin and lovastatin have been associated with abnormal liver tests.

Use with caution in patients with unstable angina or in the acute phase of MI, especially when such patients also are receiving vasoactive drugs such as nitrates, calcium channel blockers, or adrenergic-blocking agents. Use with caution in patients predisposed to gout because elevated uric acid levels have occurred with niacin therapy.

HMG-CoA reductase inhibitors cause myopathy, manifested as muscle pain or weakness associated with elevated creatine kinase. Rhabdomyolysis, with or without acute renal failure, has occurred with HMG-CoA reductase inhibitors. Risk of myopathy increased with concomitant therapy with drugs metabolized by the cytochrome P450 isoform 3A4, which increase levels of lovastatin. Niacin is excreted through kidneys and should be used with caution in patients with renal dysfunction. Niacin extended-release tablets have been associated with slight reductions in platelet counts and prolongation in PT.

Pregnancy Category X. Because of the HMG-CoA reductase inhibitor's ability to decrease synthesis of cholesterol and possibly other products of the cholesterol biosynthesis pathway, Advicor™ is contraindicated in women who are pregnant and in lactating mothers. Cholesterol and other products of the cholesterol biosynthesis pathway are essential components for fetal development. Most common adverse effect was flushing, which may be accompanied by symptoms of dizziness, tachycardia, palpitations, shortness of breath, sweating, and chills. Other common adverse reactions were headache, pain, pruritis, rash, nausea, diarrhea, and back pain.

Administration: Oral.

Patient Care Implications: Obtain liver function tests and total cholesterol profile prior to therapy. LFTs monitored every 6 to 12 weeks for the first 6 months, then at 6 month intervals. Lipid determination should be performed at intervals no less than 4 weeks and dosage adjusted according to patient's response. Monitor blood glucose. Flushing may be reduced by pretreatment with aspirin (taken up to 30 minutes prior to dose) or other NSAIDs. Flushing, pruritus, and GI distress are reduced by slowly increasing the dose of niacin and avoiding administration on an empty stomach. Advise patient of risk of myopathy and to report unexplained muscle pain, tenderness, or weakness promptly. If taking with bile acid–binding resins, 4 to 6 hours should elapse. Avoid ingestion of alcohol or hot drinks at the time of administration to minimize flushing. Do not administer with grapefruit juice because of the increase in lovastatin concentrations. Discontinue therapy, temporarily for elective major surgery, acute medical or surgical conditions, or if patient experience an acute or serious condition predisposing to renal failure secondary to rhabdomyolysis.

Preparations: Tablets, extended-release niacin and immediate-release lovastatin: niacin, 500 mg, and lovastatin, 20 mg; niacin, 750 mg, and lovastatin, 20 mg; niacin, 1000 mg, and lovastatin, 20 mg.

NIACINAMIDE, see Nicotinamide

NIASPAN, see Nicotinic acid

NICARDIPINE HYDROCHLORIDE—Cardene®, Cardene IV®

Antihypertensive and antianginal agent.

Description/Actions: A calcium channel-blocking agent that is indicated for the treatment of hypertension and for the management of chronic stable angina.

Warnings: Contraindicated in patients with advanced aortic stenosis. Adverse reactions include flushing, headache, edema of the feet, asthenia, palpitations, dizziness, tachycardia, and nausea. Some angina patients experience increased anginal symptoms.

Administration: Oral and intravenous.

Preparations: Capsules, 20 and 30 mg. Sustained-release capsules, 30, 45, and 60 mg. Ampules, 2.5 mg/ml.

NICLOSAMIDE—Niclocide®

Description/Actions: Anthelmintic indicated for the treatment of tapeworm infections caused by beef, fish, and dwarf tapeworms.

Preparations: Tablets, 500 mg.

NICODERM®, see Nicotine

NICORETTE®, see Nicotine polacrilex

NICORETTE DS®, see Nicotine polacrilex

NICOTINAMIDE—Niacinamide

Description/Actions: Vitamin analogue (of nicotinic acid) used in the prophylaxis and treatment of pellagra.

Preparations: Tablets, 50, 100, 125, 250, and 500 mg. Vials, 100 mg/ml.

NICOTINE—Habitrol®, Nicoderm®, Nicoderm CQ®, Nicotrol®, Nicotrol NS®, ProStep®

Adjunct for smoking cessation.

Description/Actions: Nicotine is contained in a multilayered transdermal system that provides systemic delivery of the drug following its application to intact skin. Indicated as an aid to smoking cessation as part of a comprehensive behavioral smoking-cessation program.

Warnings: Contraindicated during the immediate postmyocardial infarction period, and in patients with life-threatening arrhythmias or severe or worsening angina pectoris. Adverse reactions include headache, insomnia, tachycardia, erythema, pruritus, and burning at application sites.

Administration: Topical, nasal spray.

Preparations: Transdermal systems, 7, 14, and 21 mg absorbed in 24 hours (Habitrol®, Nicoderm®), 11 and 22 mg absorbed in 24 hours (ProStep®), and 5, 10, and 15 mg absorbed in 16 hours (Nicotrol). Nasal spray, 0.5 mg/spray (nicotrol NS). Inhalation system, 10 mg (4 mg delivered), contains menthol.

NICOTINE POLACRILEX— Nicorette®, Nicorette DS®

Adjunct for smoking cessation.

Description/Actions: Nicotine is bound to an ion exchange resin in a chewing gum base and is absorbed through the buccal mucosa as the gum is chewed. Indicated as a temporary aid to the cigarette smoker seeking to give up his or her smoking habit while participating in a behavioral modification program.

Warnings: Contraindicated in patients during the immediate postmyocardial infarction period, and in patients with life-threatening arrhythmias or severe or worsening angina pectoris. Should be used with caution in patients with dental problems, or with dentures, dental caps, or partial bridges to which the gum may stick and cause damage. Adverse reactions include jaw muscle ache, hiccups, nausea, vomiting, and pharyngitis.

Administration: Buccal.

Preparations: Chewing gum pieces, 2 and 4 mg.

NICOTINIC ACID—Niacin, Niaspan®, Nicobid®, Slo-Niacin®, Vitamin B_3

Description/Actions: Vitamin used to correct nicotinic acid deficiency, and in the prevention and treatment of pellagra. Has been used as adjunctive therapy in patients with significant hyperlipidemia.

Preparations: Tablets, 25, 50, 100, 125, 250, and 500 mg. Controlled-release capsules, 125, 250, 375, 400, 500, 750, and 1000 mg. Elixir, 50 mg/5 ml. Vials, 100 mg/ml.

NICOTROL®, Nicotrol® NS, see Nicotine

NIFEDIPINE—Adalat®, Adalat CC®, Procardia®, Procardia XL®

Antianginal and antihypertensive agent.

Description/Actions: Is a calcium channel-blocking agent that is indicated in the treatment of (1) vasospastic angina, (2) chronic stable angina in patients who remain symptomatic despite adequate doses of beta-adrenergic-blocking agents and/or organic nitrates or who cannot tolerate these agents, and (3) hypertension.

Warnings: Adverse reactions include hypotension, flushing, peripheral edema, dizziness, nervousness, and muscle cramps. Although usually well tolerated, concurrent therapy with a beta-adrenergic-blocking agent should be closely monitored because of an increased possibility of hypotension, congestive heart failure, or exacerbation of angina.

Administration: Oral.

Preparations: Capsules, 10 and 20 mg. Controlled-release tablets, 30, 60, and 90 mg.

NILSTAT®, see Nystatin

NIMODIPINE—Nimotop®

Agent for spasm following subarachnoid hemorrhage.

Description/Actions: A calcium channel-blocking agent that prevents or relieves the spasm following subarachnoid hemorrhage, thereby reducing the risk of severe ischemic neurologic deficits. Indicated for the improvement of neurologic deficits due to spasm following subarachnoid hemorrhage from ruptured congenital intracranial aneurysms in patients who are in good neurologic condition.

Warnings: Adverse reactions include decreased blood pressure, headache, nausea, and bradycardia.

Administration: Oral. Therapy should be initiated within 96 hours of the subarachnoid hemorrhage. If the capsules cannot be swallowed (e.g., at the time of surgery, or if the patient is unconscious), a hole should be made in both ends of the capsule with an 18 gauge needle, and the contents of the liquid-filled capsule withdrawn into a syringe. The contents should then be emptied into the patient's in situ nasogastric tube and washed down the tube with 30 ml of normal saline (0.9%).

Preparations: Capsules, 30 mg.

NIMOTOP®, see Nimodipine

NIPENT®, see Pentostatin

NISOLDIPINE—Sular®

Description/Actions: Calcium channel blocker indicated in the treatment of hypertension as monotherapy or as an adjunct to other antihypertensives.

Warnings: Use cautiously in patients with hypotension, heart failure, hepatic impairment, and coronary artery disease. Adverse reactions include peripheral edema, headache, dizziness, pharyngitis, vasodilation, sinusitis, palpitations, chest pain, nausea, rash, increased angina, and MI (rare).

Administration: Oral. Do not crush, chew, divide, or take with a high-fat meal or grapefruit juice.

Preparations: Extended-release tablets, 10, 20, 30, and 40 mg.

NITRIC OXIDE—INOmax®

Description/Actions: INOmax, in conjunction with ventilatory support and other appropriate agents, is indicated for the treatment of term and near-term (> 34 weeks) neonates with hypoxic respiratory failure associated with clinical or echocardiographic evidence of pulmonary hypertension, where it improves oxygenation and reduces the need for extracorporeal membrane oxygenation.

Precautions/Adverse Reactions: INOmax should not be used in the treatment of neonates known to be dependent on right-to-left shunting of blood. Abrupt discontinuation of INOmax may lead to worsening oxygenation and increasing pulmonary arterial pressure. Adverse reactions include hypotension, withdrawal syndrome, atelectasis, hematuria, hyperglycemia, sepsis, infection, cellulitis, and stridor. INOmax should be administered with monitoring for PaO_2, methemoglobin, and NO_2.

Administration: 20 ppm maintained up to 14 days or until the underlying oxygen desaturation has resolved and the neonate is ready to be weaned from INOmax therapy. Additional therapies should be used to maximize oxygen delivery.

Preparations: Aluminum cylinders, 100 and 800 ppm.

NITRO-BID®, see Nitroglycerin

NITRODISC®, see Nitroglycerin

NITRO-DUR®, see Nitroglycerin

NITROFURANTOIN—Furadantin®, Macrobid®

NITROFURANTOIN MACROCRYSTALS—Macrodantin®

Urinary tract antibacterial agent.

Description/Actions: Indicated for urinary tract infections caused by susceptible strains of *E. coli, Proteus* species, *Klebsiella* species, *Enterobacter* species, *S. aureus,* and enterococci.

Warnings: Contraindicated in patients with significantly impaired renal function, in pregnancy at term, and in infants under 1 month of age. Adverse reactions include nausea, vomiting, pulmonary reactions, dizziness, drowsiness, headache, peripheral neuropathy, anemia, pruritus, and urticaria.

Administration: Oral. Should be administered with food.

Preparations: Tablets, 50 and 100 mg. Suspension, 25 mg/5 ml. Capsules (macrocrystals), 25, 50, and 100 mg. Capsules (Macrobid), 100 mg (25 mg macrocrystals and 75 mg monohydrate).

NITROFURAZONE—Furacin®

Description/Actions: Anti-infective agent used topically for adjunctive therapy of patients with second- and third-degree burns, and in skin grafting where bacterial contamination may cause graft rejection and/or donor site infection.

Preparations: Cream and soluble dressing, 0.2%.

NITROGARD®, see Nitroglycerin

NITROGEN MUSTARD, see Mechlorethamine

NITROGLYCERIN (see list of preparations below for trade names)

Antianginal agent.

Description/Actions: An organic nitrate indicated for the prophylaxis and treatment of patients with angina pectoris.

Warnings: Adverse reactions include headache, dizziness, hypotension, palpitation, and cutaneous vasodilation with flushing.

Administration: Sublingual, translingual, transmucosal, oral, topical, and transdermal.

Preparations: Sublingual tablets (Nitrostat®), 0.15, 0.3, 0.4, and 0.6 mg. Translingual metered dose spray for oral use (Nitrolingual®), 0.4 mg/dose. Transmucosal (buccal) tablets (Nitrogard®), 1, 2, and 3 mg. Sustained-release capsules (Nitro-Bid®, Nitroglyn®), 2.5, 6.5, and 9 mg. Ointment (Nitro-Bid®, Nitrol®, Nitrostat®), 2%. Transdermal systems (Minitran®, Nitro-Dur®, Nitro-disc®), Transderm-Nitro®, Deponit®), 2.5, 5, 7.5, 10, and 15 mg/24 hours.

NITROGLYCERIN, INTRAVENOUS—Nitro-Bid IV®, Tridil®

Description/Actions: Administered intravenously for (1) control of blood pressure in perioperative hypertension, (2) congestive heart failure associated with acute myocardial infarction, (3) treatment of angina pectoris, and (4) production of controlled hypotension during surgical procedures.

Preparations: Ampules and vials, 0.5, 0.8, 5, and 10 mg/ml.

NITROGLYN®, see Nitroglycerin

NITROL®, see Nitroglycerin

NITROLINGUAL®, see Nitroglycerin

NITROPRESS®, see Sodium nitroprusside

NITROSTAT®, see Nitroglycerin

NITROUS OXIDE—Laughing gas

Description/Actions: Anesthetic gas usually used in conjunction with other anesthetics.

NIX®, see Permethrin

NIZATIDINE—Axid®

Antiulcer agent.

Description/Actions: A histamine H_2-receptor antagonist indicated for the treatment of active duodenal ulcer, for maintenance therapy for duodenal ulcer patients, for benign gastric ulcer, and for gastroesophageal reflux disease including erosive esophagitis.

Warnings: Adverse reactions include somnolence, sweating, urticaria. Patients receiving high doses of aspirin may experience increased salicylate levels when nizatidine is given concurrently.

Administration: Oral.

Preparations: Capsules, 150 and 300 mg.

NIZORAL®, see Ketoconazole

NODOZ®, see Caffeine

NOLAHIST®, see Phenindamine

NOLVADEX®, see Tamoxifen

NONOXYNOL-9—Emko®

Description/Actions: Spermicide used in contraceptive formulations.

Preparations: Vaginal foam, jelly, gel, cream, and suppositories.

NORCO®, see Hydrocodone bitartrate with Acetaminophen

NORCURON®, see Vecuronium

NOREPINEPHRINE BITARTRATE—Levarterenol, Levophed®

Description/Actions: Sympathomimetic agent having inotropic stimulating and peripheral vasoconstricting actions. Indicated for the restoration of blood pressure in controlling certain acute hypotensive states, and as an adjunct in the treatment of cardiac arrest and profound hypotension.

Preparations: Ampules, 1 mg/ml.

NORETHINDRONE—Micronor®, Norlutin®, Nor-QD®

NORETHINDRONE ACETATE—Norlutate®

Description/Actions: Progestin indicated in the treatment of amenorrhea, in abnormal uterine bleeding due to hormonal imbalance (e.g., uterine cancer), and in endometriosis. Used in combination with an estrogen in oral contraceptive formulations and also in progestin-only oral contraceptive formulations.

Preparations: Tablets, 0.35 mg norethindrone for use as an oral contraceptive. Tablets, 5 mg.

NORETHYNODREL

Description/Actions: Progestin used in combination with an estrogen in various oral contraceptive formulations.

NORFLEX®, see Orphenadrine citrate

NORFLOXACIN—Chibroxin®, Noroxin®

Fluoroquinolone antibacterial agent.

Description/Actions: Indicated for the treatment of adults with complicated and uncomplicated urinary tract infections caused by susceptible strains. Also indicated for uncomplicated urethral and cervical gonorrhea, and prostatitis caused by *E. coli.* Indicated for ophthalmic use for ocular infections caused by susceptible bacteria.

Warnings: Adverse reactions include nausea, headache, and dizziness. Because the drug may cause CNS effects, patients should be cautioned about engaging in activities that require mental alertness or coordination. The drug has caused arthropathy in immature animals, and it is recommended that norfloxacin not be used in children or pregnant women.

Administration: Oral and ophthalmic.

Preparations: Tablets, 400 mg. Ophthalmic solution, 0.3%.

NORGESTIMATE/ETHINYL ESTRADIOL—Ortho-Cyclen®, Ortho Tri-Cyclen®, Ortho Tri-CyclenLo®

Oral contraceptive.

Description/Actions: Is a progestin/estrogen combination that acts primarily by the suppression of gonadotropins and inhibition of ovulation. Norgestimate exhibits a highly selective progestational action and minimal androgenicity. Indicated for the prevention of pregnancy in women who elect to use oral contraceptives as a method of contraception.

Warnings: Contraindicated in women who have thrombophlebitis or a thromboembolic disorder, a past history of such disorders, cerebral vascular or coronary artery disease, known or suspected carcinoma of the breast, carcinoma of the endometrium or other known or suspected estrogen-dependent neoplasia, undiagnosed abnormal genital bleeding, cholestatic jaundice of pregnancy or jaundice with prior oral contraceptive use, hepatic adenomas or carcinomas, or known or suspected pregnancy. Adverse reactions include bleeding irregularities (e.g., breakthrough bleeding, spotting, changes in menstrual flow), gastrointestinal effects (e.g., nausea, vomiting, abdominal cramps), fluid retention, melasma, rash, reduced tolerance to carbohydrates, and vaginal candidiasis. Women should be strongly advised not to smoke because of the increased risk of cardiovascular effects.

Administration: Oral. Administered once a day at about the same time each day. Available in packages designed for a 21-day regimen (i.e., 1 tablet per day for 21 days, followed by 7 days in which medication is not taken) and a 28-day regimen (i.e., 1 tablet per day for 21 days, followed by one inactive "reminder" tablet a day for 7 days).

Preparations: Tablets (monophasic formulation), 0.25 mg of norgestimate, and 35 µg of ethinyl estradiol in 21-day and 28-day regimens. Tablets (triphasic formulation), graduated doses of 0.18, 0.215, and 0.25 mg of norgestimate with each dosage used in 7 tablets in combination with 35 µg of ethinyl estradiol, in 21-day and 28-day regimens. Tablets (triphasic formulation), graduated doses of 0.18, 0.215, and 0.25 mg of norgestimate with each dosage used in 7 tablets in combination with 25 µg of ethinyl estradiol, in a 21-day regimen.

NORGESTREL—Ovrette®

Description/Actions: Progestin used alone as an oral contraceptive and also in combination with an estrogen in various oral contraceptive formulations.

Preparations: Tablets, 0.075 mg.

NORINYL®

Description/Actions: Oral contraceptive combination of ethinyl estradiol or mestranol with norethindrone.

NORITATE®, see Metronidazole

NORLESTRIN®

Description/Actions: Oral contraceptive combination of ethinyl estradiol with norethindrone acetate.

NORLUTATE®, see Norethindrone acetate

NORLUTIN®, see Norethindrone

NORMIFLO®, see Ardeparin

NOR-MIL®, see Diphenoxylate

NORMODYNE®, see Labetalol

NOROXIN®, see Norfloxacin

NORPACE®, see Disopyramide

NORPLANT®, see Levonorgestrel implant

NORPRAMIN®, see Desipramine

NOR-QD®, see Norethindrone

NORTRIPTYLINE HYDROCHLORIDE—Aventyl®, Pamelor®

Description/Actions: Tricyclic antidepressant indicated for the relief of symptoms of depression.

Preparations: Capsules, 10, 25, 50, and 75 mg. Oral solution, 10 mg/5 ml.

NORVASC®, see Amlodipine besylate

NORVIR®, see Ritonavir

NORZINE®, see Thiethylperazine

NOSCAPINE

Description/Actions: Antitussive used in combination with other agents in the treatment of various respiratory conditions.

NOVAFED®, see Pseudoephedrine

NOVANTRONE®, see Mitoxantrone

NOVOBIOCIN SODIUM—Albamycin®

Description/Actions: Antibiotic used in selected infections when primary less toxic anti-infective agents are not effective or are contraindicated.

Preparations: Capsules, 250 mg.

NOVOCAIN®, see Procaine

NOVOLIN®, see Insulin

NOVOLOG®, see Insulin aspart

NOVOPEN®

Insulin delivery device that uses penfill insulin cartridges.

NPH INSULIN®, see Insulin

NUBAIN®, see Nalbuphine

NUMORPHAN®, see Oxymorphone

NUPERCAINAL®, see Dibucaine

NUPRIN®, see Ibuprofen

NUROMAX®, see Doxacurium chloride

NUTROPIN DEPOT®, see Somatropin

NUTROPIN®, see somatropin

NUVARING®, see Ethinyl Estradiol and Etonogestrel

NYDRAZID®, see Isoniazid

NYSTATIN—Mycostatin®, Nilstat®

Description/Actions: Antifungal agent indicated in the treatment of cutaneous, mucocutaneous, vaginal, oral, and intestinal infections caused by *Candida albicans* and other *Candida* species.

Preparations: Tablets, 500,000 units. Troches, 200,000 units. Oral suspension, 100,000 units/ml. Vaginal tablets, 100,000 units. Cream, ointment, and powder, 100,000 units/g.

NYTOL®, see Diphenhydramine

O

OCTREOTIDE ACETATE—Sandostatin®

Agent for hypersecretory disorders.

Description/Actions: Exhibits actions that are similar to those of the natural hormone somatostatin. Suppresses the secretion of growth hormone, serotonin, and the gastroenteropancreatic (GEP) peptides-gastrin, vasoactive intestinal peptide (VIP), insulin, glucagon, secretin, motilin, and pancreatic polypeptide. Indicated for the treatment of the symptoms of two types of gastroenteropancreatic carcinoma. Suppresses or inhibits the severe diarrhea and flushing episodes associated with metastatic carcinoid tumors, and is also indicated for the treatment of profuse watery diarrhea associated with vasoactive intestinal peptide-secreting tumors. Also indicated in the treatment of acromegaly.

Warnings: Adverse reactions include nausea, diarrhea, loose stools, abdominal discomfort, vomiting, cholelithiasis, and pain at the injection site. May cause hyperglycemia or hypoglycemia, and, in patients with diabetes, it may be necessary to adjust the dosage of insulin or oral hypoglycemic agent. May alter the absorption of nutrients, as well as medications that are administered orally.

Administration: Subcutaneous; intravenous bolus injections have been used under emergency conditions.

Preparations: Ampules (1 ml), 0.05, 0.1, 0.2, and 0.5 mg.

OCUCLEAR®, see Oxymetazoline

OCUFEN®, see Flurbiprofen sodium

OCUFLOX®, see Ofloxacin

OCUPRESS®, see Carteolol

OFLOXACIN—Floxin®, Floxin IV®, Floxin otic®, Ocuflox®

Fluoroquinolone antiinfective agent.

Description/Actions: Exhibits a bactericidal action against many gram-positive and gram-negative bacteria. Indicated for the treatment of lower respiratory tract infections, acute, uncomplicated urethral and cervical gonorrhea, chlamydial urethritis and cervicitis, skin and skin structure infections, urinary tract infections, and prostatitis. Also indicated for ophthalmic use in the treatment of bacterial conjunctivitis and corneal ulcers.

Warnings: Has caused arthropathy and damage to weight-bearing joints in immature animals and its use in children under the age of 18, pregnant women, and women who are nursing is best avoided. Adverse reactions include nausea, headache, diarrhea, phototoxicity reactions and hypersensitivity reactions. May cause dizziness, lightheadedness, insomnia, and other central nervous system effects, and patients should know how they tolerate the drug before they engage in activities (e.g., driving) that require mental alertness and coordination.

Administration: Oral, intravenous, and ophthalmic. The drug should not be taken with food.

Preparations: Tablets, 200, 300, and 400

mg. Vials, 200 and 400 mg. Ophthalmic solution (Ocuflox), 0.3%.

OGEN®, see Estropipate

OLANZAPINE—Zyprexa®, Zydis®

Description/Actions: Antipsychotic. Indicated in the management of the manifestations of psychotic disorders.

Warnings: Use cautiously in cardio- or cerebrovascular disease, hypovolemia, dehydration, seizures, Alzheimer's disease, hepatic impairment, prostatic hypertrophy, narrow-angle glaucoma, history of paralytic ileus, breast cancer, patients at risk of aspiration pneumonia, and the elderly and debilitated. Adverse reactions include somnolence, dizziness, constipation, weight gain, personality disorder, akathisia, rhinitis, postural hypotension, tachycardia, headache, fever, abdominal pain, cough, pharyngitis, nervousness, joint pain, and peripheral edema. May cause tardive dyskinesia or neuroleptic malignant syndrome.

Administration: Initially 5–10 mg once daily. Increase to 10 mg once daily within several days. Thereafter adjust by 5 mg/day at intervals of 1 week. Maximum dose is 20 mg/day.

Preparations: Tablets, 2.5, 5, 7.5, 10, and 15 mg. Orally disintegrating tablets, 5, 10, 15, and 20 mg.

OLOPATADINE HYDROCHLORIDE—Patanol®

Description/Actions: Antiallergic agent indicated in temporary prevention of itching of the eye due to allergic conjunctivitis.

Warnings: Adverse reactions include headache, ocular effects (including burning/stinging, dry eye, foreign body sensation, hyperemia, keratitis, lid edema, pruritis), asthenia, cold syndrome, pharyngitis, rhinitis, sinusitis and taste perversion. Use proper instillation techniques, being careful not to contaminate the dropper tip. Not for use with contact lenses.

Administration: 1–2 drops in affected eye(s) twice daily at 6–8-hour intervals.

Preparations: 0.1% ophthalmic solution containing benzalkonium chloride.

OLUX, see Clobetasol propionate

OIL OF WINTERGREEN, see Methyl salicylate

OLSALAZINE SODIUM— Dipentum®

Agent for ulcerative colitis.

Description/Actions: Is converted in the colon into 2 molecules of 5-aminosalicylic acid (5-ASA, also known as mesalamine). Exhibits a topical anti-inflammatory action in the colon. Indicated for the maintenance of remission of ulcerative colitis in patients who are intolerant of sulfasalazine.

Warnings: Contraindicated in patients who are hypersensitive to the salicylates. Adverse reactions include diarrhea, abdominal pain or cramps, nausea, dyspepsia, bloating, headache, fatigue, depression, rash, and arthralgia. Use should be monitored closely in patients with impaired renal function.

Administration: Oral. Should be administered with food to reduce the possibility of GI adverse reactions.

Preparations: Capsules, 250 mg.

OMEPRAZOLE—Prilosec®

Antisecretory agent.

Description/Actions: Inhibits the enzyme system known as the acid or proton pump at the secretory surface of the gastric parietal cell. Blocks the final step of acid production and is a potent inhibitor of gastric acid secretion. Indicated for the short-term treatment (4–8 weeks) of symptomatic gastroesophageal reflux disease; the maintenance treatment of healed erosive esophagitis; the long-term treatment of pathological hypersecretory conditions (e.g. Zollinger-Ellison syndrome); and the short-term treatment of active duodenal ulcer. Also used in treatment of active duodenal ulcer accociated with *H. pylori* infection in combination with clarithromycin.

Warnings: Adverse reactions include headache, diarrhea, abdominal pain, and nausea.

Administration: Oral. The drug should be taken before eating and capsules should be swallowed whole and not be opened, chewed, or crushed.

Preparations: Delayed-release capsules, 10, 20, and 40 mg.

OMNICEF®, see Cefdinir

OMNIPEN®, see Ampicillin

ONCASPAR®, see Pegaspargase

ONCOVIN®, see Vincristine

ONDANSETRON HYDROCHLORIDE—Zofran®, Zofran ODT

Antiemetic.

Description/Actions: Is a selective blocking agent of the serotonin 5-HT$_3$ receptor type. Indicated for the prevention of nausea and vomiting associated with initial and repeat courses of emetogenic cancer chemotherapy, including high-dose cisplatin. Also indicated for the prevention of postoperative nausea and vomiting.

Warnings: Adverse reactions include diarrhea, headache, constipation, and elevations of hepatic enzyme levels.

Administration: Oral and intravenous.

Preparations: Tablets, 4 and 8 mg. Oral disintegrating tablets 4 and 8 mg. Oral solution, 4 mg/5 ml. Vials, 2 mg/ml in 2 ml single-dose vials and 20 ml multidose vials; 32 mg/50 ml (premixed) in single-dose containers.

ONTAK®, see Denileukin Diftitox

OPHTHAINE®, see Proparacaine

OPIUM

Analgesic, antitussive, and *antidiarrheal.*

Description/Actions: Mixture of alkaloids including morphine and codeine. Various formulations are used in the management of pain, cough, and diarrhea.

Preparations: Tincture, 10% (opium tincture, deodorized).

OPTIMINE®, see Azatadine

OPTIPRANOLOL® see Metipranolol

OPTIVAR®, see Azelastine

ORALET®, see Fentanyl citrate

ORAMORPH SR®, see Morphine sulfate

ORAP®, see Pimozide

ORATROL®, see Dichlorphenamide

ORETIC®, see Hydrochlorothiazide

ORETON METHYL®, see Methyltestosterone

ORGARAN®—Danaparoid sodium

ORINASE®, see Tolbutamide

ORLAAM®, see Levomethadyl acetate hydrochloride

ORLISTAT—Xenical®

Description/Actions: Orlistat works by

inhibiting the absorption of dietary fat. It is indicated as an adjunct to a reduced calorie diet in obesity management, including weight loss and weight maintenance, to reduce the risk of weight regain after loss. Use in patients with an initial body mass index of ≥ 30 kg/m2 or ≥ 27 kg/m2 in the presence of other risk factors(e.g., hypertension, diabetes, dyslipidemia).

Precautions/Adverse Reactions: Orlistat is contraindicated in chronic malabsorption syndrome and cholestasis. Use cautiously in hypertoxaluria and calcium oxolate nephrolithiasis. Weight loss may affect doses needed for antidiabetic drugs. Pregnancy Category B. Not recommended for use in nursing mothers.

Adverse reactions may include GI effects(oily spotting, flatus with discharge, fecal urgency, fatty/oily stools, oily evacuation, increased defecation, and fecal incontinence).

Administration: Adults—120 mg 3 times daily with each of the 3 main meals. Take during or up to 1 hour after meals. If a meal is missed or has no fat, the dose may be skipped.

Patient Care Implications: Instruct patients to eat a balanced reduced calorie diet with about 30% of calories from fat. Spread daily fat intake over 3 meals. GI side effects may decrease over time. Higher doses do not add benefit. Orlistat may reduce the absorption of fat soluble vitamins.

Preparations: Capsules, 120 mg.

ORNADE®, Combination of chlorpheniramine and phenylpropanolamine

ORPHENADRINE CITRATE— Norflex®

Description/Actions: Skeletal muscle relaxant indicated as an adjunct to rest, physical therapy, and other measures for the relief of discomfort associated with acute painful musculoskeletal conditions.

Preparations: Tablets, 100 mg. Ampules, 60 mg. Extended release tablets, 100 mg.

ORTHO-CEPT®, see Desogestrel/ ethinyl estradiol

ORTHO-CYCLEN®, see Norgestimate/ethinyl estradiol

ORTHO-EVRA™, see Ethinyl Estradiol and Norelgestromin

ORTHO-NOVUM®

Description/Actions: Oral contraceptive combination of ethinyl estradiol or mestranol with norethindrone.

ORTHO TRI-CYCLEN®, see Norgestimate/ethinyl estradiol

ORTHO TRI-CYCLEN LO®, see Norgestimate/Ethinyl Estradiol

ORTHOCLONE OKT3®, see Muromonab-CD3

ORUDIS®, see Ketoprofen

ORUVAIL®, see Ketoprofen

OS-CAL®, see Calcium carbonate

OSELTAMIVIR—Tamiflu®

Description/Actions: Oseltamivir acts as a neuraminidase inhibitor for the treatment of influenza A and B.

Precautions/Adverse Reactions: Oseltamivir dosage has to be adjusted in patients with renal impairment. Also, the drug should not be administered to children under 1, pregnant women, and breast-feeding women. The most common complaints are nausea and vomiting. Other common side effects are bronchitis, insomnia, vertigo, diarrhea, abdominal pain, dizziness, headache, cough, and fatigue.

Arrythmias, confusion, and seizures have also been reported.

Administrations: Oral.

Patient Care Implications: Oseltamivir dosage should be adjusted in patients with renal impairment. For patients with creatinine clearance of 10–30 ml/min the dosage should be reduced to 75 mg PO once a day for 5 days. The drug should not be administered to children under 18, pregnant women, and breast-feeding women.

Preparations: Tablet, 75 mg. Oral suspension, 12 mg/ml.

OSMITROL®, see Mannitol

OTRIVIN®, see Xylometazoline

OVRAL®

Description/Actions: Oral contraceptive combination of ethinyl estradiol and norgestrel.

OVRETTE®, see Norgestrel

OVULEN®

Description/Actions: Oral contraceptive combination of mestranol and ethynodiol diacetate.

OXACILLIN SODIUM—Prostaphlin®

Description/Actions: Penicillin antibiotic indicated in the treatment of staphylococcal infections.

Preparations: Capsules, 250 and 500 mg. Powder for oral solution, 250 mg/5 ml when reconstituted. Vials, 250 and 500 mg, 2, 4, and 10 g.

OXAMNIQUINE—Vansil®

Description/Actions: Antiparasitic agent indicated in the treatment of infections caused by *Schistosoma mansoni.*

Preparations: Capsules, 250 mg.

OXANDRIN®, see Oxandrolone

OXAPROZIN—Daypro®

Nonsteroidal anti-inflammatory drug.

Description/Actions: Inhibits prostaglandin synthesis and exhibits analgesic, anti-inflammatory, and antipyretic actions. Indicated for acute and long-term use in the management of osteoarthritis and rheumatoid arthritis.

Warnings: Contraindicated in patients with the syndrome of nasal polyps, angioedema, and bronchospastic reactivity to aspirin or another nonsteroidal anti-inflammatory drug. May cause gastrointestinal effects including nausea, dyspepsia, constipation, diarrhea, abdominal pain/distress, anorexia, flatulence, and vomiting. Use should be avoided in patients with active gastrointestinal tract disease and closely monitored in patients with a previous history of such disorders. Use is not recommended during the third trimester of pregnancy. May prolong bleeding time and concurrent use with warfarin should be closely monitored.

Administration: Oral.

Preparations: Caplets, 600 mg.

OXAZEPAM—Serax®

Benzodiazepine antianxiety agent.

Description/Actions: A CNS depressant indicated for the management of anxiety disorders or for the short-term relief of the symptoms of anxiety. Also useful in anxiety associated with depression and in alcoholics experiencing alcohol withdrawal.

Warnings: Adverse reactions include drowsiness and other CNS effects; patients should be cautioned regarding activities such as driving and operating machinery, as well as interactions with other CNS-acting drugs including alcohol. Can cause dependence and is included in Schedule IV.

Administration: Oral.

Preparations: Capsules and tablets, 10, 15, and 30 mg.

OXCARBAZEPINE—Trileptal®

Description/Actions: Oxcarbazepine is an antiepileptic/anticonvulsant indicated for use as monotherapy or adjunctive therapy in the treatment of partial seizures in adults with epilepsy.

Precautions/Adverse Reactions: Oxcarbazepine is contraindicated in patients with a hypersensitivity to oxcarbazepine or any component of the formulation. Its use has been associated with central nervous system–related adverse events, most of which were cognitive symptoms including psychomotor slowing, difficulty with concentration, speech or language problems, somnolence or fatigue, and coordination abnormalities, including ataxia and gait disturbances. Clinically significant hyponatremia can develop while on therapy; monitoring of serum sodium levels should be considered for patients during maintenance therapy. Use with caution in patients with previous hypersensitivity to carbamazepine—a cross-sensitivity occurs in 25–30%. Concurrent use with hormonal contraceptives may render this method of contraception less effective (nonhormonal contraceptive measures are recommended). Pregnancy Category C. There are no adequate well-controlled clinical studies in pregnant women; however, oxcarbazepine is closely structurally related to carbamazepine (teratogenic in humans). Should be used during pregnancy only if the potential benefit justifies the potential risk to the fetus. Oxcarbazepine and its active metabolite are excreted in human breast milk; the decision to utilize oxcarbazepine in nursing women must be based on the potential adverse effects in the nursing infant and take into account the importance of the drug to the mother. Some adverse effects are somnolence, headache, ataxia, fatigue, vertigo, vomiting, nausea, abdominal pain, tremor, dyspepsia, abnormal gait, hyponatremia, and diplopia.

Administration: Oral.

Patient Care Implications: Inform those patients who have exhibited hypersensitivity reactions to carbamazepine that there is the possibility (25–30%) of cross-sensitivity reactions with oxcarbazepine. Inform patients of childbearing age that hormonal contraceptives may be less effective while on oxcarbazepine (see precaution section). Use caution if alcohol is taken with oxcarbazepine, due to the possible additive sedative effects. Early in therapy it may cause dizziness and somnolence—advise patients not to drive or operative heavy machinery until they have gained experience on oxcarbazepine to determine if it will adversely affect their ability to drive or operate heavy machinery.

Preparations: Suspension, oral: 300 mg/5ml (250 ml). Tablet: 150 mg, 300 mg, 600 mg.

OXICONAZOLE NITRATE—Oxistat®

Imidazole antifungal agent.

Description/Actions: A topically applied antifungal agent that is indicated for the topical treatment of tinea pedis, tinea cruris, and tinea corporis.

Warnings: Adverse reactions include itching, burning, and irritation.

Administration: Topical.

Preparations: Cream, 1%. Lotion, 1%.

OXISTAT®, see Oxiconazole

OXSORALEN®, see Methoxsalen

OXSORALEN-ULTRA®, see Methoxsalen

OXTRIPHYLLINE—Choline theophyllinate, Choledyl®

Description/Actions: Bronchodilator indicated for relief of bronchial asthma and for reversible bronchospasm associated with chronic bronchitis and emphysema.

Preparations: Tablets, 100 and 200 mg. Syrup, 50 mg/5 ml. Elixir, 100 mg/5 ml.

OXYBENZONE

Description/Actions: Sunscreen used in combination with other agents in sunscreen formulations.

OXYBUTYNIN CHLORIDE—
Ditropan®, Ditropan XL®

Description/Actions: Antispasmodic indicated for the relief of symptoms associated with voiding in patients with uninhibited neurogenic and reflex neurogenic bladder. Also indicated in the treatment of nocturia, frequent urination, urgency, and incontinence.

Preparations: Tablets, 5 mg. Extended-release tablets, 5 and 10 mg. Syrup, 5 mg/5 ml.

OXYCODONE AND ACETAMINOPHEN

Description/Actions: Acetaminophen and oxycodone are used together to treat moderate to severe pain due to cancer, dental procedures, headache, back pain, arthralgias, and myalgias. The combination of these two drugs produces additive analgesia as compared to the same doses of either agent alone.

Precautions/Adverse Reactions: Acetaminophen-oxycodone should be used cautiously in patients with GI disease, including GI obstruction or ileus, uclerative colitis, or preexisting constipation. It should not be administered to patients who are hypersensitive to oxycodone or acctaminophen. Oxycodone is contraindicated in patients who have or are suspected of having paralytic ileus. Caution should also be used in patients with asthma or severe pulmonary disease, head trauma, cardiac arrhythmias, hypotension, hypovolemia, renal impairment, hepatic disease, or anemia. Oxycodone may cause psychologic dependence, which may lead to substance abuse in a small percentage of patients. Abrupt discontinuation of prolonged acetaminophen-oxycodone therapy can result in withdrawal symptoms. Patients should be tapered off gradually to avoid a withdrawal reaction. Adverse reactions include respiratory depression, GI effects, and hepatic and renal toxicity.

Administrations: Oral.

Preparations: Tablets, 2.5/325 mg, 5/325 mg, 5/500 mg, 7.5/325 mg, 7.5/500 mg, 10/325 mg, 10/650 mg. Capsules, 5/500 mg. Oral solution, 5 ml–5/325 mg.

OXYCODONE HYDROCHLORIDE—
Oxycontin®, Oxyfast®, Roxicodone®

OXYCODONE TEREPHTHALATE

Opioid analgesic.

Description/Actions: A centrally acting analgesic indicated for the relief of moderate to moderately severe pain.

Warnings: Adverse reactions include sedation and other CNS effects; patients should be cautioned regarding activities such as driving and operating machinery, as well as interactions with other CNS-acting drugs including alcohol. Other adverse reactions include constipation, nausea, and vomiting. Can cause dependence and formulations are covered under the provisions of the Controlled Substances Act.

Administration: Oral.

Preparations: Tablets, 5 mg. Controlled-release tablets, 10, 20, 40, and 80 mg. Solution, 5 mg/5 ml. Concentrated oral solution, 20 mg/ml.

OXYFAST®, see Oxycodone

OXYGEN

Description/Actions: Gas administered by inhalation in situations in which there is insufficient oxygen available to tissues.

Preparations: Gas

OXYMETAZOLINE HYDROCHLORIDE—Afrin®, Ocuclear®

Description/Actions: Decongestant administered topically in the form of nose drops or a nasal spray, and as an ophthalmic solution for the relief of redness of the eye due to minor eye irritations.

Preparations: Drops, 0.025%. Drops and spray, 0.05%.

OXYMETHOLONE—Anadrol-50®

Description/Actions: Anabolic steroid indicated in the treatment of anemias caused by deficient red cell production.

Preparations: Tablets, 50 mg.

OXYMORPHONE HYDROCHLORIDE— Numorphan®

Description/Actions: Opioid analgesic indicated for parenteral and rectal use for the relief of moderate to severe pain.

Preparations: Ampules and vials, 1 mg/ml and 1.5 mg/ml. Suppositories, 5 mg.

OXYTETRACYCLINE HYDROCHLORIDE— Terramycin®

Description/Actions: Tetracycline antibiotic indicated for the treatment of infections caused by susceptible organisms.

Preparations: Capsules, 250 mg. Ampules and vials (for intramuscular use), 50 mg/ml and 125 mg/ml. Formulations also including polymyxin B sulfate are used topically for the treatment of ocular, dermatologic, and vaginal infections.

OXYTOCIN—Pitocin®, Syntocinon®

Description/Actions: Oxytocic hormone indicated for parenteral use to initiate or improve uterine contractions (e.g., when it is desirable to induce labor), and to produce uterine contractions during the third stage of labor and to control postpartum bleeding or hemorrhage. Also used in the form of a nasal spray for initial milk letdown.

Preparations: Ampules, 5 and 10 units. Vials, 10 units/ml. Syringes, 10 units. Nasal spray, 40 units/ml.

P

PABA, see Para-aminobenzoic acid

PACLITAXEL—Taxol®

Antineoplastic agent.

Description/Actions: Indicated for the treatment of metastatic carcinoma of the ovary and metastatic carcinoma of the breast, after failure of first-line or subsequent chemotherapy.

Warnings: Contraindicated in patients who are hypersensitive to the drug or to polyoxyethylated castor oil (Cremophor EL—a solubilizing agent included in the formulation), and in patients with a history of such reactions to other drugs that are available in formulations containing polyoxyethylated castor oil. Is also contraindicated in patients with baseline neutropenia of < 1500 cells/mm3. May cause myelosuppression (neutropenia, thrombocytopenia, anemia) and the resultant risks of infection and bleeding; frequent peripheral blood counts should be performed. Therapy must be closely monitored when other drugs causing myelosuppression are used concurrently or sequentially. Use has been associated with a high incidence of hypersensitivity reactions, and patients should be premedicated with a corticosteroid (e.g., dexamethasone), antihistamine (e.g., diphenhydramine), and a histamine H_2-receptor antagonist (e.g., cimetidine). Other adverse reactions include peripheral neuropathy, hypotension, bradycardia, severe conduction abnormalities, arthralgia/myalgia, nausea, vomiting, diarrhea, mucositis, alopecia, and hepatic effects. Metabolism may be inhibited by the concurrent administration of ketoconazole. Women of childbearing potential should be advised to avoid becoming pregnant during treatment with the drug.

Administration: The concentrated solution of paclitaxel may extract the plasticizer DEHP from plasticized polyvinyl chloride (PVC) equipment or devices used to prepare solutions for infusion. Contact of the concentrate with such equipment or devices is not recommended, and diluted solutions should be stored in bottles (glass, polypropylene) or plastic bags (polypropylene, polyolefin) and administered through polyethylene-lined administration sets. The diluted solution should be administered through an in-line filter with a microporous membrane not greater than 0.22 microns. Gloves should be worn when handling and preparing the solutions.

Preparations: Vials, 30 mg/5 ml (paclitaxel concentrate).

PALIVIZUMAB—Synagis®

Description/Actions: Palivizumab is an immunomodulator (antiviral monoclonal antibody) indicated in the prevention of serious lower respiratory tract infections caused by respiratory syncytial virus (RSV) in pediatric patients at high risk for RSV disease. RSV disease is the leading cause of pneumonia and bronchiolitis in infants.

Precautions/Adverse Reactions: Anaphylaxis and anaphylactoid reactions have occurred during therapy with palivizumab.

Have epinephrine available for treatment of acute allergic reactions.

Adverse reactions include vomiting, diarrhea, local reactions, erythma, upper respiratory infections, otitis media, rhinitis, rash, pain, hernia, SGOT increases, and pharyngitis.

Administration: Give by IM injection in the anterolateral thigh.

Patient Care Implications: Do not administer in the gluteal muscle because of the risk of sciatic nerve damage. Volumes of over 1 ml should be administered in divided doses. The 1st dose should be administered prior to the start of the season. Patients should continue to receive the medication throughout the season including those who contract RSV. This product is not indicated for the treatment of established RSV. As with all IM injections caution should be used when administering to patients with coagulation disorders.

Preparations: Vial, 50 mg for injection after reconstitution.

PAMELOR®, see Nortriptyline

PAMIDRONATE DISODIUM—Aredia®

Agent for hypercalcemia of malignancy and Paget's disease.

Description/Actions: Inhibits bone resorption; adsorbs to calcium phosphate in bone and may directly block dissolution of this mineral component of bone. Indicated in conjunction with adequate hydration (to restore the urine output to about 2 liters per day) for the treatment of moderate or severe hypercalcemia associated with malignancy, with or without bone metastases. Also indicated for the treatment of Paget's disease and management of osteolytic bone lesions associated with multiple myeloma.

Warnings: Contraindicated in patients who are hypersensitive to the drug or to etidronate. Adverse reactions include low-grade fever, infusion site reactions (redness, swelling, pain), fluid overload, generalized pain, hypertension, abdominal pain, anorexia, constipation, nausea, vomiting, urinary tract infection, bone pain, anemia, hypokalemia, hypomagnesemia, and hypophosphatemia. Serum calcium, electrolytes, phosphate, magnesium, and creatinine, and complete blood count, differential, and hematocrit/ hemoglobin must be closely monitored.

Administration: Intravenous infusion. Should not be mixed with calcium-containing infusion solutions. Adult dose: Moderate hypercalcemia of malignancy (corrected serum calcium of approximately 12–13.5 mg/dl)—60–90 mg given as a single dose, intravenous infusion over 2–24 hours. Severe hypercalcemia of malignancy (corrected serum calcium > 13.5 mg/dl)—90 mg given as a single-dose, intravenous infusion over 2–24 hours. Infusions > 2 hours may reduce the risk for renal toxicity, especially in patients with pre-existing renal insufficiency.

Preparations: Vials, 30, 60, and 90 mg.

PAMINE®, see Methscopolamine

PANADOL®, see Acetaminophen

PANCREASE®, see Pancrelipase

PANCRECARB MS-8®—
 Pancreatic Enzymes—Lipase 8000 units, amylase 40,000 units, protease 45,000 units

PANCREATIN

Description/Actions: Digestive enzyme often used in combination with other agents as a digestive aid.

PANCRELIPASE—Pancrease®, Viokase®, Zymase®

Description/Actions: Digestive enzyme representing a standardized pancreatic enzyme concentrate that is indicated as a digestive aid in the treatment of disorders associated with pancreatic insufficiency.

Preparations: Capsules, tablets, and powder.

PANCURONIUM BROMIDE—
 Pavulon®

Description/Actions: Nondepolarizing neuromuscular blocking agent indicated for parenteral use as an adjunct to general anesthesia, to facilitate tracheal intubation, and to provide skeletal muscle relaxation during surgery or mechanical ventilation.

Preparations: Ampules and vials, 1 mg/ ml and 2 mg/ml.

PANDEL®, see Hydrocortisone

PANMYCIN®, see Tetracycline

PANTOPRAZOLE SODIUM—
 Protonix

Description/Actions: Proton pump inhibitor indicated in the short-term treatment (up to 8 weeks) of erosive esophagitis associated with gastroesophageal reflux disease (GERD). For those patients who have not healed after 8 weeks of therapy, an additional 8-week course of Protonix may be considered.

Precautions/Adverse Reactions: The safety and efficacy of Protonix for maintenance therapy (e.g., beyond 16 weeks) have not been established. Protonix is contraindicated in patients with known hypersensitivity to any component of the formulation. Adverse effects include headache, diarrhea, flatulence, abdominal pain, rash, eructation, insomnia, and hyperglycemia.

Administrations: Intravenous and oral.

Patient Care Implications: Protonix delayed-release tablets should be swallowed whole, with or without food in the stomach. Patients should be cautioned that tablets should not be split, chewed, or crushed. Use in-line filter for intravenous administration.

Preparations: Delayed-release tablets, 20 and 40 mg. Powder for injection, 40 mg.

PAPAVERINE HYDROCHLORIDE—Pavabid®

Description/Actions: Vasodilator indicated for the relief of cerebral and peripheral ischemia associated with arterial spasm and myocardial ischemia complicated by arrhythmias.

Preparations: Tablets, 30, 60, 100, 200, and 300 mg. Controlled-release capsules, 150 mg. Ampules, 30 mg/ml.

PARA-AMINOBENZOIC ACID— PABA, Potaba®

Description/Actions: Has been used orally in the treatment of conditions such as scleroderma, dermatomyositis, and Peyronie's disease, and topically as a sunscreen and protectant.

Preparations: Capsules and tablets (as the potassium salt), 500 mg. Packets (as the potassium salt), 2 g. Powder.

PARA-AMINOSALICYLIC ACID, see Aminosalicylate sodium.

PARAFLEX®, see Chlorzoxazone

PARAFON FORTE DSC®, see Chlorzoxazone

PARALDEHYDE

Description/Actions: **Sedative-hypnotic and anticonvulsant** used in some patients with delirium tremens and other psychiatric states characterized by excitement. Has been used in the emergency treatment of tetanus, eclampsia, and status epilepticus.

Preparations: Liquid that has been administered orally and rectally. Ampules and vials, 1 g/ml.

PARAMETHADIONE

Description/Actions: **Anticonvulsant** indicated for the control of absence (petit mal) seizures that are refractory to treatment with other drugs.

Preparations: Capsules, 150 and 300 mg. Oral solution, 300 mg/ml.

PARAPLATIN®, see Carboplatin

PAREGORIC—Camphorated opium tincture

Description/Actions: **Analgesic and antidiarrheal.** Contains opium alkaloids and is used in the treatment of diarrhea and in conditions associated with pain.

Preparations: Liquid containing the equivalent of 2 mg of morphine per 5 ml.

PARICALCITOL—Zemplar®

Description/Actions: Paricalcitol is a synthetic vitamin D analogue. Vitamin D and paricalcitol have been shown to reduce parathyroid levels. Paricalcitol is indicated for the prevention and treatment of secondary hyperparathyroidism associated with chronic renal failure.

Precautions/Adverse Reactions: Paricalcitol should not be administered to patients with evidence of vitamin D toxicity, hypercalcemia, or with hypersensitivity to any of the components of this product.

Adverse reactions include chills, sepsis, palpitation, nausea, edema, and pneumonia.

Administration: Intravenous.

Patient Care Implications: Instruct patients about the importance of adhering to a dietary regimen of calcium supplementation and phosphorous restriction. Teach patients about the necessity of frequent follow-up blood work to ensure proper dosing of the drug is achieved.

Preparations: Vial, 5 mcg/ml.

PARLODEL®, see Bromocriptine

PARNATE®, see Tranylcypromine

PAROMOMYCIN SULFATE—Humatin®

Description/Actions: Anti-infective agent indicated in the treatment of intestinal amebiasis. Has also been used as adjunctive therapy in the management of hepatic coma.

Preparations: Capsules, 250 mg.

PAROXETINE HYDROCHLORIDE—Paxil®, Paxil CR

Antidepressant.

Description/Actions: Is a selective serotonin reuptake inhibitor. Indicated for the treatment of depression, panic disorders, social anxiety disorders, obsessive-compulsive disorders, and post-traumatic stress disorders.

Warnings: Contraindicated in patients taking a monoamine oxidase inhibitor (MAOI) or thioridazine. Adverse reactions include nausea, dry mouth, asthenia, somnolence, dizziness, insomnia, tremor, nervousness, sweating, ejaculatory disturbance, and other male genital disorders. May decrease appetite resulting in weight loss. Should not be used concomitantly with an MAOI, or during either the 14-day period following discontinuation of treatment with a MAOI or the 14-day period preceding initiation of treatment with a MAOI. Concomitant use with tryptophan is not recommended. Dosage should be tapered prior to discontinuation of therapy.

Administration: Oral, usually in the morning to reduce the possibility of insomnia.

Preparations: Tablets, 20 and 30 mg. Suspension 10 mg/5 ml, controlled-release tablet, 12.5, 25, and 37.5 mg.

PARSIDOL®, see Ethopropazine

PAS, see Aminosalicylate sodium

PATANOL®—see Olopatadine hydrochloride

PATHILON®, see Tridihexethyl chloride

PATHOCIL®, see Dicloxacillin

PAVABID®, see Papaverine

PAVULON®, see Pancuronium

PAXAREL®, see Acetylcarbromal

PAXIL®, see Paroxetine hydrochloride

PAXIL®, CR™, see Paroxetine hydrochloride

PAXIPAM®, see Halazepam

PBZ®, see Tripelennamine

PCE®, see Erythromycin base

PECTIN

Adsorbent used in combination with agents such as kaolin for the treatment of diarrhea.

PEDAMETH®, see Methionine

PEDIALYTE®

Description/Actions: Fluid and electrolyte replacement. A liter contains dextrose 25 g (fructose 5 g, in fruit flavors), sodium 45 mEq, potassium 20 mEq, chloride 35 mEq. Citrate 30 mEq with 100 calories.

Preparations: Liquid and freezer pops.

PEDIAZOLE®, Combination of erythromycin ethylsuccinate and sulfisoxazole

PEG, see Polyethylene glycol

PEGADEMASE BOVINE—Adagen®

Enzyme for replacement therapy.

Description/Actions: Also known as PEG-ADA, is prepared by attaching numerous strands of polyethylene glycol (PEG) to adenosine deaminase (ADA) of bovine origin. Indicated for enzyme replacement therapy for ADA deficiency in patients with severe combined immunodeficiency disease (SCID) who are not suitable candidates for—or who have failed—bone marrow transplantation.

Warnings: Contraindicated in patients with severe thrombocytopenia. Adverse reactions include headache and pain at injection site.

Administration: Intramuscular.

Preparations: Vials, 250 units/ml.

PEGANONE®, see Ethotoin

PEGASPARGASE—Oncaspar®

Antineoplastic agent.

Description/Actions: Is a modified form of L-asparaginase (derived from *E. coli*) that is produced by conjugating units of monomethoxypolyethylene glycol (PEG) to the enzyme. Causes a rapid depletion of asparagine resulting in the destruction of leukemic cells that are unable to synthesize asparagine. Indicated for patients with acute lymphoblastic leukemia who require L-asparaginase in their treatment regimen, but have developed hypersensitivity to the native forms of L-asparaginase. Is generally used in combination with other chemotherapeutic agents.

Warnings: Contraindicated in patients with a history of pancreatitis or who have had significant hemorrhagic events associated with prior asparaginase therapy. Is less likely than asparaginase to cause hypersensitivity reactions but may cause immediate and life-threatening anaphylaxis. May cause pancreatitis, and frequent serum amylase determinations should be obtained to detect early evidence of pancreatitis. Thrombosis may occur, and, if possible, the concurrent use of other drugs that may increase the risk of bleeding (e.g., warfarin, aspirin, NSAIDs) should be avoided. Other adverse reactions include hyperglycemia, liver function abnormalities, nausea, vomiting, fever, and malaise.

Administration: Intravenous or intramuscular. The IM route is preferred because of a lower risk of serious hypersensitivity and other adverse reactions. When administered IM, the volume of a single injection should be limited to 2 ml. When administered IV, should be given over a period of 1–2 hours in 100 ml of sodium chloride or dextrose injection 5%, through an infusion that is already running. The vials should not be shaken.

Preparations: Vials, 3,750 IU in 5 ml.

PEMIROLAST—Alamast®

Description/Actions: Pemirolast is used for the relief of ophthalmic pruritus due to allergic conjunctivitis.

Precautions/Adverse Reactions: The most frequent adverse effects associated with pemirolast ophthalmic solution were generally mild and included headache, rhinitis, cold/flu symptoms, burning, dry eye, foreign body sensation, and ocular discomfort. Other, nonocular adverse events included were back pain, bronchitis, cough, dysmenorrhea, fever, sneezing, nasal congestion, and sinusitis.

Administration: Adults: 1–2 drops in each affected eye 4 times daily for up to 4 weeks.

Patient Care Implications: Do not touch the eyelids or surrounding areas with the dropper tip to prevent contamination of the dropper tip and solution.

Keep the bottle tightly closed when not in use.

Patients should not wear contact lens if their eye is red. Patients should wait at least 10 minutes after instilling Alamast before they insert their contact lenses.

Preparations: 0.1% ophthalmic solution, in 10 ml dropper bottles.

PEMOLINE—Cylert®

Description/Actions: Central nervous system stimulant indicated in the treatment of attention-deficit disorder.

Preparations: Tablets, 18.75, 37.5, and 75 mg. Chewable tablets, 37.5 mg.

PENBUTOLOL SULFATE— Levatol®

Antihypertensive agent.

Description/Actions: A nonselective beta-adrenergic-blocking agent with mild intrinsic sympathomimetic activity. Indicated in the treatment of hypertension.

Warnings: Contraindicated in patients with bronchial asthma, cardiogenic shock, severe bradycardia, and second- and third- degree atrioventricular conduction block. Adverse reactions include headache, dizziness, fatigue, and nausea. Use is best avoided in patients with bronchospastic diseases, and therapy in diabetic patients must be closely monitored.

Administration: Oral. Patients should be cautioned about the interruption or discontinuation of therapy; exacerbation of angina pectoris has occurred following the abrupt cessation of therapy, and, when therapy is to be discontinued, the dosage should be gradually reduced over a period of 1 to 2 weeks.

Preparations: Tablets, 20 mg.

PENCICLOVIR—Denavir®

Description/Actions: Antiviral agent indicated for the treatment of topical recurrent herpes simplex labialis (cold sores) on the lips and face in adults. Topical cream form of the active component of the oral antiviral prodrug famciclovir.

Warnings: Contraindicated in patients with previous and significant adverse reactions to famciclovir. Do not use on mucous membranes or near eyes. Use cautiously in the immunocompromised patient. Adverse reactions include headache and mild skin irritation.

Administrations: Apply every 2 hours while awake for 4 days. Begin treatment at earliest sign or symptom (i.e., during prodrome or when lesions appear). Only to be used on lips and face.

Preparations: 1% cream.

PENETREX®, see Enoxacin

PENICILLAMINE—Cuprimine®, Depen®

Description/Actions: Chelating agent indicated in the treatment of Wilson's disease, cystinuria, and in patients with severe, active rheumatoid arthritis who have failed to respond to an adequate trial of conventional therapy.

Preparations: Capsules and tablets, 125 and 250 mg.

PENICILLIN G POTASSIUM

Penicillin antibiotic.

Actions and Uses: Is active against gram-positive and gram-negative cocci, gram-positive and selected gram-negative bacilli, and certain spirochetes.

Warnings: Contraindicated in patients with a history of allergic reaction to any of the penicillins. Adverse reactions include hypersensitivity reactions.

Administration: Intravenous, intramuscular, and oral.

Preparations: Tablets, 200,000, 250,000 and 400,000 units. Oral solution, 400,000 units/5 ml. Vials, 200,000, 500,000, 1, 5, 10, and 20 million units.

PENICILLIN G SODIUM

Preparations: Vials, 5 million units.

PENICILLIN V POTASSIUM— Beepen VK®, Betapen VK®, Ledercillin VK®, Pen-Vee K®, V-Cillin K®, Veetids®

248 • PENLAC NAIL LACQUER®

Penicillin antibiotic.

Description/Actions: Is primarily active against gram-positive bacteria and is commonly used in conditions such as respiratory tract infections caused by susceptible organisms (e.g., streptococci).

Warnings: Contraindicated in patients with a history of allergic reaction to any of the penicillins. Adverse reactions include hypersensitivity reactions, rash, and nausea.

Administration: Oral. May be administered without regard to meals.

Preparations: Solution, 125 mg/5 ml.

PENLAC NAIL LACQUER®, see Cicloprox

PENTAERYTHRITOL TETRANITRATE

Description/Actions: Antianginal agent used in the prophylactic treatment of angina pectoris.

Preparations: Tablets, 10, 20, and 40 mg. Controlled-release tablets, 80 mg.

PENTAGASTRIN—Peptavlon®

Description/Actions: Diagnostic agent for evaluation of gastric acid secretory function.

Preparations: Ampules, 0.25 mg/ml.

PENTAM 300®, see Pentamidine isethionate

PENTAMIDINE ISETHIONATE—
NebuPent®, Pentam 300®

Description/Actions: Antiprotozoal agent indicated for parenteral use in the treatment of *Pneumocystis carinii* pneumonia and for use via inhalation in the prevention of *Pneumocystis carinii* pneumonia in high-risk human immunodeficiency virus (HIV)–infected patients.

Preparations: Vials, 300 mg. Vials for aerosol use, 300 mg.

PENTASA®, see Mesalamine

PENTAZOCINE—Talwin®

Description/Actions: Opioid agonist-antagonist analgesic indicated for the relief of moderate to severe pain, as an analgesic during labor, as a sedative prior to surgery, and as a supplement in balanced anesthesia.

Preparations: Tablets (as the hydrochloride with naloxone hydrochloride), 50 mg (Talwin Nx®). Ampules, vials, and syringes (as the lactate), 30 mg/ml.

PENTAZOCINE HYDROCHLORIDE AND ACETAMINOPHEN—Talacen®

Description/Actions: Acetaminophen and pentazocine are used together to treat mild to moderate pain. This combination produces a greater analgesic effect than when either is used alone. Also, this combination might cause fewer adverse reactions than do equianalgesic doses of either agent alone.

Precautions/Adverse Reactions: Pentazocine is not recommended for use in the elderly due to the potential for increased CNS side effects, such as confusion and hallucinations. Adverse effects are those of the individual drug components.

Administration: Oral.

Preparations: Caplets and tablets, pentazocine 25 mg/acetaminophen 650 mg.

PENTHRANE®, see Methoxyflurane

PENTOBARBITAL SODIUM—
Nembutal®

Description/Actions: Barbiturate sedative-hypnotic used in the management of anxiety and insomnia. Also used parenterally as a preanesthetic medication and for the emergency control of acute convulsive episodes.

Preparations: Capsules, 50 and 100 mg. Elixir, pentobarbital acid equivalent to 20 mg of the sodium salt/5 ml. Suppositories, 30, 60, 120, and 200 mg. Vials and syringes, 50 mg/ml.

PENTOSAN POLYSULFATE SODIUM—Elmiron®

Description/Actions: Bladder protectant indicated in relief of bladder pain or discomfort associated with interstitial cystitis. A semisynthetic, low molecular weight, heparinlike compound that exerts both anticoagulant and fibrinolytic effects.

Warnings: Use cautiously in bleeding disorders or conditions associated with an increased risk of bleeding (e.g., surgery, coagulopathy, aneurysm, hemophilia, GI ulceration, polyps, diverticulitis), in patients with a history of heparin-induced thrombocytopenia, hepatic insufficiency, and splenic disorders. Additive effects may be expected when administered with other anticoagulant drugs, such as warfarin or heparin, and possible similar effects when administered with aspirin or thrombolytics. Adverse reactions include alopecia, GI disturbances, headache, rash, abdominal pain, liver function abnormalities, dizziness, hemorrhage, or increased bleeding times.

Administration: Take 1 hour before or 2 hours after meals with water, 100 mg 3 times daily. Reevaluate symptoms at 3 and 6 months.

Preparations: Capsules, 100 mg.

PENTOSTATIN—Nipent®

Antineoplastic agent.

Description/Actions: Indicated as a single agent treatment for adult patients with alpha-interferon-refractory hairy cell leukemia.

Warnings: May cause myelosuppression (e.g., neutropenia), and, in patients with infections, efforts should be made to control the infection before treatment is initiated or resumed. Other adverse reactions include gastrointestinal effects (e.g., nausea, vomiting, anorexia, diarrhea), respiratory effects (e.g., increased cough, upper respiratory infection), nervous system effects (e.g., fatigue, neurologic disorders), fever, infection, pain, elevated hepatic function tests, genitourinary disorders, headache, allergic reactions, chills, myalgia, and rash. May cause fetal harm if administered during pregnancy. Concurrent use with fludarabine phosphate is not recommended because of the risk of pulmonary toxicity.

Administration: Intravenous.

Preparations: Vials, 10 mg.

PENTOTHAL®, see Thiopental

PENTOXIFYLLINE—Trental®

Hemorrheologic agent.

Description/Actions: A xanthine derivative that decreases the viscosity and improves the flow properties of blood. Indicated for the treatment of intermittent claudication on the basis of chronic occlusive arterial disease of the limbs.

Warnings: Contraindicated in patients who have previously exhibited intolerance to a xanthine derivative (e.g., caffeine, theophylline). Adverse reactions include nausea.

Administration: Oral.

Preparations: Controlled-release tablets, 400 mg.

PEN-VEE K®, see Penicillin V potassium

PEPCID®, see Famotidine

PEPCID AC®, see Famotidine

PEPCID RFD®, see Famotidine

PEPTAVLON®, see Pentagastrin

PEPTO-BISMOL®, see Bismuth subsalicylate

PERCOCET®, Combination of oxycodone and acetaminophen

PERCODAN®, Combination of oxycodone and aspirin

PERGOLIDE MESYLATE—Permax®

Antiparkinson agent.

Description/Actions: An ergot derivative that acts by stimulating dopamine receptors. Indicated as an adjunctive treatment to levodopa/carbidopa in the management of Parkinson's disease.

Warnings: Adverse reactions include dyskinesia, dizziness, hallucinations, fatigue, insomnia, nausea, constipation, diarrhea, dyspepsia, rhinitis, and orthostatic hypotension. Effectiveness may be decreased by dopamine antagonists (e.g., phenothiazines, haloperidol) or metoclopramide.

Administration: Oral.

Preparations: Tablets, 0.05, 0.25, and 1 mg.

PERGONAL®, see Menotropins

PERIACTIN®, see Cyproheptadine

PERIDEX®, see Chlorhexidine gluconate

PERMAPEN®, see Benzathine penicillin G

PERMAX®, see Pergolide

PERMETHRIN—Elimite®, Nix®

Pediculicide and scabicide.

Description/Actions: A synthetic pyrethroid that is indicated for the single-application treatment of infestation with *Pediculus humanus* var. *capitis* (the head louse) and its nits (eggs), and for the single-application treatment of scabies. Also indicated for prophylaxis during epidemic (20% of an institutional population are infected or immediate household contacts).

Warnings: Contraindicated in patients with a known hypersensitivity to any synthetic pyrethroid or pyrethrin, or to chrysanthemums. Adverse reactions include itching, mild burning or stinging, tingling, numbness, or scalp rash.

Administration: Topical.

Preparations: Cream, 5%. Cream rinse, 1% (for head lice infestation). Lotion, 1%.

PERMITIL®, see Fluphenazine

PEROXIDE, see Hydrogen peroxide

PERPHENAZINE—Trilafon®

Description/Actions: Phenothiazine antipsychotic agent and antiemetic.

Preparations: Tablets, 2, 4, 8, and 16 mg. Controlled-release tablets, 8 mg. Oral concentrate, 16 mg/5 ml. Ampules, 5 mg/ml.

PERSANTINE®, see Dipyridamole

PERSANTINE IV®, see Dipyridamole

PERTOFRANE®, see Desipramine

PERUVIAN BALSAM

Description/Actions: Local irritant used topically in various dermatologic disorders.

PETROLATUM

Description/Actions: Ointment base used as a vehicle for various topically applied medications. Sometimes used topically as a protective agent.

PHAZYME®, see Simethicone

PHENACEMIDE—Phenurone®

Description/Actions: Anticonvulsant indicated for the control of severe epilepsy, particularly mixed forms of complex partial (psychomotor) seizures, refractory to other drugs.

Preparations: Tablets, 500 mg.

PHENAZOPYRIDINE HYDROCHLORIDE—Azo-Standard®, Pyridium®

Description/Actions: Urinary tract analgesic indicated for the symptomatic relief of pain, burning, urgency, frequency, and other discomforts arising from irritation of the lower urinary tract mucosa. Causes a reddish orange discoloration of the urine and patients should be advised of this effect.

Preparations: Tablets, 100 and 200 mg.

PHENDIMETRAZINE TARTRATE—Bontril®

Description/Actions: Anorexiant indicated in the management of exogenous obesity as a short-term adjunct in a regimen of weight reduction based on caloric restriction.

Preparations: Capsules and tablets, 35 mg. Controlled-release capsules, 105 mg.

PHENELZINE SULFATE—Nardil®

Description/Actions: Monoamine oxidase inhibitor indicated for the treatment of depression.

Preparations: Tablets, 15 mg.

PHENERGAN®, see Promethazine

PHENINDAMINE TARTRATE—Nolahist®

Description/Actions: Antihistamine indicated in the management of allergic disorders.

Preparations: Tablets, 25 mg.

PHENIRAMINE MALEATE

Description/Actions: Antihistamine used in combination with other agents in the management of allergic and related disorders.

PHENOBARBITAL

PHENOBARBITAL SODIUM— Luminal sodium®

Barbiturate sedative, hypnotic, and anticonvulsant.

Description/Actions: A CNS depressant indicated (1) for anxiety-tension states, (2) for insomnia, (3) as a long-term anticonvulsant for the treatment of tonic-clonic and cortical focal seizures, (4) in the symptomatic control of acute convulsions (e.g., tetanus, status epilepticus), (5) as a preanesthetic sedative, and (6) in other situations associated with anxiety.

Warnings: Adverse reactions include drowsiness and other CNS effects; patients should be cautioned regarding activities such as driving and operating machinery, as well as interactions with other CNS-acting drugs including alcohol. Can cause dependence and is included in Schedule IV.

Administration: Oral, intravenous, and intramuscular.

Preparations: Tablets, 8, 15, 30, 60, and 100 mg. Capsules, 15 mg. Elixir, 20 mg/5 ml. Injection dosage forms (phenobarbital sodium), 30, 60, 65, and 130 mg/ml.

PHENOL—Carbolic acid

Description/Actions: Antipruritic, topical anesthetic, antiseptic, and caustic. Used topically in the management of various dermatologic conditions, and in certain other formulations (e.g., throat lozenges, mouthwashes, and gargles) that are utilized for a local effect.

Preparations: Solutions and lotions (with other agents for dermatologic use), 0.5–1%. Liquefied phenol is phenol maintained in a liquid condition by the presence of 10% water; is used as a source of phenol for preparing various formulations.

PHENOLSULFONPHTHALEIN

Description/Actions: Diagnostic agent used in evaluating renal function.

Preparations: Ampules, 6 mg/ml.

PHENOXYBENZAMINE HYDROCHLORIDE—Dibenzyline®

Description/Actions: Alpha-adrenergic receptor–blocking agent indicated in the management of pheochromocytoma to control episodes of hypertension and sweating.

Preparations: Capsules, 10 mg.

PHENSUXIMIDE—Milontin®

Description/Actions: Anticonvulsant indicated for the control of absence (petit mal) seizures in conjunction with other anticonvulsants when other forms of epilepsy coexist with petit mal.

Preparations: Capsules, 500 mg.

PHENTERMINE—Adipex®, Fastin®, Ionamin®

Description/Actions: Anorexiant indicated in the management of exogenous obesity as a short-term adjunct in a regimen of weight reduction based on caloric restriction.

Warnings: Contraindicated in atherosclerosis, cardiovascular disease, hypertension, hyperthyroidism, glaucoma, agitation, drug or alcohol abuse, during or within 14 days of MAOIs. Discontinue if dyspnea, angina pectoris, syncope, lower extremity edema, or other symptoms of primary pulmonary hypertension occur. Discontinue after a few weeks as tolerance to anorectic effect occurs. Use cautiously in diabetes. Prescribe limited supply to prevent overdose. Pregnancy Category C. Use in nursing mothers not recommended.

Adverse Reactions: CNS overstimulation, dizziness, palpitation, psychosis, dry mouth, GI disturbance, urticaria, impotence, primary pulmonary hypertension, and/or regurgitant cardiac valvular disease.

Preparations: Capsules and tablets (as the hydrochloride), 8, 15, 30, and 37.5 mg. Capsules (as the resin complex), 15 and 30 mg.

PHENTOLAMINE MESYLATE—Regitine®

Description/Actions: Alpha-adrenergic–blocking agent indicated for parenteral use to prevent or control hypertensive episodes in patients with pheochromocytoma, for the prevention or treatment of dermal necrosis and sloughing following intravenous administration or extravasation of norepinephrine, and for the diagnosis of pheochromocytoma.

Preparations: Vials, 5 mg.

PHENURONE®, see Phenacemide

PHENYLEPHRINE HYDROCHLORIDE—Neo-Synephrine®

Description/Actions: Used topically in the management of nasal congestion, and in ocular conditions in which decongestant and vasoconstrictor actions are needed. Included as a decongestant in combination with other agents in orally administered formulations. Also used parenterally in the treatment of vascular failure in shock, shocklike states, drug-induced hypotension, or hypersensitivity. Is also utilized parenterally to overcome paroxysmal supraventricular tachycardia, to prolong spinal anesthesia, and as a vasoconstrictor in regional analgesia.

Preparations: Nasal drops and spray, 0.125%, 0.25%, 0.5%, and 1%. Nasal jelly, 0.5%. Ophthalmic solution, 0.12%, 2.5%, and 10%. Ampules, 1%. Injection, 10 mg/ml.

PHENYLTOLOXAMINE CITRATE

Description/Actions: Antihistamine used in combination with other agents in the management of allergic and related disorders.

PHENYTOIN—Dilantin®

Anticonvulsant.

Description/Actions: Indicated for the control of tonic-clonic and psychomotor (grand mal and temporal lobe) seizures, and prevention and treatment of seizures occurring during or following neurosurgery. Also indicated for parenteral administration in the control of status epilepticus of the grand mal type. Has also been used intravenously in the management of certain arrhythmias (e.g., digitalis-induced arrhythmias), and orally in the treatment of trigeminal neuralgia.

Warnings: Adverse reactions include nystagmus, ataxia, slurred speech, confusion, nausea, vomiting, rash, gingival hyperplasia, hirsutism, and hematologic effects. Effect may be reduced by chronic alcohol abuse and products containing calcium ions (e.g., antacids).

Administration: Oral, intravenous, and intramuscular. Oral formulations containing phenytoin sodium, extended may be used for once-a-day dosing. When therapy is to be discontinued, it should be done so gradually as the abrupt withdrawal of therapy in epileptic patients may precipitate status epilepticus.

Preparations: Capsules (phenytoin sodium, extended), 30 and 100 mg. Chewable infatabs, 50 mg. Oral suspension, 30 and 125 mg/5 ml.

PHISOHEX®, see Hexachlorophene

PhosLo®, see Calcium acetate

PHOSPHALGEL®, see Aluminum phosphate gel

PHOSPHOLINE IODIDE®, see Echothiophate iodide

PHOTOPLEX®, see Butyl methoxydibenzoylmethane/ padimate O

PHYLLOCONTIN®, see Aminophylline

PHYSOSTIGMINE—Eserine, Antilirium®

Description/Actions: Cholinesterase inhibitor indicated for ophthalmic use in the treatment of glaucoma, and for parenteral use to reverse the central nervous system effects caused by excessive dosages of anticholinergic drugs including the tricyclic antidepressants.

Preparations: Ophthalmic solution (as the salicylate), 0.25% and 0.5%. Ophthalmic ointment (as the sulfate), 0.25%. Ampules and syringes (as the salicylate), 1 mg/ml.

PHYTONADIONE—Vitamin K₁, AquaMEPHYTON®, Konakion®, Mephyton®

Description/Actions: Vitamin K analogue indicated for the management of anticoagulant-induced prothrombin deficiency, and for the management of hypoprothrombinemia secondary to other conditions or drug therapies (e.g., salicylates, antibiotics). Is also used parenterally in the prophylaxis and therapy of hemorrhagic disease of the newborn.

Precaution/Adverse Reactions: Severe reactions, including fatalities have occurred during and immediately after intravenous injection of phytonadione even when precautions have been taken to dilute the phytonadione and to avoid rapid infusion. Severe reactions (hypersensitivity or anaphylaxis including shock, and cardiac and or respiratory arrest), including fatalities, have also been reported following intramuscular administration. The intravenous and intramuscular routes of administration should be reserved for those situations where the subcutaneous route is not feasible and the potential risk is considered justified.

Administration: Whenever possible, phytonadione should be given by the subcutaneous route.

Preparations: Tablets, 5 mg. Ampules and vials, 2 mg/ml and 10 mg/ml.

PILOCARPINE HYDROCHLORIDE—Salagen®

Description/Actions: Miotic indicated for ophthalmic use in the treatment of glaucoma, and to counter the effect of cycloplegics and mydriatics. Also indicated for oral use for the treatment of symptoms of xerostomia from salivary gland hypofunction caused by radiotherapy for cancer of the head and neck.

Preparations: Ophthalmic solutions, 0.25%, 0.5%, 1%, 2%, 3%, 4%, 5%, 6%, 8%, and 10%. Ophthalmic gel, 4%. Ocular therapeutic systems, release 20 or 40 µg pilocarpine per hour for one week. Tablets (Salagen), 5 mg.

PIMECROLIMUS—ELIDEL®

Description/Actions: Pimecrolimus is indicated for short-term and intermittent long-term therapy of mild to moderate eczema (atopic dermatitis) in patients not responsive to conventional therapy or when conventional therapy is deemed inadvisable.

Precautions/Adverse Reactions: Pimecrolimus is contraindicated in patients with Netherton's syndrome. It should not be applied to areas of active cutaneous viral infections. Patients with atopic dermatitis are predisposed to superficial skin infections, thereby increasing the risk of varicella zoster, herpes simplex viral infections, and eczema herpeticum. Clinical infections at the treatment sites should be cleared first before use of pimecrolimus. It is prudent to minimize or avoid natural or artificial sunlight exposure. It is not recommended for use in pediatric patients < 2 years of age. There are no data to support its use in immunocompromised patients. There are no well-controlled studies in pregnant women. Pregnancy Category C. Use only if clearly needed. Excretion in breast milk is unknown; therefore, breastfeeding is not recommended.

The most common side effects were a temporary, mild to moderate warm feeling or burning at the application site. Most application-site reactions did not last more than 5 days. Other common adverse effects were headache and coldlike symptoms. Cases of lymphadenopathy were reported. These cases were usually related to infections and noted to resolve upon appropriate antibiotic therapy. Consider discontinuation if lymphadenopathy occurs.

Administration: Topical.

Patient Care Implications: Patients should wash their hands after applying if hands are not an area for treatment. There is low systemic exposure via topical route; systemic drug interactions are not expected. Do not use occlusive dressings; this increases moisture, thereby increasing absorption.

Preparations: Cream, topical: 1% (15, 30, 60, and 100 g).

PIMOZIDE—Orap®

Description/Actions: Neuroleptic agent indicated for the suppression of motor and phonic tics in patients with Tourette's disorder who have failed to respond satisfactorily to standard treatment.

Preparations: Tablets, 2 mg.

PINDOLOL—Visken®

Antihypertensive agent.

Description/Actions: A nonselective beta-adrenergic blocking agent with intrinsic sympathomimetic activity that is indicated in the management of hypertension.

Warnings: Contraindicated in patients with bronchial asthma, overt cardiac failure, cardiogenic shock, second- and third-degree heart block, and severe bradycardia. Adverse reactions include dizziness, fatigue, insomnia, edema, nausea, and muscle and joint pain. Use is best avoided in patients with bronchospastic diseases and therapy in diabetic patients must be closely monitored.

Administration: Oral. Patients should be cautioned about the interruption or discontinuation of therapy and, when therapy is to be discontinued, the dosage should be gradually reduced over a period of 1 to 2 weeks.

Preparations: Tablets, 5 and 10 mg.

PIOGLITAZONE—Actos®

Description/Actions: Pioglitazone is used for the treatment of NIDDM.

Precautions/Adverse Reactions: Pioglitazone should be administered with caution in patients with hepatic impairment. The drug should not be given to patients with increased baseline liver enzymes of ALT > 2.5 times the upper limit of normal. Pioglitazone should be discontinued if jaundice occurs. Pioglitazone should also be used carefully in heart failure and peripheral edema patients because the drug can cause volume expansion. Drug should not be used in pregnant women, breast-feeding women, and children. Some side effects are headache, hyperglycemia, myalgia, pharyngitis, sinusitis, tooth disorder, weight gain, upper respiratory infection, and decreases in hemoglobin and hematocrit.

Administration: Oral.

Patient Care Implications: Pioglitazone should not be used in pregnant women, breast-feeding women, and children. Patients with hepatic disease should have liver enzymes monitored before initiation of drug and every 2 months after initiation. Pioglitazone should be discontinued if jaundice occurs. Pioglitazone should also be used carefully in heart failure and peripheral edema patients.

Preparations: Tablet, 15 mg, 30 mg, 45 mg.

PIPECURONIUM BROMIDE— Arduan®

Nondepolarizing neuromuscular blocking agent.

Description/Actions: Acts by competing for cholinergic receptors at the motor end plate, resulting in a block of neuromuscular transmission. Indicated as an adjunct to general anesthesia to provide skeletal muscle relaxation during surgery. Can also be used to provide skeletal muscle relaxation for endotracheal intubation. Has a long duration of action and is only recommended for procedures anticipated to last 90 minutes or longer.

Warnings: May cause excessive skeletal muscle weakness resulting in respiratory insufficiency and apnea. Action may be antagonized by neostigmine. Must be used with caution in patients with myasthenia gravis or myasthenic syndrome, and in patients receiving other medications that may intensify or produce neuromuscular block on their own (e.g., inhalation anesthetics, aminoglycosides, quinidine, magnesium salts). Other adverse reactions include bradycardia, hypotension, and hypertension.

Administration: Intravenous.

Preparations: Vials, 10 mg.

PIPERACILLIN SODIUM— Pipracil®

Penicillin antibiotic.

Description/Actions: Is bactericidal and is active against many gram-positive and gram-negative bacteria, including *Pseudomonas aeruginosa*. Is often used in conjunction with an aminoglycoside antibiotic in the treatment of *Pseudomonas* infections. Is also used for surgical prophylaxis.

Warnings: Contraindicated in patients with a history of allergic reactions to any of the penicillins. Adverse reactions include hypersensitivity reactions, GI disturbances, and local reactions at the injection site.

Administration: Intravenous and intramuscular.

Preparations: Vials and infusion bottles, 2, 3, 4, and 40 g.

PIPERACILLIN SODIUM/ TAZOBACTAM SODIUM— Zosyn®

Antibiotic.

Description/Actions: Is a combination of the penicillin antibiotic piperacillin with a beta-lactamase inhibitor tazobactam. By inhibiting beta-lactamase enzymes, tazobactam extends the spectrum of action of piperacillin to include certain bacteria that are not susceptible to piperacillin alone. Indicated for the treatment of the following infections caused by piperacillin-resistant, beta-lactamase-producing strains of the bacteria designated: community-acquired pneumonia caused by *Haemophilus influenzae*; appendicitis (complicated by rupture or abscess), and peritonitis caused by *E. coli*, *Bacteroides fragilis*, *B. ovatus*, *B. thetaiomicron*, or *B. vulgatus*; postpartum endometritis or pelvic inflammatory disease caused by *E. coli*; and uncomplicated and complicated skin and skin-structure infections, including cellulitis, cutaneous abscesses, and ischemic/diabetic foot infections caused by *Staphylococcus aureus*.

Warnings: Contraindicated in patients with a history of allergic reaction to any of the penicillins, cephalosporins, or beta-lactamase inhibitors. Adverse reactions include diarrhea, constipation, nausea, dyspepsia, headache, insomnia, rash, pruritus, and hemolytic anemia. Should not be administered in the same solution with an aminoglycoside antibiotic.

Administration: Intravenous. Administered as an IV infusion over a period of 30 minutes.

Preparations: Vials, 2.25, 3.375, and 4.5 grams, which provide 2, 3, and 4 g of piperacillin and 0.25, 0.375, and 0.5 g of tazobactam, respectively.

PIPERAZINE CITRATE—Antepar®

Description/Actions: Anthelmintic indicated in the treatment of pinworm and roundworm infections.

Preparations: Tablets, equivalent to 250 mg of piperazine hexahydrate. Syrup, equivalent to 500 mg piperazine hexahydrate/5 ml.

PIPERAZINE ESTRONE SULFATE, see Estropipate

PIPOBROMAN—Vercyte®

Description/Actions: Antineoplastic agent indicated in the treatment of polycythemia vera and the treatment of chronic granulocytic leukemia in patients refractory to busulfan.

Preparations: Tablets, 25 mg.

PIPRACIL®, see Piperacillin

PIRBUTEROL ACETATE—Maxair®

Bronchodilator.

Description/Actions: Stimulates beta-2-adrenergic receptors and is indicated for the prevention and reversal of bronchospasm in patients with reversible bronchospasm including asthma.

Warnings: Adverse reactions include nervousness, tremor, headache, dizziness, palpitations, tachycardia, cough, and nausea. Should be used with caution in patients with cardiovascular disorders, hyperthyroidism, diabetes mellitus, or convulsive disorders. Other beta-adrenergic aerosol bronchodilators should not be used concomitantly. It should be used with caution to patients being treated with a tricyclic antidepressant or monoamine oxidase inhibitor.

Administration: Oral inhalation.

Preparations: Metered-dose inhaler. Each actuation delivers the equivalent of 0.2 mg pirbuterol.

PIROXICAM—Feldene®

Nonsteroidal anti-inflammatory drug.

Description/Actions: Inhibits prostaglandin synthesis and is indicated in the treatment of rheumatoid arthritis and osteoarthritis.

Warnings: Should not be given to patients in whom aspirin or another NSAID causes asthma, rhinitis, urticaria, or other allergic-type reactions. May cause GI effects and use should be avoided in patients with active GI tract disease, and closely monitored in patients with a previous history of such disorders. Other adverse reactions include rash, edema, and decreases in hemoglobin and hematocrit. Has a long duration of action and may accumulate with continued use; particular caution should be exercised in elderly patients.

Administration: Oral.

Preparations: Capsules, 10 and 20 mg.

PITOCIN®, see Oxytocin

PITRESSIN®, see Vasopressin

PITUITARY, POSTERIOR

Description/Actions: Hormones of the posterior pituitary administered parenterally to control postoperative ileus, to stimulate expulsion of gas prior to pyelography, as an aid to achieve hemostasis in surgery, and for treating enuresis of diabetes insipidus. Has also been used by nasal inhalation for the control of diabetes insipidus.

Preparations: Ampules, 20 units/ml. Capsules to be used for intranasal inhalation, 40 mg.

PLACIDYL®, see Ethchlorvynol

PLAQUENIL®, see Hydroxychloroquine

PLASBUMIN®, see Albumin

PLATINOL®, see Cisplatin

PLAVIX®, see Clopidogrel

PLENDIL®, see Felodipine

PLICAMYCIN—Mithramycin, Mithracin®

Description/Actions: Antineoplastic agent indicated for intravenous use in the treatment of testicular carcinoma. Also used in the treatment of symptomatic patients with hypercalcemia and hypercalciuria associated with a variety of advanced neoplasms.

Preparations: Vials, 2500 µg.

PODOFILOX—Condylox®

Description/Actions: Antimitotic agent. An active component of podophyllum resin that is indicated for the topical treatment of external genital warts.

Actions and Uses: Antimitotic indicated in the treatment of external genital warts. Not for use on mucous membrane or perianal warts. Local reactions (e.g., burning, inflammation, erosion, pain, itching, bleeding) and headache may occur.

Administration: Apply twice daily every 12 hours for 3 days, then discontinue for 4 days. May repeat if needed for a maximum of 4 treatment cycles. Use applicator with solution.

Preparations: 0.5% topical solution and gel.

PODOPHYLLIN, see Podophyllum resin

PODOPHYLLUM RESIN—
Podophyllin

258 • POLARAMINE®

Description/Actions: Resin applied topically for the removal of benign epithelial growths such as common warts, and also in certain other dermatologic disorders.

Preparations: Liquid, 25%, often in tincture of benzoin.

POLARAMINE®, see Dexchlorpheniramine

POLYCARBOPHIL—Equalactin®, FiberCon®, Mitrolan®

Description/Actions: Hydrophilic agent used in the treatment of constipation or diarrhea by regulating intestinal water and promoting well-formed stools.

Preparations: Chewable tablets, 500 mg.

POLYCILLIN®, see Ampicillin

POLYCITRA®, see Potassium citrate

POLYETHYLENE GLYCOL— Miralax

Description/Actions: Miralax is an osmotic laxative indicated in the treatment of occasional constipation. It works by causing water to be retained in the stool. Unlike stimulant laxatives, it works on the stool rather than the colon.

Precautions/Adverse Reactions: Miralax is contraindicated in a bowel obstruction. It may increase the incidence of diarrhea in the elderly. Avoid prolonged, frequent, or excessive use.

Adverse reactions include nausea, abdominal bloating, cramping, flatulence, and diarrhea.

Administration: Dissolve 17 g in 8 oz of water and drink promptly. Take once daily. The usual duration of treatment is 2 weeks. May need 2–4 days to produce a bowel movement.

Patient Care Implications: Inform patients the first bowel movement should occur in 2–4 days after taking. Report unusual cramps, bloating, or diarrhea to the prescriber. Instruct patients in lifestyle changes that promote regular bowel movements such as regular exercise, high-fiber diet, and adequate hydration. Do not exceed the recommended dose, as this may result in severe diarrhea and dehydration. Discontinue if a rash, hives, or other symptoms of allergy occur.

Preparations: Powder for reconstitution.

POLYETHYLENE GLYCOLS— PEG, Carbowax®

Description/Actions: Ointment and suppository bases used as vehicles for active medications.

POLYETHYLENE GLYCOL 3350—Colyte®, GoLYTELY®

Description/Actions: Osmotic agent used with electrolytes for bowel cleansing prior to colonoscopy and barium enema X-ray examination.

Preparations: Powder for oral solution.

POLYMYXIN B SULFATE— Aerosporin®

Description/Actions: Antibiotic used in the treatment of infections caused by gram-negative bacteria. Administered parenterally in the treatment of infections caused by bacteria such as *Pseudomonas aeruginosa* when less toxic drugs are ineffective or contraindicated. Also indicated for ophthalmic use. Is most frequently employed in combination with other antibiotics (e.g., neomycin) in the topical management of dermatologic, otic, and ophthalmic infections, and also as a genitourinary irrigant.

Preparations: Vials, 500,000 units. Powder for ophthalmic solution, 500,000 units.

POLYMYXIN E®, see Colistin sulfate

POLYTHIAZIDE—Renese®

Description/Actions: Thiazide diuretic indicated as adjunctive therapy in edema and in the management of hypertension.

Preparations: Tablets, 1, 2, and 4 mg.

PONSTEL®, see Mefenamic acid

PONTOCAINE®, see Tetracaine

PORACTANT ALFA—Curosurf®

Description/Actions: Poractant alfa is used in the treatment of neonatal respiratory distress syndrome.

Precautions/Adverse Reactions: Poractant alfa should not be administered to patients with porcine hypersensitivity or to pregnant women. Also, patients should be monitored carefully for oxygenation because the drug can cause respiratory changes and ventilatory support should be modified accordingly. Some side effects are transient episodes of hypotension, sinus bradycardia, oxygen desaturation, and endotracheal tube blockage. If these problems occur then the drug should be discontinued, the problems should be alleviated, and then the drug should be initiated again.

Administration: Intrathecal injection.

Patient Care Implications: Poractant alfa should not be used in patients with porcine hypersensitivity or in pregnant women. The drug should only be given under strict supervision of clinicians experienced in intubation, ventilators, and care of premature babies. Also, before initiation of poractant alfa, a patient should be checked for metabolic acidosis, anemia, hypoglycemia, hypotension, and hypothermia. If these problems exist then they should be corrected before the drug is started. Patient should have ABGs and chest X-rays checked while taking poractant alfa.

Preparations: Solution, 80 mg/ml, 1.5 and 3.0 ml.

POSTERIOR PITUITARY, see Pituitary, posterior

POSTURE®, see Calcium phosphate, tribasic

POTABA®, see Para-aminobenzoic acid

POTASSIUM ACETATE

Description/Actions: For intravenous potassium replacement.

Preparations: Vials, 40 mEq, 120 mEq.

POTASSIUM CHLORIDE, ORAL (see list of preparations below for trade names)

Potassium supplement.

Description/Actions: Indicated in patients with hypokalemia, in digitalis intoxication, in patients with hypokalemic familial periodic paralysis, and for the prevention of potassium depletion when the dietary intake of potassium is inadequate.

Warnings: Is contraindicated in patients with hyperkalemia; should not be used concomitantly with a potassium-sparing diuretic because of the increased risk of hyperkalemia. Solid dosage forms (e.g., tablets) have caused lesions of the small intestine and serious GI complications; these formulations should be reserved for those patients who cannot tolerate or refuse to take liquid or effervescent potassium preparations, or for patients in whom there is a problem of compliance with these preparations. Other adverse reactions include nausea and vomiting.

Administration: Oral.

Preparations: Liquid (e.g., Kay Ciel®, Klorvess®, 20 and 40 mEq/ml. Powder (e.g., Kay Ciel®, K-Lor®), 15, 20, and 25 mEq/packet. Controlled-release tablets and capsules (e.g., Slow-K®, Klotrix®, K-Tab®, Micro-K®), 8 and 10 mEq.

POTASSIUM CHLORIDE, INTRAVENOUS

Preparations: Ampules and vials, 10, 20, 30, 40, 60, and 90 mEq.

POTASSIUM CITRATE—
Polycitra®, Urocit-K®

Description/Actions: Alkalinizing agent and potassium replacement agent. Has been used to alkalinize the urine to reduce the risk of calculi in the urinary tract, as an adjunct to uricosuric agents in gout therapy, and to correct the acidosis of certain renal tubular disorders.

Preparations: Tablets, 540 mg. Syrup, 550 mg/5 ml with sodium citrate and citric acid.

POTASSIUM GLUCONATE—
Kaon®

Potassium replacement agent.

Preparations: Tablets, 5 mEq. Liquid, 20 mEq/15 ml.

POTASSIUM IODIDE

Description/Actions: Expectorant and is also used as adjunctive therapy in other respiratory conditions. Has also been used for thyroid blocking in radiation emergencies, in the treatment of thyrotoxic crisis, and as an adjunct with other antithyroid drugs in preparation for thyroidectomy.

Preparations: Enteric-coated tablets, 300 mg. Solution, 500 mg/15 ml. Saturated solution of potassium iodide (SSKI), 1 g/ml.

POTASSIUM PHOSPHATE—
Neutra-Phos-K®

Description/Actions: Phosphorus-replacement products.

Preparations: Capsules and powder concentrate are both utilized to prepare liquid for oral administration. Vials, 3 mM phosphate/ml for intravenous administration.

POVIDONE-IODINE—Betadine®

Description/Actions: Anti-infective agent utilized for topical, vaginal, and perineal application.

Preparations: Numerous formulations including topical solution and ointment.

PRALIDOXIME CHLORIDE—
Protopam®

Description/Actions: Cholinesterase reactivator indicated as an antidote in the treatment of poisoning due to pesticides and chemicals of the organophosphate class that have anticholinesterase activity, and in the control of overdosage by anticholinesterase drugs used in the treatment of myasthenia gravis. Atropine should be administered after ventilation is established.

Preparations: Vials, 1 g.

PRAMOXINE HYDROCHLORIDE—
Tronolane®, Tronothane®

Description/Actions: Local anesthetic indicated for topical use for the temporary relief of pain and itching associated with dermatologic conditions, as well as hemorrhoids and other anorectal disorders.

Preparations: Cream, 1%. Suppositories, 1%.

PRANDIN®, see Repaglinide

PRAVACHOL®, see Pravastatin

PRAVASTATIN SODIUM—
Pravachol®

Agent for hypercholesterolemia.

Description/Actions: Reduces cholesterol biosynthesis in the liver by acting as a competitive inhibitor of 3-hydroxy-3-methylglutaryl-coenzyme A (HMG-CoA) reductase. Produces a significant reduction in total and low-density lipoprotein (LDL) cholesterol concentrations, a modest reduction in triglyceride concentrations, and an increase in high-density lipoprotein (HDL) cholesterol concentrations. Indicated as an adjunct to diet for the reduction of elevated total and LDL cholesterol concentrations in patients with primary hypercholesterolemia (Type IIa and IIb) when the response to a diet restricted in saturated fat and cholesterol has not been adequate. Also indicated to reduce the risk of MI, reduce the risk of undergoing myocardial revascularization procedures, and reduce the risk of cardiavascular mortality with no increase in death from noncardiovascular causes in hypercholesterolemia without clinically evident coronary heart disease. Also indicated for the treatment of heterozygous familial hypercholesterolemia in children ages 8 and older.

Warnings: Contraindicated in patients with active liver disease or unexplained persistent elevations in liver function tests. Is also contraindicated in pregnant women and nursing mothers. Adverse reactions include headache, rash, influenza, myalgia, myopathy, and, rarely, rhabdomyolysis. Patients should be advised to promptly report unexplained muscle pain, tenderness, or weakness. Because of the possibility of an increased risk of skeletal muscle reactions, the concurrent use of clofibrate, cyclosporine, erythromycin, gemfibrozil, or niacin (in lipid-lowering doses) is best avoided. When either cholestyramine or colestipol is used concomitantly, pravastatin should be administered at least 1 hour before or at least 4 hours after the administration of the other agent. Increases in serum transaminases may occur, and it is recommended that liver function tests be performed prior to the initiation of therapy, prior to the elevation of the dose, and when otherwise clinically indicated. Should any increase in AST or ALT of 3 times the upper limit of normal or greater persist, withdrawl of pravastatin therapy is recommended.

Administration: Oral. Should be administered at bedtime.

Preparations: Tablets, 10, 20, 40, and 80 mg.

PRAZEPAM—Centrax®

Benzodiazepine antianxiety agent.

Description/Actions: A CNS depressant indicated for the management of anxiety disorders or for the short-term relief of the symptoms of anxiety.

Warnings: Contraindicated in patients with acute narrow-angle glaucoma. Adverse reactions include drowsiness and other CNS effects; patients should be cautioned regarding activities such as driving or operating machinery, as well as interactions with other CNS-acting drugs including alcohol. Can cause dependence, and is included in Schedule IV.

Administration: Oral.

Preparations: Capsules, 5, 10, and 20 mg. Tablets, 10 mg.

PRAZIQUANTEL—Biltricide®

Description/Actions: Antiparasitic agent indicated for the treatment of schistosomiasis and other trematode infections by Chinese liver fluke.

Preparations: Tablets, 600 mg.

PRAZOSIN HYDROCHLORIDE— Minipress®

Antihypertensive agent.

Description/Actions: Indicated in the treatment of hypertension. Investigational studies have suggested it to be useful in refractory congestive heart failure and in the management of Raynaud's vasospasm.

Warnings: Prazosin is contraindicated in patients with a known hypersensitivity to quinazolines, prazosin, or any component of the formulation. May cause syncope with sudden loss of consciousness, usually attributable to an excessive postural hypotensive effect; risk may be reduced by limiting the initial dose of the drug to 1 mg, and by subsequently increasing the dosage slowly. Adverse reactions include dizziness, drowsiness, and other CNS effects; patients should be cautioned regarding activities such as driving and operating machinery, as well as interactions with other CNS-acting drugs, including alcohol. Other adverse reactions include palpitations and nausea. The concurrent use of a beta-adrenergic-blocking agent may increase the risk of hypotension.

Administration: Oral.

Preparations: Capsules and tablets, 1, 2, and 5 mg.

PRECEDEX®, see Dexmedetomidine hydrochloride injection

PRECOSE®, see Acarbose

PREDNICARBATE—Dermatop®

Description/Actions: Corticosteroid applied topically for the relief of the manifestations of corticosteroid-responsive dermatoses.

Preparations: Cream, 0.1%.

PREDNISOLONE—Delta-Cortef®

Description/Actions: Corticosteroid indicated in a wide range of endocrine, rheumatic, allergic, dermatologic, respiratory, hematologic, neoplastic, and other disorders.

Preparations: Tablets, 5 mg. Syrup, 15 mg/5 ml. Oral solution, 5 mg/ml.

PREDNISOLONE ACETATE

Preparations: Vials (for IM, intralesional, intraarticular, or soft tissue injection), 25 mg/ml, 50 mg/ml, and 100 mg/ml. Ophthalmic suspension, 0.12%, 0.125%, 1%.

PREDNISOLONE SODIUM PHOSPHATE—Hydeltrasol®

Preparations: Oral liquid, 5 mg/5 ml. Vials (for IV, IM, intralesional, intraarticular, or soft tissue injection), 20 mg/ml. Ophthalmic solution, 0.125%, 0.5%, and 1%.

PREDNISOLONE TEBUTATE—Hydeltra-TBA®

Preparations: Vials (for intralesional, intraarticular, or soft tissue injection) 20 mg/ml.

PREDNISONE—Deltasone®, Meticorten®

Corticosteroid.

Description/Actions: Indicated in a wide range of endocrine, rheumatic, allergic, dermatologic, respiratory, hematologic, neoplastic, and other disorders.

Warnings: Contraindicated in patients with systemic fungal infections. Adverse reactions include sodium and fluid retention, potassium depletion, muscle weakness, osteoporosis, peptic ulcer, thin fragile skin, development of cushingoid state, glaucoma, cataracts, and negative nitrogen balance. May mask signs of infection, and new infections may appear during use. May increase requirements for hypoglycemic agents in diabetic patients.

Administration: Oral.

Preparations: Tablets, 1, 2.5, 5, 10, 20, and 50 mg. Oral solution, 5 mg/5 ml. Oral solution (concentrate), 5 mg/ml. Syrup, 5 mg/5 ml.

PREMARIN®, see Estrogens, conjugated

PREMPHASE®, Combination of conjugated estrogens and medroxyprogesterone acetate

PREMPRO®, Combination of conjugated estrogens and medroxyprogesterone acetate

PREPIDIL®, see Dinoprostone

PREVACID®, see Lansoprazole

PREVACID® SOLUTAB, see Lansoprazole

PREVPAC®—Combination agent lansoprazole, amoxicillin, and clarithromycin (pump inhibitor and antibiotics)

PRILOCAINE HYDROCHLORIDE—Citanest®

Description/Actions: Local anesthetic administered by injection for infiltration, peripheral nerve block, central neural block, and in dental procedures.

Preparations: Ampules and vials, 1%, 2%, and 3%. Dental cartridges, 4%.

PRILOSEC®, see Omeprazole

PRIMACOR®, see Milrinone lactate

PRIMAQUINE PHOSPHATE

Description/Actions: Antimalarial agent used to prevent relapses of infections caused by *Plasmodium vivax* and *P. ovale* and to prevent attack after departure from areas where *P. vivax* and *P. ovale* are endemic (often administered during the last 2 weeks of chloroquine prophylaxis).

Preparations: Tablets, 26.3 mg.

PRIMATENE MIST®, see Epinephrine

PRIMAXIN IV®, see Imipenem-cilastatin sodium

PRIMAXIN IM®, see Imipenem-cilastatin sodium

PRIMIDONE—Mysoline®

Description/Actions: Anticonvulsant indicated in the control of grand mal, psychomotor, and focal epileptic seizures.

Preparations: Tablets, 50, 125, and 250 mg. Suspension, 250 mg/5 ml.

PRINCIPEN®, see Ampicillin

PRINIVIL®, see Lisinopril

PRINZIDE®, Combination of lisinopril and hydrochlorothiazide

PRISCOLINE®, see Tolazoline

PRIVINE®, see Naphazoline

PROAMATINE®, see Midodrine Hydrochloride

PRO-BANTHINE®, see Propantheline

PROBENECID—Benemid®

Description/Actions: Uricosuric agent indicated for the treatment of hyperuricemia associated with gout and gouty arthritis and to treat the hyperuricemia secondary to thiazide therapy. Has also been used to increase the plasma levels and activity of the penicillin derivatives.

Preparations: Tablets, 500 mg.

PROCANBID®, see Procainamide HCl

PROCAINAMIDE HYDROCHLORIDE—
Procanbid®, Pronestyl®, Pronestyl-SR®, Procan SR®

Antiarrhythmic agent.

Description/Actions: Indicated in the treatment of premature ventricular contractions and ventricular tachycardia, atrial fibrillation, and paroxysmal atrial tachycardia; also useful in preventing recurrence of certain arrhythmias after conversion to sinus rhythm by other drugs or procedures.

Warnings: Contraindicated in patients with complete heart block or lupus erythematosus, and in patients sensitive to procaine or other ester-type local anesthetics. May cause worsening of symptoms in patients with myasthenia gravis. Adverse reactions include proarrhythmic effects, hypotension (particularly after parenteral administration), nausea, vomiting, diarrhea, dizziness, weakness, pruritus, flushing, lupus erythematosus-like syndrome, and positive antinuclear antibody (ANA) test.

Administration: Oral, intravenous, and intramuscular.

Preparations: Capsules and tablets, 250, 375, and 500 mg. Sustained-release tablets, 250, 500, 750, and 1000 mg. Vials, 100 and 500 mg/ml.

PROCAINE HYDROCHLORIDE—
Novocain®

Description/Actions: Local anesthetic administered by injection for infiltration anesthesia, peripheral nerve block, spinal anesthesia, and for rectal anesthesia in proctology.

Preparations: Ampules and vials, 1% and 2%. Ampules (for spinal anesthesia), 10%.

PROCAINE PENICILLIN G—
Crysticillin®, Wycillin®

Description/Actions: Penicillin antibiotic administered intramuscularly and having an extended duration of action. Used in the treatment of streptococcal, gonococcal, and selected other infections.

Preparations: Vials and syringes, 300,000, 500,000, 600,000, 1,200,000, and 2,400,000 units.

PROCAN SR®, see Procainamide

PROCARBAZINE
HYDROCHLORIDE—Matulane®

Description/Actions: Antineoplastic agent having monoamine oxidase inhibitory activity. Indicated for use in combination with other antineoplastic drugs for the treatment of Stage III and IV Hodgkin's disease.

Preparations: Capsules, 50 mg.

PROCARDIA®, see Nifedipine

PROCARDIA XL®, see Nifedipine

PROCHLORPERAZINE—
Compazine®

Phenothiazine antipsychotic agent and antiemetic.

Description/Actions: Indicated for the control of severe nausea and vomiting, and for the management of manifestations of psychotic disorders.

Warnings: Adverse reactions include drowsiness and other CNS effects; patients should be cautioned regarding activities such as driving and operating machinery, as well as interactions with other CNS-acting drugs, including alcohol. Other adverse reactions include extrapyramidal reactions, tardive dyskinesia, blurred vision, skin reactions, and hypotension. May lower the convulsive threshold necessitating dosage adjustments of anticonvulsants. May interfere with thermoregulatory mechanisms, and must be used cautiously in persons who will be exposed to extreme heat; the risk of complications is increased in patients who are also taking other medications having anticholinergic activity.

Administration: Oral, rectal, intravenous, and intramuscular.

Preparations: Tablets (as the maleate), 5, 10, and 25 mg. Sustained-release capsules (as the maleate), 10, 15, and 30 mg. Syrup (as the edisylate), 5 mg/5 ml. Suppositories, 2.5, 5, and 25 mg. Ampules, vials, and syringes (as the edisylate), 5 mg/ml.

PROCRIT®, see Epoetin alfa

PROCYCLIDINE HYDROCHLORIDE—Kemadrin®

Description/Actions: Antiparkinson agent indicated in the treatment of parkinsonism and drug-induced extrapyramidal effects.

Preparations: Tablets, 5 mg.

PODOFILOX—Condylox®

Description/Actions: Antimitotic indicated in the treatment of external genital warts. Not for use on mucous membrane or perianal warts. Local reactions (e.g., burning, inflammation, erosion, pain, itching, bleeding) and headache may occur.

Administration: Apply twice daily every 12 hours for 3 days then discontinue for 4 days. May repeat if needed for a maximum of 4 treatment cycles. Use applicator with solution.

Preparations: 0.5% topical solution and gel.

PROFENAL®, see Suprofen

PROGESTASERT®, see Progesterone

PROGESTERONE—Progestasert®

Description/Actions: Progestin used intramuscularly in the management of conditions such as amenorrhea and functional uterine bleeding. Intrauterine system has been used for contraception.

Preparations: Vials (aqueous solution and in oil), 25 mg/ml, 50 mg/ml, and 100 mg/ml. Intrauterine system, 38 mg, provides contraceptive effectiveness for a period of 1 year.

PROGLYCEM®, see Diazoxide

PROGRAF®, see Tacrolimus

PROKINE®, see Sargramostim

PROLASTIN®, see Alpha$_1$-proteinase inhibitor (human)

PROLEUKIN®, see Aldesleukin

PROLIXIN®, see Fluphenazine

PROLOPRIM®, see Trimethoprim

PROMAZINE HYDROCHLORIDE—Sparine®

Description/Actions: Phenothiazine *antipsychotic agent* indicated in the management of the manifestations of psychotic disorders.

Preparations: Tablets, 25, 50, and 100 mg. Vials and syringes, 25 mg/ml and 50 mg/ml.

PROMETHAZINE HYDROCHLORIDE—Phenergan®

Description/Actions: Phenothiazine *antihistamine* indicated for allergic disorders, motion sickness, preoperative, postoperative, or obstetric sedation, postoperative pain as an adjunct to analgesics, and the prevention and control of nausea and vomiting associated with certain types of surgery.

Preparations: Tablets and suppositories, 10, 12.5, 25, and 50 mg. Syrup, 6.25 and 25 mg/5 ml. Ampules and vials, 25 and 50 mg/ml.

PRONESTYL®, see Procainamide

PROPAFENONE HYDROCHLORIDE—Rythmol®

Antiarrhythmic agent.

Description/Actions: A class IC antiarrhythmic agent that also has local anesthetic activity, beta-adrenergic-blocking activity, and a weak calcium channel-blocking effect. Indicated for the treatment of documented life-threatening arrhythmias or prolonged recurrence of paroxysmal atrial fibrillation/flutex

266 • PROPANTHELINE BROMIDE

or paroxysmal supraventricular tachycardia (PSVT) associated with disabling symptoms, in patients without structural heart disease.

Warnings: Contraindicated in the presence of uncontrolled congestive heart failure, cardiogenic shock, sinoatrial, atrioventricular, and intraventricular disorders of impulse generation and/or conduction in the absence of an artificial pacemaker, bradycardia, marked hypotension, bronchospastic disorders, and electrolyte imbalance. Adverse reactions include proarrhythmic effects, congestive heart failure, conduction abnormalities, nausea and/or vomiting, unusual (e.g., metallic) taste, constipation, dizziness, fatigue, and dyspnea.

Administration: Oral. If a patient misses a dose, the next dose should not be doubled because of an increased risk of adverse reactions. To help achieve a constant clinical response, the drug should be administered on a consistent basis either with food or apart from food.

Preparations: Tablets, 150, 225, and 300 mg.

PROPANTHELINE BROMIDE—
Pro-Banthine®

Description/Actions: Anticholinergic agent indicated as adjunctive therapy in the treatment of peptic ulcer.

Preparations: Tablets, 7.5 and 15 mg.

PROPARACAINE HYDROCHLORIDE—
Ophthaine®

Description/Actions: Local anesthetic indicated for ophthalmic use.

Preparations: Ophthalmic solution, 0.5%.

PROPECIA®, see Finasteride

PROPINE®, see Dipivefrin

PROPIOMAZINE HYDROCHLORIDE—Largon®

Description/Actions: Phenothiazine indicated for parenteral use for relief of restlessness and apprehension, preoperatively or during surgery or during labor.

Preparations: Ampules and syringes, 20 mg/ml.

PROPOFOL—Diprivan®
Anesthetic.

Description/Actions: Has a rapid onset of action, and the recovery from anesthesia is usually prompt. Indicated as an intravenous anesthetic agent that can be used for both induction and/or maintenance of anesthesia as part of a balanced anesthetic technique for inpatient and outpatient surgery. Also indicated for continuous sedation and control of stress responses in intubated or respiratory-controlled adult patients in intensive care units.

Warnings: Adverse reactions include excitatory reactions (e.g., spontaneous movement, twitching, tremor, myoclonus), hypotension, bradycardia, apnea, nausea, vomiting, and reactions at the injection site. Other CNS depressants can increase the depression induced by propofol and may also result in more pronounced decreases in blood pressure.

Administration: Intravenous

Preparations: Vials, 10 mg/ml. Is a white, oil-in-water emulsion that is isotonic.

PROPOXYPHENE HYDROCHLORIDE—Darvon®

PROPOXYPHENE NAPSYLATE—
Darvon-N®

Analgesic.

Description/Actions: Indicated for the relief of mild to moderate pain.

Warnings: Adverse reactions include sedation and other CNS effects; patients should be cautioned regarding activities such as driving and operating machinery, as well as interactions with other CNS-acting drugs, including alcohol. Can cause dependence and is included in Schedule IV.

Administration: Oral.

Preparations: Capsules, 65 mg. Tablets (Darvon-N), 50 and 100 mg.

PROPRANOLOL HYDROCHLORIDE—Inderal®, Inderal LA®

Antihypertensive, antianginal, and antiarrhythmic agent.

Description/Actions: A nonselective beta-adrenergic-blocking agent indicated in the treatment of hypertension, angina pectoris, and cardiac arrhythmias (i.e., supraventricular arrhythmias, ventricular tachycardias, tachyarrhythmias of digitalis intoxication, and resistant tachyarrhythmias due to excessive catecholamine action during anesthesia). Also indicated to reduce cardiovascular mortality in patients who have survived the acute phase of myocardial infarction, in the management of hypertrophic subaortic stenosis, in pheochromocytoma, and for the prophylaxis of common migraine headache.

Warnings: Contraindicated in patients with cardiogenic shock, sinus bradycardia and greater than first-degree block, bronchial asthma, and congestive heart failure. Acute increases in blood pressure have occurred after insulin-induced hypoglycemia in patients on propranolol.

Adverse reactions include weakness, lightheadedness, depression, bradycardia, paresthesia of hands, arterial insufficiency (e.g., Raynaud type), nausea, and diarrhea. Use is best avoided in patients with bronchospastic diseases, and therapy in diabetic patients must be closely monitored.

Administration: Oral and intravenous. Patients should be cautioned about the interruption or discontinuation of therapy; exacerbation of angina pectoris has occurred following the abrupt cessation of therapy, and, when therapy is to be discontinued, the dosage should be gradually reduced over a period of several weeks.

Preparations: Tablets, 10, 20, 40, 60, and 90 mg. Long-acting capsules (Inderal LA), 60, 80, 120, and 160 mg. Oral solution, 4, 8, and 80 mg/ml. Ampules, 1 mg/ml.

PROPYLENE GLYCOL

Description/Actions: Solvent used as part of the vehicle in certain pharmaceutical formulations.

PROPYLHEXEDRINE— Benzedrex®

Description/Actions: Nasal decongestant administered by inhalation.

Preparations: Inhaler, 250 mg.

PROPYLTHIOURACIL

Description/Actions: Antithyroid agent used in the treatment of hyperthyroidism.

Preparations: Tablets, 50 mg.

PROSCAR®, see Finasteride

ProSom®, see Estazolam

PROSTACYCLIN®, see Epoprostenol

PROSTAGLANDIN E2, see Dinoprostone

PROSTAGLANDIN F2 ALPHA, see Dinoprost tromethamine

PROSTAGLANDIN 12® (PG 12), see Epoprostenol

PROSTAGLANDIN X® (PGX), see Epoprostenol

PROSTAPHLIN®, see Oxacillin sodium

ProStep®, see Nicotine

PROSTIGMIN®, see Neostigmine

PROSTIN E2, see Dinoprostone

PROSTIN F2 ALPHA, see Dinoprost tromethamine

PROSTIN VR PEDIATRIC®, see Alprostadil

PROSTIN 15M®, former name for Carboprost tromethamine

PROTAMINE SULFATE

Description/Actions: Heparin antagonist indicated for intravenous use in the treatment of heparin overdosage and to neutralize heparin received during dialysis, cardiopulmonary bypass, and other procedures.

Preparations: Ampules, 10 mg/ml.

PROTAMINE ZINC INSULIN, see Insulin

PROTIRELIN—Relefact TRH®, Thypinone®

Description/Actions: Thyrotropin-releasing hormone used intravenously as an adjunctive agent in the diagnostic assessment of thyroid function.

Preparations: Ampules, 0.5 mg.

PROTONIX®, see Pantoprazole Sodium

PROTOPAM®, see Pralidoxime

PROTOPIC®, see Tacrolimus

PROTRIPTYLINE HYDROCHLORIDE—Vivactil®

Description/Actions: Tricyclic antidepressant indicated in the treatment of symptoms of depression.

Preparations: Tablets, 5 and 10 mg.

PROTROPIN®, see Somatrem

PROVENTIL®—Proventil HFA®, see Albuterol

PROVERA®, see Medroxyprogesterone

PROZAC®, see Fluoxetine

PROZAC®, WEEKLY™, see Fluoxetine

PSEUDOEPHEDRINE HYDROCHLORIDE—Efidac/24®, Novafed®, Sudafed®

PSEUDOEPHEDRINE SULFATE—Afrinol®

Decongestant.

Description/Actions: A sympathomimetic agent indicated for the temporary relief of nasal congestion due to the common cold and allergic disorders.

Warnings: Should not be used concurrently with a monoamine oxidase inhibitor. Use is best avoided in patients with advanced arteriosclerosis, symptomatic cardiovascular disease, moderate to severe hypertension, hyperthyroidism, or diabetes. Adverse reactions include restlessness, dizziness, insomnia, palpitations, tachycardia, and blood pressure elevation.

Administration: Oral.

Preparations: Tablets, 30 and 60 mg. Controlled-release capsules and tablets, 120 and 240 mg. Liquid, 15 and 30 mg/5 ml. Drops, 7.5 mg/0.8 ml.

PSYLLIUM—Metamucil®

Description/Actions: Bulk laxative used in the treatment and prevention of constipation. Used in the management of chronic watery diarrhea. Contraindicated with abdominal pain, nausea, or vomiting (especially when associated with fever), serious adhesions, and dysphagia. Diabetics and cardiacs should read product labels to see which manufacturers include sugar, aspartame, and sodium in their formulations.

Preparations: Powder, effervescent powder, granules, chewable dosage form.

PULMOZYME®, see Dornase alfa

PULMICORT RESPULES™, see Budesonide

PULMICORT TURBUHALER®, see Budesonide

PURINETHOL®, see Mercaptopurine

PYRANTEL PAMOATE—Antiminth®

Description/Actions: Anthelmintic indicated for the treatment of pinworm and roundworm infections.

Preparations: Oral suspension, 50 mg/ml.

PYRAZINAMIDE

Description/Actions: Antitubercular agent used in combination with other antitubercular agents in patients in whom therapy with the primary agents has not been satisfactory.

Preparations: Tablets, 500 mg.

PYRETHRINS—A-200 Pyrinate®, RID®, Rid Mousse®

Description/Actions: Pediculicide indicated for topical use in the treatment of head lice, body lice, and pubic (crab) lice infestations.

Preparations: Liquid, gel, and shampoo, 0.17%, 0.3%, 0.33%. Topical Scalp foam.

PYRIDIUM®, see Phenazopyridine

PYRIDOSTIGMINE BROMIDE—Mestinon®

Description/Actions: Cholinesterase inhibitor used in the treatment of myasthenia gravis. Also used parenterally as a reversal agent or antagonist to nondepolarizing muscle relaxants such as the curariform drugs.

Preparations: Tablets, 60 mg. Controlled-release tablets, 180 mg. Syrup, 60 mg/5 ml. Ampules, 5 mg/ml.

PYRIDOXINE—Vitamin B$_6$

Description/Actions: Vitamin indicated for the treatment and prevention of pyridoxine deficiency resulting from inadequate diet or use of drugs (e.g., isoniazid) that deplete pyridoxine. May also be useful in certain seizure disorders and anemias that are related to pyridoxine deficiency.

Preparations: Tablets, 10, 25, 50, 100, 200, 250, and 500 mg. Extended-release tablets, 100, 200, and 500 mg. Vials, 100 mg/ml.

PYRILAMINE MALEATE

Description/Actions: Antihistamine used in the management of allergic and related disorders, and also as an aid in the relief of insomnia.

Preparations: Tablets and capsules, 25 mg.

PYRIMETHAMINE—Daraprim®

Description/Actions: Antimalarial agent indicated for the prophylaxis of malaria and in treating infections caused by chloroquine-resistant plasmodia. Also used as an adjunct to sulfonamide in the treatment of toxoplasmosis.

Preparations: Tablets, 25 mg.

Q

QUAZEPAM—Doral®

Benzodiazepine hypnotic.

Description/Actions: Indicated for the

treatment of insomnia characterized by difficulty in falling asleep, frequent nocturnal awakenings, and/or early morning awakenings. Due to accumulation, may give larger doses for 1–2 nights, then decrease.

Warnings: Contraindicated in pregnancy. Adverse reactions include daytime sedation, headache, fatigue, dizziness, dry mouth, and dyspepsia. Patients should be cautioned regarding activities such as driving and operating machinery, as well as interactions with other CNS-acting drugs, including alcohol. Can cause dependence, and is included in Schedule IV.

Administration: Oral.

Preparations: Tablets, 7.5 and 15 mg.

QUELICIN®, see Succinylcholine

QUESTRAN®, see Cholestyramine

QUESTRAN LIGHT®, see Cholestyramine

QUETIAPINE—Seroquel®

Description/Actions: Quetiapine is a dibenzepine indicated in the management of the symptoms of psychotic disorders including schizophrenia.

Warnings: Contraindicated in hypersentitivity or lactation. Use cautiously in cardiovascular disease, cerebrovascular disease, dehydration or hypovolemia (increased risk of hypotension), history of seizures, Alzheimer's dementia, ≥ 65 y/o, hepatic impairment, hypothryroidism, history of suicide attempt, pregnancy Category C, and children (safety not established). Hepatic enzyme elevations usually occurred within the first 3 weeks of treatment and promptly returned to prestudy levels with ongoing treatment. In hepatic impairment, adjust dosing downwards.

Adverse reactions include dizziness, weight gain, leukopenia, flulike syndrome, anorexia, constipation, dry mouth, dyspepsia, palpitations, peripheral edema, postural hypotension, cough, dypsnea, pharyngitis, ear pain, rhinitis, cognitive impairment, extrapyramidal symptoms, sedation, and tardive dyskinesia,

Administration: Oral.

Preparations: Tablets, 25, 100, and 200 mg.

QUINACRINE HYDROCHLORIDE

Description/Actions: Antimalarial agent that has been used in the prevention and treatment of malaria. Acts as suppressive agent and controls clinical attacks of malaria, but is not a true prophylactic agent and does not produce a radical cure. Use as an antimalarial has been largely superseded by more effective and less toxic drugs. Also used in the treatment of giardiasis and tapeworm infections. Has been utilized via intrapleural administration in patients who experience recurrent pneumothorax.

Preparations: Tablets, 100 mg.

QUINAGLUTE®, see Quinidine gluconate

QUINAMM®, see Quinine sulfate

QUINAPRIL HYDROCHLORIDE—Accupril®

Antihypertensive agent.

Description/Actions: An angiotensin converting enzyme (ACE) inhibitor that is a prodrug. Following oral administration, is converted to its active metabolite, quinaprilat. Indicated for the treatment of hypertension and may be used alone or in combination with a thiazide diuretic. Also indicated as adjunctive therapy in the management of congestive heart failure when added to conventional therapy including a diuretic or digitalis.

Warnings: Contraindicated in patients who are hypersensitive to the drug and in patients with a history of angioedema related to previous treatment with an ACE inhibitor. Adverse reactions include headache, dizziness, fatigue, cough, nausea and abdominal pain. May cause an elevation in serum potassium levels; the risk of hyperkalemia is increased in patients also taking a potassium-sparing diuretic, a potassium supplement, and/or a potassium-containing salt substitute. May cause symptomatic postural hypotension. There have been infrequent reports of angioedema of the face, extremities, lips, tongue, glottis, and larynx, especially following the first dose. Patients should be told to report immediately any symptoms suggesting angioedema and to stop taking the drug. When used during the second and third trimesters of pregnancy, ACE inhibitors have been reported to be associated with the development of neonatal hypertension, renal failure, and skull hypoplasia; use during pregnancy should be avoided. May increase serum lithium levels and concurrent therapy should be closely monitored. Absorption is reduced when administered with a high-fat meal, and the drug is best administered apart from meals.

Administration: Oral.

Preparations: Tablets, 5, 10, 20, and 40 mg.

QUINAPRIL/ HYDROCHLOROTHIAZIDE— Accuretic®

Description/Actions: Quinapril/hydrochlorothiazide are used together orally to treat hypertension.

Precautions/Adverse Reactions: Quinapril/ hydrochlorothiazide is contraindicated in patients with a history of ACE inhibitor-induced angioedema, hereditary angioedema, or idiopathic angioedema because of the drug's tendency to cause angioedema. Quinapril/hydrochlorothiazide should be used with caution in patients with hepatic disease, renal disease, renal failure, or renal impairment because thiazides may cause hepatic coma or azotemia in these patients. Quinapril/ hydrochlorothiazide should also not be given to pregnant women, breast-feeding women, or children. Patients should have magnesium, calcium, potassium, and glucose levels in normal ranges before initiating drug. Some side affects of the drug are cough, headache, somnolence, orthostatic hypotension, electrolyte disturbances, and angioedema.

Administrations: Oral.

Patient Care Implications: Quinapril/ hydrochlorothiazide should not be administered to pregnant women, breast-feeding women, or children. Also, the drug should be given with caution to patients with hepatic and renal impairment.Blood glucose, creatinine/BUN, electrolytes, and uric acid should be monitored in patients receiving drug.

Preparations: Tablets, 10/12.5 quinapril/ hydrochlorothiazide, 20/12.5, 20/25.

QUINESTROL—Estrovis®

Description/Actions: Estrogen indicated in the treatment of moderate to severe vasomotor symptoms associated with the menopause, atrophic vaginitis, kraurosis vulvae, female hypogonadism, female castration, and primary ovarian failure.

Preparations: Tablets, 100μg.

QUINETHAZONE—Hydromox®

Description/Actions: Diuretic indicated as adjunctive therapy in edema and in the management of hypertension.

Preparations: Tablets, 50 mg.

QUINIDINE GLUCONATE— Quinaglute®

Description/Actions: Antiarrhythmic agent indicated in the prevention and treatment of a number of ventricular, atrial, and junctional (nodal) arrhythmias, and in the parenteral treatment of life-threatening *Plasmodium falciparum* malaria.

Preparations: Controlled-release tablets, 324 and 330 mg. Vials, 80 mg/ml.

QUINIDINE POLYGALACTURONATE— Cardioquin®

Description/Actions: Antiarrhythmic agent indicated in the prevention and treatment of a number of ventricular, atrial, and junctional (nodal) arrhythmias.

Preparations: Tablets, 275 mg.

QUINIDINE SULFATE

Description/Actions: Antiarrhythmic agent indicated in the prevention and treatment of a number of ventricular, atrial, and junctional (nodal) arrhythmias.

Preparations: Capsules and tablets, 100, 200, and 300 mg. Controlled-release tablets, 300 mg. Ampules, 200 mg/ml.

QUININE SULFATE—Quinamm®

Description/Actions: Antimalarial agent used in the treatment of chloroquine-resistant infections. Also used in the prevention and treatment of nocturnal leg cramps.

Preparations: Capsules and tablets, 130, 200, 260, 300, and 325 mg.

QUIXIN™, see Levofloxacin

QVAR™, see Beclomethasone

R

RABEPRAZOLE—Aciphex®

Description/Actions: Rabeprazole is a gastric proton pump inhibitor indicated for the treatment of gastroesophageal reflux disease (GERD), peptic ulcer disease, Zollinger-Ellison syndrome for the treatment of daytime and nighttime heartburn, and other symptoms associated with GERD and for the eradication of *helicobacter pylori*. It has also been effective in the management of gastric ulcer.

Precautions/Adverse Reactions: Rabeprazole should be administered with caution in patients who are pregnant or breast-feeding. The safety of the drug has not been established in children. Rabeprazole could require dosage adjustments in patients with severe hepatic disease. Rabeprazole has few side effects, but some are headache, malaise, nausea/vomiting, diarrhea, dizziness, rashes, elevation of serum gastrin (which can lead to carcinoid tumors), and elevated hepatic enzymes.

Administrations: Oral.

Patient Care Implications: Rabeprazole should be administered with caution in patients who are pregnant or breast-feeding. The drug may require dosage adjustments in patients with severe hepatic disease. Liver enzymes should be checked while patient is on the medication.

Preparations: Tablets, 20 mg.

RALOXIFENE HCL—Evista®

Description/Actions: Raloxifene is a selective estrogen receptor modulator (SERM) indicated in the prevention of osteoporosis in postmenopausal women. Clinical data indicate that raloxifene has estrogen-like effects on bone (increase BMD) and on lipid (decrease in total and LDL cholesterol levels) metabolism.

Warnings: Contraindicated in pregnancy (Category X) or in women who may become pregnant and in women with active or a history of venous thrombophlebitis. Not for use in premenopausal women. Not recommended with concomitant systemic estrogen therapy. Use cautiously in hepatic dysfunction. Discontinue 72 hours before and during prolonged immobilization and resume when fully ambulatory.

Adverse reactions include hot flashes, leg cramps, and venous thromboembolic events (rare).

Instruct patients in calcium and Vitamin D rich diet and supplement if inadequate. Add weight-bearing exercise and modify other risk factors as appropriate. Inform patients to avoid prolonged restrictions of movement during travel.

Administration: 60 mg once daily.

Preparations: Tablets, 60 mg.

RAMIPRIL—Altace®

Antihypertensive agent.

Description/Actions: An angiotensin-converting enzyme (ACE) inhibitor that is a prodrug. Following oral administration, is converted to its active metabolite, ramiprilat. Indicated for the treatment of hypertension and may be used alone or in combination with a thiazide diuretic. Treatment for CHF in stabilized patients post-MI has been found to reduce mortality.

Warnings: Adverse reactions include headache, dizziness, fatigue, and cough. May cause an elevation in serum potassium levels; the risk of hyperkalemia is increased in patients also taking a potassium-sparing diuretic, a potassium supplement, and/or a potassium-containing salt substitute. May cause symptomatic postural hypotension. There have been infrequent reports of angioedema of the face, extremities, lips, tongue, glottis, and larynx, especially following the first dose. Patients should be told to report immediately any symptoms suggesting angioedema and to stop taking the drug. When used during the second and third trimesters of pregnancy, ACE inhibitors have been reported to be associated with the development of neonatal hypertension, renal failure, and skull hypoplasia; use during pregnancy should be avoided. May increase serum lithium levels and concurrent therapy should be closely monitored.

Administration: Oral. If necessary, the capsules may be opened and the contents sprinkled on a small amount of applesauce or mixed in apple juice or water.

Preparations: Capsules, 1.25, 2.5, 5, and 10 mg.

RANITIDINE HYDROCHLORIDE—Zantac®

Antiulcer agent.

Description/Actions: A histamine H2 receptor antagonist that inhibits gastric acid secretion. Indicated (1) in the short-term treatment of active duodenal ulcer; (2) for maintenance therapy for duodenal ulcer patients at reduced dosage after healing of acute ulcers; (3) for the treatment of pathological hypersecretory conditions (e.g., Zollinger-Ellison syndrome); (4) in the short-term treatment of active, benign gastric ulcer; (5) in the treatment of gastroesophageal reflux disease; and (6) in the treatment of erosive esophagitis, and in the maintenance treatment of healed erosive esophagitis.

Warnings: Adverse reactions include headache and GI effects.

Administration: Oral, intravenous, and intramuscular.

Preparations: Tablets, 75, 150 and 300 mg. Geldose capsules, 150 and 300 mg. Efferdose tablets and granules, 150 mg. Syrup, 15 mg/ml. Vials, 25 mg/ml and 50 mg/100 ml containers.

RAPACURONIUM—Raplon®

Description/Actions: Rapacuronium is used as an adjunct to general anesthesia for endotracheal intubation and surgical procedures.

Precautions/Adverse Reactions: Rapacuronium should be administered with caution in patients who have renal impairment, hepatic impairment, obesity, pulmonary disease, underlying neuromuscular disease, dehydration, electrolyte imbalance, acid/base imbalance, burns, cerebral palsy, muscle trauma, and malignant hyperthermia.

The drug should be avoided in patients who are pregnant, breast-feeding, or under 1 month of age. Also any patients with a condition that would be exacerbated by histamine release should be monitored. Some adverse effects are erythema, bronchospasm, flushing, sinus tachycardia, sinus bradycardia, muscle paralysis, apnea, dyspnea, and respiratory depression. Hypotension is the most common adverse side effect.

Administration: Intravenous.

Patient Care Implications: The drug should be avoided in patients who are pregnant, breast-feeding, or under 1 month of age. Also any patients with a condition that would be exacerbated by histamine release should be monitored. The patient should have ABGs, peripheral nerve stimulation, serum electrolytes, and serum magnesium checked while on the medication. Rapacuronium should be given only after the patient is unconscious.

Preparations: Vials, 100 mg/5 ml, 200 mg/10 ml.

RAPAMUNE®, see Sirolimus

RAPLON®, see Rapacuronium

RAUDIXIN®, see Rauwolfia serpentina

REFLUDAN®, see Lepirudan

REGITINE®, see Phentolamine

REGLAN®, see Metoclopramide

REGRANEX®, see Becaplermin

RELA®, see Carisoprodol

RELAFEN®, see Nabumetone

RELENZA®, see Zanamivir

REMERON®, see Mirtazapine

RENESE®, see Polythiazide

RENOVA®, see Tretinoin

REOPRO®, see Abciximab

REPAGLINIDE—Prandin®

Description/Actions: Antidiabetic agent chemically unrelated to the sulfonylureas. Its action is dependent upon functioning beta cells in the pancreatic islets. Compared to other oral antidiabetic agents, repaglinide has a quick onset of action and a short duration of action. Following oral administration, peak plasma levels occur within 1 hour, and it is rapidly eliminated from the blood with a half-life of about 1 hour.

It is indicated as an adjunct to diet and exercise for patients with type 2 diabetes and as monotherapy or in combination with metformin, rosiglitazone, or pioglitazone for the treatment of type 2 diabetes.

Warnings: Contraindicated in Type I diabetes and diabetic ketoacidosis. Titrate carefully in renal or hepatic dysfunction. Use cautiously in elderly, debilitated, malnourished, stressed, adrenal, or pituitary insufficiency. Increases the risk of hypoglycemia. Monitor for initial effect and for secondary failure. Pregnancy Category C. Not recommended for use in nursing mothers.

Adverse reactions include hypoglycemia, upper respiratory infection, headache, diarrhea, constipation, arthralgia, back or chest pain. Oral antidiabetics may increase the risk of cardiovascular mortality.

Instruct patients to adhere to diet and exercise programs. Test blood glucose and HbA1C regularly. Inform patients about management of hypoglycemia and explain primary vs. secondary failure.

Administration: Oral.

Preparations: Tablets, 0.5, 1, and 2 mg.

RESCRIPTOR®, see Delavirdine Mesylate

RESCULA®, see Unoprostone

RESERPINE—Serpasil®

Description/Actions: Rauwolfia alkaloid indicated in the treatment of hypertension and for the relief of symptoms in agitated psychotic states. Has been used parenterally in acute hypertensive and psychiatric conditions.

Preparations: Tablets, 0.1, 0.25, and 1 mg. Ampules, 2.5 mg/ml.

RESORCINOL

Description/Actions: Antipruritic, anti-infective, and keratolytic agent used topically with other agents in the treatment of seborrheic dermatitis, acne, and other dermatologic conditions.

RESTORIL®, see Temazepam

RETEPLASE—Retavase®

Description/Actions: Thrombolytic indicated to improve ventricular function post acute myocardial infarction (MI), to reduce the incidence of congestive heart failure.

Warnings: Contraindicated in patients with a history of cerebral vascular accident, active internal bleeding, intracranial or intraspinal surgery or trauma within the past 2 months, intracranial neoplasm, arteriovenous malformation or aneurysm, bleeding diathesis, severe uncontrolled hypertension, and history of severe allergic reactions to altaplase, anistreplase, or streptokinase. Use cautiously in patients with hypertension, recent major surgery, obstetrical delivery, organ biopsy, previous puncture of noncompressible vessel, GU or GI bleeding or trauma, high risk of left heart thrombus, subacute bacterial endocarditis, acute pericarditis, hemostatic defects, severe renal or hepatic dysfunction, cerebrovascular disease, hemorrhagic ophthalmic conditions, septic thrombophlebitis or occluded AV cannula at seriously infected sites, and patients over 75 years of age. Cholesterol embolization and/or reperfusion arrhythmias may occur. Avoid IM injections, noncompressible punctures, and unnecessary handling of patients. Minimize venipuncture. Check puncture sites.

Adverse reactions include bleeding (including intracranial hemorrhage) and reperfusion arrhythmias.

Administration: 10 units IV over 2 minutes, then 30 minutes after initiation of first dose give a second dose of 10 units IV over 2 minutes. Withhold second dose if serious bleeding or anaphylaxis occurs.

Preparations: Powder for IV injection supplied with 2 ml diluent (preservative-free). 10.8 units/vial.

RETEVASE®, see Reteplase

RETIN-A®, see Tretinoin

RETINOIC ACID, see Tretinoin

RETROVIR®, see Zidovudine

REVERSOL®, see Edrophonium

REVEX®, see Nalmefene hydrochloride

RÉV-EYES®, see Dapiprazole hydrochloride

ReVia®, see Naltrexone hydrochloride

R-GENE®, see Arginine

RHEOMACRODEX®, see Dextran

RHEUMATREX®, see Methotrexate

RHINOCORT®, see Budesonide

RHO(D) IMMUNE GLOBULIN—RhoGAM®

Description/Actions: Immune globulin administered intramuscularly to prevent Rh immunization in Rh negative individuals exposed to Rh positive red blood cells. Indicated in pregnancy and other obstetric conditions when it is known or suspected that fetal red cells have entered the circulation of an Rh negative mother unless the fetus or the father can be shown conclusively to be Rh negative. Also indicated for any Rh negative female of childbearing age who receives a transfusion of Rh positive red blood cells or whole blood, or components prepared from Rh positive blood.

Preparations: Vials and syringes.

RHOGAM®, see Rh₀(D) immune globulin

RIBAVIRIN—Virazole®

Antiviral agent.

Description/Actions: Indicated for the aerosol treatment of carefully selected hospitalized infants and young children with severe lower respiratory tract infections due to respiratory syncytial virus (RSV).

Warnings: Should not be used in infants requiring assisted ventilation because the drug may precipitate on the valves and tubing of the respirator and interfere with safe and effective ventilation. Is teratogenic in animals and, although presently indicated only in infants and young children, its potential value for viral infections in adults warrants recognition of the contraindication to its use during pregnancy.

Administration: Aerosol, delivered to an infant oxygen hood (or administered by face mask or oxygen tent if necessary). Is administered using a small-particle aerosol generator (model SPAG-2), and other aerosol-generating devices should not be used.

Preparations: Vials, 6 g.

RIBOFLAVIN—Vitamin B₂

Description/Actions: Vitamin indicated in the prevention and treatment of riboflavin deficiency.

Preparations: Tablets, 10, 25, 50, and 100 mg.

RID®, see Pyrethrins

RIDAURA®, see Auranofin

RID MOUSSE®, see Pyrethrins

RIFABUTIN—Mycobutin®

Antimycobacterial agent.

Description/Actions: Is active against *Mycobacterium avium* and *Mycobacterium intracellulare*, which comprise *Mycobacterium avium* complex (MAC). Indicated for the prevention of disseminated *Mycobacterium avium* complex (MAC) disease in patients with advanced human immunodeficiency virus (HIV) infection.

Warnings: Contraindicated in patients who are hypersensitive to rifampin. Adverse reactions include rash, gastrointestinal intolerance, neutropenia, flulike syndrome, arthralgia, hepatitis, and a brown-orange discoloration of urine, feces, saliva, sputum, perspiration, tears, and skin, as well as permanent staining of soft contact lenses. May increase the activity of hepatic enzymes and reduce the effect of other therapeutic agents that are metabolized by these enzyme systems. Patients using oral contraceptives should be advised to use nonhormonal or additional methods of birth control while taking rifabutin. Should not be administered to patients with active tuberculosis because of the possibility of the development of tuberculosis that is resistant both to rifabutin and rifampin.

Administration: Oral, once a day. For patients who experience GI intolerance, administering doses twice a day with food may avoid these effects.

Preparations: Capsules, 150 mg.

RIFADIN®, see Rifampin

RIFADIN IV®, see Rifampin

RIFAMPIN—Rifadin®, Rifadin IV®, Rimactane®

Description/Actions: Antitubercular agent indicated in the treatment of tuberculosis. Also indicated for the treatment of asymptomatic carriers of *Neisseria meningitidis*. Has a broad-spectrum of action and is also useful in the treatment of staphylococcal infections, legionnaires' disease, leprosy, and other infections.

Preparations: Capsules, 150 and 300 mg. Vials, 600 mg.

RIFAPENTINE—Priftin®

Description/Actions: Rifapentine is a drug structurally related to rifampin indicated in the treatment of susceptible pulmonary tuberculosis.

Precautions/Adverse Reactions: Perform baseline liver enzymes including bilirubin, CBC, and platelet count. Use cautiously in patients with hepatic impairment. Monitor liver functions before and every 2–4 weeks during therapy. Discontinue if signs of liver disease occur or worsen. Do periodic susceptibility tests for persistently positive cultures. Consider pyridoxine supplements in adolescents, malnourished, or those at risk for nueropathy (e.g., alcoholics, diabetics). If used in the last few weeks of pregnancy, monitor clotting parameters in the mother and infant (may need vitamin K).

Adverse reactions include hyperuricemia, proteinuria, increased serum transaminases, lymphopenia, pyuria, urinary casts, hematuria, rash, arthralgia, pruritus, neutropenia, pain, GI upset, anemia, hepatitis, hyperbilirubinemia, and pseudomembranous colitis.

Administration: Oral.

Patient Care Implications: Rifapentine must always be administered with at least one other antituberculosis drug to which the isolate is susceptible. Inform the patient that the dosing schedule must be strictly followed and that doses are not to be skipped. Explain the concepts of resistance and the role the patient plays in prevention. Caution the patient to finish out the course of therapy and not to stop treatment when symptoms subside. Instruct patient to avoid alcohol during therapy. Advise the patient that the drug may produce a reddish coloration of the urine, sweat, sputum, and tears. Contact lenses may become permanently stained. Oral contraceptives may be affected by use of this medication, and other means of pregnancy prevention should be employed.

Preparations: Tablets, 150 mg.

RILUZOLE—Rilutek®

Description/Actions: Used in the treatment of amyotrophic lateral sclerosis (ALS) to extend survival or time to tracheostomy. The etiology and pathogenesis are not known, but it has been hypothesized that motor neurons, made vulnerable through either genetic predisposition or environmental factors, are injured by glutamate. Riluzole's pharmacologic properties include an inhibitory effect on glutamate release, among others, which may account for its effect on ALS.

Warnings: Neutropenia may develop, usually within the first 2 months of treatment. Warn patients to report febrile illnesses as a trigger for prompt checking of white blood cell counts. Use cautiously in patients with a history of abnormal liver function tests. Elevation of serial LFTs (especially bilirubin) should preclude use of riluzole. Use cautiously in patients with impaired renal function. Adverse reactions include asthenia, nausea, dizziness, diarrhea, anorexia, vertigo, somnolence, circumoral paresthesia (dose-related), decreased lung function, abdominal pain, pneumonia, and vomiting.

Administration: 50 mg orally on an empty stomach every 12 hours. No increased benefit can be expected from higher doses, but adverse events are increased.

Preparations: Tablets, 50 mg.

RIMACTANE®, see Rifampin

RIMANTADINE HYDROCHLORIDE—
Flumadine®

Antiviral agent.

Description/Actions: Indicated for the prophylaxis and treatment of illness caused by various strains of influenza A virus in adults and for prophylaxis in children age 1 year and over.

Warnings: Contraindicated in patients who are hypersensitive to the drug or to amantadine. Adverse reactions include insomnia, dizziness, nervousness, fatigue, headache, nausea, vomiting, anorexia, dry mouth, and abdominal pain.

Administration: Oral.

Preparations: Tablets, 100 mg. Syrup, 50 mg/5ml.

RIMEXOLONE—Vexol®

Description/Actions: Ophthalmic preparation containing benzalkonium chloride used in the treatment of postoperative inflammation and anterior uveitis.

Warnings: Contraindicated in epithelial herpes simplex keratitis and other viral or fungal infections, including vaccinia and varicella. Do not use in the presence of ocular mycobacterial, fungal, or untreated purident infections. Use cautiously with ocular hypertension/glaucoma, optic nerve damage, and defects in visual acuity and visual fields. Posterior subcapsular cataract formation or fungal invasion may occur with prolonged use. May mask secondary ocular infections. Corneal or scleral thinning may occur. Monitor intraocular pressures. Adverse reactions include blurred vision, discharge, discomfort, ocular pain, increased intraocular pressure, foreign body sensation, hyperemia, and pruritus.

Administration: Start 1–2 drops into the conjuctival sac(s) 4 times a day 24 hours after surgery and continue through the first 2 weeks postoperatively. Uveitis: 1–2 drops in conjunctival sac(s) every hour while awake the first week and then 1 drop every 2 hours while awake for the second week, then taper until resolved.

Preparations: Ophthalmic suspension, 5 and 10 ml.

RIMSO 50®, see Dimethyl sulfoxide

RINGER'S INJECTION

Description/Actions: Intravenous electrolyte replacement solution containing sodium, potassium, calcium, and chloride.

Preparations: Solution, 500 and 1000 ml.

RIOPAN®, see Magaldrate

RISEDRONATE—Actonel®

Description/Actions: Risendronate is used for the treatment of Paget's disease in certain patients and for the prevention and treatment of postmenopausal osteoporosis.

Precautions/Adverse Reactions: Risedronate should not be administered to patients with renal failure (creatinine clearance < 30 ml/min). Hypocalcemia or other bone abnormalities should be corrected before initiating drug therapy. Risedronate should not be given or used in caution in pregnant women, breast-feeding women, children < 18 years old, or patients with GI disease.

Some adverse effects are iritis, hypocalcemia, hypophosphatemia, diarrhea, abdominal pain, bone pain, and headache.

Administrations: Oral. Take ≤ 30 minutes before first food or drink (except water). Avoid lying down for 30 minutes after taking to reduce possibility of GI side effects.

Preparations: Tablets, 5 mg, 30 mg, 35 mg.

RISPERDAL®, see Risperidone

RISPERIDONE—Risperdal®
Antipsychotic agent.

Description/Actions: Risperidone is indicated for the management of the manifestations of psychotic disorders and for delaying relapse in the long-term treatment of schizophrenia.

Warnings: Adverse reactions include extrapyramidal symptoms, insomnia, agitation, anxiety, headache, constipation, abdominal pain, tachycardia, and rhinitis. Patients should be cautioned about driving or operating hazardous machinery until they are reasonably certain that the drug does not affect them adversely. Caution should also be exercised in patients taking other centrally acting drugs, and patients should be advised to avoid the consumption of alcoholic beverages. May cause orthostatic hypotension, especially during the initial dose-titration period, and the initial dose should not exceed 1 mg twice daily to reduce the risk. May lengthen the QT interval and caution should be exercised in patients with risk factors for this complication (e.g., bradycardia, use of other drugs that prolong the QT interval). May antagonize the effects of levodopa.

Administration: Oral.

Preparations: Tablets, 0.5, 1, 2, 3, and 4 mg. Oral solution, 0.25, 0.5, 1 mg/ml.

RITALIN®, see Methylphenidate

RITALIN SR®, see Methylphenidate

RITODRINE HYDROCHLORIDE—Yutopar®

Description/Actions: Uterine relaxant indicated in the management of preterm labor in suitable patients for the purpose of prolonging gestation. Continue IV for 12–24 hours after contractions cease, and begin PO 30 minutes before IV is stopped.

Preparations: Tablets, 10 mg. Ampules, vials, and syringes, 10 mg/ml and 15 mg/ml.

RITONOVIR—Norvir®
Antiviral/protease inhibitor.

Description/Actions: Used in treatment of HIV infection, either as monotherapy or in combination with other nucleoside analogues or protease inhibitors.

Warnings: Use cautiously in patients with impaired hepatic function. Adverse reactions include GI upset, asthenia, abdominal pain, headache, anorexia, paresthesias, taste perversion, fever, hyperlipidemia, dizziness, rash, throat irritation, malaise, somnolence, insomnia, and sweating. Due to increased plasma concentrations of various agents, and also large increases in concentrations of highly metabolized sedatives and hypnotics, the coadministration of ritonovir with such agents is contraindicated, and prescribers should verify a patient's full drug profile prior to prescribing this agent.

Administration: Oral with meals.

Preparations: Capsules, 100 mg; oral solution, 80 mg/ml.

RIVASTIGMINE TARTRATE—
Exelon®

Description/Actions: Indicated in the treatment of mild to moderate dementia of the Alzheimer's type.

Precautions/Adverse Reactions: Rivastigmine is contraindicated in patients with a known hypersensitivity to rivastigmine, or other carbamate derivatives or to any other component of the product. Significant gastrointestinal adverse reactions including nausea, vomiting, anorexia, and weight loss (females > males) have been observed during therapy with rivastigmine. Cholinesterase inhibitors have been shown to increase gastric acid secretion; therefore, patients should be monitored for the development of peptic ulcers or gastrointestinal bleeding. Rivastigmine is likely to potentiate the effects of succinylcholine-type muscle relaxation during anesthesia. Use cautiously in patients with sick sinus syndrome or other supraventricular cardiac conduction conditions. Use cautiously in patients with a history of asthma or obstructive pulmonary disease. Monitor patient for urinary obstruction and or seizures due to increased cholinergic activity. Rivastigmine is metabolized through hydrolysis by esterases with minimal metabolism via the cytochrome P450 system; therefore, no significant drug interactions are expected with drugs metabolized via this system. Anticholinergics—rivastigmine has the potential to interfere with the activity of anticholinergic agents. Other cholinesterase inhibitors—rivastigmine may potentiate the effects of these agents. Pregnancy Category B. There are no adequate or well-controlled studies in pregnant women. Rivastigmine should be used during pregnancy only if the potential benefit justifies the potential risk to the fetus. Excretion in human breast milk is unknown. Rivastigmine has no indication for use in nursing mothers. There are no adequate or well-controlled studies documenting safety or efficacy of rivastigmine in children. Most common adverse reactions occurring in at least 5% of patients treated with rivastigmine include nausea, vomiting, anorexia, dyspepsia, weight loss, and asthenia. Other adverse effects observed include increased sweating, syncope, accidental trauma, fatigue, malaise, influenza-like symptoms, hypertension, headache, somnolence, tremor, abdominal pain, constipation, flatulence, insomnia, confusion, depression, hallucinations, urinary tract infections, and rhinitis. Monitor for GI effects.

Administration: Oral with food.

Preparations: Capsules, 1.5 mg, 3 mg, 4.5 mg, and 6 mg. Oral solution, 2 mg/ml.

RIZATRIPTAN BENZOATE—
Maxalt®, Maxalt MLT®

Description/Actions: A selective 5-HT 1B/1D antimigraine medication indicated for an acute migraine attack with or without an aura.

Precautions/Adverse Reactions: Rizatriptan is contraindicated in ischemic heart disease, coronary artery vasospasm, uncontrolled hypertension, other significant cardiovascular disease, basilar or hemiplegic migraine, within 24 hours of other 5-HT1 agonists or egro-type drugs and during or within 2 weeks after discontinuing MAOIs. Confirm diagnosis prior to prescribing Rizatriptan. Reevaluate if angina or ischemic symptoms occur or if no response after the first dose. Exclude underlying cardiovascular disease, supervise first dose, and consider ECG monitoring in patients with a likelihood of undiagnosed coronary disease. Monitor cardiovascular function in long-term intermittent use. Use cautiously in patients with hepatic dysfunctions and on dialysis. Pregnancy Category C.

Adverse reactions include asthenia,

somolence, dizziness, paresthesis, chest/throat pressure or other pain, dry mouth, nausea, and headache.

Administration: Adults ≥ 18: initially 5 or 10 mg; may repeat after 2 hours; max of 30 mg/day.

Concomitant propanalol use: 5 mg; max 3 doses in a day.

Patient Care Implications: Instruct patients that this medication is for use during acute attack and does not reduce the frequency or severity of attacks. Advise patients to take the medication during the aura or immediately when the attack starts. Inform the patient to notify the prescriber immediately if chest pain/tightness occurs during use and to withhold any further doses until evaluated by the prescriber. Tell the patient that lying down in a quiet, darkened room may help to further relieve the headache.

Preparations: Maxalt—tablets, 5 and 10 mg. Maxalt MLT—orally disintegrating peppermint flavored tablets, 5 and 10 mg.

RMS®, see Morphine

ROBAXIN®, see Methocarbamol

ROBIMYCIN®, see Erythromycin base

ROBINUL®, see Glycopyrrolate

ROBITUSSIN®, see Guaifenesin

ROCALTROL®, see Calcitriol

ROCEPHIN®, see Ceftriaxone

ROCURONIUM BROMIDE— Zemuron®

Nondepolarizing neuromuscular blocking agent.

Description/Actions: Indicated for inpatients and outpatients as an adjunct to general anesthesia to facilitate both rapid sequence and routine tracheal intubation and to provide skeletal muscle relaxation during surgery or mechanical ventilation.

Warnings: Must be used with caution in patients with neuromuscular disease (e.g., myasthenia gravis) and in patients receiving other medications that may increase or prolong neuromuscular block. Action may be enhanced by the prior administration of succinylcholine, and rocuronium should not be administered until recovery from succinylcholine has been observed.

Administration: Intravenous. Should not be mixed with alkaline solutions in the same syringe or administered simultaneously during intravenous infusion through the same needle.

Preparations: Vials, 10 mg/ml.

ROFECOXIB—Vioxx®

Description/Actions: A COX-2 inhibitor indicated in the treatment of osteoarthritis, rheumatoid arthritis, acute pain, and the pain of dysmenorrhea.

Precautions/Adverse Reactions: It is contraindicated in aspirin allergy and the third trimester of pregnancy. Use cautiously in advanced renal disease, fluid retention, heart failure, hypertension, asthma, alcoholism, dehydration, debilitated and the elderly. Do not use in moderate to severe hepatic insufficiency and discontinue if liver disease develops. Monitor for GI ulcer/bleed. The risk of ulcer is increased if patient is otherwise at high risk, with extended drug treatment, high doses, history of GI bleed, or ulcer.

Adverse reactions include GI upset, edema, hypertension, bronchitis, fatigue, increases in liver function tests (AST/ALT), ulcer, GI bleed, and meningitis.

Administration: Oral. In rheumatoid arthritis: 25 mg once daily (maximum recommended dose 25 mg). Chronic use of rofecoxib 50 mg daily is not recommended. Hepatic impairment: Patients with moderate hepatic impairment (Child-Pugh score 7–9) should be treated with the lowest possible dose.

Patient Care Implications: Instruct patients not to exceed dosing guidelines and not to independently increase the dose, as this will increase the risk of serious adverse events. If pain relief is not achieved, call the prescriber for other treatment options. If stomach discomfort is experienced, promptly call the prescriber.

Preparations: Tablets, 12.5, 25 and 50 mg. Oral suspension, 12.5 mg/5 ml and 25 mg/5 ml.

ROFERON-A®, see Interferon alfa-2a recombinant

ROGAINE®, see Minoxidil

ROMAZICON®, see Flumazenil

ROPIVACAINE HYDROCHLORIDE—Naropin®

Description/Actions: Long-acting local anesthetic indicated in local or regional anesthesia or surgery and management of acute pain, including the pain of obstetrical procedures.

Warnings: Contraindicated in patients with known hypersensitivity to any local anesthetic of this type (i.e., bupivacaine, lidocaine, mepivacaine). Adverse reactions include hypotension, fetal bradycardia, nausea, bradycardia, vomiting, parasthesia, and back pain. Carefully monitor vital signs including cardiovascular and respiratory status, and level of consciousness after each injection. Oxygen and resuscitative equipment should be available. Use cautiously in patients with severe hepatic or renal impairment and impaired cardiovascular function.

Administration: Administer the smallest dose and concentration required to produce desirable results. Avoid rapid administration of large volume, and use fractional (incremental) doses. Administer as infiltrate, block or epidural or intermittent bolus.

Preparations: Injection, 2, 5, 7.5, and 10 mg/ml.

ROSIGLITAZONE—Avandia®

Description/Actions: Antidiabetic agent indicated as an adjunct to diet and exercise in Type II diabetes, for monotherapy or added to metformin.

Precautions/Adverse Reactions: Do not use for treatment of Type I diabetes or diabetic ketoacidosis. Do not start therapy in active liver disease or if ALT is > 2.5 × ULN. Monitor transaminases at baseline and every 2 months for the first 12 months, then periodically. Discontinue if ALT is > 3 × ULN or if jaundice occurs. Not for use in patients with a history of troglitazone associated juandice.

Use cautiously in patients with a history of liver disease. Rosiglitazone can cause fluid retention, which may exacerbate or lead to heart failure. Not recommended for use in patients with New York Heart Association (NYHA) class 3 and 4. Patients should be monitored for signs and symptoms of heart failure.

Rosiglitazone may cause resumption of premenopausal ovulation in anovulatory patients with a risk of an unintended pregnancy. Pregnancy Category C.

Adverse reactions include upper respiratory tract infection, edema, weight gain, anemia, and changes in serum lipid levels.

Administration: Oral.

Patient Care Implications: Instruct patients to continue following their diet and exercise to control diabetes. This drug does not eliminate the need for these other measures. Tell the patient to call the physician immediately if (s)he notes darkening of the urine or yellow color to skin or the whites of the eyes.

Preparations: Tablets, 2, 4, and 8 mg.

ROWASA®, see Mesalamine

ROXANOL®, see Morphine

ROXANOL SR®, see Morphine

ROXICODONE®, see Oxycodone

RUBEX®, see Doxorubicin

RUFEN®, see Ibuprofen

RYTHMOL®, see Propafenone

S

SAFFLOWER OIL

Description/Actions: Nutritional supplement used in the management of patients requiring caloric supplementation.

Preparations: Emulsion.

SALFLEX®, see Salsalate

SALAGEN®, see Pilocarpine hydrochloride

SALICYLAMIDE

Description/Actions: Analgesic used in the management of mild to moderate pain.

Preparations: Tablets, 325 and 667 mg.

SALICYLIC ACID

Description/Actions: Keratolytic agent used topically as an aid in the removal of excessive keratin in hyperkeratotic skin disorders, including warts. Also used in combination with other agents in a number of dermatologic conditions, including acne.

Preparations: Cream, ointment, liquid, gel, and plaster in concentrations ranging from 1% to 60%.

SALMETEROL XINAFOATE— Serevent®, Serevent® Discus

Antiasthmatic agent.

Description/Actions: Is a selective beta-2-adrenergic receptor agonist that is administered by oral inhalation. Has a long duration of action that permits twice-daily administration. Indicated for long-term, twice-daily (morning and evening) administration in the maintenance treatment of asthma and in the prevention of bronchospasm in patients 12 years of age and older with reversible obstructive airway disease, including patients with symptoms of nocturnal asthma, who require regular treament with inhaled, short-acting beta-2-adrenergic agonists. Is also indicated for the prevention of exercise-induced bronchospasm and maintenance treatment of COPD-associated bronchospasm (including emphysema and chronic bronchitis). Patients must also be provided with a short-acting inhaled beta-2-adrenergic agonist (e.g., albuterol) for the treatment of symptoms that occur despite twice-daily use of salmeterol. Should not be used to treat acute symptoms.

Warnings: Adverse reactions include headache, tremor, cough, and dizziness. Should be used with caution in patients with coronary insufficiency, cardiac arrhythmias, and hypertension, and in patients being treated with a tricyclic antidepressant or a monoamine oxidase inhibitor. Should not be used to treat acute symptoms.

Administration: Oral inhalation. Is administered twice daily (morning and evening), approximately 12 hours apart). If symptoms arise in the period between doses, a short-acting inhaled beta-2-adrenergic agonist should be taken for immediate relief, and the patient should not take higher doses of salmeterol.

Preparations: Powder for inhalation, 50 mg/blister. Serevent® Discus 50 mcg/actuation.

SALSALATE—Disalcid®, Salflex®

Description/Actions: Salicylate analgesic/anti-inflammatory agent indicated for the relief of the signs and symptoms of rheumatoid arthritis, osteoarthritis, and related disorders.

284 • SALT

Preparations: Capsules and tablets, 500 and 750 mg.

SALT, see Sodium chloride

SALURON®, see Hydroflumethiazide

SANDIMMUNE®, see Cyclosporine

SANDOSTATIN®, see Octreotide

SANOREX®, see Mazindol

SANSERT®, see Methysergide

SANTYL®, see Collagenase

SAQUINAVIR—Fortovase®, Invirase

Description/Actions: Antiviral (HIV protease inhibitor) indicated in the management of advanced HIV infection in combination with zidovudine, and/or other nucleoside analogues.

Warnings: Use cautiously in patients with hepatic impairment. Adverse reactions include diarrhea, abdominal discomfort, nausea, asthenia, and rash.

Administration: Oral with food.

Preparations: Capsules, 200 mg.

SARAFEM™, see Fluoxetine hydrochloride

SARGRAMOSTIM—Leukine®, Prokine®

Colony stimulating factor.

Description/Actions: A human granulocyte-macrophage colony–stimulating factor (GM-CSF) produced by recombinant DNA technology. Accelerates bone marrow recovery after autologous bone marrow transplantation. Indicated for acceleration of myeloid recovery in patients with non-Hodgkin's lymphoma, acute lymphoblastic leukemia, and Hodgkin's disease undergoing autologous bone marrow transplantation. Also indicated for patients who have undergone allogeneic or autologous bone marrow transplantation in whom engraftment is delayed or has failed.

Warnings: Contraindicated in patients with excessive leukemic myeloid blasts in the bone marrow or peripheral blood (greater than 10%). Adverse reactions include diarrhea, asthenia, rash, malaise, transient supraventricular arrhythmias, peripheral edema, and pleural and/or pericardial effusion. May cause dyspnea and special attention should be given to respiratory symptoms during or immediately following infusion, especially in patients with preexisting lung disease. Caution must be exercised in patients with any malignancy with myeloid characteristics because of the possibility that the drug may act as a growth factor for the tumor.

Administration: Intravenous. Should be administered not less than 24 hours after the last dose of chemotherapy and 12 hours after the last dose of radiotherapy. A complete blood count with differential is recommended twice per week during therapy.

Preparations: Vials, 250 and 500 ug.

SCOPOLAMINE HYDROBROMIDE—Hyoscine, Transderm-Scojp®

Description/Actions: Anticholinergic agent indicated for parenteral use for preanesthetic medication, for obstetric amnesia in conjunction with analgesics, and for calming delirium. Also used orally and transdermally for the prevention of nausea and vomiting associated with motion sickness. Also indicated for ophthalmic use to produce cycloplegia and mydriasis.

Preparations: Capsules, 0.25 mg. Transdermal therapeutic system, 1.5 mg (used over a period of 3 days). Ampules and vials, 0.3 mg/ml, 0.4 mg/ml, 1 mg/ml. Ophthalmic solution, 0.25%.

SECOBARBITAL SODIUM—
Seconal®

Description/Actions: Barbiturate used parenterally as a preanesthetic and for the emergency control of certain acute convulsive episodes.

Preparations: Vials and syringes, 50 mg/ml.

SECONAL®, see Secobarbital

SECTRAL®, see Acebutolol

SELEGILINE HYDROCHLORIDE—Eldepryl®

Antiparkinson agent.

Description/Actions: Also known as deprenyl, it acts as a selective inhibitor of monoamine oxidase Type B. Indicated as an adjunct to levodopa/carbidopa in the management of Parkinson's disease.

Warnings: Adverse reactions include nausea, abdominal pain, dry mouth, dizziness, fainting, confusion, hallucinations, and vivid dreams. Does not inhibit monoamine oxidase Type A at the recommended dosage level, and is not likely to interact with the sympathomimetic amines and tyramine-containing foods that can cause hypertensive reactions when used concurrently with a nonselective monoamine oxidase inhibitor; however, the recommended dosage level should not be exceeded, as the selectivity of selegiline is reduced with increasing daily doses. Concomitant use of selegiline with meperidine should be avoided.

Administration: Oral. Administered in divided doses at breakfast and lunch.

Preparations: Capsules, 5 mg.

SELENIUM SULFIDE—Selsun®

Description/Actions: Antiseborrheic agent indicated for topical use in the treatment of dandruff and seborrheic dermatitis of the scalp, and also in the management of tinea versicolor.

Preparations: Lotion shampoo, 1% and 2.5%.

SELSUN®, see Selenium sulfide

SEMI-LENTE INSULIN, see Insulin

SEMPREX-D®, see Acrivastine/pseudoephedrine hydrochloride

SENNA CONCENTRATE—
Senokot®

Description/Actions: Laxative used in the prevention and treatment of constipation.

Preparations: Tablets, granules, syrup, liquid, and suppositories.

SENOKOT®, see Senna concentrate

SEPTOCAINE™, see articaine hydrochloride and epinephrine

SEPTRA®, see Trimethoprim-sulfamethoxazole

SERAX®, see Oxazepam

SERENTIL®, see Mesoridazine

SEREVENT®, see Salmeterol xinafoate

SEREVENT® DISCUS, see Salmeterol xinafoate

SEROMYCIN®, see Cycloserine

SEROPHENE®, see Clomiphene

SEROQUEL®, see Quetiapine

SEROSTIM®, see Somatropin

SERPASIL®, see Reserpine

SERTRALINE HYDROCHLORIDE—Zoloft®

Antidepressant.

Description/Actions: Is a serotonin reuptake inhibitor. Indicated for the treatment of depression, panic disorder, obsessive-compulsive disorder (OCD), post traumatic stress disorder (PTSD), premenstrual dysphoric disorder (PMDD), and for the acute and long-term treatment of social anxiety disorder.

Warnings: Adverse reactions include nausea, diarrhea, dyspepsia, dizziness, tremor, insomnia, somnolence, dry mouth, increased sweating, and sexual dysfunction in male patients (primarily ejaculatory delay). May decrease appetite resulting in significant weight loss. Concomitant use with a monoamine oxidase inhibitor (MAOI) or use within 14 days of treatment with an MAOI may result in serious, potentially fatal reactions (hyperthermia, rigidity, myoclonus, autonomic instability, with fluctuating vital signs and extreme agitation, which may proceed to delirium and coma). Sertraline should be stopped at least 14 days prior to MAOI therapy. Concomitant administration of sertraline and pimozide is contraindicated.

Administration: Oral.

Preparations: Tablets, 25, 50, and 100 mg. Oral concentrate, 20 mg/ml.

SERZONE®, see Nefazodone hydrochloride

SEVELAMER HCL—Renagel®

Description/Actions: Sevelamer is a phosphate-binding agent indicated for the reduction of serum phosphates in end-stage renal disease (ESRD).

Precautions/Adverse Reactions: This agent is contraindicated in hypophosphotemia and bowel obstruction. Use cautiously in patients with dysphagia, swallowing disorders, severe GI motility disorders, and major GI tract surgery. Monitor serum calcium, bicarbonate, and chloride. Sevelamer may cause reductions in vitamins E, K, and folic acid, and levels should be monitored. It may bind with other agents, so, when administering with drugs that have a narrow therapeutic index, separate dosing by at least 1 hour before or 3 hours after sevelamer. Adverse reactions include nausea, constipation, diarrhea, flatulence, and dyspepsia.

Administration: Oral. Swallow whole with meals; do not crush, chew, or open.

Patient Care Implications: Instruct patients that this medication is an adjunct to diet and does not eliminate the need for dietary restrictions. Sevelamer has also been associated with decreases in total serum cholesterol and low-density lipoprotein cholesterol. It is not absorbed systemically.

Preparations: Capsules, 403 mg. Tablets, 400 and 800 mg.

SEVOFLURANE®—Ultane®

Description/Actions: Halogenated volatile anesthetic that provides rapid induction and emergence from anesthesia in inpatient and outpatient surgery.

Warnings: May cause malignant hyperthermia and is contraindicated in patients who are hypersensitive to the drug or other halogenated agents. Adverse reactions include agitation, somnolence, cough, breath holding, laryngospasm, airway obstruction, tachycardia, bradycardia, hypotension, nausea, and vomiting.

Administration: Inhalation.

Preparations: Liquid, 250 ml.

SHOHL'S SOLUTION MODIFIED®, see Sodium citrate

SILDENAFIL CITRATE—Viagra®

Description/Actions: An oral tablet indicated for the treatment of erectile dysfunction (ED).

Warnings: Contraindicated with concomitant organic nitrates or nitric oxide donors. Use cautiously in anatomical penile deformation, predisposition to priapism, or patients for whom sexual activity is inadvisable or contraindicated. Avoid use in bleeding disorders, active peptic ulceration, concomitant erectile dysfunction treatment, or retinosis pigmentosa. Not indicated for use in women, children, or newborns.

Adverse reactions include headache, flushing, dyspepsia, nasal congestion, UTI, abnormal vision (color tinge to vision, increased light sensitivity, blurred vision), diarrhea, dizziness, and rash. Concomitant administration of sildenafil with alpha blockers may lead to symptomatic hypotension. Sildenafil doses above 25 mg should not be taken within 4 hours of taking an alpha blocker.

Administration: Take 1 dose as needed about 1 hour before sexual activity at a frequency of up to once daily.

Preparations: Tablets, 25, 50, and 100 mg.

SILVADENE®, see Silver sulfadiazine

SILVER NITRATE

Description/Actions: Anti-infective agent and cauterizing and caustic agent. Indicated for ophthalmic use in the prevention of gonococcal ophthalmia neonatorum. Has been used topically in the treatment of burns. Also has been used topically for its caustic and cauterizing actions in the treatment of certain dermatologic problems (e.g., warts).

Preparations: Ophthalmic solution, 1%. Ointment and solutions for topical use.

SILVER SULFADIAZINE— Silvadene®

Description/Actions: Anti-infective agent used topically as an adjunct for the prevention and treatment of wound sepsis in patients with second- and third-degree burns.

Preparations: Cream, 1%.

SIMETHICONE—Mylicon®, Phazyme®

Description/Actions: Antiflatulent indicated for relief of the painful symptoms of excess gas in the digestive tract.

Preparations: Tablets, 40, 50, 60, 80, and 95 mg. Chewable tablets, 125 mg. Capsules, 125 mg. Drops, 40 mg/0.6 ml.

SIMVASTATIN—Zocor®

Agent for hypercholesterolemia.

Description/Actions: Is a prodrug that is converted to its active form following administration. Produces a significant reduction in total and low-density lipoprotein (LDL) cholesterol concentrations, a modest reduction in triglyceride concentrations, and an increase in high-density lipoprotein (HDL) cholesterol concentrations. Indicated as an adjunct to diet for the reduction of elevated total and LDL cholesterol concentrations in patients with primary hypercholesterolemia (Type IIa and IIb) when the response to a diet restricted in saturated fat and cholesterol and other nonpharmacological measures has not been adequate. Also indicated in patients with coronary heart disease and hypercholesterolemia to reduce the risk of total mortality by reducing coronary death; reduce the risk of nonfatal myocardial infarction, and reduce the risk for undergoing myocardial revascularization procedures.

Warnings: Contraindicated in patients with active liver disease or unexplained persistent elevations of serum transaminases. Is also contraindicated in pregnant women and nursing mothers. Increases in serum transaminases may occur, and it is recommended that liver function tests be monitored before treatment begins, every 6 weeks for the first 3 months, every 8 weeks during the remainder of the first year, and periodically thereafter (at about 6-month intervals). Adverse reactions include constipation, flatulence, dyspepsia, myalgia, myopathy, and, rarely, rhabdomyolysis. Patients should be advised to promptly report unexplained muscle pain, tenderness, or weakness. The risk of myopathy/rhabdomyolysis is dose related. The risk of myopathy/rhabdomyolysis is increased by concomitant administration of amiodarone or verapamil. In patients taking amiodarone or verapamil with simvastatin, the dose should not exceed 20 mg/day. The risk of myopathy/rhabdomyolysis is increased when simvastatin is given with itraconazole, ketoconazole, erythromycin, clarithromycin, HIV protease inhibitors, nefazodone or large quantities of grapefruit juice (> 1 quart/day). If treatment with these drugs is unavoidable, simvastatin should be stopped during the course of treatment. The dose of simvastatin should not exceed 10 mg/day when given with cyclosporine, gemfibrozil, other fibrates or niacin (> 1g/day).

Administration: Oral. Should be administered at bedtime.

Preparations: Tablets, 5, 10, 20, and 40 mg.

SINEMET—Combination of levodopa and carbidopa

SINEMET—CR, Combination of levodopa and carbidopa (controlled-release)

SINEQUAN, see Doxepin

SINGULAIR, see Montelukast

SINUMIST SR CAPLETS, see Guaifenesin

SIROLIMUS—Rapamune®

Description/Actions: Sirolimus is used as an immunosuppressant in combination with cyclosporine and prednisone as prophylaxis for kidney transplant rejection.

Precautions/Adverse Reactions: Safety and efficacy of sirolimus as immunosuppressive therapy has not been established in liver transplant patients; therefore, such use is not recommended. The use of sirolimus in combination with cyclosporine or tacrolimus in de novo liver transplant recipients was associated with an increase in hepatic artery thrombosis leading to graft loss or death. Sirolimus should be administered with caution in patients with high cholesterol or triglycerides, an active infection, pregnancy, breast-feeding, or liver disease. Mild to moderate hepatic impairment require dosage adjustments. Some side effects are lymphocele, hyperlipidemia, azotemia, hypertension, rash, and epistaxis.

Administrations: Oral.

Patient Care Implications: The drug should be avoided in patients who are pregnant or breast-feeding. Sirolimus should also be given cautiously in patients with high cholesterol or triglycerides, an active infection, or liver disease. Drug should be given in a facility equipped with supportive medical services. CBC, serum cholesterol, serum creatinine/BUN, serum lipid, and serum potassium must be monitored while patient is on medication.

Preparations: Oral solution, 1 mg/ml. Tablet, 1 mg.

SKELAXIN, see Metaxalone

SKELID®, see Tiludronate

SLO-BID, see Theophylline

SLO-NIACIN, see Nicotinic acid

SLO-PHYLLIN, see Theophylline

SLOW-FE®, see Ferrous sulfate, exsiccated

SLOW-K®, see Potassium chloride

SLOW-MAG®, see Magnesium chloride

SODIUM ASCORBATE, see Vitamin C

SODIUM BENZOATE AND SODIUM PHENYLACETATE—Ucephan®

Agents for hyperammonemia.

Description/Actions: Are metabolically active compounds that decrease elevated blood ammonia concentrations in patients with inborn errors of ureagenesis. Indicated as adjunctive therapy [with dietary management (low protein diet) and amino acid supplementation] for the prevention and treatment of hyperammonemia in the chronic management of patients with urea cycle enzymopathies.

Warnings: Adverse reactions include nausea and vomiting. Because of the sodium content of the product, the possibility of hypernatremia exists and caution should be exercised in patients with congestive heart failure, severe renal insufficiency, and in clinical states in which there is sodium retention with edema.

Administration: Oral. Ucephan is a concentrated solution and must be diluted before use. Because sodium phenylacetate has a lingering odor, care should be taken in mixing and administering the drug to minimize contact with skin and clothing.

Preparations: Oral solution, 10% sodium benzoate and 10% sodium phenylacetate.

SODIUM BICARBONATE—Baking soda

Description/Actions: Antacid and alkalinizer. Used orally as a gastric antacid and urinary alkalinizer. Administered intravenously in the management of metabolic acidosis and to alkalinize the urine in the treatment of certain drug intoxications.

Preparations: Tablets, 325 and 650 mg. Vials and syringes, 4%, 4.2%, 5%, 7.5%, and 8.4%.

SODIUM BIPHOSPHATE

Description/Actions: Laxative often used in combination with sodium phosphate. Has also been used as a urinary acidifier.

SODIUM BORATE—Collyrium

Description/Actions: Antiseptic and buffer indicated for ophthalmic use for flushing or irrigating the eye to remove loose foreign material.

Preparations: Ophthalmic solution.

SODIUM CELLULOSE PHOSPHATE—Calcibind®

Description/Actions: Indicated for absorptive hypercalciuria Type I with recurrent calcium oxalate or calcium phosphate nephrolithiasis.

Preparations: Powder, 2.5 g packets.

SODIUM CHLORIDE—Salt

Description/Actions: Used intravenously to replace fluid and electrolytes, as a genitourinary irrigant, as an abortifacient, for ophthalmic use in the treatment and diagnosis of ocular conditions, and for intranasal use to restore moisture and alleviate discomfort in certain nasal conditions.

Preparations: Solutions for intravenous infusion, 0.45%, 0.9% (normal saline), 3%, 5%. Vials for intravenous admixtures, 50 mEq, 100 mEq, and 625 mEq. Solutions for genitourinary irrigation, 0.45% and 0.9%. Solutions for inducing abortion, 20%. Ophthalmic solution or ointment, 2% and 5%. Nose drops and spray, 0.4% and 0.65%.

SODIUM CITRATE—Bicitra®, Shohl's solution modified®

Description/Actions: Alkalinizing agent useful in conditions in which the main-

290 • SODIUM FLUORIDE

tenance of an alkaline urine is desirable, and in the alleviation of chronic metabolic acidosis such as results from chronic renal insufficiency.

Preparations: Solution, 500 mg/5 ml with citric acid. Also available in formulations with potassium citrate and citric acid.

SODIUM FLUORIDE—Luride®

Description/Actions: Indicated for prevention of dental caries and certain dental procedures. Has been investigated for possible value in the treatment of osteoporosis.

Preparations: Tablets, 0.25, 0.5, and 1 mg fluoride. Drops, rinse, and gel.

SODIUM HYPOCHLORITE

Description/Actions: Anti-infective agent and bleaching agent.

Preparations: Solution.

SODIUM IODIDE

Description/Actions: Used in thyroid disorders. May be used adjunctively with an antithyroid drug in certain hyperthyroid patients. Radioactive form (sodium iodide I 131) has been used in the management of hyperthyroidism and selected cases of thyroid carcinoma.

Preparations: Solution.

SODIUM LACTATE

Description/Actions: Administered intravenously in the treatment of metabolic acidosis.

Preparations: Vials, 50 mEq. Solution (for IV use), 167 mEq/l (1/6 molar).

SODIUM LAURYL SULFATE

Description/Actions: Surfactant which is used in the preparation of certain pharmaceutical formulations and to enhance the distribution/penetration of some topically applied drugs.

SODIUM MORRHUATE

Description/Actions: Sclerosing agent used in the intravenous treatment of small uncomplicated varicose veins of the lower extremities. May be useful as a supplement to venous ligation to obliterate residual varicose veins.

Preparations: Ampules and vials, 50 mg/ml.

SODIUM NITROPRUSSIDE— Nitropress®

Description/Actions: Antihypertensive agent indicated for intravenous use for the immediate reduction of blood pressure of patients in hypertensive crisis and in the treatment of cardiac pump failure or cardiogenic shock. Also used to produce controlled hypotension during anesthesia in order to reduce bleeding in surgical procedures.

Preparations: Vials, 50 mg.

SODIUM PERBORATE—Visicol™

Description/Actions: Antiseptic and cleansing agent included in some dentifrices.

SODIUM PHOSPHATE—Visicol™

Description/Actions: Laxative often used in combination with sodium biphosphate. Also administered intravenously as a source of phosphate.

Preparations: Vials, 3 mM phosphate.

Tablet, 1.5 g (total sodium phosphate)

SODIUM POLYSTYRENE SULFONATE—Kayexalate®

Description/Actions: Cation-exchange resin indicated for the treatment of hyperkalemia.

Preparations: Powder and suspension.

SODIUM SALICYLATE

Description/Actions: Salicylate analgesic

indicated for the relief of mild to moderate pain and inflammation.

Preparations: Enteric-coated tablets, 325 and 650 mg. Ampules, 1 g/10 ml.

SODIUM SULFATE

Description/Actions: Laxative sometimes used in combination with other agents.

SODIUM TETRADECYL SULFATE—Sotradecol®

Description/Actions: Sclerosing agent administered intravenously in the treatment of small uncomplicated varicose veins of the lower extremities.

Preparations: Ampules, 1% and 3%.

SODIUM THIOSALICYLATE

Description/Actions: Salicylate analgesic/ anti-inflammatory agent used parenterally in the management of acute gout, musculoskeletal disorders, and rheumatic fever.

Preparations: Ampules and vials, 50 mg/ml.

SODIUM THIOSULFATE—Tinver®

Description/Actions: Used in the topical treatment of tinea versicolor and other dermatologic conditions including acne. Has also been used parenterally as adjunctive therapy in the management of cyanide toxicity, and also in the treatment of arsenic poisoning.

Preparations: Lotion, 25%. Ampules, 1 g/10 ml.

SOLAG®, Mequinol/Tretinoin Topical Solution

SOLGANAL®, see Aurothioglucose

SOLU-CORTEF®, see Hydrocortisone (as the sodium succinate)

SOLU-MEDROL®, see Methylprednisolone sodium succinate

SOMA®, see Carisoprodol

SOMATREM—Protropin®

Growth hormone.

Description/Actions: Indicated for the long-term treatment of children who have growth failure due to a lack of adequate endogenous growth hormone secretion.

Warnings: Contraindicated in patients with closed epiphyses or when there is evidence of any progression of underlying intracranial lesion. Patients may experience glucose intolerance. Concurrent use of a glucocorticoid may inhibit the effect of somatrem. Some patients develop persistent antibodies to growth hormone.

Administration: Intramuscular.

Preparations: Vials, 5 and 10 mg.

SOMATROPIN—Humatrope®, Genotropin®, Nutropin®, Serostim®

Growth hormone.

Description/Actions: Somatropin is indicated for the long-term treatment of children who have growth failure due to Turner's Syndrome or an inadequate secretion of normal endogenous growth hormone or chronic renal insufficiency up to the time of renal transplantation, and in adults who have a deficiency in growth hormone. Indicated in AIDS wasting or cachexia (Serostim®), as somatropin has been shown to increase lean body mass and significantly increase body weight. Also indicated in growth failure in children associated with chronic renal insufficiency up to the time of renal transplant.

Warnings: Contraindicated in patients with closed epiphyses or when there is evidence of growth of intracranial lesions. Patients may experience glucose intolerance. Concurrent use of a glucocorticoid may inhibit the effect of somatropin. Some patients develop antibodies to growth hormone. Reevaluate AIDS patient if weight loss persists after 2 weeks of therapy. Give concomitant antiviral therapy. Discontinue if carpal tunnel syndrome persists after dosage reduction. Perform periodic fundoscopic exams.

Administration: Intramuscular.

Preparations: Vials, 5 and 10 mg.

SOMATROPIN—Nutropin Depot®

Description/Actions: Long-acting dosage form of recombinant human growth hormone indicated for the long-term treatment of growth failure due to a lack of adequate endogenous GH secretion.

Precautions/Adverse Reactions: Contraindicated in patients with acute critical illness due to complications following open heart or abdominal surgery, multiple accident trauma, or acute respiratory failure. Somatropin should not be used in patients with closed epiphyses or active neoplasia. Patients may experience glucose intolerance. Therefore, caution should be used in patients with diabetes mellitus or symptomatic hypoglycemia. Caution should also be used in patients with intracranial lesions or a history of scoliosis. Other adverse effects include the development of intracranial hypertension with papilledema, visual changes, headache, nausea, vomiting, and allergic reactions. Fundoscopic exams should be performed periodically.

Administration: SQ injection.

Patient Care Implications: Monitor for evidence of glucose intolerance. For patients with diabetes mellitus, the insulin dose may require adjustment when GH therapy is instituted. Patients should be informed that allergic reactions are possible and that prompt medical attention should be sought if any allergic reactions occur.

Preparations: Single-use vials, 13.5, 18, and 22.5 mg.

SOMINEX®, see Diphenhydramine

SONATA®, see Zaleplon

SORBITOL

Description/Actions: Urologic irrigant indicated for use in transurethral prostatic resection or other transurethral surgical procedures.

Preparations: Solutions, 3% and 3.3%.

SORBITRATE®, see Isosorbide dinitrate

SORIATANE®, see Acitretin

SOTALOL HYDROCHLORIDE— Betapace®, Betapace AF™

Antiarrhythmic agent.

Description/Actions: Exhibits noncardioselective beta-adrenergic-blocking activity and prolongs cardiacrepolarization. Indicated for the treatment of documented life-threatening ventricular arrhythmias such as sustained ventricular tachycardia.

Warnings: Contraindicated in patients with bronchial asthma, sinus bradycardia, second- and third- degree AV block, unless a functioning pacemaker is present, congenital or acquired long QT syndromes, cardiogenic shock, and uncontrolled congestive heart failure. May cause proarrhythmic events (e.g., torsades de pointes), the risk of which may be increased by excessive prolongation of the QT interval, history of cardiomegaly or congestive heart failure, reduction in heart rate, and reduction in serum potassium and/or magnesium. Should not be used in patients with hypokalemia or hypomagnesemia prior to the correction of the imbalance. Concurrent use with other agents known to prolong the QT interval is best avoided. Because of its beta-blocking activity, should be used with caution in patients with diabetes, bronchospastic diseases, sick sinus syndrome associated with symptomatic arrhythmias, a history of anaphylactic reactions to a variety of allergens, and patients suspected of developing thyrotoxicosis. When sotalol is administered concurrently with a beta-2-receptor agonist (e.g., terbutaline), the dosage of the latter agent may have to be increased.

Administration: Oral.

Preparations: Tablets, 80, 120, 160, and 240 mg.

SOTRADECOL®, see Sodium tetradecyl sulfate

SPARFLOXACIN—Zagam®

Description/Actions: Quinolone antibiotic indicated in the treatment of susceptible infections including community acquired pneumonia and acute bacterial exacerbation of chronic bronchitis. Although cross-resistance with other fluoroquinolones may be observed, certain bacterial isolates resistant to fluoroquinolones may be susceptible to sparfloxacin.

Warnings: Contraindicated in patients with a history of hypersensitivity to quinolones (i.e., levofloxacin, loxacin, ciprofloxacin, norfloxacin) or photosensitivity. Instruct patients to refrain from exposure to sun or UV light (direct or indirect) during or 5 days after treatment. Concomitant use of several agents may contraindicate use of sparfloxacin, and prescribers should review the patient's full profile and adjust the medication regimen accordingly. Not recommended for use in patients with hypokalemia, significant bradycardia, CHF, myocardial ischemia, atrial fibrillation, or other pro-arrhythmic conditions. Use cautiously in patients with renal insufficiency. Maintain adequate hydration. Cautious use is recommended in patients with severe cerebral arteriosclerosis, epilepsy and other conditions that predispose to seizures or that lower seizure threshold. Not rec-

ommended in children < 18 years of age due to arthropathy. Discontinue if phototoxicity, rash or tendon pain, inflammation, or rupture occur. Adverse reactions include photosensitivity, GI upset, headache, dizziness, insomnia, pruritus, taste perversion, QTc interval prolongation, flatulence, vasodilation, and convulsions.

Administration: 400 mg on day 1, then 200 mg every 24 hours on days 2–10 for a total of 10 days of therapy (11 tablets). Reduce dose as per manufacturer's guidelines for impaired renal function (CrCl < 50 ml/min).

Preparations: Tablets, 200 mg.

SPARINE®, see Promazine

SPASMOJECT®, see Dicyclomine

SPECTAZOLE®, see Econazole

SPECTINOMYCIN HYDROCHLORIDE—Trobicin®

Description/Actions: Antibiotic indicated for intramuscular use in the treatment of acute gonorrheal urethritis and proctitis in the male and acute gonorrheal cervicitis and proctitis in the female.

Preparations: Vials, 2 and 4 g.

SPECTRACEF™, see Cefditoren Pivoxil

SPECTROBID®, see Bacampicillin

SPIRONOLACTONE—Aldactone®

Description/Actions: Potassium-sparing diuretic that is an aldosterone antagonist. Indicated in the management of edematous conditions, hypertension, primary hyperaldosteronism, and hypokalemia.

Preparations: Tablets, 25, 50, and 100 mg.

SPORANOX®, see Itraconazole

SSKI®, see Potassium iodide

STADOL®, see Butorphanol

STADOL NS®, see Butorphanol

STANOZOLOL—Winstrol®

Description/Actions: Anabolic steroid indicated prophylactically to decrease the frequency and severity of attacks of angioedema in patients with hereditary angioedema and in selected cases of aplastic anemia to increase hemoglobin.

Preparations: Tablets, 2 mg.

STAPHCILLIN®, see Methicillin

STARLIX®, see Nateglinide

STATICIN®, see Erythromycin base

STAVUDINE—Zerit®

Antiviral agent.

Description/Actions: Indicated in advanced HIV infection in patients who have had prolonged prior zidovudine therapy.

Warnings: Lactic acidosis and severe hepatomegaly with steatosis, including fatal cases, have been reported with the use of nucleoside analogues alone or in combination, including stavudine and other antiretrovirals. Fatal and nonfatal pancreatitis have occurred during therapy when stavudine was part of a combination regimen that included didanosine, with or without hydroxyurea in both treatment-naïve and treatment-experienced patients, regardless of the degree of immunosuppression. Fatal lactic acidosis has been reported in pregnant women who receive the combination stavudine and didanosine with other antiretroviral agents. The combination of stavudine and didanosine should be used with caution during pregnancy and is recommended only if the potential benefit clearly outweighs the potential risk. May cause peripheral neuropathy and patients should be advised to report symptoms such as tingling, burning, pain, or numbness in the hands or feet. Other adverse reactions include diarrhea, nausea, vomiting, abdominal pain, headache, chills/fever, asthenia, myalgia, and rash.

Administration: Oral.

Preparations: Capsules, 15, 20, 30, and 40 mg. Oral solution, 1 mg/ml after reconsititution.

STELAZINE®, see Trifluoperazine

STILPHOSTROL®, see Diethylstilbestrol diphosphate

STIMATE®, see Desmopressinacetate

STOXIL®, see Idoxuridine

STREPTASE®, see Streptokinase

STREPTOKINASE—Streptase®

Description/Actions: Thrombolytic enzyme indicated for parenteral use for the lysis of thrombi in the management of pulmonary embolism, deep vein thrombosis, arterial thrombosis and embolism, arteriovenous cannulae occlusion, and coronary artery thrombosis. Also indicated for intravenous use for acute myocardial infarction.

Preparations: Vials, 250,000, 750,000, and 1,500,000 IU.

STREPTOMYCIN SULFATE

Description/Actions: Aminoglycoside antibiotic indicated in the parenteral treatment of tuberculosis and selected other infections caused by susceptible organisms.

Preparations: Vials, 1 and 5 g.

STREPTOZOCIN—Zanosar®

Description/Actions: Antineoplastic agent indicated in the management of metastatic islet cell carcinoma of the pancreas.

Warnings: Use cautiously in renal or hepatic disease, patients with active infections or bone marrow suppression. Adverse reactions include nausea, vomiting, nephrotoxicity, and phlebitis at the IV site.

Administration: Intravenous.

Preparations: Vials, 1 g.

STRONTIUM-89 CHLORIDE—Metastron®

Agent for metastatic bone pain.

Description/Actions: Is a radiopharmaceutical that decays by beta emission. Selectively concentrates in bone mineral, and greater concentrations accumulate in primary bone tumors and in areas of metastatic involvement than can accumulate in normal bone. Has a slow onset of action (7–20 days) and a long duration of action (6 months). Indicated for the relief of bone pain in patients with painful skeletal metastases.

Warnings: May suppress the bone marrow and peripheral blood cell counts should be monitored at least every two weeks. Patients should discontinue calcium medications for about 2 weeks prior to receiving the drug. May cause fetal harm, and women of childbearing potential should be advised to avoid becoming pregnant. Because the drug is radioactive, caution must be observed in handling and administering the drug, and patients should be instructed to observe appropriate cautions during the first week after the treatment.

Administration: Intravenous. Is administered by slow intravenous injection over 1–2 minutes.

Preparations: Vials, 4 millicuries (mCi).

SUBLIMAZE®, see Fentanyl citrate

SUCCIMER—Chemet®

Agent for lead poisoning in children.

Description/Actions: Is a chelating agent that binds with lead and increases the urinary excretion of lead. Indicated for the treatment of lead poisoning in children with blood lead levels above 45 mg/dl. Use should always be accompanied by identification and removal of the source of the lead exposure.

Warnings: Adverse reactions include gastrointestinal effects (e.g., nausea, vomiting, diarrhea), increases in serum transaminases, and rash. Should be used with caution in patients with compromised renal function. Patients should be adequately hydrated. Elevated blood lead levels and associated symptoms may return rapidly after discontinuation of the drug.

Administration: Oral. In young children who cannot swallow capsules, the drug can be administered by separating the capsule and sprinkling the medicated beads on a small amount of soft food or putting them in a spoon and following with fruit drink.

Preparations: Capsules, 100 mg.

SUCCINYLCHOLINE CHLORIDE—Anectine®, Quelicin®, Sucostrin®

Description/Actions: Depolarizing skeletal muscle relaxant for intravenous use as an adjunct to general anesthesia, to facilitate endotracheal intubation, and to provide skeletal muscle relaxation during surgery or mechanical ventilation.

Preparations: Ampules and vials, 20 mg/ml, 50 mg/ml, and 100 mg/ml. Vials, 500 mg and 1 g.

SUCOSTRIN®, see Succinylcholine

SUCRALFATE—Carafate®

Antiulcer agent.

Description/Actions: Is an aluminum complex of sucrose sulfate indicated in the short-term treatment of duodenal ulcer and for maintenance therapy for duodenal ulcer.

Warnings: Adverse reactions include constipation. Simultaneous administration with other agents should be separated by an interval of at least 2 hours.

Administration: Oral. Should be administered on an empty stomach.

Preparations: Tablets, 1 g. Suspension, 1 g/10 ml.

SUDAFED®, see Pseudoephedrine

SUFENTA®, see Sufentanil

SUFENTANIL CITRATE—Sufenta®

Description/Actions: Opioid analgesic/anesthetic indicated as an analgesic adjunct in the maintenance of balanced general anesthesia, and as a primary anesthetic agent for the induction and maintenance of anesthesia with 100% oxygen in patients undergoing major surgical procedures.

Preparations: Ampules, 50 μg/ml.

SULAMYD®, see Sulfacetamide

SULAR®, see Nisoldipine

SULCONAZOLE NITRATE—Exelderm®

Antifungal agent.

Description/Actions: An imidazole antifungal agent indicated for the topical treatment of tinea pedis, tinea cruris, tinea corporis, and tinea versicolor.

Warnings: Adverse reactions include itching, burning, stinging, and redness.

Administration: Topical.

Preparations: Cream, 1%. Solution, 1%.

SULFABENZAMIDE

Description/Actions: Sulfonamide anti-infective agent used in combination with other agents in the topical management of vaginal infections.

SULFACETAMIDE SODIUM—Sulamyd sodium®, Klaron®

Description/Actions: Sulfonamide anti-infective agent indicated for ophthalmic use in the treatment of conjunctivitis, corneal ulcers, and other superficial ocular infections, and as adjunctive treatment in the management of trachoma. Also used topically in certain bacterial infections of the skin and seborrheic dermatitis, and in combination with other agents in the topical management of vaginal infections.

Preparations: Ophthalmic solution, 10%, 15%, and 30%. Ophthalmic ointment, 10%. Lotion, 10%.

SULFADIAZINE

Description/Actions: Sulfonamide anti-infective agent indicated in the treatment of infections caused by susceptible organisms.

Preparations: Tablets, 500 mg.

SULFADOXINE

Description/Actions: Sulfonamide anti-infective agent used in combination (Fansidar®) with pyrimethamine to achieve a synergistic effect in the prevention and treatment of malaria caused by chloroquine-resistant plasmodia.

Preparations: Tablets, 500 mg with 25 mg of pyrimethamine.

SULFAMERAZINE

Description/Actions: Sulfonamide anti-infective agent used in combination with other sulfonamides.

SULFAMETHAZINE

Description/Actions: Sulfonamide anti-infective agent used in combination with other sulfonamides.

SULFAMETHIZOLE—Thiosulfil Forte®

Description/Actions: Sulfonamide anti-infective agent indicated for the treatment of urinary tract infections.

Preparations: Tablets, 500 mg.

SULFAMETHOXAZOLE—Gantanol®

Description/Actions: Sulfonamide *anti-infective agent* indicated for the treatment of infections caused by susceptible organisms.

Preparations: Tablets, 500 mg and 1 g. Suspension, 500 mg/5 ml.

SULFAMYLON®, see Mafenide

SULFANILAMIDE—AVC®

Description/Actions: Sulfonamide anti-infective agent used in the topical management of vaginal infections.

Preparations: Vaginal cream, 15%. Vaginal suppositories, 1.05 g.

SULFAPYRIDINE

Description/Actions: Used in the treatment of dermatitis herpetiformis.

Preparations: Tablets, 500 mg.

SULFASALAZINE—Azulfidine®

Salicylate-sulfonamide.

Description/Actions: Agent for ulcerative colitis indicated in the treatment of mild to moderate ulcerative colitis and as adjunctive therapy in severe ulcerative colitis, and for the prolongation of the remission period between acute attacks of ulcerative colitis. Also indicated in rheumatoid arthritis that has not responded adequately to salicylates or other NSAIDs.

Preparations: Tablets and enteric-coated tablets, 500 mg. Oral suspension, 250 mg/5 ml.

SULFATHIAZOLE

Description/Actions: Sulfonamide anti-infective agent used in combination with other agents in the topical management of vaginal infections.

SULFINPYRAZONE—Anturane®

Description/Actions: Uricosuric agent indicated in the treatment of chronic gouty arthritis and intermittent gouty arthritis.

Preparations: Tablets, 100 mg. Capsules, 200 mg.

SULFISOXAZOLE—Gantrisin®

SULFISOXAZOLE ACETYL

Description/Actions: Sulfonamide anti-infective agent. Primarily used in the treatment of urinary tract infections, and is also useful in certain other infections.

Preparations: Tablets, 500 mg. Suspension (acetyl), 500 mg/5 ml.

SULFISOXAZOLE DIOLAMINE—Gantrisin®

Description/Actions: Sulfonamide anti-infective agent used in the treatment of ocular infections.

Preparations: Ophthalmic solution and ointment, 4%.

SULFUR

Description/Actions: Used topically, usually in combination with other agents, in the treatment of acne, seborrheic dermatitis, and other dermatologic conditions.

SULFURATED LIME—Lime sulfur solution, Vlemasque®

Description/Actions: Used topically in the treatment of acne and other dermatologic conditions.

Preparations: Cream, 6%. Topical solution.

SULINDAC—Clinoril®

Nonsteroidal anti-inflammatory drug.

Description/Actions: Inhibits prostaglandin synthesis, and is indicated in the treatment of rheumatoid arthritis, osteo-arthritis, ankylosing spondylitis, acute painful shoulder, and acute gouty arthritis.

Warnings: Should not be given to patients in whom aspirin or another NSAID causes asthma, rhinitis, urticaria, or other allergic-type reactions. May cause GI effects, and use should be avoided in patients with active GI tract disease and closely monitored in patients with a previous history of such disorders. Other adverse reactions include dizziness, headache, edema, and rash. Should not be used concomitantly with dimethyl sulfoxide (DMSO).

Administration: Oral.

Preparations: Tablets, 150 and 200 mg.

SUMATRIPTAN SUCCINATE— Imitrex®

Agent for migraine.

Description/Actions: Is a selective 5-hydroxytryptamine$_1$ (5-HT$_1$) receptor agonist that causes vasoconstriction of intracranial blood vessels. Indicated for the acute treatment of migraine attacks with or without aura and cluster headaches.

Warnings: Contraindicated in patients with ischemic heart disease (angina pectoris, history of myocardial infarction, or documented silent ischemia), Prinzmetal's angina, signs or symptoms consistent with ischemic heart disease, or uncontrolled hypertension. Should not be used concomitantly with ergotamine-containing preparations. Adverse reactions include pain or redness at the injection site, atypical sensations (e.g., sensations of warmth, tingling or paresthesia, pressure, burning, numbness, tightness), dizziness, weakness, neck pain/stiffness, jaw discomfort, flushing, chest discomfort, and transient increases in blood pressure. May cause vasospasm that may be additive to that caused by ergot-containing drugs, and it is recommended that the two agents not be administered within 24 hours of each other.

Administration: Subcutaneous, oral and nasal spray.

Preparations: Tablets, 25 and 50 mg. Vials, 6 mg. Unit-of-use syringes, 6 mg. Imitrex SELFdose system kit that contains two unit-of-use syringes with 6 mg each and a SELFdose unit (a push button autoinjector). Nasal spray, 5 and 20 mg/spray.

SUMYCIN®, see Tetracycline

SUPPRELIN®, see Histrelin acetate

SUPRANE®, see Desflurane

SUPRAX®, see Cefixime

SUPROFEN—Profenal®

Nonsteroidal anti-inflammatory drug for ophthalmic use.

Description/Actions: Indicated for the inhibition of intraoperative miosis.

Warnings: Caution should be exercised in the treatment of patients having a history of sensitivity to aspirin or another nonsteroidal anti-inflammatory drug.

Administration: Ophthalmic.

Preparations: Ophthalmic solution, 1%.

SURMONTIL®, see Trimipramine

SURVANTA®, see Beractant

SUTILAINS—Travase®

Description/Actions: Proteolytic enzymes applied topically as an adjunct for wound debridement of second- and third-degree burns, pressure ulcers, incisional, traumatic, and pyogenic wounds, and ulcers secondary to peripheral vascular disease.

Preparations: Ointment, 82,000 casein units/g.

SYMMETREL®, see Amantadine

SYNALAR®, see Fluocinolone

SYNALGOS-DC®, Combination of dihydrocodeine, aspirin, and caffeine

SYNERCID®, see Dalfopristin/Quinupristin

SYNAREL®, see Nafarelin acetate

SYNTHROID®, see Levothyroxine

SYNTOCINON®, see Oxytocin

SYPRINE®, see Trientine

T

TACARYL®, see Methdilazine

TACE®, see Chlorotrianisene

TACRINE HYDROCHLORIDE—Cognex®

Agent for Alzheimer's disease.

Description/Actions: Also known as tetrahydroaminoacridine (THA). Is a reversible cholinesterase inhibitor that elevates acetylcholine concentrations in the cerebral cortex. Indicated for the treatment of mild to moderate dementia of the Alzheimer's type.

Warnings: Contraindicated in patients previously treated with tacrine who developed treatment-associated jaundice confirmed by elevated total bilirubin greater than 3 mg/dl. May increase serum transaminase levels (e.g., alanine aminotransferase [ALT]) and cause liver toxicity. Serum transaminase levels should be monitored every 2 weeks for the first 16 weeks, then monthly for 2 months, then every 3 months thereafter. Other adverse reactions include nausea, vomiting, diarrhea, dyspepsia, anorexia, myalgia, and ataxia.

Administration: Oral. Bioavailability is reduced by food by about 40–50%, and doses are best administered at least 1 hour before meals. However, if gastrointestinal upset occurs, the drug may be taken with food to improve tolerability, although a significant reduction in plasma concentrations should be expected.

Preparations: Capsules, 10, 20, 30, and 40 mg.

TACROLIMUS—Prograf®, Protopic®

Immunosuppressant.

Description/Actions: Indicated for the prophylaxis of organ rejection in patients receiving allogeneic liver transplants. It is recommended that it be used concomitantly with adrenal corticosteroids.

Warnings: Contraindicated in patients who are hypersensitive to the drug, or to polyoxyl 60 hydrogenated castor oil (HCO-60) that is included in the parenteral formulation as a solubilizing agent. May cause nephrotoxicity; patients with impaired renal function should receive lower doses, and caution should be exercised when it is used in patients who are also receiving other drugs that may cause nephrotoxicity (e.g., aminoglycosides). Should not be used concurrently with cyclosporine, and it is recommended that tacrolimus or cyclosprine should be discontinued at least 24 hours prior to initiating the other. May cause hyperkalemia; serum potassium concentrations should be monitored, and the concurrent use of potassium-sparing diuretics should be avoided. Other adverse reactions include tremor, headache, hypertension, hyperglycemia, diarrhea, nausea, vomiting, abdominal pain, hypomagnesemia, anemia, pain, fever, and asthenia. Anaphylactic reactions have been experienced by some patients receiving the parenteral formulation, which may be due to the castor oil derivative used as the solubilizing agent. The parenteral formulation should be used only in patients who are unable to take the capsule formulation. Patients receiving the drug intravenously should be under continuous observation for at least the first 30 minutes following the start of the intravenous infusion and at frequent intervals thereafter.

Administration: Oral and intravenous infusion. Should be administered no sooner than 6 hours after transplantation. Patients should be converted from the intravenous to the oral formulation as soon as oral therapy can be tolerated. The parenteral formulation must be diluted and the diluted infusion solution should be stored in glass or polyethylene containers and should be discarded after 24 hours. It should not be stored in a polyvinyl chloride (PVC) container due to decreased stability and the potential for extraction of phthalates.

Preparations: Capsules, 1 and 5 mg. Ampules, 5 mg/ml. Topical ointment, 0.03% and 0.1%.

TAGAMET®, see Cimetidine

TAGAMET HB®, see Cimetidine

TALACEN®, see Pentazocine hydrochloride and Acetaminophen

TALWIN®, see Pentazocine

TAMBOCOR®, see Flecainide

TAMIFLU®, see Oseltamivir

TAMOXIFEN CITRATE— Nolvadex®

Description/Actions: Antineoplastic agent indicated in the treatment of metastatic breast cancer in postmenopausal women, and in premenopausal women as an alternative to oophorectomy or ovarian radiation. Is also used in combination with cytotoxic agents following radical or modified radical mastectomy to delay recurrence of surgically curable breast cancer in postmenopausal women. Is also indicated for adjuvant treatment for axillary node-negative breast cancer. Is also indicated for adjuvant treatment for axillary node-negative breast cancer, advanced breast cancer in men and for reduction of incidence of breast cancer in high risk women. Approved for use in girls 2–10 years of age with McCune-Albright Syndrome.

Precautions/Adverse Reactions: For women with ductal carcinoma in-situ and women at high risk for breast cancer, serious and life threatening events associated with tamoxifen in the risk reduction setting include uterine malignancies, stroke and pulmonary embolism. Some of these were fatal.

Preparations: Tablets, 10 and 20 mg.

TAMSULOSIN HYDROCHLORIDE—Flomax®

Description/Actions: An alpha-adrenergic antagonist indicated in benign prostatic hyperplasia, resulting in an improvement in urine flow and a reduction in the symptoms of BPH.

Warnings: Rule out prostate cancer. Use cautiously in patients with syncope. Adverse reactions include abnormal ejaculation, postural hypotension, dizziness, rhinitis, cough, somnolence, sinusitis, amblyopia, decreased libido, insomnia, and syncope. Tamsulosin has also been associated with priapism.

Administration: Oral. Do not crush, chew, or open caps.

Take ½ hour after the same meal each day.

Preparations: Capsules, 0.4 mg.

TAO®, see Troleandomycin

TAPAZOLE®, see Methimazole

TARGRETIN®, see Bexarotene

TARKA®—Combination ACE inhibitor (trandolapril) and calcium channel blocker (verapamil)

TASMAR®, see Tolcapone

TAVIST®, see Clemastine

TAVIST-D®, Combination of clemastine and phenylpropanolamine

TAXOL®, see Paclitaxel

TAXOTERE®, see Docetaxel

TAZAROTENE—Tazorac®

Description/Actions: Tazarotene is indicated for the treatment of mild to moderate facial acne vulgaris or atable plaque psoriasis affecting up to 20% of the body surface area and as an adjunctive agent for use in the mitigation (palliation) of facial fine wrinkling, facial mottled hyperpigmentation and hypopigmentation, and benign facial lentigines in patients who use comprehensive skin care and sunlight avoidance programs.

Warnings: Contraindicated in pregnancy (Category X). Obtain a reliable negative pregnancy test within 2 weeks before starting therapy. Do not use on broken, eczematous, or sunburned skin. Warn patients about sun sensitivity. Avoid sun and UV light; use adequate sun protection. Increased irritation may occur in extreme weather (e.g., wind, cold). Discontinue if excessive irritation occurs. Adverse reactions include pruritus, burning, stinging, erythema, worsening of psoriasis, irritation, skin pain, desquamation, and other local reactions.

Administration: Cleanse and dry skin. Apply thin film to lesions, once daily in the evening. Women of childbearing potential: Begin therapy during normal menses.

Preparations: 0.05 and 0.1% aqueous gel. 0.1% cream.

TAZICEF®, see Ceftazidime

TAZIDIME®, see Ceftazidime

TAZORAC®, see Tazarotene

TECZEM®, Combination agent enalapril maleate and diltiazem maleate (ACE inhibitor and calcium channel blocker)

TEGOPEN®, see Cloxacillin

TEGRETOL®, see Carbamazepine

TELDRIN®, see Chlorpheniramine

TELMISARTAN—Micardis®

Description/Actions: Telmisartan is an angiotensin II receptor antagonist indicated as monotherapy or as an adjunct to other antihypertensives.

Precautions/Adverse Reactions: Contraindicated in pregnancy (Category C in first trimester; Category D in the second and third trimesters) and in nursing mothers. Correct hypovolemia before beginning therapy or monitor closely. Use cautiously in hepatic insufficiency, biliary obstruction, severe renal impairment, CHF, renal artery stenosis, and dialysis (monitor for orthostasis).

Adverse reactions include back pain, upper respiratory infection, sinusitis, diarrhea, and pharyngitis.

Administration: Oral.

Patient Care Implications: Instruct patient that medication controls but does not cure hypertension. Tell patients to take the medication at the same time daily even if feeling well, as hypertension frequently occurs without any perceived symptomatology. Caution patients to avoid sudden changes in position to decrease the incidence of orthostatic hypotension.

Preparations: Tablets, 40 and 80 mg.

TEMARIL®, see Trimeprazine

TEMAZEPAM—Restoril®

Benzodiazepine hypnotic.

Description/Actions: A CNS depressant indicated for the management of insomnia.

Warnings: Contraindicated during pregnancy. Adverse reactions include residual sedation and other CNS effects upon awakening; patients should be cautioned regarding activities such as driving and operating machinery, as well as interactions with other CNS-acting drugs, including alcohol. Can cause dependence, and is included in Schedule IV.

Administration: Oral.

Preparations: Capsules and tablets, 7.5, 15, and 30 mg.

TEMODAR®, see Temozolomide

TEMOVATE®, see Clobetasol propionate

TEMOZOLOMIDE—Temodar®

Description/Actions: Temozolomide is used to treat recurrent anaplastic astrocytomas.

Precautions/Adverse Reactions: Temozolomide should not be administered to patients with severe bone marrow suppression, dacarbazine hypersensitivity, pregnant women, breast-feeding women, or children under 3 years of age. The drug should be given with caution to patients with hepatic or renal impairment. Also, if the patient has a platelet count < $50,000/mm^3$ then IM injection should not be administered. Some side effects are nausea, vomiting, headache, fatigue, myelosuppression, constipation, diarrhea, abdominal pain, anorexia, infections, fever, seizures, dizziness, insomnia, paresthesias, somnolence, confusion, Cushing's syndrome, anxiety, back pain, depression, myalgia, pruritus, incontinence, and weight gain.

Administration: Oral.

Patient Care Implications: The drug should not be administered to patients with severe bone marrow suppression, dacarbazine hypersensitivity, pregnant women, breast-feeding women, or children under 3 years of age. The drug should be given with caution to patients with hepatic or renal impairment. Also, if the patient has a platelet count < $50,000/mm^3$, then IM injection should not be administered. A CBC with a differential should be checked during treatment. Contact or inhalation of temozolomide powder should be avoided. Temozolomide capsules should not be opened.

Preparations: Capsules, 5, 20, 100, and 250 mg.

TEMPRA®, see Acetaminophen

TENECTEPLASE—Tnkase™

Description/Actions: Tenecteplase is a thrombolytic agent used in the management of acute myocardial infarction for the lysis of thrombi in the coronary vasculature to restore perfusion and reduce mortality.

Precautions/Adverse Reactions: Tenecteplase is contraindicated in patients with a hypersensitivity to tenecteplase or any component of its formulation. It is also contraindicated in the following situations because of an increased risk of bleeding: active internal bleeding, history of cerebrovascular accident, intracranial or intraspinal surgery or trauma within 2 months, intracranial neoplasm, arteriovenous malformation, aneurysm, bleeding diathesis, severe uncontrolled hypertension. Bleeding is the potential complication during therapy—if serious bleeding occurs (not controlled by local pressure), concomitant heparin or antiplatelet agents should be discontinued. For the following conditions, the risk of bleeding is higher with the use of tenecteplase and should be weighed against the benefits: recent major surgery, cerebrovascular disease, recent gastrointestinal or genitourinary bleeding, recent trauma, hypertension (systolic BP ≥ 180 mm Hg and/or diastolic BP ≥ 110 mm Hg), suspected left heart thrombus, acute pericarditis, subacute bacterial endocarditis, hemostatic defects, severe hepatic dysfunction, pregnancy, diabetic hemorrhagic retinopathy, hemorrhagic ophthalmic conditions, septic thrombophlebitis, patients receiving anticoagulation therapy (i.e. warfarin sodium), recent administration of GP IIb/IIIa inhibitors, and advanced age. Coronary thrombolysis may result in reperfusion arrhythmias. Venipunctures should be performed carefully and only when necessary. Use caution with readministration of tenecteplase (possible antibody formation). Rare reports of cholesterol embolism have been reported. Pregnancy Category C. Administer to pregnant women only if the potential benefits justify the potential risk to the fetus. Excretion into the breast milk is unknown. Exercise caution when administering to a nursing woman. Safety and efficacy have not been established in pediatric patients. Some adverse effects are bleeding (minor), hematoma, stroke, gastrointestinal hemorrhage, epistaxis, genitourinary bleeding, and pharyngeal bleeding.

Administration: Intravenous.

Patient Care Implications: Tenecteplase should be reconstituted using the supplied 10 ml syringe with TwinPak™ dual cannula device and the 10 ml sterile water for injection (follow directions supplied within the kit). The reconstituted solution is incompatible with dextrose solutions. Dextrose-containing lines must be flushed with a saline solution before and after administration. Monitor for bleeding and avoid IM injections.

Preparations: Powder for injection, 50 mg.

TENEX®, see Guanfacine

TENIPOSIDE—Vumon®
Antineoplastic agent.

Description/Actions: Is a derivative of podophyllotoxin, also known as VM-26. Indicated for use in combination with other anticancer agents for induction therapy in patients with refractory childhood acute lymphoblastic leukemia.

Warnings: Contraindicated in patients who are hypersensitive to etoposide or polyoxyethylated castor oil (Cremophor EL), a solubilizing agent included in the formulation. Adverse reactions include myelosuppression (leukopenia, neutropenia, thrombocytopenia, anemia), mucositis, diarrhea, nausea, vomiting, infection, alopecia, and bleeding. Hypersensitivity reactions to the drug or to polyoxyethylated castor oil may occur, and patients should be under continuous observation for at least 60 minutes following the start of the intravenous infusion and at frequent intervals thereafter. Transient hypotension has occurred following rapid intravenous administration, and the drug should be administered only by slow intravenous infusion, lasting at least 30–60 minutes. Patients of childbearing potential should be advised to avoid becoming pregnant during treatment. Should not be used in nursing mothers.

Administration: Intravenous. Administered as an IV infusion over at least a 30- to 60-minute period; should not be given by rapid IV injection. The concentrated solution of teniposide may extract the plasticizer DEHP from plastic equipment or devices; thus, solutions of the concentrate should be prepared in non-DEHP containers such as glass or polyolefin plastic bags or containers, and teniposide solutions should be administered with non-DEHP-containing IV administration sets. Concentrated solution must be diluted with either 5% dextrose injection or 0.9% sodium chloride injection. Gloves should be worn when handling and preparing the solutions.

Preparations: Ampules, 50 mg/ml (teniposide for injection concentrate).

TENOFOVIR DISOPROXIL FUMARATE—VIREAD™

Description/Actions: Tenofovir disoproxil fumarate is indicated in combination with other antiretroviral agents for the treatment of HIV-1 infection.

Precautions/Adverse Reactions: Lactic acidosis and severe hepatomegaly with steatosis, including fatal cases, have been reported with the use of nucleoside analogues alone or in combination with other antiretrovirals. The majority of cases have been in women. Exercise caution when administering nucleoside analogues to any patient with known risk factors for liver disease. Cases have also occurred in patients with no known risk factors. Tenofovir should not be administered to patients with renal insufficiency (creatinine clearance < 60 ml/minute).

Coadministration of tenofovir with drugs that reduce renal function or compete for active tubular secretion such as cidofovir, acyclovir, valacyclovir, ganciclovir, and valganciclovir may increase serum concentrations of tenofovir and/or increase the concentration of other renally eliminated drugs.

When administered with didanosine, tenofovir should be administered 2 hours before or 1 hour after administration of didanosine. Coadministration of tenofovir and lamivudine resulted in decreased serum concentrations of lamivudine. Coadministration of tenofovir with indinavir, lopinavir, and ritonavir resulted in decreased serum concentrations of indinavir, lopinavir and ritonavir. Coadministration of lopinavir/ritonavir with tenofovir resulted in increased serum concentrations of tenofovir. Redistribution and/or accumulation of body fat including central obesity, dorsocervical fat enlargement, peripheral wasting, facial wasting, breast enlargement, and cushingoid appearance have been observed in patients receiving antiretroviral therapy. Tenofovir may cause osteomalacia.

Pregnancy Category B. No adequate and well-controlled studies in pregnant women. Use in pregnancy only if the potential benefit justifies the potential risks to the fetus. Excretion in human breast milk is unknown. Nursing mothers should be instructed not to breast-feed if they are receiving tenofovir. Safety and efficacy in pediatric patients have not been established.

Most common adverse reactions observed in patients treated with tenofovir include nausea, diarrhea, asthenia, headache, vomiting, flatulence, abdominal pain, and anorexia. Increases in triglycerides, creatinine kinase, serum amylase, AST, urine glucose, ALT, and serum glucose have been observed in patients treated with tenofovir. Decreased neutrophil counts have also been reported.

Administration: Oral—once daily taken with food.

Patient Care Implications: Take with food. If coadministered with didanosine, tenofovir shoud be administered 2 hours before or 1 hour after administration of didanosine. Monitor for changes in serum creatinine and serum phosphorus levels in patients at risk or with a history of renal dysfunction. Women should be instructed not to breast-feed while taking tenofovir.

Preparations: Tablets, 300 mg (equivalent to 245 mg of tenofovir disoproxil).

TENORETIC®, Combination of atenolol and chlorthalidone

TENORMIN®, see Atenolol

TENSILON®, see Edrophonium

TENUATE®, see Diethylpropion

TEPANIL®, see Diethylpropion

TEQUIN®, see Gatifloxacin

TERAZOL 3®; TERAZOL 7®, see Terconazole

TERAZOSIN HYDROCHLORIDE—Hytrin®

Antihypertensive agent.

Description/Actions: An alpha-1-selective adrenergic receptor blocking agent that causes vasodilatation and a reduction in blood pressure. Indicated in the treatment of hypertension, and can be used alone or in combination with other antihypertensive agents. Also indicated for the treatment of benign prostatic hyperplasia.

Warnings: May cause orthostatic hypotension, resulting in symptoms such as dizziness, lightheadedness, palpitations and, in more severe cases, syncope. Syncope has occurred most often in association with the first dose or first few doses of therapy. To reduce the likelihood of syncope, treatment should be initiated with a 1 mg dose of terazosin, given at bedtime. Patients should be informed of the possibility of syncope and other orthostatic symptoms, and advised to avoid driving or other hazardous tasks for 12 hours after the first dose, after a dosage increase, and after interruption of therapy when treatment is resumed. They should also be advised to sit or lie down when symptoms associated with orthostatic hypotension occur, and to be cautious when rising from a sitting or lying position. Other adverse reactions include weakness, tiredness, fatigue, drowsiness, blurred vision, nasal congestion, nausea, peripheral edema, and weight gain.

Administration: Oral daily at bedtime.

Preparations: Tablets 1, 2, 5, and 10 mg. Capsules, 1, 2, 5, and 10 mg.

TERBINAFINE HYDROCHLORIDE—Lamisil®

Topical antifungal agent.

Description/Actions: An allylamine derivative that exhibits a fungicidal action by inhibiting squalene epoxidase, a key enzyme in sterol biosynthesis in fungi. Indicated for the topical treatment of interdigital tinea pedis, plantar tinea pedis (moccasin type) tinea cruris, and tinea corporis caused by *Epidermophyton floccosum, Trichophyton mentagrophytes,* or *Trichophyton rubrum.* Orally indicated in treatment of onychomycosis of the toenail and fingernail due to tinea unguium. Prior to initiating treament for onychomycosis, nail specimens should be obtained to confirm the diagnosis of onychomycosis.

Warnings: Adverse reactions include irritation and burning. Patients should be advised to avoid the use of occlusive dressings unless otherwise directed by the physician. Oral formulation contraindicated with pre-existing hepatic disease or renal impairment (Cr Cl < 50 ml/min). Discontinue if hepatobiliary dysfunction or progressive skin rash or severe neutropenia occurs. Rare cases of liver failure, some leading to death or liver transplant, have occurred with the use of terbinafine for the treatment of onychomycosis. Treatment with terbinafine should be discontinued if evidence of liver toxicity develops.

Monitor CBC and liver functions.

Administration: Oral and topical.

Preparations: Tablets, 250 mg. Cream and topical solution, 1%. Spray pump solution, 1%.

TERBUTALINE SULFATE—
Brethaire®, Brethine®, Bricanyl®

Bronchodilator.

Description/Actions: Stimulates beta-adrenergic receptors. Indicated for bronchial asthma and for reversible bronchospasm that may occur in association with bronchitis and emphysema. Also used in management of preterm labor (tocolytic).

Warnings: May cause increased heart rate and palpitations, and should be used cautiously in patients with cardiovascular disorders, especially those associated with arrhythmias. Other adverse reactions include nervousness, tremor, headache, nausea, vomiting, sweating, and muscle cramps. Other sympathomimetic agents should not be used concurrently. Beta-adrenergic-blocking agents and terbutaline may inhibit the effect of each other.

Administration: Oral, oral inhalation, and subcutaneous.

Preparations: Tablets, 2.5 and 5 mg. Metered dose inhaler (Brethaire). Ampules, 1 mg/ml.

TERCONAZOLE—Terazol 3®; Terazol 7®

Antifungal agent.

Description/Actions: Indicated for the local treatment of vulvovaginal candidiasis.

Warnings: Adverse reactions include headache, and vulvovaginal burning, itching, or irritation. Use during the first trimester of pregnancy should be avoided. Base contained in the vaginal suppository formulation may interact with certain rubber or latex products, such as those used in vaginal contraceptive diaphragms; therefore, concurrent use is not recommended.

Administration: Vaginal. Vaginal cream is administered for 7 consecutive days and the vaginal suppositories for 3 consecutive days.

Preparations: Vaginal cream (Terazol 7), 0.4%; vaginal suppository (Terazol 3), 80 mg.

TERPIN HYDRATE

Description/Actions: Expectorant most frequently used with codeine in an elixir formulation indicated for respiratory symptoms.

TERRAMYCIN®, see Oxytetracycline

TESLAC®, see Testolactone

TESSALON®, see Benzonatate

TESTODERM®, see Testosterone

TESTOLACTONE—Teslac®

Description/Actions: Antineoplastic agent indicated as adjunctive therapy in the treatment of advanced or disseminated breast cancer in postmenopausal women.

Preparations: Tablets, 50 mg.

TESTOSTERONE—Androderm®, Testoderm®

Description/Actions: Androgen indicated for use in male patients for replacement therapy for conditions associated with a deficiency or absence of endogenous testosterone. Transdermal system is indicated for primary hypogonadism and hypogonadotropic hypogonadism.

Preparations: Transdermal systems (Androderm), 2.5 and 5 mg, (Testoderm), 10 and 15 mg.

TESTOSTERONE CYPIONATE— Depo-Testosterone®

Description/Actions: Longer-acting ester of testosterone administered intramuscularly.

Preparations: Vials (in oil), 50 mg/ml 100 mg/ml, and 200 mg/ml.

TESTOSTERONE ENANTHATE— Delatestryl®

Description/Actions: Longer acting ester of testosterone administered intramuscularly.

Preparations: Vials (in oil), 100 mg/ml, and 200 mg/ml.

TESTOSTERONE GEL— Androgel®

Description/Actions: Indicated for replacement therapy in males for conditions associated with a deficiency or absence of endogenous testosterone, such as primary hypogonadism and hypogonadotropic hypogonadism.

Precautions/Adverse Reactions: Adverse effects include acne, alopecia, application site reaction, depression, headache, hypertension, nervousness, breast pain, and decreased libido. Gynecomastia frequently develops, and sleep apnea may be potentiated. Edema with or without congestive heart failure may be a serious complication in patients with preexisting cardiac, renal, or hepatic disease. Androgens are contraindicated in men with carcinoma of the breast or known or suspected carcinoma of the prostate. Testosterone gel should not be used in women.

Administration: Topical. Do not apply to genitals. Hands should be washed with soap and water after application.

Preparations: Packets, 1%, 2.5 and 5 g.

TESTOSTERONE PROPIONATE

Description/Actions: Androgen indicated for intramuscular use in male patients for replacement therapy in conditions associated with a deficiency or absence of endogenous testosterone—primary hypogonadism, hypogonadotropic hypogonadism, and delayed puberty. Also used in women with advancing inoperable metastatic mammary cancer who are 1 to 5 years postmenopausal.

Preparations: Vials, 25 mg/ml, 50 mg/ml, and 100 mg/ml.

TETRACAINE HYDROCHLORIDE—
Pontocaine®

Description/Actions: Local anesthetic indicated for spinal anesthesia, for anesthesia of the nose and throat, for ocular disorders, and skin conditions.

Preparations: Ampules (for spinal anesthesia), 0.2%, 0.3%, 1%, and powder. Solution (for anesthesia of the nose and throat), 2%. Ophthalmic solution and ointment (as base), 0.5%. Cream, 1%. Ointment (as base), 0.5%.

TETRACYCLINE HYDROCHLORIDE—
Achromycin V®, Actisite®, Panmycin®, Sumycin®

Tetracycline antibiotic.

Description/Actions: Active against many gram-positive and gram-negative bacteria, mycoplasmal, chlamydial, and rickettsial organisms, and certain spirochetes. Indicated in the treatment of respiratory and urinary tract infections and a number of other types of infections. Is useful as adjunctive therapy in the management of severe acne. Also indicated (for use as a periodontal fiber) as an adjunct to scaling and root planing for reduction of pocket depth and bleeding on probing in patients with adult periodontitis.

Warnings: Use is best avoided during the last half of pregnancy and in childhood to the age of 8 years because of the risk of discoloration of the teeth. Adverse reactions include nausea, vomiting, diarrhea, rash, and fungal superinfections. May cause photosensitivity reactions and patients should be cautioned to limit their exposure to sunlight and ultraviolet light. Must be used with caution in patients with impaired renal function. Absorption may be reduced by antacids, iron, calcium, and zinc salts, and other metal-containing formulations and foods; the administration of tetracycline and one of these agents should be separated by an interval of at least 1 hour.

Administration: Oral and topical.

Preparations: Capsules and tablets, 250 and 500 mg. Oral suspension, 125 mg/5 ml. Ointment, 3%. Topical solution. Periodontal fiber (Actisite), 12.7 mg.

TETRAHYDROZOLINE HYDROCHLORIDE—Tyzine®, Visine®

Description/Actions: Decongestant: Indicated for nasal use and for ophthalmic use to provide temporary relief of burning, irritation, and discomfort associated with certain ocular conditions.

Preparations: Nasal solution, 0.05% and 0.1%. Ophthalmic solution, 0.05%.

THALIDOMIDE—Thalpmid®

Description/Actions: Thalidomide is an immunmmodulatory agent indicated in the treatment of erythema nodosum leprosum (ENL). Not indicated as monotherapy in patients with ENL with moderate to severe neuritis. Unlabeled uses include Behcet's syndrome, HIV-associated wasting syndrome, aphthous stomatitis (including HIV-associated), and Crohn's disease.

Precautions/Adverse Reactions: Contraindicated in pregnancy (Category X). Severe, life-threatening human birth defects can occur if thalidomide is taken during pregnancy. Prescribers must be registered in the STEPS program and understand the risk of teratogenicity if thalidomide is administered during pregnancy. There are strict government mandated criteria that must be met prior to prescribing thalidomide for a woman or a man of childbearing potential. Because thalidomide is present in the semen of patients receiving the drug, males receiving thalidomide must always use a latex condom during any sexual contact with women of childbearing potential.

Adverse reactions include somolence, peripheral neuropathy, dizziness, orthostatic hypotension, neutropenia, photosensitivity, hypersensitivity, bradycardia and an increase in HIV viral load. Serious dermatologic reactions including Stevens-Johnson syndrome and toxic epidermal necrolysis, which may be fatal, have been reported. Seizures, including grand mal seizures, have also been reported during therapy with thalidomide. Patients with a history of seizures should be closely monitored.

Administration: Oral.

Patient Care Implications: Perform pregnancy testing 24 hours prior to the start of thalidomide and weekly thereafter for the duration of therapy. Instruct patients to safeguard acess to this medication and not to share the drug with anyone else. Warn patients about the effects on the unborn fetus. Teach patients the symptoms of periperal neuropathies and to report them immediately to the prescriber. The medication should be discontinued if drug-induced neuropathy develops to limit the potential for further nerve damage. Caution patients to avoid sun exposure because of the risk of photosensitivity. Advise patients to avoid alcohol during the course of treatment. Inform patients dizziness and drowsiness may occur and to avoid medication that may increase either of these effects. Tell patients to avoid activities in which drowsiness may be potentially dangerous (e.g., driving a car, running machinery) until response is ascertained.

Preparations: Capsule, 50, 100, and 200 mg.

THAM®, see Tromethamine with electrolytes

THEELIN®, see Estrone

THEO-DUR®, see Theophylline

THEO-24®, see Theophylline

THEOPHYLLINE (see list of preparations below for trade names)

Bronchodilator.

Description/Actions: A xanthine derivative indicated for the relief and/or prevention of symptoms of bronchial asthma and for reversible bronchospasm associated with chronic bronchitis and emphysema.

Warnings: Adverse reactions include nausea, vomiting, diarrhea, headaches, irritability, restlessness, insomnia, palpitation, tachycardia, flushing, and hypotension.

Administration: Oral. Controlled-release formulations should not be chewed or crushed. A high-fat content meal may increase the rate and extent of absorption of theophylline from certain formulations (e.g., Theo-24); the labeling for individual formulations should be consulted for guidelines regarding administration in relationship to meals.

Preparations: Capsules and tablets (Elixophyllin®, Slo-Phyllin®), 50, 100, 125, 200, 225, 250, and 300 mg. Controlled-release capsules and tablets (Elixophyllin SR®, Slo-bid gyrocaps®, Theo-24®, Theo-Dur®, Theovent®, Uni-Dur®, Uniphyl®), 50, 100, 125, 200, 250, 300, 400, 450, 500, and 600 mg. Liquid (Elixophyllin®, Slo-Phyllin®), 80, 112.5, and 150 mg/15 ml.

THEOPHYLLINE CALCIUM SALICYLATE

Description/Actions: Bronchodilator used in combination with other agents in the treatment of asthma and other respiratory conditions.

THEOPHYLLINE ETHYLENEDIAMINE, see Aminophylline

THEOPHYLLINE SODIUM GLYCINATE

Description/Actions: Bronchodilator indicated for the relief of bronchial asthma and for reversible bronchospasm associated with chronic bronchitis and emphysema.

THEOVENT®, see Theophylline

THIABENDAZOLE—Mintezol®

Description/Actions: Anthelmintic indicated for the treatment of trichinosis, cutaneous larva migrans, visceral larva migrans, strongyloidiasis. Is also effective in numerous other helmintic infestations.

Precautions/Adverse Reactions: Thiabendazole has been associated with abnormal sensations in eyes, xanthopsia, blurred vision, drying of mucous membranes, sicca syndrome, and abdominal pain.

Preparations: Chewable tablets, 500 mg. Suspension, 500 mg/5 ml.

THIAMINE HYDROCHLORIDE— Vitamin B₁

Description/Actions: Vitamin indicated for the treatment and prevention of thiamine deficiency and prevention of Wernicke's enceph-alopathy.

Preparations: Tablets, 5, 10, 25, 50, 100, 250, and 500 mg. Ampules and vials, 100 mg/ml and 200 mg/ml.

THIAMYLAL SODIUM

Description/Actions: Barbiturate anesthetic administered intravenously for induction of anesthesia, for supplementing other anesthetic agents, as anesthesia for short surgical procedures, and for inducing hypnotic states.

Preparations: Vials, 1, 5, and 10 g.

THIETHYLPERAZINE MALEATE—Norzine®, Torecan®

Description/Actions: Phenothiazine anti-emetic indicated for the relief of nausea and vomiting.

Preparations: Tablets, 10 mg. Suppositories, 10 mg. Ampules, 10 mg/2 ml.

THIMEROSAL—Merthiolate®

Description/Actions: Antiseptic used for antisepsis of intact skin, treatment of contaminated wounds, and for preoperative and postoperative use.

Preparations: Solution and tincture, 1:1000. Aeropump tincture, 1:1000.

THIOGUANINE

Description/Actions: Antineoplastic agent indicated for the treatment of acute nonlymphocytic leukemias and chronic myelogenous leukemia.

Precautions/Adverse Reactions: Individuals with an inherited deficiency of the enzyme thiopurine methyltransferase (TPMT) may be unusually sensitive to the myelosuppressive effects of mercaptopurine and prone to developing rapid bone marrow suppression following initiation of treatment. This problem may be potentiated by coadministration of thioguanine with drugs that inhibit TPMT, such as olsalazine, mesalazine, and sulfasalazine. Use caution if these drugs must be coadministered.

Preparations: Tablets, 40 mg.

THIOLA®, see Tiopronin

THIOPENTAL SODIUM—Pentothal®

Description/Actions: Barbiturate anesthetic administered intravenously for induction of anesthesia, for supplementing other anesthetic agents, as anesthesia for short surgical procedures, for inducing hypnotic states, for control of convulsive seizures, in certain neurosurgical patients with increased intracranial pressure, and for narcoanalysis and narcosynthesis in psychiatric disorders. Has also been used in the form of a rectal suspension when preanesthetic sedation or basal narcosis by the rectal route is desired.

Preparations: Vials and syringes, 250, 400, and 500 mg, 1, 2.5, and 5 g. Rectal suspension, 400 mg/g.

THIOPLEX®, see Thiotepa

THIORIDAZINE HYDROCHLORIDE—Mellaril®

Phenothiazine antipsychotic agent.

Description/Actions: Mellaril® is now only indicated for the treatment of schizophrenic patients who fail to show an acceptable response to other antipsychotic agents.

Warnings: Adverse reactions include drowsiness and other CNS effects; patients should be cautioned regarding activities such as driving and operating machinery, as well as interactions with other CNS-acting drugs, including alcohol. Other adverse reactions include extrapyramidal symptoms, tardive dyskinesia, dry mouth, blurred vision, and dermatitis.

Mellaril® has been shown to prolong the QT_c interval and has been associated with torsades de pointes–type arrhythmias and sudden death. Mellaril® is contraindicated with fluvoxamine, propranolol, pindolol, and drugs that inhibit the cytochrome p450206 isozyme such as fluoxetine and paroxetine and agents known to prolong the QT_c interval. Mellaril® is also contraindicated in patients known to have reduced levels of the cytochrome p450206 isozyme as well as in patients with congenital long QT syndrome or a history of cardiac arrhythmias. Baseline ECG and serum potassium levels should be monitored. Patients with a QT_c interval greater than 450 msec should not receive Mellaril®. Mellaril® should be discontinued in patients who are found to have a QT_c interval greater than 500 msec.

Administration: Oral.

Preparations: Tablets, 10, 15, 25, 50, 100, 150, and 200 mg. Oral solution (concentrate), 30 and 100 mg/ml. Oral suspension (as the base), 25 and 100 mg/5 ml.

THIOSULFIL FORTE®, see Sulfamethizole

THIOTEPA—Triethylenethiophosphoramide, Thioplex®

Description/Actions: Antineoplastic agent administered parenterally in the palliative treatment of adenocarcinoma of the breast, adenocarcinoma of the ovary, and for controlling intracavitary effusions secondary to diffuse or localized neoplastic disease of various serosal cavities, superficial papillary carcinoma of the bladder, lymphosarcoma, and Hodgkin's disease.

Preparations: Vials, 15 mg.

THIOTHIXENE—Navane®

Description/Actions: Antipsychotic agent indicated in the management of the manifestations of psychotic disorders.

Preparations: Capsules, 1, 2, 5, 10, and 20 mg. Concentrate (as the hydrochloride), 5 mg/ml.

THORAZINE®, see Chlorpromazine

3TC®, see Lamivudine

THROMBIN—Thrombinar®, Thrombostat®

Description/Actions: Hemostatic agent indicated for topical use whenever oozing blood and minor bleeding from capillaries and small venules is accessible. Also used in conjunction with absorbable gelatin sponge for hemostasis in various types of surgery.

Preparations: Vials, 1000, 5000, 10,000, 20,000, and 50,000 units.

THROMBINAR®, see Thrombin

THROMBOSTAT®, see Thrombin

THYLLINE®, see Dyphylline

THYMOL

Description/Actions: Anti-infective included in combination with other agents in certain topical formulations. Has also been included in mouthwash formulations for its aromatic and antiseptic properties.

THYROID

Agent for thyroid replacement.

Description/Actions: Thyroid hormone and is indicated as replacement therapy in patients with hypothyroidism, and as a pituitary-and thyroid-stimulating hormone (TSH) suppressant in the treatment or prevention of various types of goiters.

Warnings: Must be used cautiously in patients with cardiovascular disorders and endocrine disorders such as diabetes. Adverse reactions include headache, nervousness, palpitations, tachycardia, and nausea.

Administration: Oral.

Preparations: Tablets, 15, 30, 60, 90, 120, 180, 240, and 300 mg.

THYROTROPIN—Thyroidstimulating hormone (TSH), Thytropar®

Description/Actions: Used for diagnostic purposes.

Preparations: Vials, 10 IU of thyrotropic activity.

THYROXINE, see Levothyroxine

THYTROPAR®, see Thyrotropin

TIAGABINE HYDROCHLORIDE— Gabitril®

Description/Actions: Antiepileptic agent indicated as an adjunct in partial seizures.

Warnings: Avoid abrupt cessation. Use cautiously in nursing mothers, hepatic impairment, and the elderly. Pregnancy Category C.

Adverse reactions include dizziness, asthenia, somnolence, GI upset/pain, nervousness, tremor, abdominal pain, concentration difficulties, other CNS effects, serious rash, and possible longterm opthalmologic effects. Not recommended in children < 12 years.

Administration: Oral. Take with food.

Preparations: Tablets, 2, 4, 12, 16 mg.

TIAZAC®, see Diltiazem

TICAR®, see Ticarcillin

TICARCILLIN DISODIUM—Ticar®

Penicillin antibiotic.

Description/Actions: Is bactericidal and active against many gram-positive and gram-negative bacteria, including *Pseudomonas aeruginosa.* Is usually used in conjunction with an aminoglycoside antibiotic in the treatment of *Pseudomonas* infections.

Warnings: Contraindicated in patients with a history of allergic reaction to any of the penicillins. Adverse reactions include hypersensitivity reactions, gastrointestinal effects, bleeding manifestations, and hypokalemia. Disodium salt is utilized, and the administration of high doses may cause problems in patients in whom sodium intake must be closely monitored.

Administration: Intravenous and intramuscular.

Preparations: Vials, 1, 3, 6, 20, and 30 g.

TICARCILLIN DISODIUM/ CLAVULANATE POTASSIUM— Timentin®

Description/Actions: Penicillin antibiotic with beta-lactamase inhibitor. Clavulanic acid inhibits beta-lactamase enzymes and protects ticarcillin from degradation by these enzymes; the spectrum of action of ticarcillin is extended to include additional bacteria.

Preparations: Vials, 3.1 and 3.2 g (representing 3 g of ticarcillin and 0.1 and 0.2 g of clavulanic acid, respectively).

TICLID®, see Ticlopidine

TICLOPIDINE HYDROCHLORIDE—Ticlid®

Antiplatelet agent.

Description/Actions: Is a platelet aggregation inhibitor that is thought to act primarily by inhibiting the adenosine diphosphate (ADP) pathway for platelet aggregation. Indicated to reduce the risk of thrombotic stroke in patients who have experienced stroke warning signs [e.g., transient ischemic attacks (TIAs)], and in patients who have had a complete thrombotic stroke. Use should be reserved for patients who are intolerant to aspirin therapy, or in situations in which there is a risk of stroke but aspirin is not indicated. Ticlopidine is also indicated as an adjunctive therapy with aspirin to reduce the incidence of subacute stent thrombosis in patients undergoing successful coronary stent implantation.

Warnings: Contraindicated in the presence of hematopoietic disorders such as neutropenia and thrombocytopenia. Contraindicated in the presence of a hemostatic disorder or active pathologic bleeding and in patients with severe hepatic disease. Complete blood counts and white cell differentials should be performed every 2 weeks starting from the second week to at least the end of the third month of therapy. Causes a prolongation of bleeding time, and its use has been associated with bleeding complications (e.g., ecchymosis, epistaxis, hematuria, gastrointestinal bleeding); should be used with caution in patients who may be at risk of increased bleeding from trauma, surgery, or pathological conditions, and in patients who have lesions with a propensity to bleed (e.g., ulcers). Medication may be discontinued 10–14 days prior to elective surgery. Patients should be advised that it may take them longer than usual to stop bleeding. The concomitant use of aspirin, an anticoagulant, or fibrinolytic agent with ticlopidine is best avoided. Other adverse reactions include diarrhea, nausea, dyspepsia, gastrointestinal pain, and rash. Signs and symptoms of jaundice have occurred infrequently, and patients should be advised to inform their physicians if they observe yellowing of the skin or whites of the eyes, or consistent darkening in the color of the urine, or lightening in the color of the stools. May cause severe hematologic reactions, including neutropenia, agranulocytosis, thrombotic thrombocytopenia purpura (TTP), and aplastic anemia.

Administration: Oral. Should be administered with food.

Preparations: Tablets, 250 mg.

TIGAN®, see Trimethobenzamide

TIKOSYN®, see Dofetilide

TILADE®, see Nedocromil sodium

TILUDRONATE—Skelid®

Actions and Uses: Indicated in the treatment of Paget's disease. In vitro studies indicated that tiludronate acts primarily on bone through a mechanism involving inhibition of osteoclastic activity, probably through a reduction in the enzymatic and transport process that leads to resorption of the mineralized matrix. Use in patients with severe renal failure (CrCl < 30 ml/min) not recommended. Maintain adequae calcium and vitamin D intake. Use cautiously in patients with upper GI disease.

Warnings: Adverse reactions include GI disorders (e.g., nausea, diarrhea, dyspepsia), chest pain, edema, paresthesia, hyperparathyroidism, arthrosis, rhinitis, sinusitis, cataract, conjunctivitis, and glaucoma.

Administration: Take with 6–8 oz of plain (not mineral) water at least 2 hours before or after any other beverages, food, or medication, 400 mg once daily for 3 months. May retreat after a 3 month posttreatment evaluation period.

Preparations: Tablets, 240 mg (equivalent to 200 mg tiludronic acid).

TIMENTIN®, see Ticarcillin disodium/clavulanate potassium

TIMOLOL MALEATE—Betimol®, Blocadren®, Timoptic®, Timoptic-XE®

Antihypertensive agent and agent for glaucoma.

Description/Actions: A nonselective beta-adrenergic-blocking agent indicated in the treatment of hypertension and to reduce cardiovascular mortality and the risk of reinfarction in patients who have survived the acute phase of a myocardial infarction. Also indicated for migraine headache prophylaxis. Also indicated for ophthalmic administration in the treatment of chronic open-angle glaucoma, aphakic glaucoma, and secondary glaucoma.

Warnings: Contraindicated in patients with bronchial asthma or severe chronic obstructive pulmonary disease, sinus bradycardia, second- and third-degree AV block, overt cardiac failure, and cardiogenic shock. Adverse reactions include fatigue, dizziness, bradycardia, cold hands and feet, and, when administered in the ophthalmic dosage form, ocular irritation. Adverse reactions include anaphylaxis, angioedema, urticaria, localized and generalized rash, fatigue, dizziness, bradycardia, cold hands and feet, and, when administered in the ophthalmic dosage form, ocular irritation. Use is best avoided in patients with bronchospastic diseases, and therapy in diabetic patients must be closely monitored.

Administration: Oral and ophthalmic. Patients should be cautioned about the interruption or discontinuation of therapy; exacerbation of angina pectoris has occurred following the abrupt cessation of therapy, and, when therapy is to be discontinued, the dosage should be gradually reduced over a period of 1 to 2 weeks.

Preparations: Tablets, 5, 10, and 20 mg. Ophthalmic solution, 0.25% and 0.5%. Ophthalmic gel (Timoptic-XE®), 0.25% and 0.5%.

TIMOPTIC®, see Timolol maleate

TIMOPTIC-XE®, see Timolol maleate

TINACTIN®, see Tolnaftate

TINDAL®, see Acetophenazine

TINVER®, see Sodium thiosulfate

TINZAPARIN—Innohep®

Description/Actions: Indicated for the treatment of acute symptomatic deep vein thrombosis, with or without pulmonary embolism, when administered in combination with warfarin sodium.

Precautions/Adverse Reactions: Tinzaparin is contraindicated in patients with a hypersensitivity to Tinzaparin or any component of the formulations, sulfites, benzyl alcohol, pork products, with major active bleeding, and current or history of heparin-induced thrombocytopenia. Patients with recent or anticipated neuraxial anesthesia (epidural or spinal anesthesia) are at risk of spinal or epidural hematoma and subsequent paralysis. This risk is increased by the use of indwelling epidural catheters, by the concomitant use of drugs affecting hemostasis (i.e., nonsteroidal anti-inflammatory drugs, as well as traumatic or repeated epidural or spinal puncture. Patients should be closely monitored for signs and symptoms of neurologic impairment. Health care providers should consider the potential benefit versus risk before neuraxial anesthesia intervention in patients anticoagulated or to be anticoagulated for thromboprophylaxis. Monitor patients for signs and symptoms of bleeding while on Innohep® therapy. Caution should be exercised in conditions where patients are at increased risk of hemorrhage. Risk factors for increased bleeding include bacterial endocarditis; severe or uncontrolled hypertension; congenital or acquired bleeding disorders; active ulceration or angiodysplastic GI diseases; recent GI bleed; hepatic failure, amyloidosis; gastrointestinal disease; shortly after brain, spinal, or ophthalmic surgery; in patients treated concomitantly with platelet inhibitors; hemorrhagic stroke; diabetic retinopathy; or in patients undergoing invasive procedures. Pregnancy Category B. No adequate and well-controlled studies in pregnant women. This drug should be used during pregnancy only if clearly needed. Innohep® multiple-dose vials contain benzyl alcohol as a preservative; benzyl alcohol administered to premature neonates has been associated with fatal gasping syndrome. Since benzyl alcohol may cross the placenta, Innohep® preserved with benzyl alcohol should be used with caution in pregnant women only if clearly needed. Excretion in breast milk is unknown; use caution. Safety and efficacy have not been established in pediatric patients. Use caution in the elderly. Thrombocytopenia can occur with Innohep® therapy; discontinue administration if platelets are < 100,000/ mm3. Administer subcutaneous injection only; do not mix with other injections or infusions. Due to the increased bleeding potential, use caution in patients receiving oral anticoagulants, platelet inhibitors, and thrombolytics. Some adverse effects are bleeding, injection site hematoma, increased ALT, thrombocytopenia, urinary tract infections, pulmonary embolism, angina pectoris, headache, epistaxis, nausea, and back pain.

Administration: SQ injection.

Patient Care Implications: Innohep® is administered by SC injection. It must not be administered by intramuscular or intravenous injection. SC injection technique: Patients should be lying or sitting, and Innohep® should be administered by deep SC injection. Alternate injection site daily between the left and right anterolateral and left and right posterolateral abdominal wall. The entire needle should be introduced into the skin fold formed by the thumb and forefinger. Hold the skinfold until injection is complete. To minimize bruising, do not rub the injection site. Lab monitoring should include CBC, including platelet count and hematocrit/hemoglobin. Inform patient to report immediately any unusual bleeding or bruising (i.e., mouth, nose, blood in urine, or stool) or any other adverse effects.

Preparations: Multidose 2 ml vial (20,000 anti-Xa IU per ml). Preparation contains metabisulfite and benzyl alcohol.

TIOCONAZOLE—Vagistat®

Antifungal agent.

Description/Actions: An imidazole antifungal agent indicated for use as a local single-dose treatment of vulvovaginal candidiasis.

Warnings: Adverse reactions include burning and itching.

Administration: Vaginal.

Preparations: Vaginal ointment, 6.5%.

TIOPRONIN—Thiola®

Agent for kidney stones.

Description/Actions: Indicated for the prevention of cystine (kidney) stone formation in patients with severe homozygous cystinuria with urinary cystine greater than 500 mg/day, who are resistant to treatment with conservative measures of high fluid intake, alkali and diet modification, or who have had adverse reactions to penicillamine.

Warnings: Contraindicated during pregnancy. Adverse reactions include rash, pruritus, drug fever, lupus erythematosus–like effects, reduction in taste perception, and wrinkling and friability of the skin. May cause gastrointestinal, pulmonary, neurologic, renal, and hematologic reactions.

Administration: Oral. Should be given in divided doses 3 times a day at least 1 hour before or 2 hours after meals.

Preparations: Tablets, 100 mg.

TIROFIBAN—Aggrastat®

Description/Actions: Platelet aggregation inhibitor indicated in combination with heparin for treating acute coronary syndrome.

Warnings: Contraindicated in the following conditions within previous 30 days: active internal bleeding, bleeding diathesis, stroke, major surgery, or severe trauma. Contraindicated with a history of intracranial hemorrhage, intracranial neoplasm, arteriovenous malformation, aneurysm, hemorrhagic stroke, thrombocytopenia after previous tirofiban therapy, symptoms or findings suggestive of aortic dissection, severe hypertension, acute pericarditis, and concomitant parenteral GI 11b/111a inhibitor.

Use cautiously in patients with platelet count < 150,000 /mm^3, in patients with hemorrhagic retinopathy, and in chronic hemodialysis patients. Fatal bleeding events have been reported. Properly care for femeral artery access site to minimize bleeding. Minimize other arterial and venous punctures, IM injections, catheter use, and other invasive procedures to minimize bleeding risk. Avoid use of noncompressible IV access sites. Do baseline platelet counts, hemoglobin and hematocrit, and monitor during therapy. Discontinue tirofiban if confirmed thrombocytopenia occurs. Adjust heparin to maintain aPTT at two times control.

Severe allergic reactions, including anaphylactic reactions, have occurred during the first day of tirofiban infusion, during initial treatment, and during readministration of tirofiban. Some cases have been associated with severe thrombocytopenia (platelet count < 10,000/mm^3).

Adverse reactions include bleeding, decreased hemoglobin and/or hematocrit, reduced platelet counts, edema, vasovagal reaction, and others.

Administration: Intravenous.

Preparations: Premixed, 50 µg/ml vials. Concentrate, 250 µg/ml.

TISSUE PLASMINOGEN ACTIVATOR, see Alteplase, recombinant

TITANIUM DIOXIDE

Description/Actions: Sunscreen used topically in cream, lotion, and ointment formulations.

TIZANIDINE—Zanaflex®

Description/Actions: Reduces muscle apasticity and is indicated in acute and intermittent management of increased skeletal muscle tone associated with spasticity.

Warnings: Use cautiously in impaired hepatic or renal function, in cardiovascular disease, and in the elderly. Monitor ophthalmic and liver function (aminotransferases at baseline, 1, 3, and 6 months and periodically thereafter). Adverse reactions include sedation, dry mouth, somnolence, asthenia, dizziness, constipation, elevated liver enzymes, vomiting, speech disorders, blurred vision, dyskinesia, nervousness, pharyngitis, hypotension (including orthostatic), hallucinations, and psychosis.

Administration: Recommended dosage: 2–4 mg 3 times/day. Usual intial dose is 4 mg. May increase by 2–4 mg as needed every 6–8 hours to a maximum of 3 doses in 24 hours. Maximum dose is 36 mg/day. Reduce dose in renal impairment (CrCl < 25 ml/min).

Preparations: Tablets, 2 and 4 mg (scored). Capsules, 2, 4, and 6 mg.

TMP-SMX, see Trimethoprim-sulfamethoxazole

TNKase™, see Tenecteplase

TOBRAMYCIN SULFATE— Nebcin®, Tobrex®

Aminoglycoside antibiotic.

Description/Actions: Indicated for the parenteral treatment of serious infections caused by gram-negative bacteria including *Pseudomonas aeruginosa*. Is also effective in the treatment of staphylococcal infections. Has also been used topically in the treatment of ocular infections.

Warnings: May cause nephrotoxicity, ototoxicity, and neurotoxicity, and the concurrent or serial use of other nephrotoxic or ototoxic agents should be avoided.

Administration: Intravenous, intramuscular, and ophthalmic.

Preparations: Vials and syringes, 20 mg/ 2 ml, 60 mg/1.5 ml, 80 mg/2 ml., and 1.2 g. Ophthalmic solution and ointment, 0.3%.

TOBREX®, see Tobramycin

TOCAINIDE HYDROCHLORIDE— Tonocard®

Description/Actions: Antiarrhythmic agent indicated for the suppression of symptomatic ventricular arrhythmias, including frequent premature ventricular contractions, unifocal or multifocal, couplets, and ventricular tachycardia.

Preparations: Tablets, 400 and 600 mg.

TOFRANIL®, see Imipramine

TOLAZAMIDE—Tolinase®

Sulfonylurea hypoglycemic agent.

Description/Actions: Indicated as an adjunct to diet to lower the blood glucose in patients with non-insulin-dependent diabetes mellitus whose hyperglycemia cannot be controlled by diet alone.

Warnings: May cause hypoglycemia, and patients should be advised to contact their physician if symptoms of hypoglycemia develop. Adverse reactions include nausea, heartburn, pruritus, and erythema. Oral hypoglycemic agents have been suggested to be associated with increased cardiovascular mortality as compared to treatment by diet alone or diet plus insulin.

Administration: Oral.

Preparations: Tablets, 100, 250, and 500 mg.

TOLAZOLINE HYDROCHLORIDE—Priscoline®

Description/Actions: Peripheral vasodilator indicated for intravenous use in the treatment of persistent pulmonary hypertension of the newborn when systemic arterial oxygenation cannot be satisfactorily maintained by usual supportive care.

Preparations: Ampules, 25 mg/ml.

TOLBUTAMIDE—Orinase®

Description/Actions: Sulfonylurea hypoglycemic agent indicated as an adjunct to diet to lower the blood glucose in patients with non-insulin-dependent diabetes whose hyperglycemia cannot be satisfactorily controlled by diet alone.

Preparations: Tablets, 250 and 500 mg.

TOLCAPONE—Tasmar®

Description/Actions: Anti-Parkinson agent indicated as an adjunct to carbidopa/levodopa in idiopathic Parkinson's disease.

Warnings: Contraindicated in concomitant nonselective MAOIs (e.g., phenelzine) liver disease or a previous history of elevated liver function associated with use of this agent or a history of nontraumatic rhabdomyolysis or fever or confusion possibly related to medication. Use cautiously in orthostatic hypertension/syncope, severe renal impairment (CrCl $\leq$ 25 ml/min), and severe hepatic impairment. Monitor transaminases every month for the first 3 months, then every 6 weeks for the next 3 months (more frequently if elevation occurs). Discontinue if enzyme elevations $\geq$ 5 times the upper limit of normal or jaundice occurs. Pregnancy Category C.

Adverse reactions include dyskinesias, nausea, sleep disorders, dystonia, excessive dreaming, anorexia, muscle cramps, orthostatic complaints, somnolence, diarrhea, confusion, dizziness, headache, hallucinations, vomiting, constipation, fatigue, upper respiratory or urinary tract infection, falling, increased sweating, syncope, xerostomia, urine discoloration, and others.

Administration: Oral.

Preparations: Tablets, 100 and 200 mg.

TOLECTIN®, see Tolmetin

TOLINASE®, see Tolazamide

TOLMETIN SODIUM—Tolectin®, Tolectin DS®

Nonsteroidal anti-inflammatory drug.

Description/Actions: Inhibits prostaglandin synthesis and is indicated for the treatment of rheumatoid arthritis, juvenile rheumatoid arthritis, and osteoarthritis.

Warnings: Should not be given to patients in whom aspirin or another NSAID causes asthma, rhinitis, urticaria, or other allergic-type reactions. May cause GI effects, and use should be avoided in patients with active GI tract disease and closely monitored in patients with a previous history of such disorders. Other adverse reactions include headache, weakness, edema, elevated blood pressure, weight changes, and skin irritation. Effect may be reduced by sodium bicarbonate.

Administration: Oral. Bioavailability is reduced by food or milk and is best administered apart from meals.

Preparations: Tablets and capsules, 200, 400, and 600 mg.

TOLNAFTATE—Tinactin®

Description/Actions: Antifungal agent used topically in the treatment of superficial fungal infections of the skin.

Preparations: Cream, powder, solution, gel, aerosol powder, and aerosol liquid, 1%.

TOLTERODINE TARTRATE—
Detrol®, Detrol® LA

Description/Actions: A competitive muscarinic receptor antagonist indicated in treatment of patients with symptoms of urinary frequency, urgency, or urge incontinence.

Warnings: Contraindicated in urinary retention, gastric retention, and uncontrolled narrow-angle glaucoma. Use cautiously in patients with bladder outflow obstruction, obstructive GI disease (e.g., pyloric stenosis), narrow-angle glaucoma, renal impairment, and hepatic dysfunction. Pregnancy Category C. Not recommended in nursing mothers.

Adverse reactions include dry mouth, dyspepsia, headache, constipation, xerophthalmia, hypertension, dizziness, and other anticholinergic effects. May cause blurred vision. Anaphylactoid reactions, tachycardia, and peripheral edema have also been reported with the use of tolterodine.

Administration: Oral.

Preparations: Tablets, 1 and 2 mg. Extended-release capsule, 2 and 4 mg.

TONOCARD®, see Tocainide

TOPAMAX®, see Topiramate

TOPICORT®, see Desoximetasone

TOPIRAMATE—Topamax®

Description/Actions: Anticonvulsant indicated as adjunctive therapy for partial onset seizures in adults.

Warnings: Avoid abrupt cessation as this may precipitate seizures. Use cautiously in patients with hepatic or renal impairment. The risk of kidney stone formation is about 2–4 times that of untreated population. This may be reduced by increasing fluid intake. Adverse reactions include somnolence, dizziness, ataxia, speech disorders, psychomotor slowing, nervousness, paresthesia, nystagmus, tremor, fatigue, confusion, decreased weight, language or mood problems, anorexia, and anxiety. A syndrome consisting of acute myopia associated with secondary angle-closure glaucoma has been reported in both adult and pediatric patients receiving topiramate. Symptoms include acute onset of decreased visual acuity and/or ocular pain. May be associated with supraciliary effusion resulting in anterior displacement of the lens and iris, with secondary angle-closure glaucoma. Topiramate should be discontinued if this occurs.

Administration: Oral. Halve dose in renal impairment (CrCl < 70 ml/min), and assess for slower titration.

Preparations: Tablets 25, 100, and 200 mg. Sprinkle capsules 15 and 25 mg.

TOPOTECAN HYDROCHLORIDE—Hycamtin®

Antineoplastic.

Description/Actions: Used in the treatment of patients with metastatic ovarian cancer after failure of initial or subsequent chemotherapy.

Warnings: Bone marrow suppression (primarily neutropenia) is the dose-limiting toxicity of topotecan. Administer only to patients with adequate bone marrow reserves (baseline neutrophil counts of at least 1500 cells/mm3 and platelet count of 100,000 mm3). Adverse effects include neutropenia, thrombocytopenia, and anemia.

Administration: Intravenous.

Preparations: Powder for injection, 4 mg.

TOPROL XL®, see Metoprolol succinate

TORADOL®, see Ketorolac tromethamine

TORECAN®, see Thiethylperazine

TOREMIFENE—Fareston®

Description/Actions: Indicated in metastatic breast cancer in postmenopausal women with estrogen-receptor positive or unknown tumors.

Warnings: Contraindicated in pregnancy (Category D) and nursing mothers.

Use not recommended in history of thromboembolic disorders and longterm treatment not recommended in patients with preexisting endometrial hyperplasia. If bone metastases present, monitor for hypercalcemia for first few weeks. Discontinue if severe hypercalcemia occurs. Use cautiously with leukopenia and thrombocytopenia. Monitor blood counts, calcium levels, and liver function.

Adverse reactions include hot flashes, sweating, GI upset, vaginal discharge/bleed, dizziness, edema, tumor flare, hypercalcemia, elevated liver tests, and cardiac, ocular, and thrombotic events.

Instruct patients to report vaginal bleeding and symptoms of hypercalcemia.

Administration: Oral.

Preparations: Tablets, 60 mg.

TORNALATE®, see Bitolterol

TORSEMIDE—Demadex®
Diuretic.

Description/Actions: Is a loop diuretic that is indicated for the treatment of edema associated with congestive heart failure, renal disease, or hepatic disease. Is also indicated for the treatment of hypertension and may be used alone or in combination with other antihypertensive agents.

Warnings: Contraindicated in patients who are hypersensitive to any sulfonylurea derivative. Is also contraindicated in patients who are anuric. Adverse reactions include excessive urination, headache, dizziness, and rhinitis.

May cause electrolyte imbalance and periodic monitoring of serum potassium and other electrolytes is advised.

Administration: Oral and intravenous. When given intravenously, should be administered slowly over a period of two minutes.

Preparations: Tablets, 5, 10, 20, and 100 mg. Ampules, 20 and 50 mg.

TOTACILLIN®, see Ampicillin

TPA, see Alteplase, recombinant

TRACLEER™, see Bosentan

TRACRIUM®, see Atracurium besylate

TRAMADOL HYDROCHLORIDE—Ultram®

Description/Actions: Analgesic indicated for the management of moderate to moderately severe pain.

Warnings: Contraindicated in patients with alcohol, hypnotics, centrally acting analgesics, opioids, or psychotropic drugs. Do not give to opioid dependent patients. Adverse reactions include constipation, nausea, vomiting, dizziness, somnolence, central nervous system (CNS) stimulation, asthenia, and headache. Patients should be cautioned about driving or operating machinery. May increase the risk of seizures in patients with epilepsy. Unlikely to produce dependence and is not classified as a controlled substance.

Administration: Oral.

Preparations: Tablets, 50 mg.

TRAMADOL HYDROCHLORIDE/ ACETAMINOPHEN— ULTRACET™

Description/Actions: Ultracet™ is indicated for the short-term (5 days or less) management of acute pain.

Precautions/Adverse Reactions: Ultracet™ is contraindicated in any situation where opioids are contraindicated, including acute intoxication with any of the following: alcohol, hypnotics, narcotics, centrally acting analgesics, opioids, or psychotic drugs. It may worsen CNS and respiratory depression in these patients. Tramadol should not be used in opioid-dependent patients. Serious potential consequences of overdosage with tramadol are CNS depression, respiratory depression, and death. Administer Ultracet cautiously in patients at risk for respiratory depression.

Seizures reported when taken within the recommended dosage; risk is increased in patients taking selective serotonin reuptake inhibitors, tricyclic antidepressants, other tricyclic compounds, other opioids, monamine oxidate inhibitors (MAOIs), neuroleptics, or other drugs that reduce the seizure threshold.

Use cautiously in patients with increased intracranial pressure or head injury. Not recommended in patients with liver disease. Do not coadminister with other tramadol- or acetaminophen-containing products. Safety and effectiveness have not been studied in the pediatric population. Use with caution in elderly patients, because there is a greater frequency of decreased hepatic, renal, or cardiac function, and concomitant disease, as well as multiple drug therapy. Most common side effects were somnolence, constipation, increased sweating, and dizziness.

Pregnancy Category C; no well-controlled studies in pregnant women. Should not be used in pregnant women prior to or during labor. Chronic use during pregnancy may lead to physical dependence and postpartum withdrawal symptoms in the newborn.

Administration: Oral.

Patient Care Implications: May be taken with or without food. Advise patients they may be mentally impaired and to use caution when driving or engaging in tasks requiring alertness until response to drug is known. Patients should understand the 24-hour dose limit and the time interval between doses. Advise not to take with other tramadol- or acetaminophen-containing products.

Preparations: Tablet, acetaminophen, 325 mg, and tramadol hydrochloride, 37.5 mg.

TRANCOPAL®, see Chlormezanone

TRANDATE®, see Labetalol

TRANDOLAPRIL—Mavik®

Ace Inhibitor.

Description/Actions: Inhibits angiotensin converting enzyme (ACE). Used in treatment of hypertension as monotherapy or as an adjunct to other antihypertensive agents. Also indicated in stabilized patients after MI who have LV systolic dysfunction or DHF symptoms

Warnings: Do not use in patients with a history of ACE inhibitor– associated angioedema. Monitor for neutropenia in collagen, vascular, and/or renal disease. Monitor for hyperkalemia in diabetes. Use cautiously in patients with renal impairment, cardiovascular or cerebrovascular disease, or salt/volume depletion. Adverse reactions include cough, dizziness, and diarrhea. Discontinue if laryngeal edema, angioedema, or jaundice occurs. (Black patients may have a higher risk of angioedema than non-Black patients.)

Administration: Usual range is 2–4 mg once daily to a maximum of 8 mg/day, which may be given in two divided doses. Follow manufacturer's dosaging guidelines.

Preparations: Tablets, 1 mg (scored), 2 and 4 mg.

TRANEXAMIC ACID—Cyklokapron®

Antifibrinolytic agent.

Description/Actions: Indicated in patients with hemophilia for short-term use (2 to 8 days) to reduce or prevent hemorrhage and to reduce the need for replacement therapy during and following tooth extraction.

Warnings: Contraindicated in (1) patients with acquired defective color vision, because this prohibits measuring one end point that should be followed as a measure of toxicity; and (2) patients with subarachnoid hemorrhage. Visual abnormalities have been experienced by some patients, and, for patients who are to be treated continually for longer than several days, an ophthalmological examination is advised before commencing and at regular intervals during the course of treatment. Other adverse reactions include nausea, vomiting, diarrhea, and giddiness. Hypotension has been observed when intravenous injection is too rapid, and the solution should not be injected more rapidly than 1 ml per minute.

Administration: Oral and intravenous.

Preparations: Tablets, 500 mg. Ampules, 100 mg/ml.

TRANSDERM-NITRO®, see Nitroglycerin

TRANSDERM-SCOP®, see Scopolamine

TRANXENE®, see Clorazepate

TRANYLCYPROMINE SULFATE—Parnate®

Description/Actions: Monoamine oxidase inhibitor antidepressant indicated for the treatment of major depressive episode without melancholia.

Warnings: Hypertension or hypotension, coma, convulsions and death may occur with opioids (avoid use of meperidine within 14–21 days of MAO inhibitor therapy–decrease initial dose of other agents to 25% of usual dose). Serious potentially fatal adverse reactions may occur with concurrent use of other antidepressants. Avoid using within two weeks of each other (wait 5 weeks from end of fluoxetine therapy).

Preparations: Tablets, 10 mg.

TRASTUZUMAB—Herceptin®

Description/Actions: Indicated in the treatment of patients with metastatic breast cancer with tumors overexpressing the Human epidermal growth factor receptor2 (HER2) protein. It may be used as a single agent in patients who have received ≥ 1 chemotherapy regimens or in combinations with placitaxel in patients who have not received chemotherapy for their metastatic disease. Use only in patients whose tumors have HER2 protein overexpression.

Precautions/Adverse Reactions: Trastuzumab administration can result in development of ventricular dysfunction and CHF. Evaluate the left ventricular function in all patients prior to and during treatment. Strongly consider discontinuing the trastuzumab in patients who develop a clinically significant decrease in the left ventricular function. Patients receiving trastuzumab in combination with anthracyclines and cyclophosphomide demonstrated a particularly high incidence and severity of cardiac dysfunction.

Adverse reactions include cardiotoxicity, anemia and leukopenia, diarrhea, infection, and infusion-related symptoms (during the first infusion 40% of the patients experienced chills and fever. Other infusional symptoms included nausea, vomiting, pain, rigors, headache, dizziness, dypsnea, hypotension, rash, and asthenia). Symptoms infrequently occurred with subsequent administrations of the drug.

Administration: Intravenous.

Patient Care Implications: Treat infusion-associated symptoms with acetaminophen, diphenhydramine, and meperidine as needed. Warn patients to avoid exposure to infectious sources. Teach patients to watch for early signs of an infection and to promptly report symptoms to the prescriber. Explain the need for ongoing cardiac function testing and the importance of adhering to the testing schedule.

Preparations: Powder for reconstitution, 400 mg (diluent contains benzyl alcohol).

TRASYLOL®, see Aprotinin

TRAVASE®, see Sutilains

TRAVATAN™, see Travoprost

TRAVERT®, see Invert sugar

TRAVOPROST—TRAVATAN™

Description/Actions: Travaprost is indicated for reduction of elevated intraocular pressure (IOP) in patients with open-angle glaucoma or ocular hypertension who are intolerant or unresponsive to other IOP-lowering medication.

Precautions/Adverse Reactions: Travoprost has been reported to cause changes to pigmented tissues. The most frequently reported changes have been increased pigmentation of the iris, eyelid, and eyelashes and increase in growth of eyelashes. These changes may be permanent. Use caution in patients with intraocular inflammation, aphakic patients, pseudophakic patients with a torn posterior lens capsule or patients with risk factors for macular edema.

Pregnancy Category C. It may be teratogenic and may interfere with the maintenance of pregnancy and therefore should not be used by women during pregnancy or by women attempting to become pregnant. No adequate, well-controlled studies have been performed in pregnant women.

The most common adverse effects were ocular hyperemia, conjuntival hyperemia, eyelash growth, decreased visual acuity, foreign body sensation, eye discomfort, pain, and itching.

Administration: Topical.

Patient Care Implications: Do not exceed once daily dosing; may decrease IOP-lowering effect. If used with other ophthalmic agents, separate administration by at least 5 minutes between each medication. Remove contacts prior to administration and wait 15 minutes before reinserting. Reduction of IOP starts approximately 2 hours after administration, and the maximum effect is reached after 12 hours. Patients should be informed of the possibility of iris color change. Patients should be instructed to avoid allowing the tip of the container to contact the eye or surrounding structures. This can cause tip to become contaminated. Serious damage to the eye and subsequent loss of vision may result from using contaminated solutions. Instruct patients to wash hands before instilling. Sit or lie down to instill. Discard container within 6 weeks of removing it from the sealed pouch.

Preparations: Solution, ophthalmic, 0.004% (2.5 ml and 2 × 2.5 ml).

TRAZODONE HYDROCHLORIDE—Desyrel®

Antidepressant.

Description/Actions: Indicated for the treatment of depression.

Warnings: Is not recommended for use during the initial recovery phase of myocardial infarction. Adverse reactions include drowsiness and other CNS effects; patients should be cautioned regarding activities such as driving and operating machinery, as well as interactions with other CNS-acting drugs including alcohol. May cause priapism, and patients with prolonged or inappropriate penile erection should discontinue the drug and consult with the physician. Other adverse reactions include dry mouth, blurred vision, hypotension, nausea, and vomiting.

Administration: Oral.

Preparations: Tablets, 50, 100, 150, and 300 mg.

TRECATOR-SC®, see Ethionamide

TRELSTAR® Depot, see Triptorelin pamoate

TRELSTAR™ LA, see Triptorelin pamoate

TRENTAL®, see Pentoxifylline

TRETINOIN—Retinoic acid, vitamin A acid, Avita®, Renova®, Retin-A®

Agent for acne.

Description/Actions: A vitamin A analogue indicated for topical application in the treatment of acne.

Warnings: Skin may become excessively red, edematous, blistered, or crusted in some patients. May increase susceptibility to sunlight and patients should be advised to minimize exposure to sunlight, including sunlamps.

Administration: Topical.

Preparations: Cream, 0.02%, 0.025%, 0.05%, and 0.1%. Solution, 0.05%. Gel, 0.01% and 0.025%. Microspheres aqueous gel, 0.1%, 0.04%. Capsule, 10 and 25 mg.

TREXAN®, trade name formerly used for naltrexone

TRIACETIN—Glyceryl triacetate

Description/Actions: Antifungal agent indicated for topical use in the treatment of athlete's foot and other superficial fungal infections.

Preparations: Cream, 25%.

TRIAMCINOLONE—Aristocort®, Kenacort®

Description/Actions: Corticosteroid indicated in a wide range of endocrine, rheumatic, allergic, dermatologic, respiratory, hematologic, neoplastic, and other disorders.

Preparations: Tablets, 1, 2, 4, and 8 mg.

TRIAMCINOLONE ACETONIDE— Aristocort®, Azmacort®, Kenalog®, Nasacort®, Nasacort AQ®, Tri-Nasal®

Description/Actions: Preparations: Vials (for intramuscular, intraarticular, intrabursal, and intradermal injection), 10 mg/ml and 40 mg/ml. Aerosol (for inhalation), 100 μg/actuation (Azmacort®). Cream and ointment, 0.025%, 0.1%, and 0.5%. Lotion, 0.025% and 0.1%. Aerosol (for topical use). Nasal spray, 55 μg/actuation (Nasacort®), 50 μg/actuation (Tri-Nasal™).

TRIAMCINOLONE DIACETATE— Aristocort®, Kenacort®

Preparations: Syrup, 2 mg/5 ml and 4 mg/5 ml. Vials (for intramuscular, intraarticular, intrasynovial, and intralesional injection), 25 mg/ml and 40 mg/ml.

TRIAMCINOLONE HEXACETONIDE—Aristospan®

Preparations: Vials (for intraarticular, intralesional, and sublesional injection), 5 mg/ml and 20 mg/ml.

TRIAMTERENE—Dyrenium®

Diuretic.

Description/Actions: A potassium-sparing diuretic indicated in the treatment of edema associated with congestive heart failure, cirrhosis of the liver, and the nephrotic syndrome; also used in ste-

TRIAVIL

roid-induced edema, idiopathic edema, and edema due to secondary hyperaldosteronism.

Warnings: Contraindicated in patients with anuria, severe hepatic or renal disease, or preexisting elevated serum potassium levels. Should not be used in patients receiving another potassium-sparing diuretic or potassium salts or supplements.

Administration: Oral.

Preparations: Capsules, 50 and 100 mg.

TRIAVIL®, Combination of amitriptyline and perphenazine

TRIAZOLAM—Halcion®

Benzodiazepine hypnotic.

Description/Actions: A CNS depressant indicated in the management of insomnia.

Warnings: Contraindicated during pregnancy. Adverse reactions include residual sedation, amnesic effects, and other CNS effects upon awakening; patients should be cautioned regarding activities such as driving and operating machinery, as well as interactions with other CNS-acting drugs, including alcohol. Can cause dependence, and is included in Schedule IV.

Administration: Oral.

Preparations: Tablets, 0.125 and 0.25 mg.

TRICHLOROACETIC ACID

Description/Actions: Cauterizing agent applied topically to warts and to debride callus tissue.

TRICHLORMETHIAZIDE— Metahydrin®, Naqua®

Description/Actions: Thiazide diuretic indicated as adjunctive therapy in edema and in the management of hypertension.

Preparations: Tablets, 2 and 4 mg.

TRICOR®, see Fenofibrate

TRIDESILON®, see Desonide

TRIDIL®, see Nitroglycerin

TRIDIONE®, see Trimethadione

TRIENTINE HYDROCHLORIDE— Syprine®

Agent for Wilson's disease.

Description/Actions: A chelating agent indicated in the treatment of patients with Wilson's disease who are intolerant of penicillamine.

Warnings: Adverse reactions include fever, skin eruption, and iron deficiency anemia. Mineral supplements should usually not be administered concurrently because they may reduce the absorption of trientine. Should be administered at least 1 hour before or 2 hours after meals and at least 1 hour apart from any other drug, food, or milk.

Administration: Oral.

Preparations: Capsules, 250 mg.

TRIETHYLENETHIOPHOSPHOR- AMIDE, see Thiotepa

TRIFLUOPERAZINE HYDROCHLORIDE—Stelazine®

Description/Actions: Phenothiazine antipsychotic agent indicated for the manifestations of psychotic disorders.

Preparations: Tablets, 1, 2, 5, and 10 mg. Oral concentrate, 10 mg/ml. Vials, 2 mg/ml.

TRIFLUPROMAZINE HYDROCHLORIDE—Vesprin®

Description/Actions: Phenothiazine antipsychotic agent and antiemetic indicated for parenteral use for the manifestations of psychotic disorders, and for the control of severe nausea and vomiting.

Preparations: Vials, 10 mg/ml and 20 mg/ml.

TRIFLURIDINE—Viroptic®

Description/Actions: Antiviral agent indicated for ophthalmic use for the treatment of primary keratoconjunctivitis and recurrent epithelial keratitis due to *Herpes simplex* virus, Types 1 and 2.

Preparations: Ophthalmic solution, 1%.

TRIHEXYPHENIDYL HYDROCHLORIDE—Artane®

Description/Actions: Antiparkinson agent indicated for the treatment of parkinsonism and the management of drug-induced extrapyramidal reactions.

Preparations: Tablets, 2 and 5 mg. Controlled-release capsules, 5 mg. Elixir, 2 mg/5 ml.

TRIIODOTHYRONINE, see Liothyronine

TRILAFON®, see Perphenazine

TRILEPTAL®, see Oxcarbazepine

TRILISATE®, see Choline magnesium trisalicylate

TRIMEPRAZINE TARTRATE— Temaril®

Description/Actions: Phenothiazine antihistamine indicated for the treatment of pruritic symptoms in a number of allergic and nonallergic conditions.

Preparations: Tablets, 2.5 mg. Controlled-release capsules, 5 mg. Syrup, 2.5 mg/5 ml.

TRIMETHADIONE—Tridione®

Description/Actions: Anticonvulsant indicated for the control of petit mal seizures that are refractory to treatment with other drugs.

Preparations: Tablets, 150 mg. Capsules, 300 mg.

TRIMETHOBENZAMIDE HYDROCHLORIDE—Tigan®

Description/Actions: Antiemetic indicated for the control of nausea and vomiting.

Preparations: Capsules, 100, 250, and 300 mg. Suppositories, 100 and 200 mg. Vials and syringes, 100 mg/ml.

TRIMETHOPRIM—Proloprim®, Trimpex®

Description/Actions: Antibacterial indicated in the treatment of urinary tract infections.

Preparations: Tablets, 100 and 200 mg. Oral solution, 50 mg/5 ml.

TRIMETHOPRIM— SULFAMETHOXAZOLE—TMP-SMX, Cotrimoxazole, Bactrim®, Septra®

Anti-infective agent.

Description/Actions: Combined actions of the 2 agents result in a synergistic action against many microorganisms. Is active against many gram-positive and gram-negative bacteria as well as certain other organisms. Indications include urinary tract infections, acute otitis media, acute exacerbations of chronic bronchitis, shigellosis, treatment and prophylaxis of *Pneumocystis carinii* pneumonitis, and the treatment of travelers' diarrhea in adults due to susceptible strains of enterotoxigenic *E. coli.* Is also useful in a number of other infections including prostatic infections.

Warnings: Should not be used in pregnancy at term or during the nursing period. Adverse reactions include nausea, vomiting, rash, and urticaria. Because serious reactions such as the Stevens-Johnson syndrome have occurred in some individuals, therapy should be discontinued at the first appearance of skin rash or other adverse effects.

Administration: Oral and intravenous.

Preparations: Tablets, 80/400 and 160/800 mg. Suspension, 40/200 mg/5 ml. Ampules and vials, 16/80 mg/ml.

TRIMETREXATE GLUCURONATE—NeuTrexin®

Anti-infective agent.

Description/Actions: Is a structural analogue of folic acid. Exhibits a folic acid antagonist (antifolate) action that leads to cell death of certain microorganisms such as *Pneumocystis carinii* that require folate metabolism for continued cell viability. Indicated with concurrent leucovorin administration (leucovorin protection) as alternative therapy for the treatment of moderate to severe *Pneumocystis carinii* pneumonia in immunocompromised patients, including patients with AIDS, who are intolerant of, or are refractory to trimethoprim/sulfamethoxazole (TMP/SMX) therapy or for whom TMP/SMX is contraindicated.

Warnings: Contraindicated in patients with a known hypersensitivity to trimetrexate or methotrexate. It is also contraindicated in patients with severe myelosuppression. It is essential that leucovorin be used concurrently to reduce the risk of bone marrow suppression, oral and gastrointestinal mucosal ulceration, and renal and hepatic dysfunction. It is recommended that blood tests be performed at least twice a week to assess absolute neutrophil counts and platelets, as well as renal function (serum creatinine) and hepatic function (AST, ALT, alkaline phosphatase). Adverse reactions include neutropenia, thrombocytopenia, anemia, increased AST and ALT, fever, rash, pruritus, nausea, and vomiting. It is recommended that zidovudine not be used during the period of trimetrexate therapy. May cause fetal harm if administered during pregnancy.

Administration: Intravenous. Administered once daily by IV infusion over 60–90 minutes. Leucovorin must be administered daily (every 6 hours) during treatment with trimetrexate and for 72 hours past the last dose of trimetrexate. The recommended course of treatment is 21 days of trimetrexate and 24 days of leucovorin. Trimetrexate must not be reconstituted or mixed with solutions containing either chloride ion or leucovorin because precipitation occurs instantly. The intravenous line must be flushed thoroughly with at least 10 ml of 5% dextrose injection before and after administering trimetrexate.

Prepartion: Vials, 25 mg trimetrexate.

TRIMIPRAMINE MALEATE— Surmontil®

Description/Actions: Tricyclic antidepressant indicated for the relief of symptoms of depression.

Preparations: Capsules, 25, 50, and 100 mg.

TRIMOX®, see Amoxicillin

TRIMPEX®, see Trimethoprim

TRINALIN®, Combination of azatidine and pseudoephedrine

TRI-NASAL®, see Triamcinolone acetonide

TRIOSTAT®, see Liothyronine

TRIOXSALEN—Trisoralen®

Description/Actions: Photoactive agent indicated for repigmentation of idiopathic vitiligo, enhancing pigmentation, and increasing tolerance to sunlight in blond persons and those with fair complexions who suffer painful reactions when exposed to sunlight.

Preparations: Tablets, 5 mg.

TRIPELENNAMINE—PBZ®

Description/Actions: Antihistamine indicated for the management of allergic disorders.

Preparations: Tablets (as the hydrochloride), 25 and 50 mg. Controlled-release tablets (as the hydrochloride), 100 mg. Elixir (as the citrate), equivalent to 25 mg of the hydrochloride/5 ml.

TRIPLE SULFAS, see Trisulfapyrimidines

TRIPROLIDINE HYDROCHLORIDE

Description/Actions: Antihistamine used in combination with pseudoephedrine

TRIPTORELIN PAMOATE— Trelstar® Depot, Trelstar™ LA

Description/Actions: Indicated in the palliative treatment of advanced prostate cancer. It offers an alternative to orchiectomy or estrogen therapy.

Precautions/Adverse Reactions: Triptorelin is contraindicated in patients with hypersensitivity to triptorelin or to any other component of the product, other LH-RH agonists, or LH-RH. Initial increase in testosterone levels may lead to the temporary worsening of symptoms of prostate cancer. Cases of spinal cord compression have been reported. Cases of anaphylactic shock and angioedema have been reported. Chronic administration of triptorelin results in suppression of the pituitary-gonadal axis. Diagnostic tests to access pituitary function performed during therapy or up to 8 weeks after discontinuation of therapy may be misleading. No formal drug interaction studies have been conducted. Coadministration with hyperprolactinemic drugs is not recommended because hyperprolactinemia decreases the number of pituitary gonadotropin releasing hormone receptors. Pregnancy Category X. Triptorelin is contraindicated in pregnancy. Triptorelin may cause fetal harm when administered to pregnant women. Excretion in human breast milk is unknown. It should not be used by nursing mothers. Safety and efficacy in children have not been established. Most common adverse reactions observed in patients treated with triptorelin include hot flashes (59%), bone pain (12%), impotence (7.1%), headache (5%), injection site pain (3.6%), and hypertension (3.6%).

Administration: IM injection.

Patient Care Implications: Worsening of symptoms may occur during the first few weeks of therapy. Reconstitute each vial with 2 ml of sterile water for injection. Do not use any other diluent. Shake well and withdraw the entire reconstituted suspension into the syringe, and use immediately.

Preparations: Powder for injection, Trelstar®Depot 3.75 mg single-dose vials. Trelstar™ LA 11.25 mg single-dose vials.

TRISENOX®, see Arsenic trioxide

TRISORALEN®, see Trioxsalen

TRISULFAPYRIMIDINES—Triple sulfas

Description/Actions: Anti-infective agents (sulfadiazine, sulfamerazine, sulfamethazine) indicated in the treatment of infections caused by susceptible organisms.

Preparations: Tablets, 500 mg. Suspension, 500 mg/5 ml.

TRITEC®—Combination of ranitidine and bismuth citrate

TRIVAGIZOLE 3™, see Clotrimazole

TRIZIVIR™, see Abacavir, Lamivudine, and Zidovudine

TROBICIN®, see Spectinomycin

TROLAMINE SALICYLATE— Aspercreme®, Myoflex®

328 • TROLEANDOMYCIN

Description/Actions: Salicylate analgesic indicated for topical use for the temporary relief of minor aches and pains of muscles and joints. Also used as a topical adjunct in arthritis.

Preparations: Cream, 10%.

TROLEANDOMYCIN—Tao®

Description/Actions: Antibiotic indicated for infections caused by susceptible gram-positive bacteria.

Preparations: Capsules, 250 mg.

TROMETHAMINE—Tham®

Description/Actions: Alkalinizing agent indicated for parenteral use for the prevention and correction of systemic acidosis in selected patients.

Preparations: Bottles, 18 g/500 ml.

TRONOLANE®, see Pramoxine

TRONOTHANE®, see Pramoxine

TROPICAMIDE—Mydriacyl®

Description/Actions: Anticholinergic agent indicated for ophthalmic use to provide mydriasis and cycloplegia for diagnostic purposes.

Preparations: Ophthalmic solutions, 0.5% and 1%.

TRUSOPT®, see Dorzolamide hydrochloride

TRYPSIN

Description/Actions: Proteolytic enzyme used in combination with other agents for enzymatic debridement and to promote normal healing.

TUBOCURARINE CHLORIDE—Curare

Description/Actions: Nondepolarizing neuromuscular blocking agent indicated as an adjunct to anesthesia to induce skeletal muscle relaxation.

Preparations: Vials, 3 mg/ml.

TUMS®, see Calcium carbonate

TUSSI-ORGANIDIN®NR, Combination of codeine and guaifenesin

TYLENOL®, see Acetaminophen

TYLOX®, Combination of oxycodone and acetaminophen

TYZINE®, see Tetrahydrozoline

U

UCEPHAN®, see Sodium benzoate and Sodium phenylacetate

ULTANE®, see Sevoflurane

ULTRA-LENTE INSULIN, see Insulin

ULTRACET™, see Tramadol Hydrochloride/Acetaminophen

ULTRAM®, see Tramadol hydrochloride

ULTRAVATE®, see Halobetasol propionate

UNASYN®, see Ampicillin sodium/sulbactam sodium

UNDECYLENIC ACID AND SALTS—Desenex®

Description/Actions: Antifungal agent applied topically in the management of superficial fungal infections.

Preparations: Powder, cream, ointment, liquid, foam, and soap.

UNI-DUR®, see Theophylline

UNIPEN®, see Nafcillin

UNIPHYL®, see Theophylline

UNIRETIC®, Combination agent of moexipril hcl and hydrochlorothiazide (ACE inhibitor and diuretic)

UNISOM®, see Doxylamine

UNIVASC®, see Moexipril hydrochloride

UNOPROSTONE—Rescula®

Description/Actions: Unoprostone is indicated for the lowering of intraocular pressure in patients with open-angle glaucoma or ocular hypertension; it should be used in patients who are intolerant of other intraocular pressure (IOP) medications or failed therapy on other IOP-lowering medications.

Precautions/Adverse Reactions: Utilization is contraindicated in patients with known hypersensitivity to unoprostone isopropyl, benzalkonium chloride, or any other formulation components. Permanent changes in eye pigmentation have been reported with usage; long-term effects and consequences from the changes in eye coloration for potential injury to the eye are currently not known. Bacterial keratitis has been reported and associated with the inadvertent contamination of multiple-dose ophthalmic solutions. Safety and efficacy have not been established in patients with active intraocular inflammation, angle closure, inflammatory or neovascular glaucoma, hepatic or renal impairment, and pediatrics. Rescula® contains benzalkonium chloride, which may be adsorbed by contact lenses; contact lenses should be removed prior to instillation, and lenses may be reinserted 15 minutes following administration. Pregnancy Category C. Unoprostone should be used during pregnancy only if the potential benefit justifies the potential risk to the fetus. Excretion into the breast milk is unknown; use with caution if administering to a nursing woman.

Because the drug acts locally in the eye, it has limited systemic side effects. Some adverse effects are burning/stinging (upon instillation), dry/itching eyes, increased length of eyelashes, abnormal vision, eyelid disorder, foreign body sensation, and lacrimation disorder.

Administration: Ophthalmic, adults: Instill 1 drop into affected eye(s) twice daily.

Patient Care Implications: Inform patients to avoid allowing the tip of the dispensing container to contact the eye or surrounding structures because this could cause the tip to become contaminated by bacteria. If more than one ophthalmic drug is being used, the drugs should be administered at least 5 minutes apart. Patients should be informed of the warnings regarding the possibility of eye color changes and to remove contact lenses before instilling the solution (see precautions).

Preparations: Solution, ophthalmic: 0.15% (5 ml).

URACIL MUSTARD

Description/Actions: Antineoplastic agent indicated for the treatment of chronic lymphocytic leukemia, non-Hodgkin's lymphomas, chronic myelogenous leukemia, polycythemia vera, and mycosis fungoides.

Preparations: Capsules, 1 mg.

UREA—Carbamide, Aquacare®, Ureaphil®

Description/Actions: Osmotic agent administered intravenously to reduce intraocular pressure and to reduce intracranial pressure in the control of cerebral edema. Also used topically to promote hydration and removal of excess keratin in dry skin and hyperkeratotic conditions.

Preparations: Bottles (for intravenous use), 40 g. Cream, 2%, 10%, 20%, 30%, and 40%. Lotion, 2%, 10%, 15%, and 25%.

UREA PEROXIDE, see Carbamide peroxide

UREAPHIL®, see Urea

URECHOLINE®, see Bethanechol

URISPAS®, see Flavoxate

UROCIT-K®, see Potassium citrate

UROFOLLITROPIN—Metrodin®

Description/Actions: Gonadotropin administered intramuscularly and given sequentially with human chorionic gonadotropin for the induction of ovulation in selected patients with polycystic ovarian disease.

Preparations: Ampules, 0.83 mg.

UROKINASE—Abbokinase®

Description/Actions: Thrombolytic enzyme indicated for parenteral use in the management of pulmonary embolism and coronary artery thrombosis. Also used for the restoration of patency to intravenous catheters.

Preparations: Vials, 250,000 IU.

URSODIOL—Actigall®, URSO®

Gallstone solubilizing agent.

Description/Actions: A bile acid that decreases hepatic synthesis and secretion of cholesterol. Used for dissolving gallstones and is indicated for patients with radiolucent, noncalcified gallbladder stones less than 20 mm in greatest diameter in whom elective cholecystectomy would be undertaken except for the presence of increased surgical risk due to systemic disease, advanced age, idiosyncratic reaction to general anesthesia, or for those patients who refuse surgery. Prevention of gallstone formation in obese patients experiencing rapid weight loss.

Warnings: Contraindicated in patients with a history of allergy to bile acids, chronic liver disease, or with gallstones of a type (e.g., calcified) against which ursodiol is not active. Adverse reactions include diarrhea. May cause hepatotoxicity and patients should have liver function tests performed. Cholestyramine, colestipol, and aluminum-containing antacids may reduce the absorption and efficacy of ursodiol; therefore, doses should be separated from doses of these other medications by as long an interval as possible.

Administration: Oral. Therapy is usually continued for 6 to 24 months.

Preparations: Tablets, 250 mg. Capsules, 300 mg.

UTICORT®, see Betamethasone benzoate

V

VAGIFEM®, see Estradiol/Ethinyl estradiol

VAGISTAT®, see Tioconazole

VALACYCLOVIR—Valtrex®

Description/Actions: Antiviral agent indicated for the treatment of herpes zoster (shingles) in immunocompetent adults, for initial and recurrent episodes of genital herpes, and for the treatment of cold sores in adults and adolescent patients 12 years of age and older.

Warnings: Thrombotic thrombocytopenic purpura (TTP)/hemolytic uremic syndrome (HUS) has been reported in patients with advanced human immunodeficiency virus (HIV) disease and also in bone marrow transplant and in renal transplant recipients; this reaction has not been reported in immunocompetent patients, and valacyclovir is not indicated for the treatment of immunocompromised patients. Other adverse reactions include headache and nausea.

Administration: Oral.

Preparations: Capsules, 500 mg.

VALCYTE™, see Valganciclovir

VALDECOXIB—BEXTRA™

Description/Actions: Valdecoxib is indicated for the relief of signs and symptoms of osteoarthritis, adult rheumatoid arthritis, and the treatment of the acute pain of primary dysmenorrhea.

Precautions/Adverse Reactions: Valdecoxib should not be taken by patients who have experienced asthma, urticaria, or other allergic reactions after taking aspirin or NSAIDs. Severe, rarely fatal, anaphylactic-like reactions to NSAIDs are possible in such patients. Valdecoxib should not be given to patients who have demonstrated allergic-type reactions to sulfonamides. Serious skin reactions including exfoliative dermatitis, Stevens-Johnson Syndrome, and toxic epidermal necrolysis have been reported. As these reactions can be life threatening, valdecoxib should be discontinued at the first appearance of skin rash or any other sign of hypersensitivity. Cases of hypersensitivity reactions (anaphylactic reactions and angioedema) have been reported in patients receiving valdecoxib. These cases have occurred in patients with and without a history of allergic-type reactions to sulfonamides. Valdecoxib should not be given to patients with the aspirin triad (typically occurs in asthmatic patients who experience rhinitis with or without nasal polyps or who exhibit severe, potentially fatal bronchospasm after taking aspirin or other NSAIDs). Use with caution in patients with a history of GI disease (bleeding or ulcers) or risk factors for GI bleeding; use lowest dose for shortest time possible. Use caution in patients with decreased renal function, hepatic disease, dehydration, or asthma. Use caution in patients with fluid retention, hypertension, or heart failure.

Valdecoxib should not be given to patients who are in their third trimester of pregnancy; it may cause premature closure of the ductus arteriosus. Pregnancy Category C. There are no studies in pregnant women. Use only if potential benefit justifies potential risk to the fetus.

Common adverse events were nausea, diarrhea, dyspepsia, headache, and abdominal pain.

Administration: Oral.

Patient Care Implications: May be taken with or without food. Although valdecoxib has an improved safety profile compared to other NSAIDs, serious GI ulcerations can occur without warning. Inform patients about signs and symptoms of serious GI toxicity. It should not be used for cardiovascular prophylaxis instead of aspirin because it does not alter platelet function. Avoid alcohol, aspirin, and over-the-counter medications unless approved by prescriber. Inform patients they may experience dizziness, headache, abdominal pain, nausea, and vomiting. They can eat small, frequent meals or chew gum to alleviate gastric distress. Patients should stop taking medication and immediately report stomach pain, cramping, and any unusual bleeding or bruising.

Preparations: Tablets, 10 and 20 mg.

VALGANCICLOVIR—VALCYTE™

Description/Actions: Valganciclovir is indicated in the treatment of cytomegalovirus retinitis in patients with acquired immunodeficiency syndrome (AIDS).

Precautions/Adverse Reactions: Valganciclovir is contraindicated in anyone with a known hypersensitivity to valganciclovir, ganciclovir, or any component of the formulation. Valganciclovir should not be administered if the absolute neutrophil count is less than 500 cells/ l, the platelet count is less than 25,000/ l, or the hemoglobin is less than 8 g/dl. Severe leukopenia, neutropenia, anemia, thrombocytopenia, pancytopenia, bone marrow depression, and aplastic anemia have occurred with the use of valganciclovir. Use with caution in patients with preexisting cytopenias, prior or current use of myelosuppressive drugs, or irradiation. The clinical toxicity of valganciclovir includes granulocytopenia, anemia, and thrombocytopenia. It is considered probable that in humans, valganciclovir at the recommended doses may cause temporary or permanent inhibition of spermatogenesis. Suppression of fertility in females may also occur.

Pregnancy Category C. No adequate and well-controlled studies in pregnant women. Use during pregnancy only if the potential benefit justifies the potential risk to the fetus. Women of childbearing age are advised to use effective contraception during treatment with valganciclovir. Men should also be advised to practice barrier contraception during and for at least 90 days following treatment with valganciclovir. Excretion in human breast milk is unknown. Women should be instructed not to breast-feed while receiving valganciclovir. Safety and efficacy in pediatric patients have not been established.

Strict adherence to dosage recommendations is necessary to avoid overdose. Valganciclovir tablets cannot be substituted for ganciclovir capsules on a one-to-one basis.

Zidovudine and ganciclovir each have the potential to cause neutropenia and anemia, and some patients may not tolerate concomitant therapy at full dosage. Coadministration of ganciclovir and probenecid resulted in increased ganciclovir blood levels and decreased clearance of ganciclovir. Patients with renal impairment should be monitored carefully when ganciclovir and mycophenolate are coadministered, as levels of metabolites of both drugs may increase.

Major adverse effects associated with valganciclovir include diarrhea, nausea, fever, neutropenia, anemia, headache, vomiting, insomnia, abdominal pain, retinal detachment, peripheral neuropathy, paresthesia, and thrombocytopenia. Adverse effects occurring in less than 5% of patients treated with valganciclovir include pancytopenia, bone marrow depression, aplastic anemia, decreased creatinine clearance, local and systemic infections and sepsis, potentially life-threatening bleeding associated with thrombocytopenia, convulsions, psychosis, hallucinations, confusion, and agitation.

Administration: Oral.

Valganciclovir should not be prescribed to patients receiving hemodialysis. For patients on hemodialysis (creatinine clearance < 10 ml/minute), it is recommended that ganciclovir be used with dosage adjustments as recommended in ganciclovir product labeling.

Patient Care Implications: Complete blood counts, platelet counts, and renal function should be monitored. Patients should be instructed to take valganciclovir with food.

Patients should be informed that ganciclovir has caused decreased sperm production in animals and may cause decreased fertility in humans. Women of childbearing potential should be instructed to use effective contraception during treatment. Men should be advised to practice barrier contraception during and for at least 90 days following treatment with valganciclovir.

Patients should be told that valganciclovir is not a cure for cytomegalovirus retinitis and that progression of disease may occur. Patients should be informed to have ophthalmogic examinations every 4–6 weeks while receiving treatment.

Patients should be instructed to observe caution when driving, operating machinery, or performing tasks requiring alertness due to the potential for valganciclovir to cause convulsions, sedation, dizziness, ataxia, and/or confusion.

Valganciclovir tablets should be handled and disposed of properly. Tablets should not be broken or crushed. Avoid direct contact of broken or crushed tablets with skin or mucous membranes. If contact occurs, wash thoroughly wih soap and water, and rinse eyes thoroughly with plain water.

Preparations: Tablets, 450 mg (496.3 mg of valganciclovir HCL corresponding to 450 mg of valganciclovir).

VALISONE®, see Betamethasone valerate

VALIUM®, see Diazepam

VALPROIC ACID—Depacon®, Depakene®

DIVALPROEX SODIUM— Depakote®, Depakote® ER

Description/Actions: Anticonvulsant indicated for use in the treatment of simple (petit mal) and complex absence seizures. Also used adjunctively in patients with multiple seizure types, including absence seizures. Also indicated for the treatment of manic episodes associated with bipolar disorder and prophylaxis against migraine headaches.

Contraindicated in patients with a known hypersensitivity to divalproex sodium or to any component of the formulation. Contraindicated in patients with hepatic disease or significant hepatic dysfunction. Hepatic failure resulting in fatalities has occurred in patients receiving valproic acid and its derivatives. Children under 2 years of age are at an increased risk of developing hepatotoxicity. Use with extreme caution in these individuals. Cases of life-threatening pancreatitis have been reported in both children and adults. Contraindicated in patients with urea cycle disorders. Hyperammonemic encephalopathy, sometimes fatal, has been reported following initiation of valproate therapy in patients with urea cycle disorders. Pregnancy Category D. Valproic acid and its derivatives have been shown to produce teratogenic effects such as neural tube defects. Use only if the benefits outweigh the potential risk of injury to the fetus. Excreted in breast milk. Nursing is not recommended.

Preparations: Capsules (as valproic acid), 250 mg. Syrup (as sodium valproate), 250 mg/5 ml. Enteric-coated tablets (divalproex sodium—representing a stable coordination compound comprised of sodium valproate and valproic acid in a 1:1 molar relationship), 125, 250, and 500 mg, extended release tablet, 250 and 500 mg. Sprinkle capsules (divalproex sodium), 125 mg, 100 mg/ml solution for IV infusion.

VALRELEASE®, see Diazepam

VALRUBICIN—Valstar®

Description/Actions: Indicated for intravesical therapy of BCG refractory carcinoma in situ (CIS) of the urinary bladder in patients for whom immediate cystectomy would be associated with unacceptable morbidity or mortality.

Precautions/Adverse Reactions: Valrubicin is contraindicated with a known hypersensitivity to this agent or Cremophor EI (polypoxyethyleneglycol tricinoleate), concurrent urinary tract infection, small bladder capacity.

Inform patients that valrubicin includes complete response in only about 1 out of 5 patients and that delaying cystectomy could lead to development of metastatic bladder cancer, which is lethal. If there is not a complete response to valrubicin or CIS recurs within 3 months, reconsider cystectomy. Do not administer to patients with a perforated bladder or to those in whom the integrity of the bladder mucosa has been compromised. Adverse reactions include irritable bladder symptoms. These reactions usually occur during or shortly after installation and resolve within 1–7 days post instillation.

Administration: 800 mg intravesically once a week for 6 weeks. Empty the bladder, instill the medication via catheter under aseptic conditions, withdraw the catheter, and have patient retain the medication for 2 hours before voiding.

Patient Care Implications: Instruct patients to void at the end of the 2 hour period. Patients should be told to maintain adequate hydration postadministration of the medication. Use appropriate cytotoxic precautions when handling the agent for administration. May not be administered via IV/IM route.

Preparations: Solution for intravesical administration, 40 mg/ml.

VALSARTAN—Diovan®

Description/Actions: Angiotensin II receptor antagonist indicated in the treatment of hypertension either as monotherapy or in combination with other antihypertensives for the treatment of heart failure in patients who are intolerant of angiotensin-converting enzyme inhibitors.

Warnings: Contraindicated in pregnancy, hyperaldosteronism, and biliary cirrhosis. Correct hypovolemia before beginning therapy or monitor closely. Use cautiously in severe CHF, renal artery stenosis, hepatic dysfunction, or severe renal impairment. Adverse reactions include viral infection, fatigue, and abdominal pain. In clinical studies comparing valsartan to ACE inhibitors, the incidence of dry cough was significantly greater in the ACE inhibitor group.

Administration: Oral.

Preparations: Tablets, 40, 80, 160, and 320 mg.

VALTREX®, see Valacyclovir

VANCENASE®, see Beclomethasone dipropionate

VANCENASE AQ®, see Beclomethasone dipropionate

VANCERIL®, see Beclomethasone dipropionate

VANCOCIN®, see Vancomycin

VANCOLED®, see Vancomycin

VANCOMYCIN HYDROCHLORIDE—Lyphocin®, Vancocin®, Vancoled®

Description/Actions: Antibiotic used primarily for the intravenous treatment of staphylococcal infections. Also used orally for the treatment of staphylococcal enterocolitis and antibiotic-associated pseudomembranous colitis produced by *Clostridium difficile*.

Preparations: Vials, 500 mg. Capsules, 125 and 250 mg. Powder for oral solution, 1 and 10 g when reconstituted.

VANIQA™, see Eflornithine (topical)

VANSIL®, see Oxamniquine

VANTIN®, see Cefpodoxime proxetil

VASCOR®, see Bepridil hydrochloride

VASERETIC®, see Enalapril/ Hydrocholorothiazide

VASODILAN®, see Isoxsuprine

VASOPRESSIN—Pitressin®

Description/Actions: Hormone indicated for parenteral use in the prevention and treatment of postoperative abdominal distention, in abdominal roentgenography to dispel interfering gas shadows, and in diabetes insipidus.

Preparations: Ampules, 10 and 20 units.

VASOTEC®, see Enalapril

VASOXYL®, see Methoxamine

V-CILLIN K®, see Penicillin V potassium

VECURONIUM BROMIDE— Norcuron®

Description/Actions: Nondepolarizing neuromuscular blocking agent indicated as an adjunct to general anesthesia, to facilitate endotracheal intubation and to provide skeletal muscle relaxation during surgery or mechanical ventilation.

Preparations: Vials, 10 mg.

VEETIDS®, see Penicillin V potassium

VELBAN®, see Vinblastine

VELOSEF®, see Cephradine

VELOSULIN®, see Insulin

VENLAFAXINE HYDROCHLORIDE—Effexor®, Effexor XR®

Antidepressant.

Description/Actions: Is extensively metabolized, and one of its metabolites, O-desmethylvenlafaxine (ODV), is also pharmacologically active. Inhibits the neuronal reuptake of both serotonin and norepinephrine. Indicated for the treatment of depression, generalized anxiety disorder, and the prevention of recurrence of depression and relapse of depression. Effexor XR® is also indicated for the short-term treatment of social anxiety disorder.

Warnings: Adverse reactions include somnolence, dizziness, insomnia, nervousness, anxiety, tremor, dry mouth, nausea, constipation, anorexia, weight loss, vomiting, asthenia, sweating, blurred vision, and, in men, abnormal ejaculation and impotence. Patients should be advised to avoid the consumption of alcoholic beverages and cautioned about driving or operating machinery until they are certain that the drug does not adversely affect their ability to engage in such activities. May cause sustained increases in blood pressure, and blood pressure should be monitored regularly. It is recommended that it not be used in combination with a monoamine oxidase inhibitor (MAOI) or within 14 days of discontinuing treatment with an MAOI. There should be at least a 7 day interval after stopping venlafaxine before starting therapy with an MAOI.

Administration: Oral. Administered with food for the purpose of reducing the occurrence of gastrointestinal side effects.

Preparations: Tablets, 25, 37.5, 50, 75, and 100 mg. Release capsules, 37.5, 75, and 150 mg.

VENTOLIN®, see Albuterol

VEPESID, see Etoposide

VERAPAMIL HYDROCHLORIDE—Calan®, Calan SR®, Covera HS®, Isoptin®, Isoptin SR®, Verelan®

Antianginal, antiarrhythmic, and antihypertensive agent.

Description/Actions: Is a calcium channel-blocking agent that is indicated in the treatment of (1) hypertension, (2) vasospastic and unstable angina, (3) chronic stable angina, (4) in association with digitalis for the control of ventricular rate at rest and during stress in patients with chronic atrial flutter and/or atrial fibrillation, and (5) prophylaxis of repetitive paroxysmal supraventricular tachycardia. Also indicated for intravenous use in the treatment of supraventricular tachycardia.

Warnings: Contraindicated in patients with hypotension or cardiogenic shock, sick sinus syndrome, second- or third-degree AV block, and certain other cardiovascular disorders. Adverse reactions include constipation, dizziness, headache, and edema. May increase serum digoxin levels. Should not be administered IV to a patient also receiving a beta-adrenergic-blocking agent IV; the concurrent oral administration of these agents may be beneficial in some patients, but therapy must be closely monitored. Concomitant use with disopyramide is not recommended. Coadministration of verapamil with aspirin has led to increased bleeding times greater than that observed with aspirin alone. Coadministration of verapamil and grapefruit juice may lead to increased levels of verapamil.

Administration: Oral and intravenous.

Preparations: Tablets, 40, 80, and 120 mg. Sustained-release tablets 120, 180, and 240 mg. Sustained-release capsules 120, 180, 240 and 360 mg. Ampules, vials, and syringes, 5 mg/2 ml.

VERCYTE®, see Pipobroman

VERELAN®, see Verapamil

VERMOX®, see Mebendazole

VERSED®, see Midazolam

VERSENATE CALCIUM DISODIUM®, see Edetate calcium disodium

VERTEPORFIN—Visudyne®

Description/Actions: Verteporfin is a light-activated drug used in photodynamic therapy. It is indicated for the treatment of age-related macular degeneration in patients with predominantly classic subfoveal choroidal neovascularization. It is also indicated for the treatment of predominantly classic subfoveal choroidal neovascularization secondary to either pathologic myopia or presumed ocular histoplasmosis.

Precautions/Adverse Reactions: Verteporfin is contraindicated in patients with porphyria. Avoid exposure of skin or eyes to direct sunlight or bright indoor light for 5 days following injection with verteporfin. Avoid extravasation. If extravasation occurs, stop the infusion immediately and apply cold compresses. The extravasation area must be protected from direct sunlight until the swelling and discoloration have faded in order to prevent a burn that could be severe. It is recommended that the largest arm vein possible, preferably the antecubital, be used for the injection. If surgery is required within 48 hours after verteporfin therapy, as much of the internal tissue as possible should be protected from intense light. Patients who experience a severe decrease of vision of 4 lines or more within 1 week after treatment should not be retreated until their vision returns to pretreatment levels and the potential benefits and risks of future treatments are carefully considered by the physician. Use only approved lasers. Use of incompatible lasers may cause undertreatment, overtreatment, or damage to the surrounding normal tissue. Calcium channel blockers, polymixin B, or radiation therapy may enhance the rate of verteporfin uptake by the vascular endothelium. Photosensitizing drugs such as tetracyclines, sulfonamides, phenothiazines, sulfonylurea hypoglycemic agents, thiazide diuretics, and griseofulvin could increase the potential for skin photosensitivity reactions. Drugs or compounds that quench active oxygen species or scavenge radicals such as dimethyl sulfoxide, betacarotene, ethanol, formate, and mannitol may decrease verteporfin's efficacy. Drugs that decrease clotting, vasoconstriction, or platelet aggregation such as thromboxane A_2 inhibitors could also decrease the efficacy of verteporfin therapy. Pregnancy category C. Verteporfin has been shown to be embryotoxic in animals. There are no adequate and well-controlled studies in pregnant women. Verteporfin should be used in pregnancy only if the benefit justifies the potential risk to the fetus. Excretion in human breast milk is unknown. Safety and efficacy in pediatric patients have not been established. Most common adverse reactions include headache, injection site reactions, and visual disturbances. These occur in 10–20% of patients. Adverse reactions occurring in 1–10% of patients include ocular treatment site (cataracts, conjunctivitis/conjunctival injection, dry eyes, itching, severe vision loss, subconjunctival subretinal or vitreous hemorrhage), asthenia, back pain during infusion, fever, flulike syndrome, photosensitivity reactions in the form of sunburn following exposure to sunlight, atrial fibrillation, hypertension, peripheral vascular disorder, varicose veins, eczema, constipation, gastrointestinal cancers, nausea, anemia, decreased or increased white blood cell count, increased liver function tests, albuminuria, increased creatinine, arthralgias, hypesthesia, sleep disorder, vertigo, pharangitis, pneumonia, decreased hearing, diplopia, lacrimation disorder, and prostatic disorder. Severe vision decrease equivalent to 4 lines or more within 7 days after treatment has been reported in 1–4% of patients. Partial recovery of vision was observed in many patients.

Administration: IV with light activation via laser.

Patient Care Implications: Avoid extravasation. Use the largest vein possible, preferably the antecubital. Avoid small veins. Avoid contact with the eyes and skin during the preparation and administration of verteporfin. Any exposed person must be protected from bright light. Use of rubber gloves and eye protection is recommended. Wipe any spills with a damp cloth, and dispose of properly. Reconstituted vials must be protected from light and used within 4 hours. Patients should be instructed to avoid direct sunlight or bright light such as tanning salons, bright halogen lights, and high-power lighting during the first 5 days after treatment. If direct sunlight or bright light cannot be avoided, patients should be instructed to protect all parts of their skin and eyes by wearing protective clothing and sunglasses. Ultraviolet sunscreens are not effective in protecting against photosensitivity reactions. Ambient light is encouraged to help inactivate the drug.

Preparations: Injection, single-use glass vial containing 15 mg of verteporfin.

VESPRIN®, see Triflupromazine

VIACTIV®—Combination drug of Calcium carbonate 500 mg with vitamin D 100 units, vitamin K 400 μg in soft chewable tablets

VIADUR™, see Leuprolide Acetate

VIAGRA®, see Sidenafil citrate

VIBRAMYCIN®, see Doxycycline

VIBRA-TABS®, see Doxycycline

VICODIN®, Combination of hydrocodone and acetaminophen

VICOPROFEN®, Combination agent of hydrocodone bitartate and ibuprofen (opiod and NSAID)

VIDARABINE—Vira-A®
Description/Actions: **Antiviral agent** indicated for ophthalmic use for the treatment of acute keratoconjunctivitis and recurrent epithelial keratitis due to herpes simplex virus Types 1 and 2.
Preparations: Ophthalmic ointment, 3%.

VIDEX®, see Didanosine

VIDEX® EC, see Didanosine

VINBLASTINE SULFATE—
Velban®
Description/Actions: **Antineoplastic agent** administered intravenously in the treatment of Hodgkin's disease, lymphocytic lymphoma, histiocytic lymphoma, mycosis fungoides, advanced carcinoma of the testes, Kaposi's sarcoma, choriocarcinoma resistant to other agents, and carcinoma of the breast that is not responsive to other therapy.
Preparations: Vials, 10 mg.

VINCASAR PFS®, see Vincristine

VINCRISTINE SULFATE—
Oncovin®, Vincasar PFS®
Description/Actions: **Antineoplastic agent** administered intravenously in the treatment of acute leukemia, Hodgkin's disease, lymphosarcoma, reticulum cell sarcoma, rhabdomyosarcoma, neuroblastoma, and Wilms' tumor.
Preparations: Vials and syringes, 1, 2, and 5 mg.

VINORELBINE TARTRATE—
Navelbine®
Description/Actions: **Antineoplastic agent** indicated as monotherapy or in combination with cisplatin for the first-line treatment of ambulatory patients with unresectable advanced non-small-cell lung cancer.
Warnings: Contraindicated in patients with pretreatment granulocyte counts of less than 1000 cells/mm^3. Cautious use is recommended in patients with previous irradiation or chemotherapy because of increased risk of myelosuppression. Granulocytopenia is the major dose-limiting toxicity. Sepsis has occurred and patients should be taught to immediately report the occurrence of fever or chills. Adverse reactions include fatigue, peripheral neuropathy, alopecia, constipation, diarrhea, nausea and vomiting, chest pain, shortness of breath, and elevation of liver enzymes. Observe vesicant precautions.
Administration: Intravenous.
Preparations: Vials, 10 mg/ml.

VIOFORM®, see Clioquinol

VIOKASE®, see Pancrelipase

VIOXX®, see Rofecoxib

VIRA-A®, see Vidarabine

VIRACEPT®, see Nelfinavir

VIRAMUNE®, see Nevirapine

VIRAZOLE®, see Ribavirin

VIREAD™, see Tenofovir Disoproxil Fumarate

VIROPTIC®, see Trifluridine

VISICOL™, see Sodium phospates

VISINE®, see Tetrahydrozoline

VISKEN®, see Pindolol

VISTARIL®, see Hydroxyzine

VISTIDE®, see Cidofovir

VISUDYNE®, see Verteporfin

VITACARN®, see L-carnitine

VITAMIN A—Aquasol A®

Description/Actions: Vitamin indicated for the treatment of vitamin A deficiency.

Preparations: Capsules, 10,000, 25,000, 50,000 IU. Drops, 5000 IU/0.1 ml. Vials, 50,000 IU/ml.

VITAMIN A ACID, see Tretinoin

VITAMIN B1, see Thiamine

VITAMIN B2, see Riboflavin

VITAMIN B3, see Nicotinic acid

VITAMIN B6, see Pyridoxine

VITAMIN B12, see Cyanocobalamin

VITAMIN B COMPLEX

Description/Actions: Vitamin mixture usually including thiamine, riboflavin, niacin, pantothenic acid, pyridoxine, and cyanocobalamin.

VITAMIN C—Ascorbic acid, Sodium ascorbate, Cevalin®

Description/Actions: Vitamin indicated in the prevention and treatment of scurvy. Has been suggested to be of benefit in high doses in the prevention and treatment of colds. Has been used as a urinary acidifier.

Preparations: Tablets, 25, 50, 100, 250, and 500 mg. Chewable, controlled-release, and effervescent tablets. Solution, syrup, powder, and crystals. Ampules and vials, 100 mg/ml, 250 mg/ml, and 500 mg/ml.

VITAMIN D, see Cholecalciferol and Ergocalciferol

VITAMIN D2, see Ergocalciferol

VITAMIN D3, see Cholecalciferol

VITAMIN E—Aquasol E®

Description/Actions: Vitamin indicated for the treatment and prevention of vitamin E deficiency. Has been used in certain premature infants to reduce the toxic effects of oxygen therapy on the lung parenchyma and to decrease the severity of hemolytic anemia in infants.

Preparations: Capsules, 50, 100, 200, 400, 500, 600, and 1000 IU. Drops, 15 IU/0.3 ml.

VITAMIN K, see Menadiol sodium diphosphate

VITAMIN K1, see Phytonadione

VIVACTIL®, see Protriptyline

VIVELLE®, see Estradiol

VLEMASQUE®, see Sulfurated lime

VOLMAX®, see Albuterol sulfate

VOLTAREN®, see Diclofenac

VONTROL®, see Diphenidol

VOSOL®, see Acetic acid

VP-16®, see Etoposide

VUMON®, see Teniposide

W

WARFARIN SODIUM—Coumadin®
Coumarin anticoagulant.

Description/Actions: Indicated for (1) the prophylaxis and treatment of venous thrombosis and its extension, (2) the treatment of atrial fibrillation with embolization, (3) the prophylaxis and treatment of pulmonary embolism, (4) as an adjunct in the treatment of coronary occlusion, (5) for the prevention and treatment of thromboembolic complications associated with cardiac valve replacements, and (6) to reduce the risk of death, recurrent myocardial infarction and thromboembolic events such as stroke or systemic embolization after myocardial infarction.

Warnings: Contraindicated during pregnancy, in patients with bleeding tendencies associated with active ulceration, hemorrhagic tendencies, or blood dyscrasias or in patients who have recently undergone or are to undergo surgery of the CNS or eye, or other surgery that has resulted in large open surfaces. Adverse reactions include hemorrhage and therapy must be closely monitored. Effect may be increased by the concurrent administration of allopurinol, antibiotics, cimetidine, erythromycin, monoamine oxidase inhibitors, phenylbutazone, quinidine, salicylates, sulfonylurea hypoglycemic agents, and trimethoprim-sulfamethoxazole, as well as other agents. Effect may be reduced by barbiturates, carbamazepine, griseofulvin, and other agents.

Administration: Oral, intravenous, and intramuscular.

Preparations: Scored tablets, 1, 2, 2.5, 3, 4, 5, 6, 7.5, and 10 mg. Vials, 2 mg/ml, 5 mg/ml.

WELCHOL™, see Colesevelam

WELLBUTRIN®, see Bupropion

WELLBUTRIN® SR, see Bupropion

WELLCOVORIN®, see Leucovorin

WHITFIELD'S OINTMENT, see Benzoic acid

WINSTROL®, see Stanozolol

WINTERGREEN OIL, see Methyl salicylate

WOOL FAT, see Lanolin

WYAMINE®, see Mephentermine

WYCILLIN®, see Procaine penicillin G

WYDASE®, see Hyaluronidase

WYMOX®, see Amoxicillin

WYTENSIN®, see Guanabenz

X

XALATAN®, see Latanoprost

XANAX®, see Alprazolam

XELODA®, see Capecitabine

XIGRIS™, see Drotrecogin Alfa

XYLOCAINE®, see Lidocaine

XYLOMETAZOLINE HYDROCHLORIDE—Otrivin®

Description/Actions: Decongestant used topically for the relief of nasal congestion.

Preparations: Nose drops, 0.05% and 0.1%. Nose spray, 0.1%.

Y

YASMIN®, see Ethinyl Estradiol and Drospirenone

YODOXIN®, see Iodoquinol

YOHIMBINE HYDROCHLORIDE

Description/Actions: Has been suggested to have an aphrodisiac effect

Preparations: Tablets, 5 mg.

YUTOPAR®, see Ritodrine

Z

ZADITOR®, see Ketotifen

ZAFIRLUKAST—Accolate®

Description/Actions: Antiasthmatic (leukotriene receptor antagonist) indicated for the prophylaxis and chronic treatment of asthma in adults and children 5 years of age and older.

Warnings: Not for primary treatment of acute asthma attacks. Use cautiously in cirrhosis. Adverse reactions include headache, infection (respiratory tract), and nausea. Remind patients that this drug should be taken regularly as prescribed and not to make changes in dosing on their own. This drug is not a bronchodilator. While it may be used during an acute episode, it is not indicated for the reversal of acute bronchospasm.

Administrations: Take twice daily on an empty stomach.

Preparations: Tablets, 20 mg.

ZAGAM®, see Sparfloxacin

ZALCITABINE—Hivid®

Antiviral agent.

Description/Actions: Also known as dideoxycytidine or ddC. Inhibits the replication of the human immunodeficiency virus (HIV). Is converted by cellular enzymes to the active antiviral metabolite that inhibits viral replication, in part, by interfering with reverse transcriptase. Indicated for use in combination with zidovudine for the treatment of adult patients (i.e., 13 years of age and older) with advanced HIV infection (CD4 cell count less than or equal to 300 cells/mm^3) who have demonstrated significant clinical or immunologic deterioration. Also indicated for second-line monotherapy in HIV-infected patients who experience disease progression with zidovudine or are intolerant to zidovudine.

Warnings: May cause peripheral neuropathy which may become severe and potentially irreversible if the drug is not stopped promptly; patients should be advised to report symptoms such as tingling, burning, pain, or numbness in the hands or feet. Use should be avoided in patients with moderate or severe peripheral neuropathy, and the concurrent use with other drugs that have the potential to cause peripheral neuropathy (e.g., didanosine) should be avoided where possible. May cause pancreatitis and, if a patient develops abdominal pain and nausea, vomiting, or elevated amylase levels, the use of the drug should be interrupted until the possibility of pancreatitis is excluded. Other adverse reactions include esophageal ulcers, cardiomyopathy, congestive heart failure, anaphylactoid reactions, oral ulcers, nausea, dysphagia, anorexia, abdominal pain, vomiting, rash, pruritus, headache, dizziness, myalgia, fatigue, pharyngitis, anemia, leukopenia, and elevation of hepatic enzymes. May cause fetal harm and women of childbearing potential should not receive the drug unless they are using effective contraception.

Administration: Oral.

Preparations: Tablets, 0.375 and 0.75 mg.

ZALEPLON—Sonata®

Description/Actions: Zaleplon is used in the treatment for insomnia.

342 • ZANAFLEX®

Precautions/Adverse Reactions: Zaleplon dosage should be reduced in patients with mild hepatic impairment and not given to patients with severe hepatic disease. The drug should not be administered to pregnant women, breast-feeding women, or children. Some adverse effects are anorexia, colitis, constipation, dyspepsia, nausea, vomiting, abdominal pain, back pain, fever, headache, malaise, conjunctivitis, hyperacusis, otalgia, pruritus, migraine, angina, hypertension, syncope, anxiety, depression, dizziness, hallucination, vertigo, bronchitis, epistaxis, and myalgia.

Administrations: Oral.

Patient Care Implications: The drug should be administered in reduced doses to patients with mild hepatic impairment and not given to patients with severe hepatic disease.

Preparations: Capsule, 5 and 10 mg.

ZANAFLEX®, see Tizanidine

ZANAMIVIR—Relenza®

Description/Actions: Zanamivir is an inhaler that is used in the treatment of influenza A and B.

Precautions/Adverse Reactions: Zanamivir should be used with caution in patients with COPD, asthma, pregnant women, and breast-feeding women. The drug should not be administered to children < 7 years of age. Some side effects are bronchospasm, headache, diarrhea, nausea, vomiting, sinusitis, bronchitis, cough, nasal congestion, and dizziness.

Administration: Oral inhalation.

Patient Care Implications: Patients with respiratory disease should be careful using the inhaler, and the drug should not be administered to children < 12 years of age. If patient is on a bronchodilator, then it should be administered before zanamivir.

Preparations: Diskhaler, 5 mg (4 blister pack).

ZANTAC®, see Ranitidine

ZARONTIN®, see Ethosuximide

ZAROXOLYN®, see Metolazone

ZEBETA®, see Bisoprolol fumarate

ZEMURON®, see Rocuronium bromide

ZEPHIRAN®, see Benzalkonium chloride

ZERIT®, see Stavudine

ZESTORETIC®, Combination of lisinopril and hydrochlorothiazide

ZESTRIL®, see Lisinopril

ZEVALIN™, see Ibritumomab Tiuxetan

ZIAC®, Combination of bisoprolol and hydrochlorothiazide

ZIDOVUDINE—AZT, Retrovir®

Antiviral agent.

Description/Actions: Also known as azidothymidine (AZT), it inhibits the replication of certain retroviruses including human immunodeficiency virus (HIV), which causes acquired immunodeficiency syndrome (AIDS). Indicated for the management of adult patients with symptomatic HIV infection [AIDS and advanced AIDS-related complex (ARC)] who have a history of cytologically confirmed pneumonia (PCP) or an absolute CD4 (T4 helper/inducer) lymphocyte count of less than 200/mm^3 in the peripheral blood before therapy is begun. Also indicated for the management of patients with HIV infection who have evidence of impaired immunity, and for HIV-infected children who have HIV-related symptoms or who are asymptomatic with abnormal laboratory values indicating significant HIV-related immunosuppression. Also indicated for the prevention of maternal-fetal HIV transmission.

Warnings: Hematologic toxicity (e.g., granulocytopenia, anemia) is the adverse event reported most frequently and may require dose adjustment, discontinuation of the drug, and/or blood transfusions. Frequent (at least every 2 weeks) blood counts are strongly recommended in patients taking the medication. Other adverse reactions include headache, nausea, insomnia, and myalgia. Caution must be exercised in patients taking other medications that are nephrotoxic, cytotoxic, or that interfere with the number or function of red blood cells and/or white blood cells, because the risk of toxicity may be increased. Probenecid may increase the activity of zidovudine.

Administration: Oral and intravenous.

Preparations: Capsules, 100 mg. Tablets, 300 mg. Syrup, 50 mg/5 ml. Vials, 10 mg/ml.

ZILABRACE®, see Benzocaine

ZILADENT®, see Benzocaine

ZILEUTON—Zyflo®

Description/Actions: Antiasthmatic indicated in the prophylaxis and chronic treatment of asthma.

Warnings: Contraindicated in acute liver disease. Do not administer if transaminase levels are greater than or equal to 3 times the upper limit of normal. Evaluate liver function before initiation of and during therapy (discontinue if signs of liver disease occur). Use cautiously in patients with a history of liver disease or alcohol consumption. Adverse reactions include dyspepsia, pain, nausea, asthenia, headache, and myalgia. Documented drug interactions require a full drug profile review and adjustment of the regimen accordingly.

Administration: 600 mg, 4 times a day without regard to meals.

Preparations: Tablets, 600 mg (scored).

ZINACEF®, see Cefuroxime sodium

ZINC CHLORIDE

Description/Actions: Trace metal supplement to intravenous solutions given for total parenteral nutrition.

ZINC GLUCONATE

Description/Actions: Dietary supplement to prevent or treat deficiencies of zinc.

Preparations: Tablets, 35, 50, and 105 mg.

ZINC OXIDE

Description/Actions: Protectant and antiseptic applied topically in the treatment of various dermatologic conditions.

Preparations: Ointment, 25%. Paste, 25% with 25% starch.

ZINC SULFATE

Description/Actions: Trace metal supplement to intravenous solutions given for total parenteral nutrition. Also used as a dietary supplement to prevent or treat deficiencies of zinc. Has been investigated in dermatologic and arthritic disorders, and also in situations in which there is delayed wound healing associated with zinc deficiency. Also used in an ophthalmic solution for the relief of minor eye irritation.

Preparations: Vials, 1 mg/ml and 5 mg/ml. Capsules and tablets, 110 and 220 mg. Ophthalmic solution, 0.25%.

ZINECARD®, see Dexrazoxane

ZIPRASIDONE—Geodon™

Description/Actions: Ziprasidone is an antipsychotic agent used for the treatment of schizophrenia.

Precautions/Adverse Reactions: Usage is contraindicated in patients with a hypersensitivity to ziprasidone or any component of the formulation, history of (or current) QT prolongation, congenital long QT interval, recent acute myocardial infarction, or uncompensated heart failure. Ziprasidone is contraindicated with concurrent use of other QT_c-prolonging agents, including amiodarone, dofetilide, class A antiarrythmics, cisapride, pimozide, moxifloxacin, sparfloxacin, chlorpromazine, droperidol, halofantrine, levomethadyl acetate, dolasetron mesylate, probucol, or tacrolimus. Ziprasidone usage may result in a dose-related prolongation QT_c, which has been associated with the development of malignant ventricular arrhythmias (torsades de pointes) and sudden death. The observed QT_c prolongation was greater than with other atypical antipsychotic agents. Avoid hypokalemia and hypomagnesemia, and use caution in patients with bradycardia—these circumstances may increase the risk of the occurrence of torsades de pointes. Discontinue therapy in patients found to have persistent QT_c intervals > 500 msec. Patients who exhibited symptoms of dizziness, palpitations, or syncope should receive further cardiac evaluation. Antipsychotic therapy may cause extrapyramidal reactions and neuroleptic malignant syndrome (NMS). Use with caution in patients with a history of seizures or with conditions that lower the seizure threshold. May induce orthostatic hypotension; use with caution in patients at risk of this effect. May cause cognitive and motor impairment. Use with caution in patients with Parkinson's disease, Alzheimer's disease, breast cancer, or other prolactin-dependent tumors. Ziprasidone is associated with high incidence of rash; discontinue if alternative etiology is not identified. Safety and efficacy have not been established in pediatric patents. Pregnancy Category C. Use only if potential benefit justifies risk to the fetus. Excretion in breast milk is unknown; breast-feeding is not recommended.

Some adverse effects are somnolence, QT_c prolongation, tachycardia, postural hypotension, dizziness, akathisia, extrapyramidal symptoms, dystonia, rash, nausea, constipation, dyspepsia, diarrhea, weight gain, dry mouth, respiratory disorders, and abnormal vision.

Administration: Oral.

Patient Care Implications: Inform patients that they may experience drowsiness, lightheadedness, impaired coordination, dizziness, or blurred vision (use caution when driving or engaging in hazardous tasks until response to the drug is known). Patients should report to their physician any signs of cardiac arrhythmias (fainting or loss of consciousness, or palpitations).

Preparations: Capsule, 20, 40, 60, and 80 mg. Injection, 20 mg.

ZITHROMAX®, see Azithromycin

ZITHROMAX® TRI-PAK, see Azithromycin

ZOCOR®, see Simvastatin

ZOFRAN®, see Ondansetron

ZOLADEX®, see Goserelin acetate

ZOLEDRONIC ACID—ZOMETA®

Description/Actions: Zolendronic acid is indicated for hypercalcemia of malignancy (HCM), a common life-threatening metabolic complication of cancer, multiple myeloma, and bone metastases of solid tumors. It is also indicated for the treatment of patients with multiple myeloma and patients with bone metastasis from solid tumors along with standard antineoplastic agents.

Precautions/Adverse Reactions: Renal function should be assessed prior to and after treatment; additional treatments should be held until renal function returns to baseline. Because of risk of significant deterioration in renal function, which may progress to renal failure, single doses should not exceed 4 mg, and the duration of infusion should not be less than 15 minutes. Use is not recommended in patients with severe renal impairment (serum creatinine > 3.0 mg/dl). Use caution when bisphosphonates are administered with aminoglycosides, because these agents may have an additive effect to lower serum calcium level for prolonged periods. Exercise caution when zolendronic acid is used in combination with loop diuretics because of the increased risk of hypocalcemia. In multiple myeloma patients, the risk of renal dysfunction may be increased when zalendronic acid is used with thalidomide.

Pregnancy Category D. May cause fetal harm. Excretion in human breast milk is unknown; not recommended. Adverse reactions are usually mild and similar to some seen with other bisphosphonates, such as conjunctivitis and hypomagnesemia. Fever is common, and occasionally a flulike syndrome (chills, fever, bone pain, arthralgia, and myalgia) occurs.

Administration: Intravenous.

Patient Care Implications: Vigorous saline hydration should be initiated. Urine output should be about 2 L per day throughout treatment. Reconstitute 4 mg vial with 5 ml sterile water for injection. Zolendronic acid must not be mixed with calcium-containing solutions, such as lactated Ringer's solution. Patients with diagnosis of multiple myeloma or metastatic bone lesions from solid tumors should take a daily calcium (500 mg) and daily multivitamin (with 400 IU vitamin D); however, patients should avoid taking vitamins during infusion or for 2–3 hours after completion of zolendronic acid.

Preparations: Injection, powder for reconstitution, 4 mg (as monohydrate 4.264 mg).

ZOLICEF®, see Cefazolin

ZOLMITRIPTAN—Zomig®, Zomig-ZMT®

Description/Actions: Indicated in the acute treatment of migraine headache with or without auras.

Warnings: Use not recommended in children. Contraindicated in ischemic heart disease, coronary artery vasospasm, uncontrolled hypertension, other significant cardiovascular disease, or basilar or hemiplegic migraine, within 24 hours of other 5-HT1 agonists or ergot-type drugs, during or within 2 weeks after discontinuing MAOIs.

Confirm diagnosis and exclude underlying cardiovascular disease. Supervise first dose and consider monitoring ECG in patients with likelihood of unrecognized coronary disease (e.g., postmenopausal women, men over age 40), hypertension, hyperocholesterolemia, obesity, diabetes, smokers, strong family history). Monitor cardiovascular function in longer-term intermittent use. Use not recommended in Wolff-Parkinson-White syndrome or arrhythmias associated with other cardiac accessory conduction pathway disorders. Use cautiously in hepatic dysfunction, elderly, and nursing mothers. Pregnancy Category C.

Adverse reactions include paresthesia, asthenia, nausea, dizziness, pain, chest or neck tightness/heaviness, somnolence, anaphylaxis or anaphylactoid reactions and warm feeling.

Administration: Initially 2.5 mg or lower (may break 2.5 mg tablet by hand).

If headache returns, may repeat after 2 hours; max 10 mg/day. Reevaluate if no response.

The safety of treating more than 3 headaches in a 30-day period has not been established.

ZOLOFT®

Use low dose in hepatic impairment.
Preparations: Tablets, 2.5 mg and 5 mg. Orally disintegrating tablet, 2.5 and 5 mg.

ZOLOFT®, see Sertraline

ZOLPIDEM TARTRATE—Ambien®
Hypnotic.

Description/Actions: Is an imidazopyridine derivative that is indicated for the short-term treatment of insomnia.

Warnings: Adverse reactions include drowsiness, dizziness, drugged feelings, and diarrhea. Patients should be cautioned against engaging in activities requiring complete mental alertness or motor coordination, including potential impairment of the performance of such activities the following day. Patients should also be warned about the risk of additive depressant effects when other agents with central nervous system depressant activity (including alcohol) are used concurrently. Has a potential for causing problems of dependence and abuse, and is classified in Schedule IV.

Administration: Oral. For faster sleep onset, should not be administered with or immediately after a meal. Use should generally be limited to a period of 7 to 10 days.

Preparations: Tablets, 5 and 10 mg.

ZOMETA®, see Zoledronic acid

ZOMIG®, see Zolmitriptan

ZONALON®, see Doxepin hydrochloride

ZONASAR®, see Streptozocin

ZONEGRAN®, see Zonisamide

ZONISAMIDE—Zonegran®

Description/Actions: Indicated as adjunctive treatment of partial and tonic-clonic seizures.

Precautions/Adverse Reactions: Major adverse reactions include nephrolithiasis, impaired memory, drowsiness, ataxia, nystagmus, diplopia, tremors, psychosis, Stevens-Johnson syndrome, and leukopenia. Zonegram is contraindicated in patients who have demonstrated hypersensitivity to sulfonamides or zonisamide. Pediatric patients appear to be at an increased risk for zonisamide associated oligohydrosis and hyperthermia. Monitor patients closely for evidence of decreased sweating and increased body temperature, especially in warm/hot weather. Safety and efficacy in pediatric patients have not been established.

Administration: Oral.

Preparations: Capsules, 100 mg.

ZORPRIN®, see Aspirin

ZOSTRIX®, see Capsaicin

ZOSTRIX—HP®, see Capsaicin

ZOSYN®, see Piperacillin sodium/tazobactam sodium

ZOVIRAX®, see Acyclovir

Z-PAK®, see Azithromycin

ZYBAN®, see Bupropion

ZYFLO®, see Zileuton

ZYLOPRIM®, see Allopurinol

ZYMASE®, see Pancrelipase

ZYPREXA®, see Olanzapine

ZYPREXA ZYDIS®, see Olanzapine

ZYRTEC®, see Cetirizine hydrochloride

ZYRTEC-D 12 HOUR™, see Cetirizine and Pseudophedrine

ZYVOX®, see Linezolid

PART II

New Drugs

ADALIMUMAB

HUMIRA™

DESCRIPTION/ACTIONS

Adalimumab is a recombinant monoclonal antibody specific for tumor necrosis factor alpha (TNF-alpha). The body makes TNF-alpha, a naturally occurring cytokine involved in normal inflammatory and immune responses. People with rheumatoid arthritis (RA) have too much TNF-alpha in their bodies; increased levels can attack normal healthy body tissues and cause inflammation in the tissues in bones, cartilage and joints. Adalimumab is indicated for reducing signs and symptoms and inhibiting the progression of structural damage in adult patients with moderately to severely active RA who have had an inadequate response to one or more disease-modifying antirheumatic drugs (DMARDS).

PRECAUTIONS/ADVERSE REACTIONS

Adalimumab is contraindicated in patients with a hypersensitivity to adalimumab or any component of the formulation. The needle cover of the syringe contains latex, and should not be handled by persons sensitive to this substance. Serious infections and sepsis, including fatalities have been reported. Many serious infections have occurred in patients on concomitant immunosuppressive therapy; that in addition to their RA could predispose them to infections. Tuberculosis has been reactivated and opportunistic fungal infections have been observed. Most cases reported within the first 8 months of treatment. Patients should be evaluated for latent tuberculosis infection with a tuberculin skin test prior to therapy. Use caution in patients with chronic infection, history of recurrent infection or predisposition to infections. Do not give to patients with a clinically-important, active infection. Use caution in patients who have resided in regions where histoplasmosis is endemic. Patients who develop a new infection while undergoing treatment with adalimumab should be monitored closely. If a patient develops a serious infection or sepsis, adalimumab should be discontinued. It may exacerbate pre-existing or recent-onset central nervous system demyelinating disorders. Lymphomas have been observed; patients with RA, especially those with highly active disease, may be at a higher risk for the development of lymphoma. The role of TNF blockers in the development of malignancies is not fully known. Treatment with adalimumab may result in the formation of autoantibodies and, rarely, in the development of a lupus-like syndrome. If patient develops symptoms suggestive of a lupus-like syndrome, treatment should be discontinued. Pregnancy category B. There are no adequate and well-controlled studies in pregnant women. Use during pregnancy only if clearly needed. It is not known if adalimumab is excreted in human milk; breastfeeding not recommended. The most serious adverse reactions were serious infections, neurologic events and malignancies. The most common adverse reactions were injection site reactions, upper respiratory infection, sinusitis, nausea, headache, rash and accidental injury.

ADMINISTRATION

Adults: subcutaneous 40 mg every other week. May be administered with other DMARDs. Patients not taking methotrexate may increase dose to 40 mg/ week.

PATIENT CARE IMPLICATIONS

Patients may self-inject after proper training in injection technique. Do not use syringe if solution is cloudy, discolored or has particles in it. Adalimumab does not contain preservatives; discard the unused portion remaining in syringe. Rotate injection sites and never give in areas where the skin is tender, bruised, red or hard. If you choose your abdomen, you should avoid the area 2 inches around your navel. Each new injection should be given at least one inch from the site used before. Do not rub site. Do not use beyond expiration date on the container. If you forget to take medication when you are supposed to, inject the next dose right away. Then take your next dose when your next scheduled dose is due. May cause headache or dizziness; use caution when engaging in potentially hazardous tasks.

PREPARATIONS

Injection, solution (preservative free): 40 mg/ 0.8 ml prefilled glass syringe. Store at 2–8°C (36–46°F). Do not freeze. Protect from exposure to light. Store in original carton until time of administration.

ADEFOVIR DIPIVOXIL

HEPSERA™

DESCRIPTION/ACTIONS

Adefovir dipivoxil, is a diester prodrug of adefovir. Adefovir is an acyclic nucleotide reverse transcriptase inhibitor which interferes with hepatitis B virus (HBV) viral RNA dependent DNA polymerase resulting in inhibition of viral replication. Adefovir is indicated for the treatment of chronic hepatitis B in adults with evidence of active viral replication and either evidence of persistent elevations in serum aminotransferases or histologically active disease.

PRECAUTIONS/ADVERSE REACTIONS

Adefovir is contraindicated in patients hypersensitive to the drug or any component of the formulation. Severe acute exacerbations of hepatitis have been reported in patients who have discontinued anti-hepatitis B therapy, including adefovir. Monitor hepatic function closely in patients who discontinue therapy. If appropriate, resumption of therapy may be warranted. Chronic administration of adefovir may result in nephrotoxicity in patients at risk of or having underlying renal dysfunction. These patients should be monitored closely for renal function and may require dose adjustment. HIV resistance may emerge in chronic hepatitis B patients with unrecognized or untreated HIV infection. Prior to initiating therapy, HIV antibody testing should be offered to all patients. Lactic acidosis and severe hepatomegaly with steatosis, including fatal cases, have been reported with the use of nucleoside analogs alone or in combination with other antiretrovirals. Caution should be exercised when administering nucleoside analogs to any patient with known risk factors for liver disease. Since adefovir is eliminated by the kidneys, co-administration with drugs that reduce renal function or compete for active tubular secretion may increase serum concentration of either adefovir and/or the co-administered drugs. Pregnancy category C. No adequate and well-controlled studies in pregnant women. It is not known whether adefovir is excreted in human milk; breastfeeding is not recommended. Most common adverse effects were asthenia, headache, abdominal pain and nausea.

ADMINISTRATION

Patients with adequate renal function: 10 mg once daily.

Dosage adjustment in renal impairment:

cl_{cr} 20–49 ml/minute: 10 mg every 48 hours

cl_{cr} 10–19 ml/minute: 10 mg every 72 hours

hemodialysis: 10 mg every 7 days

PATIENT CARE IMPLICATIONS

It may be taken without regard to food. Avoid ethanol. Maintain adequate hydration (2–3L/day). You may be more susceptible to infection (avoid crowds and exposure to infection and do not have any vaccinations without consulting your physician). Report any unusual bleeding, persistent fatigue, muscle weakness or other persistent adverse effects. Inform patient if he/she acquires or has HIV that is not currently being treated with medicines, that adefovir may increase the chances that HIV infection cannot be helped with usual HIV medications. All patients should get an HIV test prior to initiating therapy. Inform patient adefovir will not cure chronic hepatitis B and that it does not prevent patient from spreading hepatitis B to others by sex or sharing needles. Instruct patient to practice safe sex and needle use. If you forget to take your dose, take it as soon as you remember that day. Do not take more than 1 dose in a day. Do not take 2 doses at the same time. Inform patient that hepatitis may get worse if dose is changed or stopped.

PREPARATIONS

Tablet: 10 mg

ATOMOXETINE HYDROCHLORIDE

STRATTERA™

DESCRIPTION/ACTIONS

Atomoxetine is the first nonstimulant medication approved for the treatment of attention deficit/hyperactivity disorder (ADHD) in children, adolescents, and adults. The exact mechanism by which atomoxetine produces its effects on ADHD is unknown, but it is thought to be related to it being a potent inhibitor of the presynaptic norepinephrine transporter. Atomoxetine is not a controlled substance; it was not associated with a pattern of response that suggested stimulant or euphoriant properties.

PRECAUTIONS/ADVERSE REACTIONS

Atomoxetine is contraindicated in individuals hypersensitive to atomoxetine or any of its components, those with narrow-angle glaucoma, or those who have used MAO inhibitors in the past 14 days. There have been reports of serious and fatal reactions (hyperthermia, rigidity, myoclonus, autonomic instability with possible rapid fluctuations of vital signs, and mental status changes that include extreme agitation progressing to delirium and coma) when taken in combination with an MAOI. Use caution in patients with hypertension, tachycardia, cardiovascular, or cerebrovascular disease because blood pressure and heart rate can be increased. Monitor pulse and blood pressure at baseline and during therapy. Use with caution in any condition that may predispose patients to hypotention; orthostatic hypotension has been reported. Monitor children for adequate growth and weight gain; children given atomoxetine during clinical trials exhibited slightly less growth in height and weight than did placebo-treated patients. Safety and efficacy have not been evaluated in pediatric patients under 6 years of age. May cause urinary retention and urinary hesitation; use caution in patients with history of urinary retention or bladder outlet obstruction. Allergic reactions such as angioneurotic edema, urticaria, and rash may occur. Metabolism is primarily through the CYP2D6-enzymatic pathway. A fraction of the population are poor metabolizers (PMs) of CYP2D6 metabolized drugs. These individuals have reduced activity in this pathway, resulting in higher peak plasma concentrations and slower elimination of atomoxetine. Use with caution in these patients. When given with CYP2D6 inhibitors (e.g., paroxetine, fluoxetine, quinidine), may increase concentrations in extensive metabolizers. Atomoxetine given with albuterol and sympathomimetics may increase heart rate and blood pressure. Use caution with pressor agents. Most common adverse effects were headache, abdominal pain, insomnia, xerostomia, decreased appetite, dyspepsia, nausea, vomiting, dizziness, and mood swings. Pregnancy Category C. No adequate and well-controlled studies in pregnant women; use only if potential benefit to mother outweighs possible risk to fetus. Breast feeding not recommended.

ADMINISTRATION

Children and adolescents, up to 70 kg: 0.5 mg/kg/day. Increase after a minimum of 3 days to a target dose of approximately 1.2 mg/kg/day. May be administered as a single daily dose in the morning or in divided doses in the morning and late afternoon. Maximum daily dose: 1.4 mg/kg or 100 mg, whichever is less.

Children, adolescents and adults over 70 kg: Initial: 40 mg/day. Increase after a minimum of 3 days to a target daily dose of approximately 80 mg/day. After 2–4 additional weeks, may increase dose to a maximum of 100 mg in patients who have not achieved an optimal response.

Dosing adjustments for use with strong CYP2D6 inhibitors (paroxetine, fluoxetine, and quinidine): In children and adolescents up to 70 kg: Initiate at 0.5 mg/kg/day and increase to the usual target dose of 1.2 mg/kg/day only if symptoms fail to improve after 4 weeks and the initial dose is well tolerated. In children, adolescents, and adults over 70 kg: Initiate at 40 mg/day and only increase to the usual target dose of 80 mg/day only if symptoms fail to improve after 4 weeks and the initial dose is well tolerated.

Dosing adjustment for hepatically impaired: Moderate hepatic insufficiency (Child–Pugh Class B): All doses reduced to 50% of normal dose. Severe hepatic insufficiency (Child–Pugh Class C): All doses reduced to 25% of normal dose.

PATIENT CARE IMPLICATIONS

Atomoxetine can be taken with or without food. Take as directed at same time of day. If a dose is missed, it should be taken as soon as remembered, but the total daily dose should not be exceeded within a 24-hour period. May cause dizziness: instruct patient not to drive or operate heavy machinery until response to drug is known. Avoid alcohol. Atomoxetine can be discontinued without being tapered. Monitor patient's growth, attention, hyperactivity, anxiety, blood pressure, and pulse. Patients should be instructed to call physician if they have any allergic reaction, if there is a change in how much or how often they urinate, and if there is an increase in heart rate or light headedness.

PREPARATIONS

Capsules, 10, 18, 25, 40, and 60 mg.

BUPRENORPHINE

SUBUTEX®

DESCRIPTION/ACTIONS

Buprenorphine is a partial agonist at the mu-opioid receptor. It is one of the first medications approved for office-based induction treatment of opioid dependence. Prescribing is limited to physicians who have met the qualification criteria and have received a DEA number specific to prescribing this product. It is part of a complete addiction treatment program that includes counseling or behavior therapy. Buprenorphine is available through pharmacies and wholesalers that normally provide controlled substances.

PRECAUTIONS/ADVERSE REACTIONS

Buprenorphine is contraindicated in individuals with a hypersensitivity to the product or any component of the formulation. May cause respiratory depression: use caution in patients with compromised respiratory function or preexisting respiratory depression. When taken with other narcotic analgesics, general anesthetics, benzodiazepines, tranquilizers, sedatives, hypnotics, or other CNS depressants, patients may exhibit increased CNS depression. A number of deaths have occurred when addicts have intravenously misused buprenorphine with a benzodiazepine, alcohol, and other opioids concomitantly. Buprenorphine is a partial agonist at the mu-opioid receptor, and chronic administration produces dependence of the opioid type, marked by withdrawal upon abrupt discontinuation or rapid taper. Cytolytic hepatitis and hepatitis with jaundice have been seen in the addict population receiving buprenorphine. Buprenorphine may elevate cerebrospinal fluid pressure and should be used with caution in patients with head injury, intracranial lesions, and other circumstances where cerebrospinal pressure may be increased. Miosis and changes in the level of consciousness that may interfere with patient evaluation may occur. In general, buprenorphine should be administered with caution in elderly or debilitated patients and those with severe impairment of hepatic, pulmonary, or renal function; myxedema or hyperthyroidism; adrenal cortical insufficiency; CNS depression or coma; toxic psychoses; prostatic hypertrophy or urethral stricture; acute alcoholism; delirium tremens; or kyphoscoliosis. Most common adverse reactions are headache, pain, insomnia, depression, nausea, back pain, abdominal pain, and constipation. Pregnancy Category C. Withdrawal has been reported in infants of women receiving buprenorphine during pregnancy. Enters breast milk; not recommended while nursing.

ADMINISTRATION

Sublingual: Children ≥ 16 years and adults: 8 mg on day 1, followed by 16 mg on day 2. Range 12–16 mg/day. The first dose should be given at least 4 hours after the patient last used opioids or preferably when early signs of opioid withdrawal appear. It is usually used under a doctor's direct supervision. The physician may supply medication himself. Titrating dose to clinical effectiveness should be done as rapidly as possible to prevent undue withdrawal symptoms and patient drop-out. Maintenance treatment is started with Suboxone on day 3. The use of buprenorphine for unsupervised administration should be limited to patients who cannot tolerate Suboxone, such as those who are hypersensitive to naloxone.

PATIENT CARE IMPLICATIONS

Caution patient if self-administered to use exactly as directed and not to use alcohol, other prescriptions, or OTC medications (especially sedatives, tranquilizers, antihistamines, or analgesics) without consultation. May cause dizziness, drowsiness, confusion, or blurred vision; use caution when driving or changing position from sitting or lying to standing, or when engaging in tasks requiring alertness until response to drug is known. Patients may experience nausea or vomiting; frequent mouth care, small frequent meals, sucking lozenges or chewing gum may help. Patients should inform their family members that in the event of an emergency, the treating physician or emergency room staff should be informed that the patient is physically dependent on narcotics and is being treated with buprenorphine. Caution patient that there have been a number of post-marketing experiences of coma and death associated with the misuse of the drug by the self-injecting of crushed buprenorphine tablets when taken with benzodiazepines. Tablet should be placed under the tongue until dissolved; it should not be swallowed or chewed. May cause liver problems; patients should call their physician right away if the skin or the whites of their eyes turn yellow, their urine is dark, bowel movements turn light in color, their appetite diminishes for several days or longer, or they have lower stomach pain or nausea.

PREPARATIONS

Sublingual tablets: 2 and 8 mg.

BUPRENORPHINE AND NALOXONE

SUBOXONE®

DESCRIPTION/ACTIONS

Suboxone® is one of two drugs first approved for office-based treatment of opioid dependence (e.g., morphine, heroine, or methadone). It contains buprenorphine, which produces typical opioid agonist effects, which are limited by a ceiling effect. Suboxone® is indicated for maintenance treatment due to naloxone in the formulation. Naloxone is an antagonist at the mu-opiod receptor; it is intended to deter intravenous abuse by individuals dependent on other opiates. Prescribing is limited to physicians who have met the qualification criteria and have received a DEA number specific to prescribing this product.

PRECAUTIONS/ADVERSE REACTIONS

Suboxone® is contraindicated in patients with a hypersensitivity to buprenorphine, naloxone, or any component of the formulation. Because Suboxone® may cause respiratory depression, use caution in patients with compromised respiratory function or pre-existing respiratory depression. In the presence of other narcotic analgesics, general anesthetics, benzodiazepines, tranquilizers, sedative/hypnotics, or other CNS depressants, patients may exhibit increased CNS depression. A number of deaths have occurred when addicts have intravenously misused buprenorphine, usually with a benzodiazepine, alcohol, and other opioids concomitantly. Buprenorphine is a partial agonist at the mu-opiod receptor, and chronic administration produced dependence of the opioid type, characterized by withdrawal upon abrupt discontinuation or rapid taper. Withdrawal syndrome is milder than seen with full agonists. Because Suboxone® contains naloxone, it is highly likely to produce intense withdrawal symptoms if misused parenterally by individuals dependent on opioid agonists such as heroin, morphine, or methadone and when administered before opioid effects have subsided. Cytolytic hepatitis and hepatitis with jaundice have been observed in the addict population receiving buprenorphine. Suboxone®, like other opioids, may elevate cerebrospinal fluid pressure and should be used with caution in patients with head injury, intracranial lesions, and other circumstances where cerebrospinal pressure may be increased. Suboxone® can produce miosis and changes in the level of consciousness that may interfere with a patient's evaluation. In general, it should be administered with caution in elderly or debilitated patients and those with severe impairment of hepatic, pulmonary, or renal function; CNS depression or coma; toxic psychoses; prostatic hypertrophy or urethral stricture; acute alcoholism; delirium tremens; or kyphoscoliosis. Most common adverse reactions are headache, pain, nausea, constipation, abdominal pain, vasodilation, and vomiting. Pregnancy Category C. There are no adequate and well-controlled studies in pregnant women. Give only during pregnancy if the potential benefit justifies the potential risk to the fetus. Withdrawal has been reported in infants of women receiving buprenorphine during pregnancy. Buprenorphine enters breast milk; breast feeding not recommended.

ADMINISTRATION

Children = 16 years and adults: Opioid dependence: **NOTE:** This combination product is not recommended for use during the induction period; initial treatment should begin using buprenorphine oral tablets. Patients should be switched to the combination product for maintenance and unsupervised therapy on day 3 with a dose of 16 mg/day. Dosage of Suboxone® should be progressively adjusted in increments/decrements of 2 mg or 4 mg to a level that holds the patient in treatment and suppresses opioid withdrawal effects. Target dose (based on buprenorphine content): 16 mg/day; range 4–24 mg/day. Both gradual and abrupt discontinuation have been used; no controlled trials have been undertaken to determine the best method of dose taper at the end of treatment.

PATIENT CARE IMPLICATIONS

Caution patient if self-administering to use exactly as directed, and not to use alcohol, other prescriptions, or OTC medications (especially sedatives, tranquilizers, antihistamines, or pain medications) without consultation. May cause dizziness, drowsiness, confusion, or blurred vision; use caution when driving or changing position from sitting or lying to standing, or when engaging in tasks requiring alertness until response to drug is known. Patients may experience nausea or vomiting; frequent mouth care, small frequent meals, sucking lozenges, or chewing gum may help. Patients should inform their family members that in the event of an emergency, the treating physician or emergency room staff should be informed that the patient is physically dependent on narcotics and is being treated with Suboxone®. Patients should be cautioned that a serious overdose and death may occur if benzodiazepines, sedatives, tranquilizers, antidepressants, or alcohol are taken at the same time. Tablet should be placed under the tongue until dissolved; it should not be swallowed or chewed. If dose requires more than 2 tablets, patients should take all tablets at the same time together under the tongue or take 2 tablets at a time, putting them under the tongue and letting them melt. They should put the next tablet or tablets under the tongue right away. If they miss a dose, they should take it as soon as possible. If it is almost time for the next dose, patients should skip the missed dose and go back to the regular dosing schedule. Inform patient that Suboxone® may cause liver problems; pateints should call their physician right away if their skin or the whites of their eyes turn yellow, their urine is dark, bowel movements turn light in color, appaetite is diminished for several days or longer, or if they have lower stomach pain or nausea.

PREPARATIONS

Sublingual tablet, 2 mg buprenorphine with 0.5 mg naloxone, 8 mg buprenorphine with 2 mg naloxone.

CLINDAMYCIN AND BENZOYL PEROXIDE

DUAC™

DESCRIPTION/ACTIONS

Duac™ is a topical skin product used for the treatment of acne vulgaris. Clindamycin binds to the 50S ribosomal subunits of susceptible bacteria, which eventually suppresses protein synthesis. Benzoyl peroxide is a potent oxidizing agent that oxidizes bacterial proteins in the sebaceous follicles, decreasing the number of anaerobic bacteria and decreasing irritating-type free fatty acids.

PRECAUTIONS/ADVERSE REACTIONS

Duac™ topical gel is contraindicated in individuals who have shown hypersensitivity to benzoyl peroxide, lincomycin, clindamycin, or any component of the formulation. Also contraindicated in individuals with a history of regional enteritis, ulcerative colitis, pseudomembranous colitis, or antibiotic-associated colitis; or with concurrent use of erythromycin and clindamycin. Diarrhea, bloody diarrhea, and colitis have been reported with topical clindamycin use; stop the drug if significant diarrhea occurs. Orally and parenterally administered clindamycin has been associated with severe colitis that can result in patient death. Concomitant topical acne therapy should be used with caution; possible cumulative irritancy may occur. Products containing clindamycin and erythromycin should not be used in combination; it may lead to antagonism of antimicrobial effects. Concurrent use with tretinoin increases adverse reactions. Most common adverse reactions were erythema, peeling, and dry skin. Pregnancy Category C. Animal reproductive studies have not been conducted. Give only if clearly needed to a pregnant woman. It is not known if Duac™ is secreted into human milk. Breast feeding not recommended.

ADMINISTRATION

Children = 12 years and adults: After skin has been cleansed gently and patted dry, apply to affected areas in the evening or as directed by physician. **To the pharmacist:** Prior to dispensing, store in refrigerator, between 2° and 8° C. Do not freeze. Once dispensed, clindamycin may be stored at room temperature by the patient. Dispense with a 60-day expiration date and specify "store at room temperature up to 25° C (77° F), do not freeze."

PATIENT CARE IMPLICATIONS

Skin should be clean and dry before applying. Avoid applying to inside of nose, mouth, eyes, and mucous membrane. Duac™ may bleach hair or colored fabrics. Protect skin from sun. Patients should notify prescriber if severe diarrhea, dryness, redness, or peeling occurs. Inform patient not to use any other topical acne preparation unless otherwise directed by their physician. Duac™ topical gel should be stored at room temperature and any unused product should be discarded after 60 days.

PREPARATIONS

Gel, topical: clindamycin 1% and benzoyl peroxide 5%.

ELETRIPTAN HYDROBROMIDE

RELPAX®

DESCRIPTION/ACTIONS

Eletriptan binds with high affinity to $5\text{-}HT_{1B}$, $5\text{-}HT_{1D}$, and $5\text{-}HT_{1F}$ receptors. The exact mechanism of how eletriptan has efficacy in migraines is not known. One theory is activation of $5\text{-}HT_1$ receptors on intracranial blood vessels leads to vasoconstriction. The other theory is activation of $5\text{-}HT_1$ receptors on sensory nerve endings results in the inhibition of pro-inflammatory neuropeptide release. Eletriptan is indicated for the acute treatment of migraines with or without aura in adults. It is not intended for the prophylactic therapy of migraine or for use in the management of hemiplegic or basilar migraine. Safety and effectiveness have not been established for cluster headaches, which occur in an older, predominantly male population.

PRECAUTIONS/ADVERSE REACTIONS

Eletriptan is contraindicated in patients hypersensitive to eletriptan or any component of the formulation; patients with ischemic heart disease (e.g., angina pectoris, history of myocardial infarction, or documented silent ischemia, or patients who have symptoms or findings consistent with ischemic heart disease, coronary artery vasospasm, or other significant underlying cardiovascular disease. Eletriptan should not be given to patients with cerebrovascular syndromes including (but not limited to) strokes of any type as well as transient ischemic attacks. It should not be given to patients with peripheral vascular disease including (but not limited to) ischemic bowel disease. Eletriptan may elevate blood pressure. It should not be given to patients with uncontrolled hypertension. Do not give to patients with hemiplegic or basilar migraine. Do not use within 24 hours of treatment with another $5\text{-}HT_1$ agonist, ergotamine-containing or ergot-type medication such as dihydroergotamine (DHE) or methysergide. Eletriptan should not be used in patients with severe hepatic impairment. Safety and effectiveness in pediatric patients have not been established; not recommended in patients under 18 years of age. Eletriptan should not be used within at least 72 hours of treatment with the following potent CYP3A4 inhibitors: ketoconazole, itraconazole, nefazodone, troleandomycin, clarithromycin, ritonavir, and nelfinavir. $5\text{-}HT_1$ agonists have the potential to cause coronary vasospasm; therefore, eletriptan should not be given to patients with documented ischemic or vasospastic coronary artery disease (CAD). Strongly not recommended to be given to patients in whom unrecognized CAD is predicted by presence of risk factors (hypertension, hypercholesterolemia, smoker, obesity, diabetes, strong family history of CAD, female with surgical or physiological menopause, or male over 40 years of age) unless a cardiovascular evaluation provides satisfactory clinical evidence that the patient is reasonably free of coronary artery and ischemic myocardial disease or other significant underlying cardiovascular disease. For patients with risk factors predictive of CAD, who are determined to have a satisfactory cardiovascular evaluation, it is strongly recommended that the first dose of eletriptan take place in the setting of a physician's office or similar medically staffed and equipped facility unless the patient has previously received eletriptan. Because cardiac ischemia can occur in the absence of clinical symptoms, consideration should be given to obtaining on the first occasion of use an electrocardiogram during the interval immediately following administration of eletriptan. Serious adverse cardiac events, including acute myocardial infarction, life-threatening disturbances of cardiac rhythm, and death have been reported within a few hours after the administration of other 5-HT$_1$ agonists. 5-HT$_1$ agonists may cause vasospastic reactions other than coronary artery vasospasm. Peripheral vascular ischemia and colonic ischemia with abdominal pain and bloody diarrhea have been reported with 5-HT$_1$ agonists. Significant blood pressure elevation, including hypertensive crisis, has been reported in patients with and without a history of hypertension. Because 5-HT$_1$ agonists may cause coronary artery vasospasm, patients who experience signs or symptoms suggestive of angina following dosing should be evaluated for the presence of CAD or a predisposition to Prinzmetal's variant angina before receiving additional doses of eletriptan and should be monitored electrocardiographically if dosing is resumed and similar symptoms recur. Pregnancy Category C. No adequate, well-controlled studies in pregnant women. Teratogenic effects were observed in animal studies. Use only if potential benefit to the mother outweighs the possible risk to the fetus. Eletriptan enters breast milk; use caution. Ergot-containing drugs have been reported to cause prolonged vasospastic reactions; use of ergotamine-containing or ergot-type medications (like DHE or methysergide) within 24 hours of eletriptan is not recommended. CYP3A4 inhibitors increase serum concentration and half-life of eletriptan. Eletriptan should not be used within at least 72 hours of taking potent CYP3A4 inhibitors. Most common adverse reactions are pain or pressure sensation in chest or throat, dizziness, somnolence, nausea, xerostomia, and weakness.

ADMINISTRATION

Acute migraine: 20–40 mg; if the headache improves but returns, dose may be repeated after 2 hours have elapsed after the first dose. The maximum recommended single dose is 40 mg. The maximum daily dose should not exceed 80 mg. The safety of treating an average of more than 3 headaches in a 30-day period has not been established. If the initial dose is ineffective, controlled clinical trials have not shown a benefit of a second dose to treat the same attack. Also, if the first dose is ineffective, diagnosis needs to be reevaluated. A greater proportion of patients had a response following a 40 mg dose than following a 20 mg dose.

PATIENT CARE IMPLICATIONS

Make sure patient knows eletriptan is ineffective for the prevention of migraines. Instruct patient to call physician immediately if experience severe chest pains or shortness of breath. Blood pressure may be increased to a greater extent in the elderly. Monitor for increased blood pressure.

PREPARATIONS

Tablet (film coated), 20 and 40 mg.
Store at 25° C (77° F); excursions permitted to 15°–30° C (59°–86° F).

EPLERENONE

INSPRA™

DESCRIPTION/ACTIONS

Eplerenone is a blocker of aldosterone binding at the mineralocorticoid receptor. Aldosterone binds to mineralocorticoid receptors in both epithelial (kidney) and nonepithelial tissues (heart, blood vessels, and brain) and increases blood pressure by causing sodium reabsorption and possibly other mechanisms. It is indicated for the treatment of hypertension either alone or in combination with antihypertensive agents.

PRECAUTIONS/ADVERSE REACTIONS

Eplerenone is contraindicated in patients with a known hypersensitivity to it or to any component of the formulation. It is contraindicated in patients with the following conditions: serum potassium > 5.5 meq/L, type 2 diabetes with microalbuminuria, serum creatinine > 2.0 mg/dL in males and 1.8 mg/dL in females, and in patients with creatinine clearances < 50 mL/min. Eplerenone is also contraindicated in patients treated concomitantly with the following medications: potassium supplements or potassium-sparing diuretics (amiloride, spironolactone, or triamterene) and strong inhibitors of CYP450 3A4 (ketoconazole, itraconazole). The principle risk of eplerenone is hyperkalemia, which can cause serious, sometimes fatal arrhythmias. Monitor potassium levels every 2 weeks for the first 1–2 months and then monthly thereafter. Pregnancy Category B. No adequate and well-controlled studies in pregnant women. Concentration of eplerenone in human breast milk is unknown. Use during pregnancy and lactation only if the potential benefit justifies the potential risk to the fetus. Safety and efficacy in pediatric patients has not been established. Eplerenone metabolism is primarily mediated via cytochrome 3A4. Concomitant administration of eplerenone and ACE inhibitors or Angiotensin receptor antagonists has led to clinically significant hyperkalemia. Caution should be used and serum potassium levels should be monitored if administering eplerenone with these drugs. Concomitant administration of eplerenone and inhibitors of CYP450 3A4 (ketoconazole, itraconazole) has led to a 5.4 fold increase in AUC of eplerenone. Eplerenone should not be used with ketoconazole or itraconazole. Concomitant administration with other CYP450 3A4 inhibitors (erythromycin, verapamil, saquinavir, or fluconazole), resulted in a 2.0 to 2.9 fold increase in the AUC of eplerenone. Concomitant administration of lithium and eplerenone has not been studied; however, serum lithium levels should be monitored. Concomitant administration of eplerenone and NSAIDs has not been studied; however, NSAIDs have been shown to reduce the antihypertensive effect in some patients and result in severe hyperkalemia in patients with impaired renal function. Blood pressure should be monitored closely if NSAIDs are administered with eplerenone. Concomitant administration of grapefruit juice resulted in a 25% increase in eplerenone's AUC. Concomitant administration of eplerenone and St.John's Wort resulted in a 30% decrease in eplerenone's AUC. No clinically significant drug interactions were observed when eplerenone was administered with digoxin, warfarin, midazolam, cisapride, cyclosporine, simvastatin, glyburide, or oral contraceptives. Increases in serum triglycerides (dose-related effect) were observed in approximately 15% of patients treated with eplerenone. Most common adverse reactions observed during therapy with eplerenone include dizziness (3%), diarrhea (2%), coughing (2%), fatigue (2%), influenza-like symptoms (2%), and albuminuria (1%). Hypercholesterolemia occurred in approximately 0.3% of patients treated with eplerenone (dose-related effect). Gynecomastia occurred in 0.5%–1% of patients treated with eplerenone. Abnormal vaginal bleeding occurred in 0.6%–2.1% of female patients treated with eplerenone. Increases in AST, ALT, GGT, BUN, serum creatinine, and uric acid levels were observed during therapy with eplerenone. Hyperkalemia (dose-related) was observed in < 1% of patients and increased with decreasing renal function. Hyponatremia was observed in approximately 2.3% of patients receiving eplerenone.

ADMINISTRATION

Adults: 50 mg orally once a day (may increase up to 50 mg orally twice a day) alone or in combination with other antihypertensive agents. Full antihypertensive effect may not be seen for 4 weeks. Doses higher than 100 mg/day are not recommended. For patients receiving weak CYP450 3A4 inhibitors such as erythromycin, saquinavir, verapamil, and fluconazole, the starting dose should be reduced to 25 mg orally once daily.

Dosage adjustment in renal impairment: eplerenone is contraindicated in patients with serum creatinine > 2.0 mg/dL in males and 1.8 mg/dL in females and in patients with creatinine clearances < 50 mL/min.

Dosage adjustment in hepatic impairment (mild to moderate hepatic insufficiency): no dosage adjustment is necessary. Use of eplerenone in severe hepatic impairment has not been evaluated.

PATIENT CARE IMPLICATIONS

Patients should be informed not to use potassium supplements, salt substitutes, or contraindicated drugs without consulting with their doctor.

PREPARATIONS

Tablets, 25, 50, and 100 mg.

ESCITALOPRAM OXALATE

LEXAPRO™

DESCRIPTION/ACTIONS

Escitalopram is the S-enantiomer of citalopram, which selectively inhibits the reuptake of serotonin with minimal effects on norepinephrine and dopamine reuptake. Escitalopram is indicated for the treatment of major depressive disorder.

PRECAUTIONS/ADVERSE REACTIONS

Escitalopram is contraindicated in individuals with a hypersensitivity to escitalopram, citalopram, or any component of the formulation. It should not be administered with or within 2 weeks of use of monoamine oxidase inhibitors (MAOIs). There have been reports of serious, sometimes fatal reactions including hyperthermia, rigidity, myoclonus, autonomic instability with possible rapid fluctuations of vital signs, and mental status changes that include extreme agitation progressing to delirium and coma when serotonin reuptake inhibitors are given in combination with MAOIs. At least 14 days should be allowed to pass after stopping escitalopram before starting an MAOI. May precipitate a shift to mania/hypomania; use cautiously in patients with a history of mania. Psychoactive drugs may impair judgment, thinking, or motor skills. Use caution in patients with a previous seizure disorder or condition predisposing to seizures such as brain damage, alcoholism, or concurrent therapy with other drugs that lower the seizure threshold. May cause hyponatremia/SIADH (syndrome of inappropriate antidiuretic hormone secretion). Use caution if suicidal risk may be present; the possibility of a suicide attempt is inherent in major depressive disorder. Close supervision of these high-risk patients should accompany initial drug therapy. Caution is advisable when used with concomitant illness due to limited experience. Safety and efficacy in pediatric patients have not been established. Pregnancy Category C. Teratogenic effects have been reported in animal studies. There are no adequate and well-controlled studies in pregnant women. Use only if potential benefit to mother outweighs the possible risk to the fetus. Enters breast milk; breast feeding not recommended. Most common adverse reactions were nausea, insomnia, somnolence, diarrhea, xerostomia, and ejaculation disorder. Escitalopram use with buspirone, linezolid, MAOI, meperidine, moclobemide, nefazodone, selegiline, SSRIs, sumatriptan, trazodone, and venlafaxine may cause serotonin syndrome; avoid concurrent use.

ADMINISTRATION

Initial: 10 mg/day. May be increased to 20 mg/day after a minimum of 1 week.
Dosage adjustment in hepatic impairment and elderly: 10 mg/day.
Mild to moderate renal impairment: No adjustment needed.
Severe renal impairment: Creatinine clearance < 20 mL/minute: Use caution; no information is available about the pharmacokinetics in patients with severely reduced renal function.

PATIENT CARE IMPLICATIONS

Administer once daily (morning or evening), with or without food. Patients should inform physician of all prescriptions, OTC medications, or herbal products they are taking. Take exactly as directed. Do not discontinue without consulting physician. Inform patient it may take up to 3 weeks for effects to occur. May cause dizziness, lightheadedness, or impaired concentration; use caution when driving or engaging in tasks requiring alertness until response to drug is known. Small, frequent meals, frequent mouth care, and chewing gum or sucking lozenges may help with nausea, vomiting, or loss of appetite. Report CNS changes (confusion, impaired concentration, severe headache, insomnia, or irritability). Patients should be made aware that escitalopram is the active isomer of Celexa® (citalopram) and that the 2 medications should not be taken concomitantly. Avoid caffeine or alcohol. Physician should be informed if patient is or intends to become pregnant.

PREPARATIONS

Solution (oral), 1 mg/ml (240 ml).

Tablet (film coated), 5, 10, and 20 mg.

EZETIMIBE

ZETIA™

DESCRIPTION/ACTIONS

Ezetimibe belongs to a class of lipid-lowering compounds that selectively inhibit the intestinal absorption of cholesterol and related phytosterols. Ezetimibe acts at the brush border of the small intestine and inhibits the absorption of cholesterol, leading to a decrease in the delivery of cholesterol to the liver. It may be used alone or in combination with an HMG-CoA reductase inhibitor (atorvastatin, fluvastatin, lovastatin, pravastatin, or simvastatin) or as adjunctive therapy to diet for the reduction of elevated total cholesterol, LDL-C, and APo B in patients with primary heterozygous familial and nonfamilial hypercholesterolemia and homozygous sitosterolemia.

PRECAUTIONS/ADVERSE REACTIONS

Ezetimibe is contraindicated in patients with a known hypersensitivity to any component of the formulation. It is contraindicated in combination with an HMG-CoA reductase inhibitor in patients with active liver disease or unexplained persistent elevations in serum transaminases. Not recommended for use in patients with moderate or severe hepatic insufficiency. Pregnancy Category C. No adequate or well-controlled studies in pregnant women. Ezetimibe should be used during pregnancy only if the potential benefit justifies the potential risk to the fetus. Excretion in human breast milk is unknown. All HMG-CoA reductase inhibitors are contraindicated in pregnancy/nursing. When ezetimibe is administered with an HMG-CoA reductase inhibitor in a woman of childbearing potential, refer to the pregnancy category and package labeling for the HMG-CoA reductase inhibitor used. Not recommended for use in children under 10 years of age. Most common adverse effects observed during treatment with ezetimibe (as monotherapy or in combination with an HMG-CoA reductase inhibitor) include headache, diarrhea, abdominal pain, fatigue, pharyngitis, sinusitis, arthralgias, back pain, coughing, chest pain, and dizziness. When ezetimibe is used in combination with an HMG-CoA reductase inhibitor, liver function tests should be performed at initiation of therapy and according to the package labeling for the HMG-CoA reductase inhibitor. Prior to initiation of therapy with ezetimibe, secondary causes of hypercholesterolemia (i.e., diabetes hypothyroidism, obstructive liver disease, chronic renal failure, and drugs that affect cholesterol levels) should be excluded. Baseline lipid panel should be obtained prior to initiation of therapy and periodically thereafter. Ezetimibe does not appear to be an inducer or inhibitor of the cytochrome P450 enzyme system. Coadministration of ezetimibe and fibrates has not been studied; therefore, it is not recommended. Coadministration of ezetimibe and cyclosporine may lead to increased serum levels of ezetimibe. Coadministration of ezetimibe with cholestyramine (bile acid sequestrant) may lead to decreased bioavailability of ezetimibe. Administer ezetimibe ≥ 2 hours before or ≥ 4 hours after administration of a bile acid sequestrant.

ADMINISTRATION

Adults and children ≥ 10 years of age: 10 mg once daily; may be administered with or without food.

Renal impairment: No dosage adjustment

Hepatic impairment: No dosage adjustment necessary in patients with mild hepatic insufficiency. Use of ezetimibe is not recommended in patients with moderate to severe hepatic impairment.

PATIENT CARE IMPLICATIONS

Patients should be placed on a standard cholesterol-lowering diet before receiving ezetimibe and should continue on this diet during therapy with ezetimibe.

PREPARATIONS

Tablets, 10 mg.

FULVESTRANT

FASLODEX®

DESCRIPTION/ACTIONS

Fulvestrant is an estrogen receptor antagonist. Many breast cancers have estrogen receptors (ER); growth of these tumors is stimulated by estrogen. Fulvestrant binds to the ER in a competitive manner, with affinity comparable to that of estradiol. Fulvestrant down-regulates the ER protein in human breast cancer cells. Fulvestrant is indicated for the treatment of hormone receptor–positive metastatic breast cancer in postmenopausal women with disease progression following antiestrogen therapy. It is approved for use only in postmenopausal women.

PRECAUTIONS/ADVERSE REACTIONS

Fulvestrant is contraindicated in individuals hypersensitive to fulvestrant or any component of the formulation and in pregnant women. It should not be used in patients with bleeding diathesis or thrombocytopenia or in patients on anticoagulants. Metabolism is primarily in the liver; use with caution in patients with liver disease, and monitor closely. Pregnancy Category D. Antiestrogenic compounds have been associated with embryo toxicity and abnormalities in fetal development. Excretion into breast milk is unknown/contraindicated. Most common adverse reactions were nausea, vomiting, constipation, diarrhea, abdominal pain, headache, back pain, vasodilation (hot flushes), and pharyngitis. Three of the most serious common effects were anemia, leukopenia and thrombocytopenia.

ADMINISTRATION

Intramuscular injection: 250 mg once a month. Administer slowly into a large muscle (buttocks). Refrigerate (2°- 8°C). Protect from light and store in original container until time of use. Do not give intravenously, subcutaneously, or intra-arterially.

PATIENT CARE IMPLICATIONS

If self-administered, follow directions for injection and syringe/needle disposal. Inform patient that severe fetal damage can occur with use of this drug. Patient may experience dizziness and should use caution when driving or engaging in tasks requiring alertness until response to drug is known. Small, frequent meals, frequent mouth care, sucking lozenges, or chewing gum may help with vomiting, nausea, and loss of appetite.

PREPARATIONS

Injection, solution (prefilled syringe): 50 mg/ml (2.5 ml, 5 ml).

GALANTAMINE

REMINYL®

DESCRIPTION/ACTIONS

Galantamine is a reversible, competitive acetylcholinesterase inhibitor. Exact mechanism of action is unknown; however, it is thought to exert its therapeutic effect by enhancing cholinergic function. It enhances cholinergic activity by increasing the concentration of acetylcholine through reversible inhibition of its hydrolysis by cholinesterase. It is indicated for the treatment of mild to moderate dementia of the Alzheimer's type.

PRECAUTIONS/ADVERSE REACTIONS

Galantamine is contraindicated in patients with a known hypersensitivity to it or to any component of the formulation. Galantamine may exaggerate the neuromuscular blocking effects of succinylcholine-type and similar blocking agents during anesthesia. Due to its vagotonic effects on the sinoatrial and atrioventricular nodes, bradycardia and heart block have been reported in patients both with and without known underlying cardiac conduction abnormalities. Galantamine may increase gastric acid secretion due to increased cholinergic activity. Monitor patients closely for symptoms of active or occult gastrointestinal bleeding, especially in those at high risk for developing ulcers (patients with a history of ulcer disease or patients on NSAID therapy). Galantamine may cause bladder outflow obstruction and seizures. Use with caution in patients with a history of severe asthma or obstructive pulmonary disease. Use of galantamine in patients with severe hepatic and or severe renal impairment is not recommended.

Galantamine is metabolized by the cytochrome P450 enzyme system 2D6 and 3A4. Concomitant administration of galantamine and cimetidine resulted in a 16% increase in the bioavailability of galantamine. Coadministration of galantamine and ketoconazole resulted in a 30% increase in the AUC of galantamine. Concomitant administration of galantamine and erythromycin resulted in a 10% increase in the AUC of galantamine. Coadministration of galantamine and paroxetine resulted in approximately a 40% increase in the bioavailability of galantamine. Clearance of galantamine was decreased by about 25%–33% by concurrent administration of amitriptyline, fluoxetine, fluvoxamine, and quinidine. Galantamine had no effect on the pharmacokinetics of digoxin and warfarin or on the prothrombin time. A synergistic effect is expected when galantamine is given concurrently with succinylcholine, other cholinesterase inhibitors, similar neuromuscular blocking agents, or cholinergic agonists such as bethanecol. Pregnancy Category B. No adequate and well-controlled studies in pregnant women. Use in pregnancy only if the potential benefit justifies the potential risk to the fetus. Galantamine has no indication for use by nursing mothers. Safety and efficacy in pediatrics have not been established; therefore, use of galantamine in children is not recommended. Major adverse reactions reported during therapy with galantamine include nausea, vomiting, diarrhea, dizziness, headache, weight loss, anorexia, fatigue, abdominal pain, dyspepsia, depression, insomnia, somnolence, anemia, rhinitis, urinary tract infections, hematuria, tremor, syncope, and bradycardia. Other reported adverse reactions include chest pain, postural hypotension, hypotension, edema, cardiac failure, vertigo, convulsions, paresthesia, ataxia, flatulence, gastritis, melena, dysphagia, rectal hemorrhage, dry mouth, increased saliva, hiccup, AV block, palpitation, atrial fibrillation, QT prolonged, bundle branch block, supraventricular tachycardia, ventricular tachycardia, hyperglycemia, increased alkaline phosphatase, epistaxis, thrombocytopenia, apathy, paranoid reaction, delirium, increased libido, incontinence, hematuria, micturition frequency, cystitis, urinary retention, nocturia, renal calculi, dehydration, aggression, upper and lower GI bleeding, and hypokalemia.

ADMINISTRATION

Adults: recommended starting dose is 4 mg orally twice a day for 4 weeks with the morning and evening meal. The dose should be increased to the initial maintenance dose of 8 mg orally twice a day for 4 weeks. If the 8 mg orally twice a day dose is tolerated, the dose should be increased to 12 mg orally twice a day. If therapy is interrupted for several days or longer, the patient should be restarted at the lowest dose and the dose titrated to the current dose.

Dosage adjustment in renal impairment: for moderate renal impairment, dose should not exceed 16 mg/day. For severe renal impairment (creatinine clearance < 9 mL/min), use of galantamine is not recommended.

Dosage adjustment in hepatic impairment: For moderate hepatic impairment (Child-Pugh score 7–9), dose should not exceed 16 mg/ day. For severe hepatic impairment (Child-Pugh score 10–15), use of galantamine is not recommended.

PATIENT CARE IMPLICATIONS

Administering with food, using antiemetics, and ensuring adequate fluid intake may help reduce the GI side effects of galantamine. If using the oral solution, mix with 3–4 ounces of any nonalcoholic beverage, stir well, and drink right away.

PREPARATIONS

Tablets, 4, 8, and 12 mg. Oral solution, 4 mg/mL 100 mL bottle.

GLIPIZIDE AND METFORMIN

METAGLIP™

DESCRIPTION/ACTIONS

The combination of glipizide and metformin, two antidiabetic agents, is used for initial therapy for management of type 2 diabetes mellitus when hyperglycemia cannot be managed with diet and exercise alone. Metaglip™ is indicated as second-line therapy for the management of type 2 diabetes when hyperglycemia cannot be managed with a sulfonylurea or metformin along with diet and exercise. Glipizide is an antihyperglycemic drug of the sulfonylurea class; it lowers blood glucose by stimulating the release of insulin from the pancreas. Metformin, a biguanide, decreases hepatic glucose production, decreases intestinal absorption of glucose, and improves insulin sensitivity by increasing peripheral glucose uptake and utilization.

PRECAUTIONS/ADVERSE REACTIONS

Metaglip™ is contraindicated in individuals with a known hypersensitivity to glipizide, other sulfonamides, metformin, or any component of the formulation. Not to be used in patients with renal disease or renal dysfunction (serum creatinine ≥ 1.5 mg/dL in males or ≥ 1.4 mg/dL in females, or creatinine clearance < 60 ml/minute). Metaglip™ is contraindicated in patients with congestive heart failure requiring pharmacologic treatment and in acute or chronic metabolic acidosis, including diabetic ketoacidosis, with or without coma. Temporarily discontinue in patients undergoing radiologic studies involving intravascular administration of iodinated contrast materials, because use of such products may result in acute alteration of renal function. Discontinue Metaglip™ prior to the procedure and hold for 48 hours subsequent to the procedure. Reinstitute only after renal function has been reevaluated and found to be normal. Use should also be suspended temporarily for any surgical procedure (except minor procedures not associated with restricted intake of food and fluids). Restart when the patient's oral intake has resumed and renal function has been evaluated as normal.

Use caution in patients with hepatic impairment, malnourished or debilitated conditions, or adrenal or pituitary insufficiency. Lactic acidosis is a rare but serious metabolic complication that can occur due to metformin accumulation. When it occurs, it is fatal in approximately 50% of cases. Lactic acidosis may also occur in association with a number of pathophysiologic conditions, such as diabetes mellitus and significant tissue hypoperfusion and hypoxemia. The reported incidence of lactic acidosis in patients receiving metformin is very low; reported cases have occurred primarily in diabetic patients with significant renal insufficiency, including both intrinsic renal disease and renal hypoperfusion, often in the setting of multiple concomitant medical/surgical problems and multiple concomitant medications. Patients with congestive heart failure requiring pharmacologic management, in particular those with unstable or acute congestive heart failure who are at risk of hypoperfusion and hypoxemia, are at increased risk of lactic acidosis. The risk of lactic acidosis increases with the degree of renal dysfunction and the patient's age. The risk of lactic acidosis may be significantly decreased by regular monitoring of renal function in patients taking metformin and by use of the minimum effective dose of metformin. Treatment of the elderly should be accompanied by careful renal function monitoring. Treatment should not be initiated in patients 80 years of age or older unless measurement of creatinine clearance demonstrates that renal function is not reduced.

Metaglip™ should be promptly withheld in the presence of any condition associated with hypoxemia, dehydration, or sepsis. Impaired hepatic function may significantly limit the ability to clear lactate; generally avoid in patients with clinical or laboratory evidence of hepatic disease. Caution against excessive alcohol intake; alcohol potentiates the effects of metformin on lactate metabolism. Lactic acidosis should be suspected in any diabetic patient with metabolic acidosis lacking evidence of ketoacidosis (ketonuria and ketonemia). Lactic acidosis is a medical emergency that must be treated in a hospital setting. Metaglip™ should be discontinued immediately and supportive measures given promptly. Hemodialysis is recommended to correct the acidosis and remove the accumulated metformin.

The administration of oral hypoglycemic drugs has been reported to be associated with increased cardiovascular mortality as compared with treatment with diet alone or diet plus insulin. Metaglip™ can produce hypoglycemia; proper patient selection, dosing, and instructions are important to avoid potential hypoglycemic episodes. Hypoglycemia risk is increased when caloric intake is deficient, when strenuous exercise is not compensated by caloric supplementation, or during concomitant use with other glucose-lowering agents or ethanol. Renal insufficiency may cause elevated levels of glipizide and may diminish gluconeogenic capacity, both of which increase the risk of hypoglycemic reactions. Elderly, debilitated, or malnourished patients and those with adrenal or pituitary insufficiency or alcohol intoxication are particularly susceptible to hypoglycemic effects. Patients previously well controlled on metformin who develop laboratory abnormalities or clinical illness should be evaluated promptly for evidence of ketoacidosis or lactic acidosis. If acidosis of either form occurs, stop Metaglip™ immediately and initiate appropriate corrective measures. A decrease to subnormal levels of previously normal serum Vitamin B_{12} (without clinical manifestations) was observed and appears to be rapidly reversible with discontinuation of metformin or with Vitamin B_{12} supplementation. Hypoglycemic action of sulfonylureas may be potentiated by certain drugs, including nonsteroidal anti-inflammatory agents, some azoles, drugs that are highly protein-bound, salicylates, sulfonamides, chloramphenicol, coumarins, MAOI, and beta adrenergic blocking agents. When such drugs are withdrawn from a patient receiving Metaglip™, the patient should be observed closely for loss of blood glucose control. Drugs that tend to produce hyperglycemia are thiazides, diuretics, corticosteroids, phenothiazines, thyroid products, estrogens, oral contraceptives, phenytoin, sympathomimetics, nicotinic acid, calcium channel blocking agents, and isoniazid. When these drugs are withdrawn from a patient receiving Metaglip™, the patient should be observed closely for hypoglycemia. Cationic drugs (e.g., amiloride, digoxin, morphine, procainamide, quinidine, quinine, ranitidine, triamterene, trimethoprim, or vancomycin) that are eliminated by renal tubular secretion theoretically have the potential for interaction with metformin by competing for common renal tubular transport systems. Careful monitoring and dose adjustment is recommended.

Pregnancy Category C. Insulin is the drug of choice for the control of diabetes during pregnancy. Gipizide and metformin both cross the placenta; use during pregnancy only if clearly needed. Severe prolonged hypoglycemia has been reported in neonates whose mothers were taking sulfonylureas at the time of delivery. If Metaglip™ has been decided for use during pregnancy, it should be discontinued at least 1 month prior to delivery. Not recommended while breast feeding. Most common adverse reactions were upper respiratory tract infection, headache, hypoglycemia, musculoskeletal pain, nausea, vomiting, and diarrhea. Once patient is stabilized on Metaglip™, GI symptoms, which are common during initiation of the therapy, are unlikely to be drug-related. Later occurrence of GI symptoms could be due to lactic acidosis or other serious disease.

ADMINISTRATION

Type 2 diabetes, first-line therapy: start with 2.5 mg/250 mg once a day. Dose adjustment: increase by 1 tablet/day, every 2 weeks. Maximum: 10 mg/1000 mg. For fasting plasma glucose (FPG) of 280 to 320 mg/dL, consider 2.5 mg/500 mg twice a day. Dose adjustment: Increase by 1 tablet/day, every 2 weeks. Maximum: 10 mg/2000 mg daily in divided doses. Efficacy in FPG exceeding 320 mg/dL has not been established.

Type 2 diabetes, second-line therapy: 2.5 mg/500 mg or 5 mg/500 mg 2 times a day with morning and evening meal. Starting dose should not exceed the current daily dose of glipizide (or sulfonylurea equivalent) or metformin. Dose adjustment: Titrate in increments of no more than 5 mg/500 mg up to a maximum dose of 20 mg/2000 mg per day.

Conservative doses are recommended in the elderly due to potentially decreased renal function. Do not titrate to maximum dose. Do not use in patient 80 years of age or older unless renal function has been verified as normal.

PATIENT CARE IMPLICATIONS

Patient should take with meals to decrease GI upset. Patient must be able to recognize symptoms of hypoglycemia (palpitations, sweaty palms, and lightheadedness). Inform of increase in hypoglycemic symptoms when meals are skipped, too much alcohol is consumed, or heavy exercise occurs without enough food. Patient should be aware that onset of lactic acidosis is subtle and accompanied by nonspecific symptoms such as malaise, myalgias, respiratory distress, increasing somnolence, and nonspecific abdominal distress, and patient should be instructed to notify physician immediately if they occur. Before initiation of therapy and annually thereafter, hematologic parameters and renal function should be assessed and verified as normal. Periodic fasting blood glucose and glycosylated hemoglobin measurements should be performed to monitor therapeutic response.

PREPARATIONS

Tablet (film coated), 2.5 mg/250 mg (glipizide 2.5 mg and metformin 250 mg), 2.5/500 mg (glipizide 2.5 mg and metformin 500 mg), and 5/500 mg (glipizide 5 mg and metformin 500 mg).

NITAZOXANIDE

ALINIA™

DESCRIPTION/ACTIONS

Nitazoxanide is a synthetic antiprotozoal, indicated in the treatment of diarrhea caused by *Cryptosporidum parvum* and *Giardia lamblia* in pediatric patients from 1–11 years of age. Antiprotozoal activity of nitazoxanide is believed to be due to the interference with the pyruvate: ferredoxin oxidoreductase (PFOR) enzyme-dependent electron transfer reaction that is essential to anaerobic energy metabolism. Safety and effectiveness of nitazoxanide have not been established in HIV-positive patients or patients with immunodeficiency, pediatric patients less than 1 year of age, pediatric patients greater than 11 years of age, and adults.

PRECAUTIONS/ADVERSE REACTIONS

Nitazoxanide is contraindicated in patients hypersensitive to nitazoxanide or any of the formulation's components. Pharmacokinetics of nitazoxanide in patients with compromised renal or hepatic function have not been studied; therefore, nitazoxanide must be administered with caution to patients with hepatic, biliary, or renal disease and to patients with combined renal and hepatic disease. The active metabolite tizoxanide is highly bound to plasma protein. Use with caution when administering concurrently with other highly plasma protein-bound drugs with narrow therapeutic indices. Pregnancy Category B. No adequate and well-controlled studies in pregnant women. It is not known whether nitazoxanide is excreted in human milk; use caution when given to a nursing woman. Most common adverse events were abdominal pain, diarrhea, vomiting, and headache.

ADMINISTRATION

Age 12–47 months: 5 ml (100 mg) every 12 hours for 3 days.

Age 4–11 years: 10 ml (200 mg) every 12 hours for 3 days.

Directions for Mixing Oral Suspension: need 48 ml of water for preparation of suspension. Tap bottle until all powder flows freely. Add approximately one-half of the total water required (24 ml) and shake vigorously to suspend powder. Add remainder of water and again shake vigorously.

PATIENT CARE IMPLICATIONS

Shake well each time before taking medication and administer with food. Store at room temperature and discard any unused portion after 7 days. Diabetic patients should be aware that the oral suspension contains 1.48 grams of sucrose per 5 ml. Contact physician if severe or persistent headache, abdominal pain, diarrhea, or vomiting occur.

PREPARATIONS

Powder for oral suspension, 100 mg/5 ml (60 ml).

NITISINONE

ORFADIN®

DESCRIPTION/ACTIONS

Nitisinone inhibits 4-hydroxyphenylpyruvate dioxygenase, used for the treatment of hereditary tyrosinemia type 1 (HT-1). HT-1 is a disease of the pediatric population. This disorder is characterized by progressive liver failure, increased risk of hepatocellular carcinoma, coagulopathy, painful neurologic crises, and renal tubular dysfunction resulting in rickets. Nitisinone inhibits the normal catabolism of tyrosine in patients with HT-1, preventing the accumulation of catabolic metabolites responsible for the observed liver and kidney toxicities.

PRECAUTIONS/ADVERSE REACTIONS

Nitisinone is contraindicated in patients with a hypersensitivity to nitisinone or any component of the formulation. Since it inhibits tyrosine catabolism, it must be used with dietary restriction of tyrosine and phenylalanine. Inadequate restriction can result in toxic effects to the eyes, skin, and nervous system. Plasma tyrosine levels should be kept below 500 µmol/L to avoid toxic effects to the eyes (corneal ulcers, corneal opacities, keratitis, conjunctivitis, eye pain, and photophobia), skin (painful hyperkeratotic plaques on the soles and palms), and nervous system (variable degrees of mental retardation and developmental delay). Slit-lamp exam of the eyes should be performed prior to initiation of treatment. Patients who develop photophobia, eye pain, or signs of inflammation such as redness, swelling, or burning of the eyes during treatment with nitisinone should undergo slit-lamp reexamination and immediate measurement of the plasma tyrosine concentration. Regular liver monitoring by imaging (ultrasound, computerized tomography, magnetic resonance imaging) and laboratory tests is recommended. An increase in serum alpha-fetoprotein concentration may be a sign of inadequate treatment, but patients with increasing alpha-fetoprotein or signs of nodules of the liver during treatment should always be evaluated for hepatic malignancy. Platelet and white blood cell (WBC) counts should be monitored regularly because of the risk of transient thrombocytopenia and leucopenia. Serum alpha-fetoprotein concentrations are elevated at the time of diagnosis and gradually decrease during the course of nitisinone treatment; increases during therapy may be a sign of inadequate therapy. Pregnancy Category C. Safety and efficacy have not been established in pregnant women. Excretion in breast milk unknown; use caution. Most frequent adverse reactions were hepatic neoplasm, liver failure, conjunctivitis, corneal opacity, thrombocytopenia, and leucopenia. Leucopenia and thrombocytopenia are dose-dependent; decreasing dose resulted in normalization of platelet and WBC counts.

ADMINISTRATION

Initial: 1 mg/kg/day, divided into morning and evening dosing. Effect of food is unknown; nitisinone should be taken at least 1 hour before a meal. If biochemical parameters are not normalized within 1 month, the dose should be increased to 1.5 mg/kg/day. For plasma succinylacetone (one of the metabolites responsible for kidney and liver toxicity), it may take up to 3 months before the level is normalized. Maximum: 2 mg/kg/day. Doses do not need to be divided evenly. For young children, capsules may be opened and the contents suspended in a small amount of water, formula, or applesauce immediately before use. Store under refrigeration.

PATIENT CARE IMPLICATIONS

Patients should have slit-lamp exam prior to beginning treatment. Carefully monitor liver, platelet, WBC count, plasma tyrosine, and urine succinylacetone levels. Patients and parents should be counseled that HT-1 is a hereditary metabolic disease that is treated with nitisinone and dietary restriction to avoid the need for liver transplantation. Patients and parents should monitor for all symptomatic changes; they should report immediately rashes, excessive bleeding, eye pain, sensitivity to light, skin changes on feet or hands, and yellowing of skin or eyes.

PREPARATIONS

Capsule, 2, 5, and 10 mg.

OLMESARTAN MEDOXOMIL

BENICAR™

DESCRIPTION/ACTIONS
Olmesartan is a selective AT_1 subtype angiotensin II receptor antagonist. Angiotensin II is the principal pressor agent of the renin-angiotensin system, with effects that include vasoconstriction, stimulation and release of aldosterone, cardiac stimulation, and renal reabsorption of sodium. Olmesartan blocks the vasoconstrictor effects of angiotensin II by selectively blocking the binding of angiotensin II to the AT_1 receptor in vascular smooth muscle. Olmesartan is used in the treatment of hypertension. It may be used alone or with concurrent use of other antihypertensive agents.

PRECAUTIONS/ADVERSE REACTIONS
Olmesartan is contraindicated in individuals with a hypersensitivity to olmesartan or any component of the formulation and in those with hypersensitivity to other angiotensin II receptor antagonists. Also contraindicated in patients with primary hyperaldosteronism or bilateral renal artery stenosis and in women who are in their second and third trimester of pregnancy. Hypotension may occur in patients with volume and/or salt depletion (those being treated with high doses of diuretics). Treatment should start under close medical supervision. Deterioration in renal function can occur. Use with caution in unilateral renal artery stenosis, preexisting adrenal insufficiency, and significant aortic/mitral stenosis. Treatment with angiotensin receptor antagonists has been associated with oliguria and/or progressive azotemia and rarely with acute renal failure and/or death. Pregnancy Category C (first trimester) and D (second and third trimesters). The drug should be discontinued as soon as possible when pregnancy is detected. Drugs that act directly on the renin-angiotensin system can cause injury and even death to the developing fetus when used in pregnancy during the second and third trimesters. NSAIDs may decrease olmesartan efficacy; monitor blood pressure. There is an increased risk of hyperkalemia when taken with potassium-sparing diuretics. If given with lithium, the risk of lithium toxicity may be increased; monitor lithium levels. Most common adverse reactions were dizziness, headache, hyperglycemia, diarrhea, and back pain.

ADMINISTRATION
Initial: 20 mg once a day. May be increased to 40 mg daily after 2 weeks. Doses above 40 mg do not appear to have greater effect. Patients with possible depletion of intravascular volume should be started at a lower dose.

PATIENT CARE IMPLICATIONS
Inform patient that he/she may experience headache or dizziness and to use caution when driving or engaging in tasks that require alertness until response to drug is known. Unrelieved headaches, flulike symptoms, or other persistent adverse events should be reported. Monitor blood pressure. Monitor glucose levels if diabetic. May take with or without food.

PREPARATIONS
Tablet (film coated), 5, 20, and 40 mg.

OXALIPLATIN

ELOXATIN™

DESCRIPTION/ACTIONS

Oxaliplatin is an antineoplastic agent that undergoes nonenzymatic conversion to several active derivatives that covalently bind with macromolecules and thus inhibit DNA replication and transcription. Cytotoxicity is cell-cycle nonspecific. Oxaliplatin is indicated for use in combination with 5-fluorouracil (5-FU) and leucovorin (LV) for the treatment of metastatic carcinoma of the colon or rectum when disease has recurred or progressed during or within 6 months of completion of first-line therapy with the combination of bolus 5-FU/LV and irinotecan.

PRECAUTIONS/ADVERSE REACTIONS

Oxaliplatin should not be administered to patients with a known allergy to platinum compounds or oxaliplatin. It should be administered under the supervision of a qualified physician experienced in the use of cancer chemotherapeutic agents. Anaphylactic-like reactions have been reported and may occur within minutes of administration. Manage with appropriate supportive therapy. Drug-related deaths associated with platinum compounds from this reaction have been reported. Oxaliplatin has been associated with pulmonary fibrosis, which may be fatal. If unexplained respiratory symptoms such as nonproductive cough, dyspnea, crackles, or radiological pulmonary infiltrates occur, oxaliplatin should be discontinued until further pulmonary investigation excludes interstitial lung disease or pulmonary fibrosis. The safety and effectiveness of the combination of oxaliplatin and 5-FU/LV in patients with renal impairment have not been evaluated. Oxaliplatin and 5-FU/LV combination should be used with caution in patients with preexisting renal impairment since the primary route of platinum elimination is renal. Safety and effectiveness in pediatrics have not been established. Oxaliplatin is associated with two types of neuropathy. One is an acute, reversible, primarily peripheral, sensory neuropathy that occurs within hours or 1 to 2 days. It resolves within 14 days and frequently recurs with further dosing. Symptoms may be precipitated or exacerbated by exposure to cold temperature or cold objects. Symptoms present as transient paresthesia, dysesthesia, and hypoesthesia in the hands, feet, perioral area, or throat. The second type of neuropathy is a persistent (> 14 days), primarily peripheral, sensory neuropathy that is usually characterized by paresthesias, dysethesias, or hypoesthesias but may also include deficits in proprioception that can interfere with daily activities. The most common adverse effects were peripheral sensory neuropathies, fatigue, neutropenia, nausea, emesis, and diarrhea. Pregnancy Category D. Oxaliplatin may cause fetal harm when administered to a pregnant woman. It is not known if oxaliplatin or its derivatives are excreted in milk; breast feeding not recommended.

ADMINISTRATION

Recommended dose schedule is every 2 weeks as follows:

Day 1: Oxaliplatin 85 mg/m^2 IV infusion in 250–500 ml D5W and LV 200 mg/m^2 IV infusion in D5W. Give both drugs over 120 minutes, at the same time, in separate bags using a Y-line. Follow with 5-FU 400 mg/m^2 IV bolus given over 2–4 minutes, followed by 5-FU 600 mg/m^2 IV infusion in 500 ml D5W as a 22-hour continuous infusion.

Day 2: LV 200 mg/m² IV infusion over 120 minutes, followed by 5-FU 400 mg/m² IV bolus given over 2–4 minutes. Follow with 5-FU 600 mg/m² IV infusion in 500 ml D5W as a 22-hour continuous infusion.

Repeat cycle every 2 weeks. Administration does not require prehydration. Premedicate with antiemetics. Neuropathy was graded using a study-specific neurotoxicity scale. For patients who experience persistent Grade 2 neurosensory events that do not resolve, a dose reduction to 65 mg/m² should be considered. For patients with persistent Grade 3 neurosensory events, discontinuing therapy should be considered. A dose reduction of oxaliplatin to 65 mg/m² and infusional 5-FU by 20% (300 mg/m² bolus and 500 mg/m² via 22-hour infusion) is recommended for patients after recovery from Grade 3/4 gastrointestinal events (despite prophylactic treatment) or Grade 3/4 hematologic toxicity (neutrophils < 1.5 X 10⁹/L, platelets < 100 X 10⁹/L).

Preparation of infusion solution: Reconstitution or final dilution must never be performed with a sodium chloride solution or other chloride-containing solutions. Lyophilized powder is reconstituted by adding 10 ml (50 mg vial) or 20 ml (100 mg vial) of water for injection, USP, or D5W. DO NOT ADMINISTER RECONSTITUTED SOLUTION WITHOUT FURTHER DILUTION. The reconstituted solution must be further diluted in 250–500 ml of D5W. After reconstituting in the original vial, the solution may be stored up to 24 hours in refrigerator. After final dilution with D5W, the shelf life at room temperature is 6 hours, or up to 24 hours under refrigeration.

Oxaliplatin is incompatible in solution with alkaline medications or media (such as basic solutions of 5-FU) and must not be mixed with these or administered simultaneously through the same infusion line. The infusion line should be flushed with D5W prior to administration of any concomitant medication. Inspect visually for particulate matter and discoloration prior to administration and discard if present. Needles or intravenous administration sets containing aluminum parts that may come in contact with oxaliplatin should not be used for the preparation or mixing of the drug. Aluminum has been reported to cause degradation of platinum compounds.

PATIENT CARE IMPLICATIONS

Inform patient he/she will be monitored closely during and after infusion. Patient should report immediately any pain, burning, swelling at infusion site or any signs of allergic reaction. Patient should maintain adequate nutrition and adequate hydration (2–3 L/day of fluids) unless instructed to restrict fluid intake. Patient will be susceptible to infection (avoid crowds and exposure to infection). Contact physician immediately should fever, particularly if associated with persistent diarrhea or evidence of infection, develops. Patient should not have any vaccinations without consulting prescriber. Inform patient of common adverse effects, especially the neurologic adverse effects. Instruct to avoid cold drinks and use of ice and to cover exposed skin prior to exposure to cold temperature or cold objects. Inform patient to contact physician if persistent vomiting, diarrhea, signs of dehydration, cough or breathing difficulties, or signs of allergic reaction appear. Prior to subsequent therapy cycles, patient should be evaluated for clinical toxicities and laboratory tests.

PREPARATIONS

Injection, preservative-free lyophilized powder for reconstitution: 50 and 100 mg.

PEGINTERFERON ALFA-2A

PEGASYS®

DESCRIPTION/ACTIONS

Interferons bind to specific receptors on the cell surface, initiating intracellular signaling via a complex cascade of protein-protein interactions leading to rapid activation of gene transcription. Interferon-stimulated genes modulate many biological effects, such as inhibition of viral replication in infected cells, inhibition of cell proliferation, and immunomodulation. Peginterferon alfa-2a is indicated for the treatment of chronic hepatitis C, alone or in combination with ribavirin, in patients who have compensated liver disease and have not been previously treated with interferon alpha.

PRECAUTIONS/ADVERSE REACTIONS

Peginterferon alfa-2a is contraindicated in patients with a known hypersensitivity to peginterferon alfa-2a or any of its components, interferon alfa, or polyethylene glycol (PEG). It should not be used in patients with autoimmune hepatitis, hepatic decompensation (Child-Pugh class B and C), or previous treatment with interferon, and in neonates and infants because it contains benzyl alcohol. Life-threatening or fatal neuropsychiatric reactions such as suicide, suicide ideation, depression, relapse of drug addiction, and drug overdose may manifest in patients. Avoid use in severe psychiatric disorders; must use caution in patients with a history of depression. Neuropsychiatric adverse events observed with alpha interferon treatment include aggressive behavior, mania, psychoses, hallucinations, and bipolar disorders. Physicians should monitor all patients for evidence of depression and other psychiatric symptoms. Serious and severe bacterial infections, some fatal, have been observed. Some infections have been associated with neutropenia; use caution in patients with baseline neutrophil counts < 1500 cells/mm^3, baseline platelet counts < 90,000 cells/mm^3, or baseline hemoglobin < 10 g/dL. Peginterferon alfa-2a should be discontinued in patients who develop severe infections and appropriate antibiotic therapy instituted.

Peginterferon alfa-2a suppresses bone marrow function and may result in severe cytopenia. It is advised that complete blood counts be obtained pretreatment and monitored during therapy. Hypertension, supraventricular arrhythmias, chest pain, and myocardial infarction have been observed; administer with caution to patients with preexisting cardiac disease. Peginterferon causes or aggravates hypothyroidism and hyperthyroidism. Hyperglycemia, hypoglycemia, and diabetes have been observed; patients who develop these conditions during treatment and can't be controlled with medication may require discontinuation of therapy. Use with caution in patients with autoimmune disorders; exacerbation of autoimmune disorders including myositis, hepatitis, psoriasis, rheumatoid arthritis, interstitial nephritis, and systemic lupus erythematosus have been reported. Dyspnea, pulmonary infiltrates, pneumonia, bronchiolitis obliterans, interstitial pneumonitis, and sarcoidosis, some resulting in respiratory failure and/or patient deaths, may be induced or aggravated by peginterferon alfa-2a. Patients who develop persistent or unexplained pulmonary infiltrates or pulmonary function impairment should discontinue peginterferon alfa-2a. Ulcerative colitis and hemorrhagic/ischemic colitis, sometimes fatal, have been observed; discontinue immediately if abdominal pain, bloody diarrhea, and fever develop. Treatment should be suspended if signs of pancreatitis are seen.

Peginterferon may induce or aggravate decrease or loss of vision, retinopathy including macular edema, retinal artery or vein thrombosis, retinal hemorrhages and cotton wool spots, optic neuritis, and papilledema. Patients with preexisting ophthalmic disorders should receive periodic ophthalmology exams during treatment. Patients who develop ocular symptoms should receive a prompt and complete eye exam and treatment should be discontinued in patients who develop new or worsening ophthalmologic disorders. Use caution in geriatric patients. Safety and efficacy have not been established in children or in patients who have failed other alpha interferon therapy, received organ transplants, have been infected with HIV or hepatitis B, or for treatment beyond 48 weeks. Pregnancy Category C. There are no adequate or well-controlled studies in pregnant women. Very high doses are abortifacient in Rhesus monkeys and are assumed to have abortifacient potential in humans. Excretion into breast milk is unknown; breast feeing not recommended during treatment. Most common adverse reactions are headache, fatigue, pyrexia, insomnia, depression, dizziness, nausea, diarrhea, abdominal pain, neutropenia, myalgia, impaired concentration and arthralgia.

ADMINISTRATION

Monotherapy: 180 µg subcutaneously once weekly for 48 weeks.

Combination therapy with ribavirin: 180 µg subcutaneously once weekly.

Duration of therapy based on genotype:

Genotype 1, 4: Treat for 48 weeks.

Genotype 2, 3: Treat for 24 weeks.

Dose modification: Moderate to severe adverse reactions: Initial: 135 µg/week, may need to decrease to 90 µg/week.

Dose modification based on depression:

Mild depression: no adjustment required.

Moderate depression: 90–135 mcg once a week. Evaluate once weekly with an office visit at least every other week. If depression remains stable, consider psychiatric consultation and continue with reduced dose. If symptoms improve and are stable for 4 weeks, resume normal visit schedule and continue reduced dosing or return to normal dose.

Severe depression: discontinue permanently.

Hematologic parameters:

ANC < 750/mm^3: 135 µg/week.

Platelet count < 50,000/mm^3: 90 µg/week.

Platelet count < 25,000/mm^3: discontinue.

Renal failure adjustment: for end-stage renal disease requiring hemodialysis:135 µg/week. Monitor for toxicity.

Hepatic impairment adjustment: ALT progressively rising above baseline: Decrease to 135 µg/week. If ALT continues to rise or is accompanied by increased bilirubin or hepatic decompensation, discontinue therapy immediately.

PATIENT CARE IMPLICATIONS

Administer in the abdomen or thigh by subcutaneous injection; rotate site. Do not use if solution contains particulate matter or is discolored. Discard unused solution. Avoid ethanol use. If self-administering, patient should follow exact instructions for injection and syringe/needle disposal. Inform patient he/she will need laboratory and ophthalmic exams prior to and during therapy. May cause dizziness; advise patient to use caution when engaged in potentially hazardous tasks until response to drug is known. Advise patient to report any severe or persistent adverse effects, including nausea, vomiting, abdominal pain, severe depression, anxiety, suicidal ideation, chest pain, palpitations, or breathing difficulty. Inform patient that due to difference in dosage, patients should not change brand of interferon.

PREPARATIONS

Injection, solution: 180 µg/ml (1.2 ml).

Store in refrigerator (2°C to 8°C). Do not freeze or shake; protect from light. Vials are for single use only. Discard any unused portion.

RASBURICASE

ELITEK™

DESCRIPTION/ACTIONS

Rasburicase is a recombinant urate-oxidase enzyme. It acts at the end of the purine catabolic pathway, where it converts uric acid into allantoin, an inactive and insoluble metabolite. It is indicated for the initial management of plasma uric acid levels in pediatric patients with leukemia, lymphoma, and solid tumor malignancies who are receiving anticancer therapy expected to result in tumor lysis and subsequent elevation of plasma uric acid.

PRECAUTIONS/ADVERSE REACTIONS

Rasburicase is contraindicated in patients with a known hypersensitivity to it or to any component of the formulation. It is contraindicated in individuals with glucose-6-phosphate dehydrogenase (G6PD) deficiency and in patients with a known history of anaphylaxis or hypersensitivity reactions, hemolytic reactions, or methemoglobinemia. Patients at high risk for G6PD deficiency should be screened prior to initiation of therapy with rasburicase. Rasburicase should be immediately and permanently discontinued in any patient developing a serious hypersensitivity reaction, hemolysis, or methemoglobinemia. Rasburicase is immunogenic and can elicit antibodies that inhibit the activity of rasburicase. Time to detection of antibodies ranged from 1–6 weeks after rasburicase exposure and lasted up to 494 days. Pregnancy Category C. No adequate and well-controlled studies have been conducted in pregnant women. Excretion in human breast milk is unknown. Use in pregnancy and lactation only if the potential benefit justifies the potential risk to the fetus. Most serious adverse reactions caused by rasburicase were allergic reactions including anaphylaxis (<1%), rash (1%), hemolysis (<1%), and methemoglobinemia (<1%). Most commonly observed serious adverse reactions include fever (5%), neutropenia (2%), neutropenia with fever (4%), respiratory distress (3%), sepsis (3%), and mucositis (2%). Other serious adverse reactions observed in = 1% of patients include acute renal failure, arrhythmias, cardiac arrest, cardiac failure, cellulitis, cerebrovascular disorder, chest pain, convulsions, cyanosis, dehydration, diarrhea, hemorrhage, hot flashes, ileus, infection, intestinal obstruction, myocardial infarction, pancytopenia, paresthesia, pneumonia, pulmonary edema, pulmonary hypertension, retinal hemorrhage, rigors, thrombophlebitis, and thrombosis. Less serious adverse reactions include vomiting (50%), fever (46%), nausea (27%), headache (26%), abdominal pain (20%), constipation (20%), diarrhea (20%), mucositis (15%), and rash (13%). Safety and efficacy of rasburicase have been established only for a single course of treatment. No drug interaction studies have been conducted in humans; however, rasburicase does not appear to be an inducer or inhibitor of the cytochrome P450 enzyme system.

ADMINISTRATION

Children: I.V. Infusion 0.15 mg/kg or 0.20 mg/kg once daily for 5 days in 50 mL of 0.9% sodium chloride infused over 30 minutes.

Do not administer as a bolus infusion. Do not filter. Do not shake or vortex. IV infusion is stable for 24 hours.

Dosing beyond 5 days or administration of more than one course of rasburicase is not recommended. Chemotherapy should be initiated 4 to 24 hours after the first dose of rasburicase. Efficacy in adults and geriatric patients has not been established.

PATIENT CARE IMPLICATIONS

Patients on rasburicase should receive hydration according to standard practice for the management of high uric acid levels in patients at risk for tumor lysis syndrome. Rasburicase will cause enzymatic degradation of the uric acid within blood samples left at room temperature, resulting in spuriously low uric acid levels. To ensure adequate measurements of uric acid levels, blood must be collected into prechilled tubes containing heparin anticoagulant and immediately immersed and maintained in an ice water bath and analyzed within 4 hours of collection.

PREPARATIONS

Powder for injection, 3 x 1.5 mg rasburicase vials with 3 x 1.0 mL ampules of diluent.

ROSIGLITAZONE AND METFORMIN

AVANDAMET™

DESCRIPTION/ACTIONS

Avandamet™ contains two oral antihyperglycemic drugs used in type 2 diabetes management. Rosiglitazone is a thiazolidinedione that lowers blood glucose by improving insulin sensitivity without increasing pancreatic insulin secretion. Metformin, a member of the biguanide class, decreases hepatic glucose production, decreases intestinal glucose absorption, and increases peripheral glucose uptake and utilization. Avandamet™ is indicated as an adjunct to diet and exercise to improve glycemic control in patients with type 2 diabetes who are already treated with combination rosiglitazone and metformin or who are not adequately controlled on metformin alone. Avandamet™ is not appropriate for initial therapy of type 2 diabetes.

PRECAUTIONS/ADVERSE REACTIONS

Avandamet™ is contraindicated in patients with a known hypersensitivity to rosiglitazone or metformin; patients with congestive heart failure (CHF) requiring pharmacologic treatment; patients with renal disease or renal dysfunction (serum creatinine levels = 1.5 mg/dL [males], = 1.4 mg/dL [females], or abnormal creatinine clearance); and in patients with acute or chronic metabolic acidosis, including diabetic ketoacidosis, with or without coma. Lactic acidosis is a rare but serious metabolic complication that can occur due to metformin accumulation. When it occurs, it is fatal in approximately 50% of cases. Lactic acidosis may also occur in association with diabetes mellitus and with there significant tissue hypoperfusion and hypoxemia. Lactic acidosis is characterized by elevated blood lactate levels (> 5 mmol/L), decreased blood pH, electrolyte disturbances with an increased anion gap, and an increased lactate/pyruvate ratio. Reported cases occurred primarily in diabetic patients with significant renal insufficiency, including both intrinsic renal disease and renal hypoperfusion, often in the setting of multiple concomitant medical/surgical problems and multiple concomitant medications. Patients with CHF requiring pharmacologic management, in particular those with unstable or acute CHF who are at risk of hypoperfusion and hypoxemia, are at increased risk of lactic acidosis. The risk increases with the degree of renal dysfunction and the patient's age. Treatment of the elderly should be accompanied with careful renal function monitoring.

Avandamet™ should not be initiated in patient 80 years of age or older unless creatinine clearance measurement demonstrates that renal function is not reduced. Stop treatment in the presence of any condition associated with hypoxemia, dehydration, or sepsis. Because impaired hepatic function may significantly limit the ability to clear lactate, Avandamet™ should be avoided in patients with clinical or laboratory evidence of hepatic disease. Caution against excessive alcohol intake, since alcohol potentiates the effects of metformin on lactate metabolism. Lactic acidosis should be suspected in any diabetic patient with metabolic acidosis lacking evidence of ketoacidosis (ketonuria and ketonemia). Lactic acidosis is a medical emergency that must be treated in a hospital setting. In patients with lactic acidosis, discontinue drug immediately. Hemodialysis is recommended to correct the acidosis and remove the accumulated metformin. Use with caution in patients with edema. Rosiglitazone, like other thiazolidinediones, can cause fluid retention, which may exacerbate or lead to heart failure. Observe for signs and symptoms of heart failure; discontinue Avandamet™ if any deterioration in cardiac status occurs. Metformin is known to be substantially excreted by the kidneys, and the risk of metformin accumulation and lactic acidosis increases with the degree of renal function impairment. Patients with serum creatinine levels above the upper limit of normal for their age should not receive Avandamet™. In patients with advanced age, carefully titrate to establish the minimum dose for adequate glycemic effect. Before initiation of therapy and at least annually thereafter, renal function should be assessed and verified as normal. In patients in whom renal dysfunction development is anticipated, renal function should be assessed more frequently and if evidence of renal impairment is present, therapy should be discontinued. Intravascular contrast studies with iodinated materials can lead to acute alteration of renal function and have been associated with lactic acidosis in patients receiving metformin. Temporarily discontinue Avandamet™ prior to any intravascular radiocontrast study and for any surgical procedure (except minor procedures not associated with restricted intake of food and fluids) and hold for 48 hours subsequent to the procedure. Reinstate drug after renal function has been reevaluated and found to be normal.

Impaired hepatic function has been associated with some cases of lactic acidosis. Avandamet™ should not be initiated if the patient exhibits clinical evidence of active liver disease or increased serum transaminase levels (ALT > 2.5 times upper limit of normal) at baseline. Liver enzymes should be checked prior to initiation of therapy and every 2 months for the first year and periodically thereafter in patients with normal baseline liver enzymes. Patients with mildly elevated liver enzymes should proceed with caution and include close clinical follow-up. If at any time ALT levels increase to more than 3 times the upper limit of normal, liver enzymes should be rechecked as soon as possible. If ALT levels remain more than 3 times the upper limit of normal, therapy should be discontinued. If the patient develops symptoms suggesting hepatic dysfunction, liver enzymes should be checked; if jaundice is observed, discontinue drug therapy.

Hypoglycemia doesn't occur in patients receiving metformin alone under usual circumstances of use but could occur when caloric intake is deficient, when strenuous exercise is not compensated by caloric supplementation, or during concomitant use with hypoglycemic agents (sulfonylureas or insulin) or ethanol. Elderly, debilitated, or malnourished patients and those with adrenal or pituitary insufficiency or alcohol intoxication are particularly susceptible to hypoglycemic effects. Hypoglycemia may be difficult to recognize in the elderly and in people who are taking beta-adrenergic blocking agents. When a patient stabilized on any diabetic regimen is exposed to stress such as fever, trauma, infection, or surgery, a temporary loss of glycemic control may occur. It may be necessary to hold Avandamet™ at such times and temporarily administer insulin. Use caution in patients with anemia or depressed leukocyte count. Decreases in hemoglobin, hematocrit, and white blood cell counts were observed.

Therapy with rosiglitazone may result in ovulation in some premenopausal anovulatory women. These patients may be at an increased risk for pregnancy. Adequate contraception in premenopausal women is recommended. Most common adverse reactions were diarrhea, upper respiratory tract infection, headache, anemia, and sinusitis. Pregnancy Category C. Abnormal blood glucose levels are associated with a higher incidence of congenital abnormalities, as well as increased neonatal morbidity and mortality. Insulin is the drug of choice for the control of diabetes during pregnancy. Safety in pregnant women has not been established. Use during pregnancy if clearly needed. Excretion in breast milk is unknown; breast feeding is not recommended. Drugs that tend to produce hyperglycemia (thiazides or diuretics, corticosteroids, phenothiazines, estrogens, oral contraceptives, phenytoin, nicotinic acid, sympathomimetics, and isoniazid) may lead to loss of glycemic control.

ADMINISTRATION

Selection of the dose should be based on the patient's current doses of rosiglitazone and/or metformin.

For patients inadequately controlled on metformin monotherapy: Usual starting dose is 4 mg rosiglitazone (total daily dose) plus the dose of metformin already being taken (see below).

For patients inadequately controlled on rosiglitazone: 1000 mg metformin (total daily dose) plus the dose of rosiglitazone already being taken (see below).

PRIOR THERAPY TOTAL DAILY DOSE	USUAL AVANDAMET TABLET STRENGTH	STARTING DOSE NUMBER OF TABLETS
METFORMIN		
1000 mg/day	2 mg/500 mg	1 tablet b.i.d.
2000 mg/day	1 mg/500 mg	2 tablets b.i.d.
ROSIGLITAZONE		
4 mg/day	2 mg/500 mg	1 tablet b.i.d.
8 mg/day	4 mg/500 mg	2 tablets b.i.d.

If additional glycemic control is needed, the daily dose of Avandamet™ may be increased by increments of 4 mg rosiglitazone and/or 500 mg metformin. Maximum recommended total daily dose is 8 mg/2000 mg. Give in divided doses with meals, with gradual dose escalation. This reduces GI side effects and permits determination of the minimum effective dose for the individual patient. Sufficient time should be given to assess adequacy of response. Fasting plasma glucose should be used to determine the therapeutic response. Metformin dose titration is recommended in patients who are not adequately controlled after 1–2 weeks. After an increase in rosiglitazone, dose titration is recommended if patients are not adequately controlled after 8–12 weeks.

The elderly: initial and maintenance dosing should be conservative, due to the potential for decreased renal function. Do not titrate to maximum dose. Do not use in patients 80 years of age or older unless normal renal function has been established.

PATIENT CARE IMPLICATIONS

Make patient aware that the onset of lactic acidosis is often subtle and accompanied by nonspecific symptoms such as malaise, myalgias, respiratory distress, increasing somnolence, and nonspecific abdominal distress; they should be instructed to notify their physician immediately if these symptoms occur. Once a patient is stabilized on any dose level, GI symptoms, which are common during initiation of therapy, are unlikely to be drug-related. Later occurrence of GI symptoms could be due to lactic acidosis or other serious disease. Patients should be counseled against excessive alcohol intake. Inform patients of the importance of adhering to dietary instructions, weight loss, and a regular exercise program. This medication is used to control diabetes; it is not a cure. Patients should not take other medication within 2 hours of taking Avandamet™. Use alternate means of contraception.

PREPARATIONS

Tablets, 1 mg/500 mg (rosiglitazone 1 mg and metformin 500 mg), 2 mg/500 mg (rosiglitazone 2 mg and metformin 500 mg), 4 mg/500 mg (rosiglitazone 4 mg and metformin 500 mg).

Store at 25° C (77°F); excursions permitted to 15–30° C (59–86°F). Dispense in a tight, light-resistant container.

SODIUM OXYBATE

XYREM®

DESCRIPTION/ACTIONS

Sodium oxybate is gamma hydroxybutyric acid (GHB), a known drug of abuse. Nonmedical uses are classified under Schedule I. Sodium oxybate is classified as a Schedule III controlled substance by federal law. It is a psychoactive drug that produces a wide range of pharmacological effects; it is a sedative-hypnotic that produces dose- and concentration-dependent central nervous system effects in humans. Onset of effect is rapid, enhancing its desirability as a drug of abuse or misuse. Sodium oxybate is indicated for the treatment of cataplexy in patients with narcolepsy. The exact mechanism for the efficacy is not known. Sodium oxybate oral solution is available only to prescribers and patients enrolled in the Xyrem® Patient Success Program. It will NOT be stocked in retail pharmacies.

PRECAUTIONS/ADVERSE REACTIONS

Sodium oxybate is contraindicated in individuals with a hypersensitivity to sodium oxybate or any component of the formulation. It should not be used with ethanol and other CNS depressants, or in patients with succinic semialdehyde dehydrogenase deficiency. Sodium oxybate may impair respiratory drive; use caution with compromised respiratory function. Most patients in clinical trials were also treated with stimulants; therefore, an independent assessment of the effects of sodium oxybate is lacking. Sodium oxybate may cause confusion, psychosis, paranoia, hallucinations, agitation, and depression; use caution in patients with a history of depression or suicide attempt.

Sodium oxybate contains significant amounts of sodium; use caution with heart failure, hypertension, or compromised renal failure. Abuse has been associated with seizures, respiratory depression, and profound decreases in level of consciousness, with instances of coma and death. Also may cause urinary/fecal incontinence and sleepwalking, confused behavior occurring at night and at times associated with wandering. Instances of significant injury or potential injury were associated with sleepwalking.

Pregnancy Category B. No well-controlled studies in pregnant women. Use only if clearly needed in pregnancy. Past use during labor and delivery as an anesthetic has shown a slight decrease in Apgar scores due to sleepiness in the neonate. Excretion in breast milk is not known; use caution. Safety and effectiveness in patients under 16 years of age and over 65 years have not been established. Most common adverse reactions were headache, nausea, dizziness, pain, somnolence, pharyngitis, infection, viral infection, accidental injury, diarrhea, urinary incontinence, vomiting, confusion, sleepwalking, depression, abnormal dreams, and abdominal pain.

ADMINISTRATION

Starting dose: 4.5 g/day divided into 2 equal doses of 2.25 grams. Increments can be made after 2 weeks to evaluate clinical response and minimize adverse effects. Increase by 1.5 g/day to a maximum of 9 g/day. Efficacy and safety at doses higher than 9 g/day have not been investigated and should not be administered.

Hepatic insufficiency: starting dose should be 2.25 g/day divided into 2 equal doses. Dose increments should be titrated to effect while closely monitoring potential adverse events.

Take on am empty stomach; separate last meal and first dose by several hours. Try to take at same time each day. Each dose of sodium oxybate must be diluted with 2 ounces of water in the child-resistant dosing cups. Once diluted, solutions should be used within 24 hours to minimize bacteria growth and contamination. Both doses should be prepared prior to bedtime. This medication will cause sleep immediately; it must be taken at bedtime and only after getting in bed. The first dose is to be taken at bedtime while in bed and the second dose taken 2.5–4 hours later while sitting in bed. Patients will need to set an alarm to awaken for the second dose. The second dose should be placed in close proximity to the patient's bed. After ingesting each dose, the patient should lie down and remain in bed.

PATIENT CARE IMPLICATIONS

Sodium oxybate should be used only by patient. Keep out of the reach of children and pets. The Xyrem® Patient Success Program consists of a videotape and printed educational material. The central pharmacist will not fill the first prescription unless the patient has confirmed to the pharmacist that he or she has read the educational materials. Patients should inform their physician of trouble breathing while asleep, confusion, abnormal thinking, depression, loss of consciousness, and other persistent adverse effects. Apprise patients that abuse of drug can cause serious medical problems, including trouble breathing, seizures, loss of consciousness, coma, and death; it can lead to dependence, craving for medicine, and severe withdrawal symptoms. Sodium oxybate may cause dizziness or confusion, which carries over into daytime. Patients should not perform any activity that requires mental alertness for at least 6 hours after taking sodium oxybate and should use extreme caution when driving or engaging in tasks requiring alertness until response to drug is known. Patients should not take alcohol or other sedative/hypnotic substances.

PREPARATIONS

Solution, oral: 500 mg/ml (180 ml). Kit contains 2 dosing cups and a measuring device.

TEGASEROD MALEATE

ZELNORM™

DESCRIPTION/ACTIONS

Tegaserod is a 5-HT$_4$ receptor partial agonist that binds with high affinity at human 5-HT$_4$ receptors. Serotonin has been shown to be involved in regulating motility, visceral sensitivity, and intestinal secretion, suggesting an important role of serotonin type-4 receptors in maintenance of GI functions in humans. Activation of 5-HT$_4$ receptors in the GI tract stimulates the peristaltic reflex and intestinal secretion, as well as inhibits visceral sensitivity. Tegaserod is indicated fro the short-term treatment of women with irritable bowel syndrome (IBS) whose primary bowel symptom is constipation. Women with this medical condition suffer from abdominal pain or discomfort, bloating, and constipation. Safety and effectiveness of tegaserod in men and patients below the age of 18 have not been established.

PRECAUTIONS/ADVERSE REACTIONS

Contraindicated in individuals who are hypersensitive to tegaserod or any component of its formulation or who have severe renal impairment, moderate or severe hepatic impairment, a history of bowel obstruction, symptomatic gallbladder disease, suspected sphincter of Oddi dysfunction, or abdominal adhesions. Do not give to patients who are currently experiencing or frequently experience diarrhea. It should be discontinued immediately in patients with new or sudden worsening of abdominal pain. Pregnancy Category B. Safety and efficacy have not been established in pregnant women, use only if clearly needed. Excretion in breast milk is unknown; breast feeding is not recommended. Most common adverse reactions were headache, abdominal pain, dizziness, and diarrhea. A majority of patients reported diarrhea as a single episode. Diarrhea occurred during the first week of therapy and resolved with continued therapy.

ADMINISTRATION

Adults: 6 mg 2 times a day for 4 to 6 weeks. If patient responds to therapy, an additional 4–6-week course can be considered. Not recommended in patients with severe renal impairment. Use caution in patients with mild hepatic impairment. Tegaserod has not been adequately studied in patients with moderate and severe hepatic impairment and is therefore not recommended in this population.

PATIENT CARE IMPLICATIONS

Take as directed on an empty stomach, 30 minutes before meals. If a dose is missed, skip that dose and continue with regular schedule. DO NOT DOUBLE THE DOSE. May cause headache or dizziness; patients should use caution when driving or operating heavy machinery until response to drug is known. May cause nausea and vomiting; small frequent meals, frequent mouth care, and gum chewing may help. Patients should be made aware of possibility of diarrhea and that they should consult their physician if they experience severe diarrhea or if the diarrhea is accompanied by severe cramping, abdominal pain, or dizziness.

PREPARATIONS

Tablets, 2 and 6 mg. Protect from moisture. Store at 25°C (77°F); excursions permitted to 15–30°C (59–86°F).

TERIPARATIDE

FORTEO™

DESCRIPTION/ACTIONS

Teriparatide is a parathyroid hormone (PTH) analogue manufactured by using a strain of *Escherichia coli* modified by recombinant DNA technology. Endogenous 84–amino-acid PTH is the primary regulator of calcium and phosphate metabolism in bone and kidney. Physiological actions of PTH include regulation of bone metabolism, renal tubular reabsorption of calcium and phosphate, and intestinal calcium absorption. The biological actions of PTH and teriparatide are mediated through binding to specific high-affinity cell-surface receptors. Treatment with teriparatide stimulates new bone formation on trabecular and cortical bone surfaces by preferential stimulation of osteoblastic activity over osteoclastic activity. There is an increase in skeletal mass, an increase in markers of bone formation and resorption, and an increase in bone strength. Use of teriparatide is indicated in the treatment of osteoporosis, in postmenopausal women at high risk of fracture; and to increase bone mass in men with primary or hypogonadal osteoporosis who are at high risk for fracture. Teriparatide reduces the risk of vertebral fractures in postmenopausal women with osteoporosis; decreases the risk of nonvertebral fractures in postmenopausal women with osteoporosis, and increases vertebral and femoral neck BMD in postmenopausal women with osteoporosis and in men with primary or hypogonadal osteoporosis. The effects of teriparatide on fracture risk have not been studied.

PRECAUTIONS/ADVERSE REACTIONS

Teriparatide is contraindicated in individuals hypersensitive to teriparatide or any of the formulation's components. **WARNING:** In rats, teriparatide caused an increase in the incidence of osteosarcoma that was dependent on dose and treatment duration. Because of the uncertain relevance of the rat osteosarcoma finding to humans, teriparatide should be prescribed only to patients for whom the potential benefits are considered to outweigh the potential risk. Not to be prescribed for patients who are at increased baseline risk for osteosarcoma, including those with Paget's disease of bone or unexplained elevations of alkaline phosphatase, open epiphyses, or prior radiation therapy involving the skeleton.

Not to be used in pediatric patients or young adults with open epiphyses. Patients with bone metastases or a history of skeletal malignancies and patients with metabolic bone diseases other than osteoporosis should be excluded from treatment with teriparatide. The safety and efficacy have not been evaluated beyond 2 years of treatment; use for more than 2 years is not recommended. Teriparatide should be used with caution in patients with active or recent urolithiasis because of the potential to exacerbate this condition. Transient episodes of symptomatic orthostatic hypotension were observed infrequently within the first several doses. It was relieved by placing the person in a reclining position. Use caution in patients at risk of orthostasis (including concurrent antihypertensive therapy) or in patients who may not tolerate transient hypotension. Because teriparatide increases serum calcium, it should be used with caution in patients taking digitalis; it has been suggested that hypercalcemia may predispose patients to digitalis toxicity. Pregnancy Category C. Effect on human fetal development has not been studied; not indicated for use in pregnancy. Not recommended for women who are breast-feeding. Most common adverse events were dizziness, leg cramps, and nausea.

ADMINISTRATION

Adults: 20 µg once daily, subcutaneously, into the thigh or abdominal wall. Administer initially under circumstances in which the patient can sit or lie down if symptoms of orthostatic hypotension occur.

PATIENT CARE IMPLICATIONS

Use injector pen and dispose of pen as directed. Rotate injection sites in thigh or abdominal wall. Patient should sit when administering to reduce the possibility of falling or injury. May cause dizziness; patient should use caution when driving or engaged in potentially hazardous tasks until response to drug is known. Do not use if solution has solid particles in it or if it is cloudy or colored—it should be clear and colorless. Do not use after the expiration date printed on the pen and pen packaging. Throw away pen after 28 days of use, even if it still has medicine in it. Inject teriparatide shortly after taking the pen out of the refrigerator. Recap the pen and put it back into the refrigerator right after use to protect cartridge from physical damage and light. Do no freeze the pen. If patient forgets to take a dose, he/she should take it as soon as possible on that day. Do not administer more than 1 injection in the same day. If patient becomes lightheaded or experiences fast heartbeats after injection, he/she should sit or lie down until feeling better. If he/she doesn't feel better, the doctor should be called before continuing treatment. Patient should contact physician if he/she has continuing nausea, vomiting, constipation, low energy, or muscle weakness; these may be signs there is too much calcium in the blood. Avoid ethanol; may increase risk of osteoporosis. Patient should receive appropriate training and instruction on the proper use and disposal of pen.

PREPARATIONS

Injection, solution: 250 µg/ml (3 ml). Prefilled pen delivery device. Store under refrigeration at 2–8°C (36–46°F). Protect from light. Do not freeze.

TREPROSTINIL

REMODULIN™

DESCRIPTION/ACTIONS

Treprostinil is a tricyclic benzidene analogue of prostacyclin (PGI_2). It produces direct vasodilation of pulmonary and systemic arterial vascular beds and inhibition of platelet aggregation. The vasodilatory effects reduce right and left ventricular afterload and increase cardiac output and stroke volume. It is indicated as a continuous subcutaneous infusion for the treatment of pulmonary arterial hypertension (PAH) in patients with NYHA class II–IV symptoms to diminish symptoms associated with exercise.

PRECAUTIONS/ADVERSE REACTIONS

Treprostinil is contraindicated in patients with a known hypersensitivity to it or to any component of the formulation. It should be used only by clinicians experienced in the treatment of PAH. Avoid abrupt withdrawl or sudden large reductions in dosage of treprostinil as this may result in worsening of PAH. Pregnancy Category B. No adequate and well-controlled studies in pregnant women. Excretion in human breast milk is unknown; use in pregnancy and lactation only if the potential benefit justifies the potential risk to the fetus. Safety and efficacy in pediatrics have not been established. Adverse reactions include infusion site pain (85%); infusion site reaction—erythema, induration, and rash (83%); headache (27%); diarrhea (25%); nausea (22%); rash (14%); jaw pain (13%); vasodilation (11%); dizziness (9%); edema (9%); pruritis (8%); and hypotension (4%). Treprostinil does not appear to be an inhibitor of the cytochrome P450 enzyme system. Whether or not it induces these enzymes has not been studied. Diuretics, antihypertensive agents, and/or vasodilators may enhance the hypotensive effects of treprostinil. Due to its inhibition of platelet aggregation, concomitant administration of treprostinil with anticoagulants may lead to an increased risk of bleeding.

ADMINISTRATION

Adults: continuous subcutaneous infusion—Initiate at 1.25 ng/kg/min. If this initial dose is not tolerated, the infusion rate should be reduced to 0.625 ng/Kg/min. The infusion rate should be increased in increments of no more than 1.25 ng/Kg/min per week for the first 4 weeks and then no more than 2.5 ng/kg/min per week for the remaining duration of infusion, depending on clinical response. Little experience with doses greater than 40 ng/kg/min. Abrupt discontinuation of infusion should be avoided.

Dosage adjustment for renal impairment: no specific recommendations. Use caution in these patients.

Dosage adjustment in mild or moderate hepatic impairment: initiate therapy at 0.625 ng/kg/min (use ideal body weight). Use caution with further dosage increases.

Severe hepatic impairment: has not been studied.

PATIENT CARE IMPLICATIONS

Goal of dose titration is to maximize efficacy (PAH symptoms are improved—dyspnea and fatigue) while minimizing side effects. Treprostinil is administered by subcutaneous infusion via a self-inserted subcutaneous catheter using an infusion pump designed for subcutaneous drug delivery. To avoid potential interruptions in drug delivery, the patient must have immediate access to a backup infusion pump and subcutaneous infusion set. During use, a single reservoir (syringe) can be administered up to 72 hours at 37^0 C. Patients should be informed that therapy with treprostinil will be needed for prolonged periods, possibly years.

PREPARATIONS

Injection: solution 1 mg/mL (20 mL), 2.5 mg/mL (20 mL), 5 mg/mL (20 mL), and 10 mg/mL (20 mL).

VORICONAZOLE

VFEND®

DESCRIPTION/ACTIONS

Voriconazole is a triazole antifungal agent. It inhibits fungal cytochrome P450 mediated 14 alpha-lanosterol demethylation, an essential step in the synthesis of ergosterol. Its antifungal activity is due to the loss of ergosterol in the fungal cell wall. Voriconazole has shown activity against *Aspergillus fumigatus, Aspergillus flavus, Aspergillus niger, Aspergillus terreus, Scedosporium apiospermum,* and *Fusarium* species including *Fusarium solani*. It is indicated for use in the treatment of serious fungal infections caused by *Scedosporium apiospermum* and *Fusarium* species including *Fusarium solani* in patients intolerant of, or refractory to, other therapy.

PRECAUTIONS/ADVERSE REACTIONS

Voriconazole is contraindicated in patients with a known hypersensitivity to voriconazole or to any component of the formulation. There is no information regarding cross-sensitivity between voriconazole and other azole antifungal agents. Use caution when administering voriconazole to patients with a hypersensitivity to other azoles. Coadministration of voriconazole and terfenadine, astemizole, cisapride, pimozide, or quinidine are contraindicated because increased plasma concentrations of these drugs can lead to QT interval prolongation and rare occurrences of torsade de pointes. Coadministration of voriconazole with sirolimus is contraindicated because voriconazole significantly increases sirolimus concentrations. Coadministration of voriconazole with rifampin, carbamazepine, and long-acting barbiturates (phenobarbital, mephobarbital) is contraindicated because these drugs are likely to significantly decrease plasma levels of voriconazole. Coadministration of voriconazole with rifabutin is contraindicated because voriconazole significantly increases rifabutin plasma concentrations and rifabutin significantly decreases voriconazole plasma concentrations. Coadministration of voriconazole with ergot alkaloids (ergotamine, dihydroergotamine) is contraindicated because voriconazole may increase the plasma concentration of the ergot alkaloid, which may lead to ergotism.

Voriconazole causes visual disturbances including altered/enhanced visual perception, blurred vision, color vision change, and/or photophobia. Patients should be instructed not to drive at night and to avoid potentially hazardous tasks such as driving or operating machinery while receiving voriconazole. Serious hepatic reactions including clinical hepatitis, cholestasis, and fulminant hepatic failure including fatalities have occurred during therapy with voriconazole. These reactions occurred most often in patients with serious underlying medical conditions, predominantly with hematologic malignancy. Hepatic reactions including hepatitis and jaundice have occurred in patients with no identifiable risk factors. Liver dysfunction has usually been reversible upon discontinuation of therapy. Liver function tests should be monitored at the start of therapy and during the course of therapy. May need to discontinue voriconazole if clinical signs and symptoms consistent with liver disease develop.

Voriconazole tablets contain lactose and should not be given to patients with rare hereditary problems of galactose intolerance, Lapp lactase deficiency, or glucose-galactose malabsorption. Voriconazole has been associated with prolongation of the QT interval. Rare cases of torsade de pointes have been reported in patients receiving voriconazole. These events occurred most often in seriously ill patients with multiple confounding risk factors, such as a history of cardiotoxic chemotherapy, cardiomyopathy, hypokalemia, and concomitant medications that may have been contributory. Voriconazole should be administered with caution to patients with potentially proarrhythmic conditions. Electrolyte abnormalities (hypokalemia, hypomagnesemia, and hypocalcemia) should be corrected prior to starting voriconazole. Anaphylactoid-type reactions including flushing, fever, sweating, tachycardia, chest tightness, dyspnea, faintness, nausea, pruritis, and rash have occurred during infusion of the intravenous formulation of voriconazole. Infusion should be stopped if this occurs. Patients should be instructed to avoid strong, direct sunlight while receiving voriconazole.

Accumulation of the intravenous vehicle sulfobutyl ether beta-cyclodextrin sodium (SBECD) occurs in patients with moderate to severe renal impairment (creatinine clearance < 50 mL/min). Serum creatinine should be monitored in these patients and oral voriconazole should be administered to these patients unless the benefits/risk to the patient justifies the use of the intravenous formulation. Pregnancy Category D. Voriconazole can cause fetal harm when administered to a pregnant woman. Women of childbearing potential should use effective contraception during treatment. Excretion in human breast milk is unknown. Voriconazole should not be used by nursing mothers unless the benefits clearly outweigh the risk to the baby. Safety and efficacy in pediatric patients less than 12 years of age have not been established.

Voriconazole is metabolized by the cytochrome P450 enzyme system CYP2C19, CYP2C9, and CYP3A4. Inhibitors or inducers of these enzymes may increase or decrease voriconazole plasma concentrations. Coadministration of cimetidine and ranitidine did not appear to affect plasma concentrations of voriconazole. Coadministration of voriconazole and erythromycin or azithromycin did not appear to affect serum levels of voriconazole. Coadministration of voriconazole and cyclosporine resulted in increased serum concentrations of cyclosporine. When initiating therapy with voriconazole in patients already receiving cyclosporine, decrease cyclosporine dosage by 50%. Monitor levels and when voriconazole is discontinued, readjust the dose as warranted. Coadministration of voriconazole and tacrolimus resulted in increased serum levels of tacrolimus. When initiating therapy with voriconazole in patients already receiving tacrolimus, decrease tacrolimus dosage to one-third of the original dose. Monitor levels and readjust dose as necessary once voriconazole is discontinued. Coadministration of voriconazole and warfarin resulted in increased prothrombin time. Prothrombin time and INR should be monitored. Coadministration of voriconazole and statins (HMG-CoA reductase inhibitors) is likely to result in increased serum levels of the statin. Increased levels of statins have been associated with myopathy/rhabdomyolysis. Coadministration of voriconazole and benzodiazepines (midazolam, triazolam, and alprazolam) resulted in increased plasma levels of the benzodiazepine and a prolonged sedative effect. Dosage adjustment of the benzodiazepine may be warranted. Coadministration of voriconazole and dihydropyridine calcium channel blockers may result in increased serum concentrations of the calcium channel blocker. Monitor patient for adverse effects and toxicity related to the calcium channel blocker. Dosage adjustment of the calcium channel blocker may be needed.

Voriconazole may increase plasma levels of sulfonylureas (tolbutamide, glyburide, and glipizide) and lead to hypoglycemia. Blood glucose levels should be monitored and the dose of the sulfonylurea adjusted accordingly. Voriconazole may increase the plasma concentration of vinca alkaloids (vincristine and vinblastine) and lead to neurotoxicity. Consider dosage adjustment of the vinca alkaloid. No significant interactions were observed when voriconazole was coadministered with prednisolone, indinavir, digoxin, or mycophenolic acid; therefore, no dosage adjustments are necessary. Coadministration of voriconazole and phenytoin resulted in decreased plasma levels of voriconazole. Dosage of voriconazole should be increased. Monitor phenytoin levels and adjust dose as needed. Coadministration of voriconazole and omeprazole (> 40 mg/day) resulted in increased serum concentrations of omeprazole. When coadministering with voriconazole, decrease the dose of omeprazole by 50%. Metabolism of other proton pump inhibitors may also be affected.

Voriconazole may inhibit the metabolism of HIV protease inhibitors (saquinavir, ritonavir, and amprenavir), and the metabolism of voriconazole may also be inhibited by HIV protease inhibitors. Patients should be monitored for drug toxicity when these agents are coadministered. The metabolism of voriconazole may be inhibited when coadministered with Non-Nucleoside Reverse Transcriptase Inhibitors (delavirdine and effavirenz), resulting in increased serum concentrations of voriconazole. The metabolism of voriconazole may be induced by effavirenz or nevirapine, resulting in decreased serum levels of voriconazole. Voriconazole may also inhibit the metabolism of delavirdine. Patients should be monitored for drug toxicity.

Most common adverse reactions observed in patients treated with voriconazole include visual disturbances, fever, rash, vomiting, nausea, diarrhea, headache, sepsis, peripheral edema, abdominal pain, and respiratory disorder. Adverse reactions that most often led to discontinuation of voriconazole were elevated liver function tests, rash, and visual disturbances. Other less common side effects (< 1% of patients) include anaphylactoid reaction, allergic reactions, enlarged abdomen, arrhythmias, complete AV block, bigeminy, bradycardia, bundle branch block, cardiomegaly, cardiomyopathy, cerebral hemorrhage, cerebral ischemia, CVA, CHF, deep thrombophlebitis, endocarditis, extrasystoles, heart arrest, MI, palpitation, phlebitis, postural hypotension, pulmonary embolus, QT interval prolongation, syncope, ascites, asthenia, back pain, cellulitis, edema, facial edema, flank pain, graft versus host reaction, granuloma, infection, bacterial infection, injection site pain/inflammation, mucous membrane disorder, multi-organ failure, pain, pelvic pain, peritonitis, substernal chest pain, anorexia, cholecystitis, constipation, dyspepsia, dysphagia, esophageal ulcer, flatulence, gastroenteritis, GI hemorrhage, elevated GGT/LDH, gum hemorrhage/ hyperplasia, hematemesis, hepatic coma, melena, pancreatitis, parotid gland enlargement, proctitis, pseudomembranous colitis, tongue edema, stomatitis, adrenal cortex insufficiency, diabetes insipidus, hyper/hypothyroidism, agranulocytosis, anemia, aplastic anemia, hemolytic anemia, cyanosis, DIC, echymosis, eosinophilia, hypervolemia, lymphadenopathy, marrow depression, thrombocytopenia purpura, albuminuria, increased BUN, CPK, hyper/hypocalcemia, hyper/hyponatremia, hyper/hypoglycemia, hypermagnesemia, hypophosphatemia, uremia, arthralgia, myalgia, osteomalacia, osteoporosis, agitation, amnesia, abnormal dreams, depression, brain edema, coma, confusion, convulsions, encephalitis, euphoria, Guillain-Barré Syndrome, nystagmus, alopecia, angioedema, discoid lupus erythematosis, eczema, erythema multiforme, exfoliative dermatitis, herpes Simplex, melanosis, photosensitivity, skin discoloration, Stevens-Johnson Syndrome, sweating, urticaria, blepharitis, deafness, ear pain, eye pain, keratoconjunctivitis, midriasis, night blindness, optic neuritis, retinal hemorrhage, taste loss/perversion, anuria, dysmenorrhea, decreased creatinine clearance, dysuria, hemorrhagic cystitis, hematuria, hydronephrosis, impotence, kidney tubular necrosis, metorrhagia, nephritis, nephrosis, oliguria, scrotal edema, urinary incontinence, urinary retention, UTI, and uterine/vaginal hemorrhage.

ADMINISTRATION

Adults and children 12 years of age or older: For the treatment of invasive *Aspergillosis* and infections due to *Fusarium* species and *Scedosporium apiospermum*.
Loading dose: 6 mg/kg intravenously every 12 hours x 2 doses.
Maintenance dose: 4 mg/kg every 12 hours.
Infuse over 1–2 hours at a maximum rate of 3 mg/kg. Not for bolus injection. May switch to oral therapy once patient can tolerate oral therapy.
Oral dose: Patients over 40 kg—200 mg orally every 12 hours. Patients under 40 kg—100 mg orally every 12 hours. If patient response is inadequate, oral maintenance dose may be increased as follows: patients over 40 kg—300 mg orally every 12 hours. Patients under 40 kg—150 mg orally every 12 hours.
If patients are unable to tolerate treatment, decrease the intravenous maintenance dose to 3 mg/kg every 12 hours. Decrease oral maintenance dose in 50 mg increments to a minimum of 200 mg orally every 12 hours (for patients over 40 kg) or to 100 mg orally every 12 hours (for patients under 40 kg).

Dosage adjustment in renal impairment: moderate or severe renal impairment (creatinine clearance < 50 mL/min)—oral voriconazole should be administered to these patients unless an assessment of the benefit/risk to the patient justifies the use of the intravenous voriconazole. Closely monitor serum creatinine levels.

Dosage adjustment in hepatic impairment: mild to moderate hepatic impairment (Child-Pugh Class A and B)—use loading dose and decrease maintenance dose by 50%.

Severe hepatic impairment (Child-Pugh Class C)—has not been studied.

Dosage adjustment with concomitant administration of phenytoin: Increase IV maintenance dose of voriconazole to 5 mg/kg every 12 hours. Increase oral maintenance dose from 200 mg to 400 mg orally every 12 hours in patients over 40 kg and from 100 mg to 200 mg orally every 12 hours in patients under 40 kg.

PATIENT CARE IMPLICATIONS

Tablets should be taken 1 hour before or 1 hour after a meal. Electrolyte abnormalities such as hypokalemia, hypomagnesemia, and hypocalcemia should be corrected prior to initiation of therapy with voriconazole. Women of childbearing potential should use effective contraception during treatment with voriconazole. Patients should be instructed not to drive at night while taking voriconazole. Patients should avoid potentially hazardous tasks, such as driving or operating machinery if they perceive any change in vision. Patients should avoid strong, direct sunlight during therapy with voriconazole. Renal and hepatic function should be monitored. Voriconazole IV must not be infused into the same line or cannula concomitantly with other drug infusions, including parenteral nutrition (e.g., aminofusin 10% plus). Do not simultaneously administer with blood products. May be simultaneously administered with total parenteral nutrition. Voriconazole must NOT be diluted with 4.2% sodium bicarbonate infusion.

PREPARATIONS

Lyophilized powder for injection, 200 mg voriconazole and 3200 mg SBECD. Tablets, 50 and 200 mg.

PART III

Glossary of Side Effects

Agranulocytosis—Severe acute shortage of certain types of blood cells (neutrophils) as a result of damage to the bone marrow by toxic drugs or chemicals.

Akathesia—A syndrome characterized by an inability to remain in a sitting posture with motor restlessness and a feeling of muscular quivering. May appear as a side effect of antipsychotic and neuroleptic medication.

Akinesia—Loss of normal muscle tonicity or responsiveness.

Allergic reactions—A response caused by sensitization to a particular antigen that provokes the release of histamine. Symptoms present as local or systemic effects ranging from local rash to respiratory wheezing.

Alopecia—Absence of hair from where it normally grows; baldness.

Amenorrhea—Stopping of menstrual flow.

Anaphylactic shock—An extreme and generalized allergic reaction in which widespread release of histamine causes swelling (edema), constriction of the bronchioles, heart failure, circulatory collapse, and sometimes death.

Anaphylaxis—An abnormal reaction to a particular antigen in which histamine is released from the tissues and causes either local or widespread symptoms typical of an allergic response. This response may be characterized by hives, itching, nasal congestion, abdominal cramping, diarrhea, dypsnea, hypotension, fainting, and choking sensation.

Angioedema (Angioneurotic edema) —An allergic condition producing transient or persistent swelling of areas of the skin accompanied by itching, which may be severe.

Anorexia—Loss of appetite.

Anticholinergic effects—Dry mouth, blurred vision.

Aphakic—Absence of the crystalline lens.

Apnea—Temporary cessation of breathing.

Arrhythmias—Any alteration from the normal sinus rhythm of the heart.

Arthralgia—Joint pain.

Asthenia—Weakness or loss of strength.

Atony—A state in which the muscles are floppy or lacking in normal tone.

AV block—Atrial-ventricular heart block.

Blepharitis—Inflammation of the eyelids.

Blepharospasm—Involuntary contraction of the eyelid.

Blood dyscrasias—Abnormal state found in the blood cells.

Bradycardia—Slowing of the heart beat to less than 50 beats per minute.

Cardiogenic shock—Shock that originates from a cardiac source.

Catabolism—The breaking down in the body of complex chemical compounds into simpler ones.

Cataplexy—A transient attack of extreme generalized muscle weakness.

Chemosis—Swelling (edema) of the conjunctiva of the eye.

Chloasm—Patchy brown discoloration of the skin, mainly on the forehead, temples, and cheeks. Usually associated with pregnancy or use of birth control pills (oral contraceptives).

Conjunctivitis—Inflammation of the conjunctiva (delicate mucous membrane that covers the front of the eyes and lines the inside of the eyelids) that becomes red and swollen and produces a watery or pus-containing discharge.

Constipation—A condition in which bowel evacuation occurs irregularly or in which the feces are hard and small or where passage of feces is difficult or painful.

Diarrhea—Frequent bowel evacuation or the passage of abnormally soft or liquid feces.

Disulfiram-like reactions—Disulfiram is a drug used in treatment of alcoholism, which, when taken in combination with alcohol, produces unpleasant reactions such as flushing, difficulty breathing, headache, palpitations, nausea, and vomiting. Drugs that produce these same unpleasant effects are classified as disufiram-like reactions.

Dyesthesia—A condition in which a disagreeable sensation is produced by ordinary stimuli.

Dysgeusia—Taste perversion;, bad taste in the mouth.

Dysmenorrhea—Painful menstruation.

Dyspepsia—Refers to pain or discomfort in the lower chest or abdomen after eating; may sometimes be accompanied by nausea and vomiting.

Dyspnea—Labored or difficult breathing.

Dystonia—A postural disorder caused by an effect on the basal ganglia of the brain characterized by muscle spasms of the shoulder, neck, and trunk.

Dysuria—Difficult or painful urination.

Ecchymosis—A bruise ("black-and-blue mark") resulting from release of blood into the tissues.

Edema—Excessive accumulation of fluid in the body tissue.

Emotional lability—Emotionally unstable.

Eosinophilia—An increase in the number of eosinophils (a variety of white blood cells) in the blood stream.

Epiphyses—Part of a long bone developed from a center of ossification distinct from that of the shaft and separated at first from the latter by a layer of cartilage.

Epistaxis—Severe nosebleed.

Erythema—Abnormal flushing of the skin caused by dilation of the blood capillaries.

Erythema multiforme—An acute inflammatory skin disease caused by an adverse reaction to medication(s) and characterized by lesions consisting of concentric circles of erythema, usually appearing on the neck, face, and legs. Occasionally blisters are observed. Often accompanied by fever, malaise, arthralgia, and gastric distress.

Extrapyramidal side effects—Reactions seen when the nerve tracts and pathways connecting the cerebral cortex, basal ganglia, thalmus, cerebellum reticular function, and spinal neurons are affected by a drug. Reactions are characterized by akinesia, fixed positioning of the limbs (rigidity), sudden violent movement of the arms and head (dystonias), akathesia, and rhythmic, clonic muscular activity(tremor).

Gynecomastia—Enlargement of the breasts in males.

Heart block—A condition in which the normal electrical conduction of the heart is disrupted so that the pumping action of the heart slows down.

Hematuria—Presence of blood in the urine.

Hepatomegaly—Enlargement of the liver so that it can be felt below the margin of the rib.

Hyperbilirubinemia—Presence in the blood of an abnormally high amount of bilirubin.

Hyperemia—Excess blood in vessels supplying a part of the body(e.g., hyperemia of the eye presents as redness of the white of the eye).

Hyperkalemia—Presence in the blood of an abnormally high amount of potassium.

Hypernatremia—Presence in the blood of an abnormally high amount of sodium.

Hypersalivation—Presence in the mouth of an abnormally high amount of saliva; excessive salivation.

Hypersensitivity reactions—Abnormal response to a particular antigen that may cause a variety of tissue reactions such as serum sickness and allergy (including anaphylaxis).

Hypertension—Elevation of the blood pressure above the normal range (high blood pressure).

Hypertonia—Exceptionally high tension in the muscles.

Hypertrophy—Increase in the size of a tissue or an organ by enlargement of the cells as opposed to an increase in the number of cells.

Hyperuricemia—Presence in the blood of an abnormally high amount of uric acid.

Hypoesthesia—Diminished sensitivity to stimulation.

Hypoglycemia—A deficiency of glucose in the blood stream that causes muscular weakness, incoordination, mental confusion, and sweating.

Hypokalemia—Presence in the blood of an abnormally low amount of potassium.

Hyponatremia—Presence in the blood of an abnormally low amount of sodium.

Hypotension—Reduction in the blood pressure below the normal range(low blood pressure).

Ichthyosis—Skin condition characterized by dry, rough, scaly appearance.

Impotence—Inability of a man to have intercourse.

Insomnia—Inability to fall asleep or stay asleep for an adequate duration.

Keratitis—Inflammation of the cornea of the eye.

Kyphoscoliosis—Lateral and posterior curvature of the spine.

Lactic acidosis—Lactic acid is the end product of glucose metabolism in the absence of oxygen. Lactic acidosis is the buildup of these products to an excessive level that results in the pH of the bloodstream becoming more acidic.

Laryngospasm—Involuntary closure of the larynx, obstructing the flow of the air to the lungs.

LV hypertrophy—Left ventricular hypertrophy of the heart.

Lupus-like syndrome—Symptoms characteristic of lupus caused by an adverse drug reaction.

Lymphopenia—A decrease in the number of lymphocytes in the blood.

Malignant hyperthermia—Rare condition most commonly precipitated by exposure to anesthetic or neuromuscular blocking agents. It is characterized by excessive muscle contraction, severe skeletal muscle rigidity, lactic acidosis, sharply elevated body temperature, tachycardia, tachypnea, and cyanosis.

Miosis—Constriction of the pupil.

Myalgia—Muscle pain.

Mydriasis—Widening of the pupil.

Myelosuppression—A reduction in the blood cell production by the bone marrow.

Nausea—A feeling that one is about to vomit.

Neuropathy—Disease of the peripheral nerves causing weakness and numbness.

Neutropenia—A decrease in the number of neutrophils in the blood.

Nystagmus—Rapid involuntary movement of the eyes that may be from side to side, up and down, or rotary.

Orthostatic hypotension—Abrupt lowering of the blood pressure in response to a position change from lying to sitting or standing.

Paresthesia—An abnormal sensation, such as burning, pricking, tickling, or tingling, described as "pins and needles.".

Peripheral neuropathy—See Neuropathy.

Petechiae—Small, round dark spots caused by bleeding into the skin.

Pharynigitis—Inflammation of the part of the throat behind the pharynx.

Phlebitis—Inflammation of the wall of the vein, most commonly seen in the legs. A segment of the vein becomes swollen and tender, and the surrounding skin becomes reddened and warm to the touch.

Photophobia—Abnormal intolerance of light in which exposure to light causes intense discomfort to the eyes.

Photosensitivity—Abnormal and severe reaction of the skin when exposed to sunlight.

Polyuria—Production of large amounts of urine, which is dilute and pale in color.

Postprandial—Occurring after eating.

Postural hypotension—See Orthostatic hypotension.

Proteinuria—Presence of protein in the urine.

Pruritis—Itching caused by skin irritation.

Pseudomembranous colitis—Inflammation of the colon caused by use of antibiotics. It is characterized by severe foul-smelling diarrhea, sometimes accompanied by blood, mucous, and abdominal pain.

Pseudophakic—An eye in which a natural lens is replaced with an intraocular lens.

Psychosis—Mental disorder in which the patient loses contact with reality.

Psychotomimetic effects—Reactions that mimic the effects seen with psychoactive drugs.

Ptosis—Drooping of the upper eyelid.

Punctate keratitis—Puncture injury of the cornea which causes inflammation.

Purpura—Skin rash that results from bleeding of the small blood vessels (capillaries) into the skin.

Pyuria—Presence of pus in the urine.

QT interval prolongation—QT interval on an electrocardiogram represents ventricular contraction. Prolongation indicates the ventricle is taking a longer time contracting.

Rhinitis—Inflammation of the mucous membranes of the nose. Frequently presents as a runny nose.

Serum sickness—A delayed hypersensitivity reaction that sometimes occurs 7–12 days after ingesting a drug. The usual symptoms are rash, fever, joint pain, and enlargement of the lymph nodes. The reaction is due to the presence of antigenic material still circulating at the time the body is forming antibodies against it.

SIADH (sudden inappropriate antidiuretic hormone)—The stimulation of production of antidiuretic hormone, which results in water retention and water intoxication.

Somnolence—Sleepiness.

Steatosis—Fatty degeneration.

Stevens-Johnson syndrome—The most severe form of erythema multiforme characterized by high fever, headache, and inflammatory lesions of the mouth, eyes, and genitalia. Frequently the bronchial and visceral mucosa are involved. Death may occur from renal failure.

Stomatitis—Inflammation of the mucous lining of the mouth.

Superinfection—An infection arising in the course of treatment of another infection, caused by a different organism and which is usually resistant to the drug used to treat the primary infection.

Syncope—Loss of consciousness caused by temporary decrease in blood flow to the brain (fainting).

Tachycardia—An above-normal increase in the heart rate.

Thrombophlebitis—See Phlebitis.

Thrombocytopenia—A reduction in the number of platelets in the blood.

Turbinate edema—Swelling of the bones that form the nasal cavity.

Urticaria—An allergic reaction on which round red wheels form on the skin, ranging in size from very small spots to several inches in diameter.

Uveitis—Inflammation of any part of the uveal tract of the eye.

Vertigo—A disabling sensation in which the affected individual feels the ground is swirling or the surroundings are in constant motion. Most commonly associated with disorders of the inner ear.

Vitreitis—Inflammation involving the vitreous humor of the eye.

PART IV

REFERENCES

1. Abbott Laboratories. Package literature for Humira™. January 2003.
2. Gilead Sciences Inc. Package literature for Hepsera™. September 2002.
3. Otsuka America Pharmaceutical Inc. Package literature for Abilify™. November 2002.
4. Eli Lilly and Company. Package literature for Strattera™. December 2002.
5. Reckitt Benckiser Pharmaceuticals Inc. Package literature for Subutex®. October 2002.
6. Reckitt Benckiser Pharmaceuticals Inc. Package literature for Suboxone®. October 2002.
7. Stiefel Laboratories Inc. Package literature for Duac™. October 2002.
8. Pfizer Inc. Package literature for Relpax®. December 2002.
9. Forest Pharmaceuticals Inc. Package literature for Lexapro™. August 2002.
10. Astra Zeneca Pharmaceuticals LP. Package literature for Faslodex®. July 2002
11. Bristol-Myers Squibb Company. Package literature for Metaglip™. October 2002.
12. Romark Laboratories. Package literature for Alinia™. April 2002.
13. Swedish Orphan International AB. Package literature for Orfadin®. January 2002.
14. Sankyo Pharma Inc. Package literature for Benicar™. April 2002.
15. Sanofi-Synthelabo Inc. Package literature for Eloxatin™. August 2002.
16. Hoffman-LaRoche Inc. Package literature for Pegasys®. December 2002.
17. Glaxo Smith Kline. Package literature for Avandamet™. October 2002.
18. Orphan Medical Inc. Package literature for Xyrem®. May 2002.
19. Novartis Pharmaceuticals Corp. Package literature for Zelnorm™. July 2002.
20. Eli Lilly and Company. Package literature for Forteo™. November 2002.
21. G. D. Searle LLC. Package literature for Inspra™. January 2003.
22. Merck/Schering-Plough Pharmaceutical. Package literature for Zetia™. March 2003.
23. Janssen Pharmaceutica N.V. Package literature for Reminyl®. August 2002.
24. Sanofi-Synthelabo. Package literature for Elitek™. July 2002.

25. United Therapeutics Corp. Package literature for Remodulin™. March 2002.
26. Pfizer Inc. Package literature for Vfend®. January 2003.
27. www.fda.gov
28. www.lexi.com (Lexi-comp Inc. 1978–2003).

Springer Publishing Company

From the Springer Series on Social Work...

A Guide for Nursing Home Social Workers

Elise M. Beaulieu, MSW, ACSW, LICSW

"In this excellent volume on social work practice in nursing homes, the author presents an in-depth discussion of all aspects of nursing home practice. ...The book is essential reading for beginning and experienced social workers alike. It is also an outstanding text for courses that include content on practice in long term care."

—**Patricia Brownell,** PhD, CSW
Fordham University Graduate School of Social Service

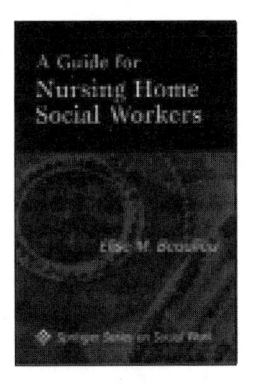

This book clearly distinguishes the function of beginning nursing home social workers and provides information and resources essential for them. Topics include the following: the assessment, intake, and discharge processes; interventions; resource allocation; medication; diagnosis and treatment of depression; dementias; and legal issues, ethics, and confidentiality agreements. Making the volume still more practical are a glossary of commonly used terms and abbreviations, as well as a section of standardized forms and charts.

Contents:
- Basic Orientation
- Social Work in Nursing Facilities
- The Nursing Facility
- Surveys
- Diagnoses and Treatment
- Legal Representatives for Residents
- Ethics
- Community Liaisons
- Problems and Solutions
- Sample Forms

2002   304pp   0-8261-1533-0   soft

**536 Broadway, New York, NY 10012 • (212) 431-4370 • Fax (212) 941-7842
Order Toll-Free: 877-687-7376 • Order on-line: www.springerpub.com**